D1538313

EQUIPMENT THEORY FOR RESPIRATORY CARE
FOURTH EDITION

Gary C. White, M.Ed., RRT, RPFT
Program Director
Spokane Community College
Spokane, Washington

THOMSON
DELMAR LEARNING

Australia Canada Mexico Singapore Spain United Kingdom United States

THOMSON

DELMAR LEARNING

Equipment Theory for Respiratory Care, Fourth Edition
by Gary C. White, M.Ed., RRT, RPFT

Vice President, Health Care Business Unit:
William Brottmiller

Editorial Director:
Cathy L. Esperti

Acquisitions Editor:
Rhonda Dearborn

Developmental Editors:
Mary Ellen Cox and
Sarah Duncan

Marketing Director:
Jennifer McAvey

Channel Manager:
Tamara Caruso

Marketing Coordinator
Kimberly Duffy

Editorial Assistant:
Debra Gorgos

Art & Design Specialist:
Jay Purcell

Project Editor:
Natalie Wager

Production Editor:
John Mickelbank

Technology Project Coordinator:
Carolyn Fox

COPYRIGHT © 2005 by Thomson Delmar Learning, a part of the Thomson Corporation. Thomson, the Star logo, and Delmar Learning are trademarks used herein under license.

Printed in the United States of America
1 2 3 4 5 XXX 08 07 06 05 04

For more information contact Thomson Delmar Learning,
5 Maxwell Drive,
Clifton Park, NY 12065
Or find us on the World Wide Web at
http://www.delmarlearning.com

ALL RIGHTS RESERVED. Portions of this book copyrighted 1999, 1996, and 1993. No part of this work covered by the copyright hereon may be reproduced or used in any form or by any means—graphic, electronic, or mechanical, including photocopying, recording, taping, Web distribution, or information storage and retrieval systems—without written permission of the publisher.

For permission to use material from this text or product, contact us by
Tel (800) 730-2214
Fax (800) 730-2215
www.thomsonrights.com

Library of Congress Cataloging-in-Publication Data

White, Gary C., 1954–
Equipment theory for respiratory care / Gary C. White.—4th ed.
p. ; cm.
Includes bibliographical references and index.
ISBN 1-4018-5223-8
1. Respiratory therapy—Equipment and supplies. 2. Respirators (Medical equipment)
[DNLM: 1. Respiratory Therapy—instrumentation. WB 26 W584e 2005] I. Title.

RC735.I5W48 2005
615.8'36—dc22
2004015051

NOTICE TO THE READER

Publisher does not warrant or guarantee any of the products described herein or perform any independent analysis in connection with any of the product information contained herein. Publisher does not assume, and expressly disclaims, any obligation to obtain and include information other than that provided to it by the manufacturer.

The reader is expressly warned to consider and adopt all safety precautions that might be indicated by the activities described herein and to avoid all potential hazards. By following the instructions contained herein, the reader willingly assumes all risks in connection with such instructions.

The publisher makes no representations or warranties of any kind, including but not limited to, the warranties of fitness for particular purpose or merchantability, nor are any such representations implied with respect to the material set forth herein, and the publisher takes no responsibility with respect to such material. The publisher shall not be liable for any special, consequential, or exemplary damages resulting, in whole or part, from the reader's use of, or reliance upon, this material.

Dedication

To my wife, Carolyn,

and

my two sons, "A2" (Andrew, age eighteen, and Austin, age fourteen), who consistently remind their father just who and what are important.

CONTENTS

LIST OF EQUIPMENT

PREFACE

CHANGES TO THE FOURTH EDITION

The three previous editions of *Equipment Theory for Respiratory Care* have been very well received texts. The features that made the first three editions a success have been retained for the fourth edition. Many reviewers and fellow educators have requested that the book be expanded to include more equipment and to include the American Association for Respiratory Care (AARC) Clinical Practice Guidelines. The AARC Clinical Practice Guidelines have been incorporated into the text where appropriate when discussing the equipment required for the procedure.

Several of my reviewers requested that older equipment be eliminated. I have done so in this edition. Many of the permanent non-disposable nebulizers, humidifiers, manual resuscitators and other equipment are no longer in use. Several ventilators that are no longer manufactured or supported with parts or service have also been eliminated from this edition.

Many educators have commented that they like the self-assessment quizzes at the end of each chapter; these have been retained. In addition, requests have been made for more clinical scenarios or critical thinking activities.

The "Clinical Corner" feature has been retained for the fourth edition. The purpose of this feature is to let the student dialog with his or her instructor using these activities as a template or guide. Additionally, they may be used for in-class discussion. Answers are not provided in the text; instead, the student should seek out the instructor. Alternatively, an instructor may choose to use these as written assignments.

The troubleshooting sections of the third edition have been well received and have been retained. The troubleshooting flowcharts and assembly and troubleshooting boxes have been made more generic rather than brand specific. Each box and troubleshooting algorithm is specific to the type and category of equipment. When required due to specifics of a particular piece of equipment, a more specific coverage is retained.

Troubleshooting flowcharts or algorithms are provided to guide the student through the steps of troubleshooting the equipment. The algorithms include decision making, process, and connection nodes in a similar way in which therapy-drive protocols are presented. The goal of these algorithms is to teach the critical thinking process of troubleshooting and to assist the student in the development of a systematic method of problem solving.

FORMAT

This text uses a comprehensive, competency-based approach to describe the equipment employed in the practice of respiratory care. The text emphasizes the physical and engineering principles employed in the operation of this equipment. These principles are then related to a representative sample of equipment; assembly and troubleshooting of the equipment is presented. Selection, assembly and troubleshooting accounts for 25% of the National Board for Respiratory Care (NBRC) written exams.

It is imperative that the student be thoroughly knowledgeable on equipment selection and application to be clinically competent. To assist in the student's understanding of the material, each chapter concludes with a self-assessment quiz using NBRC-type questions. By studying the chapter objectives, reading the text, following the assembly and troubleshooting guides, and completing the self-assessment quiz, the student will encounter important concepts and principles in many different ways, thus facilitating their retention.

HIGHLIGHTS

Highlights of this text include the use of a competency-based approach to facilitate the learning of the material. The text headings are keyed to the objectives. This simplifies finding specific areas within each chapter. The physical and engineering principles of operation are illustrated in numerous computer-aided design drawings. Those same principles are applied to a representative sample of equipment. Assembly drawings and a written assembly guide will help the student to correctly prepare the equipment for clinical use. A troubleshooting algorithm provides a logical method for the student to follow when attempting to restore a piece of equipment to operation once its performance has failed or diminished. The "Clinical Corner" feature further helps to bridge the gap from theory to practice. The self-assessment quiz provides students with another opportunity to test their knowledge of the concepts contained within the chapter.

The major priority in the development of the fourth edition continues to be its readability and student-centered focus. Reading level studies have shown that the reading level of many texts in the field of respiratory care is too high for many of the students studying respiratory care. This text has been made more readable by the elimination of reference citations within the text. Instead, references and suggested readings are listed at the conclusion of each chapter. The use of objectives, format, simplified language, and artwork all help to make this complex subject easier to comprehend.

INSTRUCTIONS TO THE STUDENT

Seven steps are listed below that will enable you, the student, to more effectively use this text. If you follow these steps it will be easier for you to understand and apply this seemingly difficult material. Ultimately it will be the application of your knowledge and skill that will enable you to be a good respiratory care practitioner.

1. Read the introduction to the chapter and, though you may not understand all of the terms or concepts, try to visualize what it is you will be learning.

2. Read and study the objectives. The objectives form the core of what will be presented in the chapter. Rephrase the objectives into questions and write them on a piece of paper. As you read the text, answer the questions you have written.

3. Read the text. Relate what you read to the artwork, forming a mental picture of how the equipment works or how the parts fit together to make a whole.

4. In the laboratory or clinical setting, work with the equipment discussed in the chapter you read. Take the equipment apart and assemble it again using the assembly guide. Troubleshoot it by deliberately rendering it inoperational or marginally effective. Follow the troubleshooting algorithms when you are troubleshooting the equipment. Hands-on practice is the fastest way to gain confidence and experience.

5. Dialog with your instructor using the "Clinical Corner" feature.

6. Read the objectives one more time and take the Self-Assessment Quiz to assess your knowledge.

7. Use the Selected Bibliography to expand your knowledge of the subject. Most references may be found in a hospital medical library or respiratory care department.

USE OF THE TROUBLESHOOTING ALGORITHMS

At first it may seem that the algorithms are difficult to follow and appear to have little to do with troubleshooting. Visualize the algorithm as a map that will illustrate the potential problems, what needs to be checked, and the steps required to resolve the problem. One step on the algorithm flows to another step until the end is reached.

The symbol shapes denote specific steps or action required by the student, as you progress through an algorithm. The circle-shaped symbol is termed a terminal symbol (Figure 1). This symbol denotes the start or end of an algorithm. The diamond-shaped symbols are decision symbols. Within a decision symbol, a question is asked. The answer to the question may only be "yes" or "no." The rectangular-shaped symbols are process symbols. These require action on your part. You must perform the steps called out in the process symbol(s) before proceeding. Arrows guide you from one place to another within the troubleshooting algorithm to another or, if the algorithm is split between two pages, it connects one page to another. Simply match the number between the two nodes (i.e., 1 to 1, 2 to 2, etc.).

Gary C. White
2004

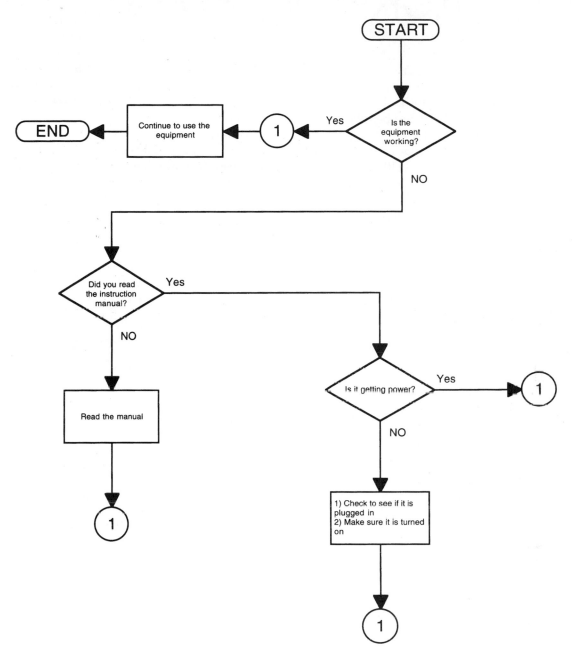

Figure 1

ACKNOWLEDGMENTS

This type of technical text could not be created without the help and support of respiratory care equipment manufacturers and vendors. The companies listed below all contributed toward the development of this text. Many provided technical manuals, technical drawings, and photographs. Others provided equipment or technical advice. I owe a great deal of thanks to these companies, their product managers, marketing managers, engineers, technical support personnel, and respiratory care practitioners.

AMBU, Inc.
Aequitron Medical, Inc.
Allied Healthcare Products, Inc.
Bear Medical Systems
BCI International
Bird Products Corporation
CAIRE, Inc.
Chad Therapeutics, Inc.
DeVilbiss Health Care, Inc.
DHD Medical, Inc.
Hamilton Medical, Inc.
ICN Pharmaceuticals, Inc.
Impact Medical Corporation
Infrasonics, Inc.
J. H. Emerson Company
Laerdal Medical Corporation
Lifecare
Life Support Products, Inc.
Medical Molding Corporation of America
MEDICO, Ogden, Utah
Monaghan Medical
Nellcor, Inc.
Newport Medical Instruments, Inc.
Novametrix Medical Systems
Nonin Medical, Inc.
Ohmeda
Omni-Tech Medical, Inc.
Pegasus Research Corporation
Puritan-Bennett Corporation
Respironics, Inc.
Sechrist Industries, Inc.
Siemens Life Support Systems
Utah Welders Supply, Salt Lake City, Utah
Viasys Healthcare, Virginia
Whitmore Medical, Ogden, Utah

REVIEWERS

In addition to the manufacturers and vendors, other individuals have helped in the creation of this text by reviewing specific content areas. These individuals include Carl G. Wood, PhD., Assistant Professor, Automotive and Mechanical Engineering Technology, Weber State University, and Leonard G. Nielsen, MS, MT (ASCP), Associate Professor, Clinical Laboratory Sciences, Weber State University.

I would like to acknowledge the reviewers who read the entire manuscript. Their insight, comments, and suggestions helped me to refine the text and produce a better book. They include:

Randall W. Anderson, R.R.T., C.R.T.T., R.C.P.
Respiratory Care Program Coordinator
Spartanburg Technical College
Spartanburg, South Carolina

Kerry Jean Connor, M.S., R.R.T.
Director of Clinical Education
Associate Professor of Respiratory Care
Manchester Community-Technical College
Manchester, Connecticut

Cynthia Smathers, M.Ed., R.R.T.
Respiratory Care Program Director
Pima Medical Institute
Mesa, Arizona

Theresa Winschel, R.R.T.
Clinical Coordinator
Hinds Community College–Jackson Branch
Nursing/Allied Health Center
Jackson, Mississippi

I would also like to thank Clark Taylor, Instructional Technology, Weber State University. Mr. Taylor provided tremendous help and suggestions toward improving my abilities as a technical photographer.

I owe special thanks to Colton Grigsby. When Colton had finished play time with my son Austin, he introduced me to his mother Becky Grigsby. It was then that I learned of Becky's talent as a technical illustrator. She has demonstrated the ability to accurately render pieces of equipment while communicating concepts and ideas simultaneously. Her art work tremendously enhances the effectiveness of this fourth edition. Thank you, Becky!

Lastly, I owe thanks to my wife Carolyn, who provided countless hours for me to create yet another edition! As my children grow, the demands placed upon my wife, so that I have time to work, also grow. Without her help and support, this fourth edition would not be possible. Thank you for believing in what I do.

Gary C. White
2004

CHAPTER 1

MEDICAL GAS SUPPLY EQUIPMENT

INTRODUCTION

Administration of medical gases is involved in most of the tasks performed by a respiratory care practitioner. It is important to understand how the supply equipment for oxygen therapy and mixed-gas therapy operates and how to troubleshoot these devices when problems arise.

In this chapter you will study the physics of equipment operation, focusing especially on gas supply systems. Only by thoroughly understanding the equipment and its components can you safely use it and troubleshoot it if it fails to function properly.

OBJECTIVES

After completing this chapter, the student will accomplish the following objectives:

PHYSICS OF THE PRINCIPLES

- Describe the kinetic theory of gases.
- Define the term *gas pressure*; explain what causes it and how it is measured.
- Explain Pascal's law.
- Explain what causes gases to flow from one place to another and how gas flow is measured.
- Explain Bernoulli's principle.
- Describe the principle of viscous shearing and vorticity.
- Explain how ejectors work:
  — in conjunction with venturi tubes
  — with constant area ducts
- Describe choked flow and the conditions under which it occurs.
- Explain the significance of Reynolds' number.
- Apply the following laws to solve for volume, temperature, or pressure:
  — Boyle's law
  — Charles' law
  — Dalton's law
  — Gay-Lussac's law
  — Combined or ideal gas law
  — Fick's law
  — Henry's law
  — Graham's law

MEDICAL GAS SUPPLY EQUIPMENT

- Differentiate between the following supply systems; describe their construction and their principles of operation:
  — cylinders
  — liquid reservoirs, including calculation of oxygen duration based on weight
  — piping systems
  — compressors
  — concentrators
- Identify the contents of a medical gas cylinder, using the U.S. and international color code system, for the following gases:
  — oxygen
  — carbon dioxide
  — nitrous oxide
  — cyclopropane
  — helium
  — carbon dioxide and oxygen
  — helium and oxygen
  — air
- Given an oxygen "E" or "H" cylinder, gauge pressure and liter flow, calculate how long the cylinder will last.

- Identify the markings stamped on the cylinder shoulder.
- List fifteen rules established by the Compressed Gas Association and the National Fire Protection Association for the safe storage and handling of compressed medical gas cylinders.
- Differentiate between the following oxygen regulation devices; describe their construction and principles of operation:
  — direct-acting cylinder valve
  — indirect-acting cylinder valve
  — single-stage reducing valve

  — modified single-stage reducing valve
  — multiple-stage reducing valve
  — regulator
  — oxygen proportioner
  — demand pulse-flow regulators
- Differentiate between the following oxygen flowmeters; describe their construction and principles of operation:
  — Bourdon gauge
  — uncompensated Thorpe tube
  — compensated Thorpe tube
  — fixed orifice flowmeter

KEY TERMS

Absolute temperature	Choked flow	Henry's law	Pressure
Adsorption	Combined gas law	Kinetic theory	Reducing valve
Aneroid barometer	Compressors	Laminar gas flow	Regulator
Bernoulli's principle	Dalton's law	Manifold	Reynolds' number
Blender	Diaphragm compressors	Mechanical manometer	Thorpe tube flowmeter
Bourdon gauge	Direct acting cylinder valve	Membrane enricher	Torr
Bourdon gauge flowmeter	Ducted ejector	Mercury barometer	Turbulent gas flow
Boyle's law	Fick's law	Molecular sieve concentrator	Venturi mask
Brownian motion	Fixed orifice flowmeter	Oxygen concentrator	Viscous shearing
Centrifugal compressor	Gay-Lussac's law	Oxygen conserving device (OCD)	Zone valves
Charles' law	Graham's law	Poiseuille's law	

PHYSICS OF THE PRINCIPLES

BEHAVIOR OF GASES

Gases behave according to the **kinetic theory.** The kinetic theory describes the behavior of ideal gases, and it incorporates five important points. These points are: (1) gases are composed of discrete molecules; (2) the molecules are in random motion; (3) all molecular collisions are elastic, causing no energy transfer between molecules; (4) the molecular activity is directly dependent upon the temperature; and (5) there is no physical attraction between the molecules composing the gas.

Gases are composed of very small, discrete molecules. The distance between molecules is much greater than the actual diameter of the individual molecules. Therefore, gases consist of large amounts of open space between the

gas molecules. The volume of the molecules (if they could be gathered together) is very small when compared to the total volume of the molecules and space as a whole.

Gas molecules are in constant, random motion. The molecules travel in a straight line or path. This motion continues until they collide with something else. These collisions can occur with other molecules, the walls of the container holding the gas, or other particles. Evidence of these collisions was first described by Robert Brown in 1827. He described the motion of larger particles that moved as a result of the smaller molecules of the gas colliding with them. This random movement can be observed today by watching the behavior of cigarette smoke under a microscope. The random motion of the larger particles is termed **Brownian motion**.

The collisions between molecules are completely elastic. This means that there is no energy transferred as a result of these collisions. Energy is not lost or gained by the molecules as a result of this process. Therefore, the total energy of the gas remains constant.

The kinetic activity or speed of the molecules is largely determined by the temperature. As the temperature of a gas increases, so does the kinetic activity. Conversely, as the temperature of a gas decreases, its kinetic activity decreases.

In ideal gas behavior, the gas molecules do not attract or repel one another. There is no physical attractive force between individual molecules. The molecules move about freely without any significant attractive forces between them.

GAS PRESSURE

Causes

Gas **pressure** (force per unit area) is caused by the individual gas molecules colliding with one another and the walls of a container. This exerts a force on the container walls. Even gas molecules have mass and a velocity, and thus possess a certain momentum (momentum = mass $\times$ velocity). The momentum transferred from these multiple collisions is what creates pressure, or the force on the walls of a container. The temperature of a gas influences the level of kinetic activity and therefore the velocity of the molecules.

Pascal's Law

Blaise Pascal, a seventeenth-century investigator, described how force is transmitted in a fluid. Pascal discovered that a fluid confined in a container will transmit force or pressure uniformly in all directions and that the pressure, or force at the walls of the container, acts perpendicular to that surface.

Since gases behave according to fluid properties, Pascal's law also applies. Pressure at any point in a closed container is equal to the pressure at any other point in the same container. If you take a long, closed tube and pressurize it with a gas, the pressure at one end will be equal to the pressure at the opposite end. Also, the pressure acts equally in all directions, with the force applied perpendicular to all surfaces of the tube.

Measurement of Gas Pressure— Barometers

The atmospheric pressure is measured with an instrument called a barometer. There

are two types of barometers, mercury and aneroid.

The **mercury barometer** uses the weight of a column of mercury opposing the force of the atmosphere to measure atmospheric pressure (Figure 1-1). The barometer consists of a closed column of mercury inverted in a shallow reservoir open to the atmosphere. When the column is inverted in the reservoir, a vacuum is created as gravity pulls the column of mercury down from the top of the closed tube. Atmospheric pressure against the open reservoir balances the gravitational force, pushing the mercury upward in the closed tube. The level of the mercury column rises or falls, depending upon the atmospheric pressure exerted against the open reservoir. A calibrated scale adjacent to the mercury column provides a method to measure the height of the column of mercury. For medical and scientific purposes, atmospheric pressure is measured in millimeters of mercury. This measurement is also referred to as **torr** (named after Evangelista Torricelli, the inventor of this barometer).

The **aneroid barometer** (Figure 1-2) consists of an evacuated metal container that has a pressure lower than atmospheric pressure. A spring is attached between the container and a pointer mechanism. This indicates the pressure. As gas pressure increases, the container is compressed. This causes the pointer to move, indicating an increased pressure. The pointer moves adjacent to a scale calibrated in millimeters of mercury.

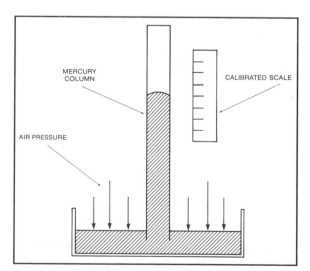

Figure 1-1 *A full section of a mercury barometer. Note how air pressure causes the mercury column to rise in the vertical tube.*

Figure 1-2 *A functional diagram of an aneroid barometer. As air pressure causes the evacuated container to expand or contract, the pointer moves adjacent to the scale.*

Measurement of Gas Pressure—Other Devices

In addition to barometers, mechanical manometers and Bourdon gauges can be used to measure gas pressure. A **mechanical manometer** (Figure 1-3) is similar in construction to an aneroid barometer. A diaphragm or evacuated container is exposed to the area where pressure measurement is desired. As gas exerts a force against the diaphragm or container, it causes the pointer's position to change, indicating the pressure. Note that these instruments are calibrated so that atmospheric pressure measures zero on the instrument's scale. The majority of manometers in respiratory care are calibrated in centimeters

(A)

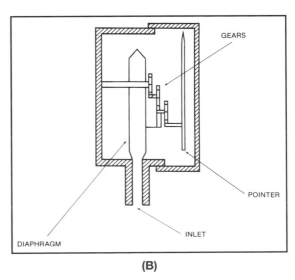

(B)

Figure 1-3 *A photograph and functional diagram of an inspiratory force manometer. As pressure causes the evacuated container to expand or contract, the pointer moves adjacent to its scale.*

of water pressure or Kilopascals (KPa) (le Système International d'Unités [si], or metric units). Table 1-1 lists standard units of pressure measurement.

A **Bourdon gauge** (Figure 1-4) consists of a hollow coiled metal tube with an elliptical cross section that is exposed to an area where gas pressure measurement is desired. Attached to the coiled tube are a gear mechanism and a pointer. As pressure increases, the tube begins to straighten, causing the gears to turn and the position of the pointer to change. The tube straightens because the pressure causes the cross section of the tube to become rounder. As the cross section changes, the outside of the tube is stretched while the inside becomes compressed. These gauges are commonly found on medical gas cylinders, indicating the pressure inside of the cylinder, and are calibrated in pounds per square inch (psi).

GAS FLOW

Cause

Gas flows from one point to another due to a difference in pressure between the two points. Gas will flow from an area of greater pressure to an area of lower pressure. The area of greater pressure contains gas molecules with greater kinetic activity. As a result of the increased kinetic activity (energy), the molecules push

TABLE 1-1 Units of Pressure Measurement

Unit		Equivalent
1 Atm	=	760 mm Hg
		29.921 in Hg
		1034 cm H_2O
		101.325 KPa
		14.7 lb/in²
1 cm H_2O	=	.735 mm Hg
		.0142 lb/in²
1 mmHg	=	1.36 cm H_2O
		.019 lb/in²
1 KPa	=	.133 mm Hg
		.098 cm H_2O
		6.895 lb/in²
1 lb/in²	=	51.7 mm Hg
		70.34 cm H_2O

Figure 1-4 *A functional diagram of a Bourdon gauge. As the coiled tube expands, the gear mechanism rotates, causing the pointer to move.*

one another, moving from the area of higher energy to the area of lower energy.

The rate of gas flow, or velocity, is dependent on two factors: the difference in pressure (energy) and the size of the opening between the two areas. If the pressure difference is large, gas flow will be faster. If the pressure difference is small, gas flow will be slower. If the opening between the two areas is large, more gas can pass through and the flow will be greater than if the opening is small (Figure 1-5).

Bernoulli's Principle

During the eighteenth century, Daniel Bernoulli studied the flow of gas through tubes. He discovered that as the velocity of a gas increases, the lateral pressure within the tube decreases. This is due to the fact that the total energy content of the gas is constant. The total energy of the gas results from the kinetic energy created by the velocity and pressure energy. As velocity increases, the pressure must decrease for the total energy to remain constant (conservation of energy). As gas flow increases, more of the gas's energy is contained in kinetic energy, causing a further reduction in lateral pressure (Figure 1-6). In this application, **Bernoulli's principle** applies to the flow of gas within a tube that changes in

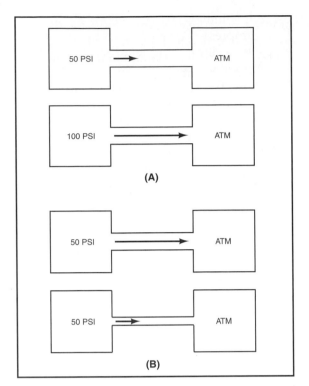

Figure 1-5 *Factors influencing gas flow: (A) two different pressures; (B) two different orifice sizes.*

area along its length. A cross-sectional change is required to change the velocity. Bernoulli's equation assumes that the fluid is incompressible, that is, that the specific weight (weight

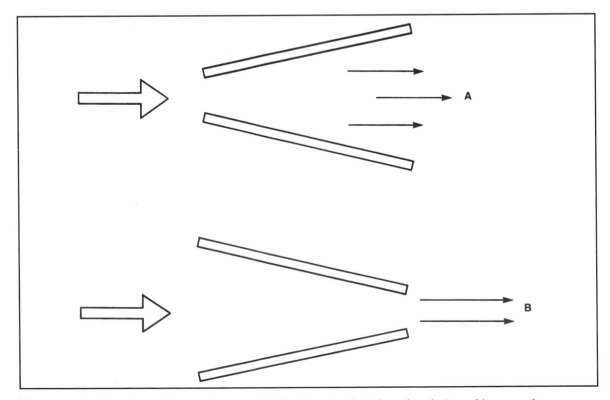

Figure 1-6 *Diverging and converging ducts: (A) the diverging duct slows the velocity and increases the pressure; (B) the converging duct increases the velocity and decreases the pressure.*

per unit volume) is constant. If the fluid were to be compressed, volume would decrease while the weight would remain constant, increasing the specific weight. Keep in mind that gases will remain incompressible at low velocities, generally less than 100 meters per second.

This principle is commonly applied in respiratory care equipment. The reduced pressure within the tube may be used to introduce gases (usually air) or liquids into a low-pressure region of gas flow.

VISCOUS SHEARING, VORTICITY, AND EJECTORS

Viscous shearing is another means by which oxygen is mixed with ambient or stationary air. **Viscous shearing** occurs when a high-velocity jet is injected into a quiescent gas. The high-velocity gas from the jet forms a thin boundary layer, where frictional forces develop between the high-velocity gas and the stationary surrounding air, cleaving it (Figure 1-7). The rapidly flowing gas accelerates the stationary gas, while the stationary gas decreases the velocity of the jet. Shear forces develop along the boundary layer between the two gases. The decelerating, high-velocity jet forms vortices, which envelop the ambient air, along the boundary layer. The viscous shearing effect entrains the room air into the vortices, mixing the oxygen with it. By varying the size of the oxygen jet and the entrainment ports, differing oxygen concentrations can be obtained. Manufacturers have developed specific combinations of entrainment ports and jet sizes to deliver precise F_iO_2 levels. This principle is applied in *High Air Flow with Oxygen Enrichment (HAFOE)* masks, commonly called "**venturi masks**."

Venturi's Principle

Venturi expanded Bernoulli's principle by adding a specially shaped tube downstream from the jet. This tube has an increasing radius such that the angle of the walls does not exceed 15 degrees (Figure 1-8A). Note the pressure curve as gas passes through the tube. Pressure is reduced in the center and, due to the Bernoulli effect, progressively increases as the diameter of the tube increases near the outlet (Figure 1-8B). The high velocity of the gas from the nozzle causes ambient air to be mixed with the gas from the nozzle (by viscous shearing and vorticity, described earlier in this chapter), adding to the total quantity of gas flowing through the tube. As the tube expands, gas velocity slows and pressure increases. Venturi tubes are often employed where gas flow can be increased through entrainment of ambient air. Due to the Bernoulli effect, gas velocities through venturi tubes are generally low.

Constant Area Duct

This type of **ducted ejector** is similar to a venturi tube except that instead of restoring lateral pressure, the tube's purpose is to maintain a high velocity following the jet or restriction.

The ejector consists of a straight-walled tube that does not change in diameter downstream from the jet. Gas is entrained at the entrance to the tube (due to viscous shearing and vorticity between the source gas and ambient air) increasing total flow through the device. The tube downstream from the jet shields the flow of gas from entrainment without significantly slowing the velocity of the gas through the device (Figure 1-9). Velocity remains high and pressure remains constant

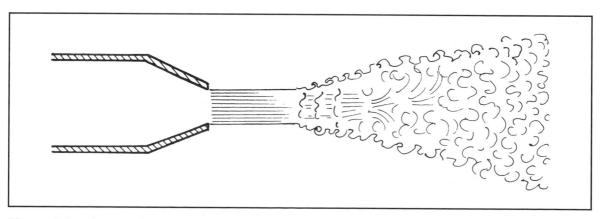

Figure 1-7 *The principle of viscous shearing. Note how the quiescent gas reduces the high velocity of the gas stream through the formation of vortices.*

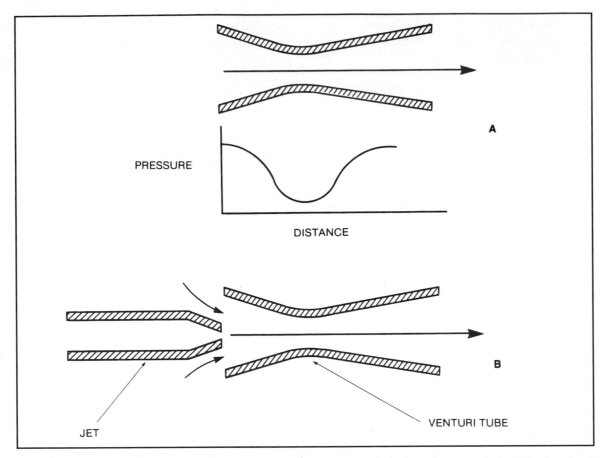

Figure 1-8 *Venturi's principle: (A) an illustration of the pressure gradient through a venturi tube; (B) a functional diagram of a nozzle combined with a venturi tube to form an ejector.*

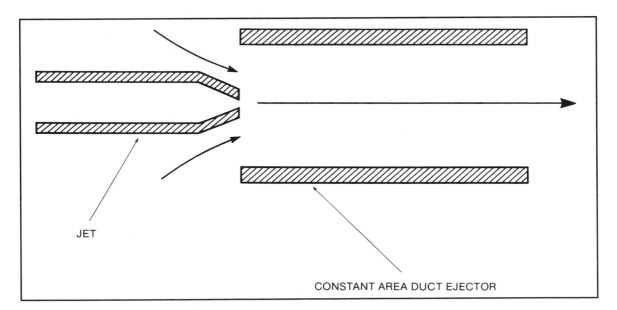

Figure 1-9 *A functional diagram of a constant-area duct ejector.*

because the diameter of the tube is constant (unlike the venturi tube). An advantage of this device is that an increased pressure downstream from the straight-walled tube has less effect on gas entrainment than with a venturi tube. These devices are employed in nebulizers and oxygen/air entrainment devices where there is moderate resistance downstream from the tube.

Effects of Increased Distal Pressure on Venturi and Constant Area Ducts

An increase in pressure downstream from an ejector will decrease the amount of ambient air entrainment. An increase in pressure may be caused by a kink in the delivery tubing or an obstruction distal to the point of air entrainment. This increase in pressure distal to the jet results in less ambient air entrainment because the total flow through the tube decreases as the back pressure increases. The flow through the jet's nozzle is constant; thus, the entrainment must decrease (Figure 1-10).

CHOKED FLOW OR COMPRESSIBLE FLOW

When a gas is flowing through an orifice or nozzle, the velocity of the gas increases as the pressure upstream (head pressure) of the nozzle increases. When the head reaches pressure 1.893 times the atmospheric pressure for air, the velocity of the gas no longer increases and the flow is choked. This corresponds to sonic flow at the orifice of the jet, which for air at room temperature is approximately 347 meters per second. This velocity corresponds to the speed of sound in air at room temperature. Once the gas reaches sonic velocity, the gas's velocity can no longer increase. Increasing the head pressure will not result in an increased flow when the flow is choked. The behavior of **choked flow** may be predicted using the choked flow equation, but this is beyond the scope of this text.

Choked flow is used in nebulizers when the head pressure driving the jet exceeds 26 psi, making the gas velocity out of the nozzle's exit sonic. Liquids are drawn into the gas flow from the reservoir via the capillary tube at the boundary layer by shear forces and vorticity.

When these high-velocity jets are used in ventilators, the gas flow downstream from the nozzle at a distance of approximately three times the diameter of the nozzle exit ceases to be well behaved or laminar. At this point a shear layer develops and ambient gas may be entrained by vorticity. When used in this application, these jets are sometimes referred to as injectors, although the term ejector is technically more correct. If designed properly, the flow output from an ejector will exceed the flow provided by the nozzle alone.

Reynolds' Number

Reynolds' number is used to determine if gas flow through a tube is laminar or turbulent. **Laminar gas flow** is a smooth, uniform flow that requires less energy (pressure) to sustain. **Turbulent gas flow** is more erratic and irregular, requiring more energy to sustain. Figure 1-11 compares turbulent and laminar

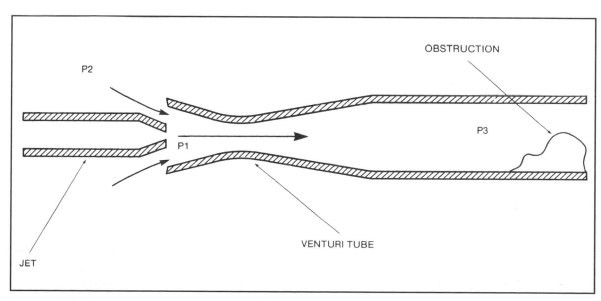

Figure 1-10 *An obstruction can result in decreased air entrainment through a venturi tube. P1 is less than P2 (atmospheric), and the obstruction causes P3 to be greater than P2. Note that the obstruction increases pressure distal to the entrainment ports, thus decreasing gas entrainment.*

Figure 1-11 *(A) Laminar and (B) turbulent gas flow.*

gas flow. The Reynolds' number formula is as follows:

$$R_e = \frac{(Velocity)(Density)(Diameter)}{Viscosity}$$

R_e = Reynolds' number

Note that if you include the correct units in the calculation of Reynolds' number, the units cancel one another, resulting in a number that is dimensionless. As a general rule, if the Reynolds' number is greater than 2000, flow will be turbulent. If the Reynolds' number is less than 2000, flow will be laminar.

Poiseuille's Law

Poiseuille described the resistance to the flow of gas or liquid through a tube when the flow is laminar. He determined that it is directly related to volumetric flow, length of the tube and viscosity of the gas, and inversely related to the radius of the tube to the fourth power. This law is generally expressed in the following formula:

$$\dot{V} = \frac{\Delta P(\pi)(r^4)}{8(l)(\mu)}$$

$\dot{V}$ = volumetric flow rate (velocity × area)
ΔP = pressure gradient
π = 3.1415
r = radius of the tube
μ = viscosity of the gas
l = length of the tube

Resistance is equal to the change in pressure divided by the volumetric flow rate.

Solving Poiseuille's law for resistance:

$$R = \frac{\Delta P}{\dot{V}}$$

$$R = \frac{8(l)(\mu)}{(\pi)(r^4)}$$

This formula is often simplified for clinical applications to the following:

$$\Delta P = \dot{V}(R)$$

$$\dot{V} = \frac{\Delta P}{R}$$

ΔP = pressure gradient
$\dot{V}$ = volumetric flow rate
R = resistance

Simply stated, as the radius of a tube decreases by one-half, resistance increases sixteen times. As gas velocity increases, resistance to gas flow also increases. Increasing the length of a tube also will increase resistance to flow. These relationships will become very important when studying mechanical ventilation of the lungs. For example, if secretions within the airways increase, the effective radius of the airway decreases and resistance to gas flow increases dramatically. This will require higher pressures within the airway to maintain a constant flow.

For turbulent flow, the relationship between flow rate, pressure gradient, and the radius of the tube is more complex. This is because the flow is affected by the shape of the tube, viscous forces that dissipate energy, and the Reynold's number. Generally, the volumetric flow rate is proportional to the radius to the 2.7th power, expressed as the following:

$$\dot{V} = r^{2.7}$$

The effect of radius on volumetric flow rate is not as great for turbulent flow as it is for laminar flow, but the effect is still quite pronounced. If the radius decreases by one-half, the volumetric flow rate is decreased by a factor of sixteen for laminar flow, and by a factor of between six and seven for turbulent flow. Generally, the flow of gas through most respiratory care equipment is turbulent rather than laminar. Laminar flow occurs physiologically within the lungs after several branches in the bronchial system.

GAS LAWS

An understanding of the gas laws is important in the practice of respiratory care. During mechanical ventilation, volumes, pressures, flows and the temperature of the gas delivered to a patient are routinely manipulated to better match changes in the patient's condition. It is important to be able to predict how these changes will affect gas delivery to the patient.

When performing mathematical calculations, it is important to use consistent units in all equations. For example, one can not mix cmH_2O and psi and expect correct results. It will be necessary to convert temperatures, and sometimes pressures, depending on the circumstances under which the gas laws are applied.

When converting temperature scales, you will need to apply the formulas listed in Table 1-2.

The two new temperature scales introduced are called the **absolute temperature** scales. Both scales are referenced to absolute zero. Therefore, neither scale will have negative numbers since the lowest temperature is zero.

Boyle's Law

Boyle's law relates the volume of a gas to its pressure. With temperature remaining constant, the volume of a gas varies inversely

TABLE 1-2 Temperature Conversion

Degrees Fahrenheit to Degrees Celsius

$\frac{5}{9}$ (Fahrenheit Temperature − 32)
= Degrees Celsius

Degrees Celsius to Degrees Fahrenheit

$\frac{9}{5}$ (Celsius Temperature) + 32
= Degrees Fahrenheit

Degrees Celsius to Degrees Kelvin

Celsius Temperature + 273 = Degrees Kelvin

30 C + 273 = 303 K

Degrees Fahrenheit to Degrees Rankine

Fahrenheit Temperature + 460
= Degrees Rankine

70 F + 460 = 530 R

with the pressure. Boyle's law is described in the following formula:

$$P_1(V_1) = P_2(V_2)$$

P_1 = original pressure
V_1 = original volume
P_2 = new pressure
V_2 = new volume

This formula is commonly rearranged as follows to solve for the original pressure (P_1) or the new pressure (P_2).

$$P_1 = \frac{P_2(V_2)}{V_1}$$

$$P_2 = \frac{P_1(V_1)}{V_2}$$

For example:

Given the following, V_1 = 500 ml, P_1 = 700 mmHg and P_2 = 300 mmHg, find the new volume.

$$\frac{P_1(V_1)}{V_2} = V_2$$

$$\frac{700 \text{ mmHg}(500 \text{ mL})}{300 \text{ mmHg}} = 1,167 \text{ mL}$$

This law is often applied in the mechanics of ventilation of the lungs and calculating residual volume using a body plethysmograph.

Charles' Law

Charles' law states that if pressure remains constant, the volume of a gas varies directly with the temperature (in degrees Kelvin). As the temperature increases, the volume of the gas also will increase. As the temperature of the gas decreases, volume will decrease. Charles' law is summarized in the following formula:

$$\frac{V_1}{T_1} = \frac{V_2}{T_2}$$

Before beginning this calculation, the temperature must first be converted to Kelvin, or absolute, temperature. To convert from Celsius to Kelvin, add 273 degrees. For example, given an original volume of 400 mL, an original temperature of 20 degrees Celsius and a new temperature of 40 degrees Celsius, find the new volume.

$$V_2 = \frac{T_2(V_1)}{T_1}$$

Converting Celsius to Kelvin:

$$20° + 273° = 293 \text{ K}$$
$$40° + 273° = 313 \text{ K}$$

$$V_2 = \frac{313°K(400 \text{ mL})}{293°K}$$

$$= 427.3 \text{ mL}$$

An easy way to demonstrate this law is to attach an inflated balloon to a small narrow-necked chemistry flask, then heat the flask with a Bunsen burner. As the gas warms, it expands, causing the balloon to become larger.

Dalton's Law

Dalton's law is sometimes referred to as the law of partial pressures. Dalton described how the pressure of a gas composed of a mixture of gases is equal to the sum of the partial pressures of all the discrete gases. That is, the total is equal to the sum of the parts. Furthermore, he stated that the partial pressure each gas exerts would be the same as if the gas occupied the total volume alone. Lastly, the partial pressure of each gas is proportional to its volumetric percentage.

For example:

Gas mixture D is composed of 15 mmHg gas A, 25 mmHg gas B and 200 mmHg gas C. What is the total pressure?

Gas A =	15 mmHg	
Gas B =	25 mmHg	
Gas C =	+ 200 mmHg	
Total Pressure =	240 mmHg	

What is the percentage of each gas in the mixture?

Gas A percentage
= 15 mmHg/240 mmHg = 6.3%

Gas B percentage
= 25 mmHg/240 mmHg = 10.4%

Gas C percentage
= 200 mmHg/240 mmHg = 83.3%

Another example of this law's use is the calculation of the partial pressures of the various gases in the atmosphere. Air is composed of nitrogen, oxygen, argon, and other gases sometimes referred to as trace gases.

Nitrogen	78.08%
Oxygen	20.95%
Argon	.93%
Carbon Dioxide	.03%
Trace Gases	.01%

At an atmospheric pressure of 640 mmHg (Denver, Colorado), what is the partial pressure of oxygen and how does that compare to the partial pressure of oxygen in Seattle, Washington (atmospheric pressure of 760 mmHg)?

Denver, Colorado:
640 mmHg × .2095 = 134.08 mmHg

Seattle, Washington:
760 mmHg × .2095 = 159.22 mmHg

There is a partial pressure difference of 25.14 mmHg for oxygen between the two cities due to a difference in atmospheric pressure.

Gay-Lussac's Law

Gay-Lussac described the relationship between pressure and temperature of a gas. He found that as temperature increases pressure will increase as long as volume is constant. This is known as **Gay-Lussac's law**. This relationship is described in the following formula:

$$\frac{P_1}{T_1} = \frac{P_2}{T_2}$$

For example:

A gas at 30° C and 700 mmHg is compressed to 900 mmHg. What is the new temperature?

$$\frac{P_2(T_1)}{P_1} = T_2$$

$$30°C + 273 = 303 \text{ K}$$

$$\frac{900 \text{ mmHg}(303 \text{ K})}{700 \text{ mmHg}} = 389.6 \text{ K}$$

$$389.6 \text{ K} - 273° = 117.6°C$$

This law can be illustrated when a bicycle tire is inflated using a manual tire pump. As the air is compressed in the pump, its temperature increases. After the tire is inflated, the tire pump is noticeably warmer. In respiratory care equipment, air compressors have external fins that conduct and dissipate the heat generated when the ambient air is compressed.

Combined Gas Law

The **combined gas law**, or general gas law, is a combination of Boyle's, Charles' and Gay-Lussac's laws. It is useful in determining pressure, volume or temperature changes. The law is summarized in the following formula:

$$\frac{P_1(V_1)}{T_1} = \frac{P_2(V_2)}{T_2}$$

For example:

A gas at a pressure of 200 mmHg, 300° K, and occupying 6 liters has its temperature increased to 400° K while occupying the same volume. Find the new pressure.

$$\frac{P_1(V_1)(T_2)}{T_1(V_2)} = P_2$$

$$\frac{200 \text{ mmHg}(6 \text{ liters})(400 \text{ K})}{300 \text{ K}(6 \text{ liters})} = 389.6 \text{ K}$$

GAS DIFFUSION

Besides pressure, volume and temperature relationships, it is important to understand gas diffusion. Gas diffusion is important physiologically in that gases constantly move from the atmosphere into our bodies, and then from our cells into our blood, by means of diffusion. There are three important laws of gas diffusion: Fick's, Henry's and Graham's laws.

Fick's Law

Fick's law describes how a gas diffuses into another gas. Fick's law states that the rate of diffusion of a gas into another gas is proportional to its concentration. That is, as the concentration gradient between the gases increases, the rate of diffusion will increase. Given two gases, where Gas A has a higher concentration than Gas B, Gas A will diffuse more rapidly than Gas B due to its greater concentration.

Henry's Law

Henry's law describes how gases diffuse into and out of liquids. Henry's law states that the rate of a gas's diffusion into a liquid is proportional to the partial pressure of that gas at a given temperature. Applying Henry's law, observe what happens when you open a bottle of soda pop. Once the cap is removed, bubbles can be seen moving toward the surface of the liquid and bursting once they reach the surface. The partial pressure of carbon dioxide is greater in the liquid than in the atmosphere. Therefore, carbon dioxide gas diffuses from the dissolved state (liquid) to a gaseous state and escapes into the atmosphere.

Graham's Law

Gas diffusion in the blood is more complex than what occurs as described in Henry's law. Other factors, such as the gram molecular weight and solubility of the gases, must be accounted for when understanding diffusion across the alveolar capillary membrane.

Graham's law states that the rate of gas diffusion through a liquid is proportional to the solubility of a gas and inversely proportional to the gram molecular weight. Comparing oxygen and carbon dioxide, oxygen's solubility is .023, while carbon dioxide's solubility is .510.

$$\text{Solubility of } CO_2 = \frac{0.510}{0.023}$$

$$= \frac{22}{1}$$

This relationship shows that carbon dioxide is over 20 times more soluble in the blood than oxygen. Once the gases are dissolved, they must diffuse through the blood. In determining the rate of diffusion, you must now account for the gram molecular weight.

$$Solubility = \frac{(Sol\ Coef\ CO_2)(\sqrt{gmw}\ O_2)}{(Sol\ Coef\ O_2)(\sqrt{gmw}\ CO_2)}$$

$$= \frac{(0.510)(\sqrt{32})}{(0.023)(\sqrt{44})}$$

$$= \frac{19}{1}$$

This relationship shows that carbon dioxide is 19 times more diffusible in the blood than oxygen. This relationship is true, assuming that the partial pressures for the two gases are equal. Normally in the alveolus, the partial pressure of oxygen is greater than that for carbon dioxide, resulting in a slightly greater rate of diffusion for oxygen.

MEDICAL GAS SUPPLY EQUIPMENT

COMPRESSORS

Medical **compressors** provide oil-free compressed air to power equipment and also to mix with pure oxygen to provide lower oxygen concentrations. The compressed air must be oil free for two primary reasons: (1) oil particles, when inhaled, are not healthy, (2) oil droplets, when mixed with oxygen, may result in spontaneous combustion. (Spontaneous combustion is the ignition of a substance without the addition of heat.) There are three types of compressors: piston, diaphragm and centrifugal.

Piston Compressor

A piston compressor utilizes a piston driven by an electric motor (Figure 1-12). Carbon or Teflon® piston rings seal the piston against the cylinder wall, eliminating the need for oil. The compressed air is fed into a storage reservoir providing a large supply of air to meet high flow demands. A filter at the outlet removes any particles from the compressed air. The pressure is then reduced to 50 psi by means of a reducing valve before the air is fed into a piping system.

Diaphragm Compressor

Diaphragm compressors utilize a flexible diaphragm driven by an electric motor to compress the air. Diaphragm compressors are typically employed to power small nebulizers. They are not capable of providing the large amounts of compressed air needed for large

Figure 1-12 *A functional diagram of a piston compressor.*

ASSEMBLY AND TROUBLESHOOTING

Assembly—Compressors

To prepare a compressor for use, complete the following steps.

1. Connect the power cord to the correct electrical outlet—115 volts, alternating current (VAC).

2. Attach equipment requiring compressed air to the threaded outlet.

3. Check inlet filter for obstruction and, if required, clean or replace it.

4. Turn on the compressor with the on/off switch.

5. Verify correct outlet pressure (50 psi) with the gauge provided.

Troubleshooting

Troubleshooting compressors is very easy. Unfortunately, if the unit fails to operate, little can be done other than to take the compressor to an authorized repair center. When troubleshooting this equipment, please follow the suggested troubleshooting algorithm (ALG 1-1).

---

equipment. Figure 1-13 depicts a typical diaphragm compressor suitable for home use.

Centrifugal Compressor

The **centrifugal compressor** utilizes an electrically powered impeller mounted eccentrically within the compressor housing. As the impeller rotates, it compresses the air. Centrifugal force and the decreasing size of

the chamber compress the gas as the impeller turns (Figure 1-14). These compressors are incorporated in some adult mechanical ventilators such as the Bennett MA-1.

A larger version of this type of compressor is used to provide a compressed air source for hospitals and other institutions. These rotary compressors use similar principles of operation, except that a working fluid (usually water) is used between the impeller and the

Figure 1-13 *A functional diagram of a diaphragm compressor.*

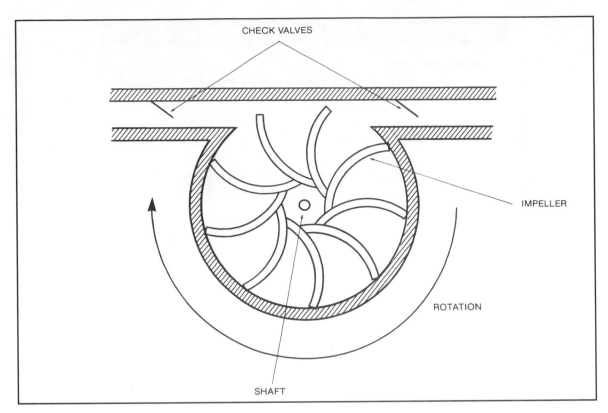

Figure 1-14 *A functional diagram of a centrifugal compressor.*

compressor housing. The working fluid allows tolerances to be greater between the impeller and the compressor housing, reducing wear and eliminating the need for lubrication. A water separator and particle filters purify the air prior to delivery to the hospital piping system.

Water traps should be used with all ventilators powered by compressed gases. Water can become condensed as air or oxygen is pressurized. A contemporary ventilator's pneumatic, electronic control and monitoring system can be damaged by water that may be contained in the high pressure supply lines. To avoid this potential problem, the use of water traps is recommended by most manufacturers.

CONCENTRATORS

Oxygen concentrators are electrically powered devices that separate the oxygen from the atmosphere and deliver it under pressure for medical use. There are two types of oxygen concentrating devices, molecular sieve and membrane types.

The **molecular sieve concentrator** is more effective than the membrane type. Inlet air to a compressor is passed through a particle filter to remove large particles from the air. Then the gas is passed through a bacteria filter that removes particles as small as 0.3 microns. The filtered air is then compressed by a compressor to approximately 20 psi, and conducted to molecular sieves containing Zeolite. The compressed gas alternately charges one sieve and then the other. The Zeolite in the sieve adsorbs some of the nitrogen and passes the oxygen contained in the ambient air, thus increasing the oxygen concentration.

The process of **adsorption** is a surface phenomenon in which the gas molecules are forced under pressure into the pores of the Zeolite. As the nitrogen oxygen mixture (air) flows through the pores of the Zeolite, the nitrogen molecules stick or adhere to the surface and the oxygen molecules pass through. When the sieve is depressurized, the nitrogen is released to the atmosphere and exhausted, separating it from the oxygen-enriched gas.

Oxygen concentrators use some of the oxygen-rich gas flowing from one sieve to purge the other sieve. This is done prior to pressurization to improve oxygen percentage levels. The purge cycle helps to rid the canister of nitrogen before it is again pressurized with room air.

Oxygen concentration will vary between 50% to greater than 90% depending on the

START

Is the compressor operating OK?

Yes → 1 → Continue to operate the equipment and monitor the patient → END

ON

Does it work when turned on?

Yes

Is the output low?

Yes → 1

Yes → Inlet filter dirty?

Yes → Clean or replace inlet filter

NO

Are any connecting tubing or hoses obstructed?

Yes → 1) Clear obstruction or 2) Replace tubing or hose

NO

Are there any leaks at fittings or connections?

Yes → Tighten all connections

NO → Send to bio-medical repair facility → END

Does it work when turned on?

NO → Is the electrical outlet OK?

NO → Check the outlet with a lamp or test indicator

Yes → Is a fuse blown or a circuit breaker tripped?

Yes → 1) Replace fuse or 2) Reset circuit breaker

NO → 1

ALG 1-1 *An algorithm describing how to troubleshoot a compressor.*

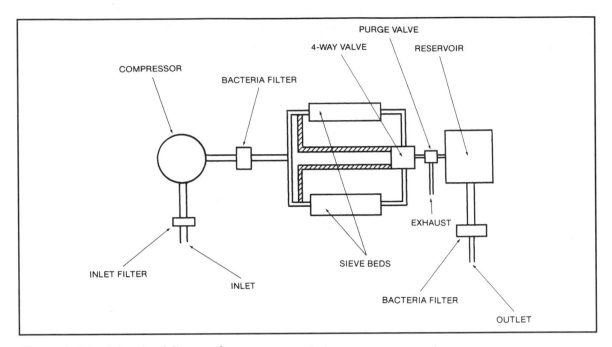

Figure 1-15 *A functional diagram of an oxygen concentrator.*

flow rate out of the concentrator. If the flow rate is set for 2 liters (L) per minute or less, the oxygen concentration will be 90% or sometimes higher. If flow is increased to 10 liters per minute, the oxygen concentration drops to 50%. Figure 1-15 shows a schematic of a typical oxygen concentrator and its component parts.

The **membrane enricher**, commonly called an enricher, uses a semipermeable polymer membrane to remove the nitrogen from the air. An air compressor forces the air through the one-micron-thick membrane, allowing the smaller oxygen molecules to pass. A membrane enricher can provide a concentration of 40% oxygen at flow rates between 1 and 10 liters per minute.

Invacare® Platinum™ 5 Oxygen Concentrator

The Invacare® Platinum™ 5 oxygen concentrator is a unit that uses molecular sieve technology to separate oxygen from room air (Figure 1-16).

The unit is capable of providing low-flow oxygen at concentrations between 95.6% to 87% from flows between 0.5 to 5 L/min. These concentrators allow patients to receive continuous oxygen without the use of liquid oxygen systems or compressed gas cylinders. Power consumption averages 400 watts during continuous operation.

Figure 1-16 *A photograph of the Invacare® Platinum™ 5 oxygen concentrator.*

Invacare® Venture® HomeFill™ II Oxygen Filling System

Invacare® Venture® HomeFill™ II oxygen filling system is a small multistage compressor that is designed to interface with the Invacare® 5-liter oxygen concentrators (Figure 1-17). The oxygen filling system allows patients to transfill small ambulatory cylinders from the oxygen concentrator's output. The unit is

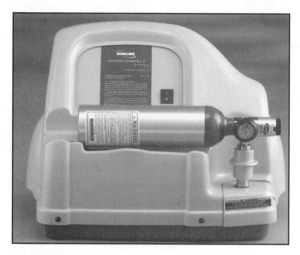

Figure 1-17 *A photograph of the Invacare® Venture® HomeFill™ II oxygen filling system. This unit is a multi-stage pump designed to fill portable oxygen cylinders.*

designed to interface with the Invacare® ML6 (164 liter) and M9 (248 liter) capacity portable oxygen cylinders. It takes approximately 1½ to 2½ hours to fill a cylinder (ML6 and M9, respectively). The filling system provides patient independence from their home care provider delivering filled portable oxygen cylinders for ambulatory use, as well as long-term cost savings.

Liter flow from the concentrator during transfilling is limited to 0 to 3 L/min. The input to the transfilling compressor during operation is 2 L/min. Power consumption averages 200 watts when transfilling the cylinders. An electrical outlet separate from the concentrator must be available for the Home-Fill II® oxygen filling system, in that each unit has its own independent power supply.

Puritan Bennett Companion 492a

The Puritan Bennett Companion 492a oxygen concentrator operates using two molecu-

Figure 1-18 *A photograph of the Puritan Bennett Companion 492a oxygen concentrator. (Courtesy Puritan Bennett Corporation, Lenexa, KS)*

lar sieves to separate oxygen from room air (Figure 1-18). The unit is capable of providing 95% oxygen concentration ± 3% at flows between 1 and 3 L/min. If the oxygen flow is 4 L/min, oxygen concentrations are 92% ± 3%. During normal operation the Companion 492a will consume an average of 330 watts electrical power. Ideally, the concentrator should be the only item connected to the electrical outlet and on that electrical circuit.

ASSEMBLY AND TROUBLESHOOTING

Oxygen Concentrators

1. Position the oxygen concentrator in the room where your patient will spend the majority of his or her time. Be sure to choose a location away from heaters, radiators, and hot-air registers. Place the unit so that the back and sides are at least 6 inches away from any objects to ensure adequate air flow through the unit.

2. Concentrators incorporate a particle filter. Remove the filter from its housing or holder. Inspect the particle filter for lint or other debris. The patient should be instructed to wash this filter at least once a week. The filter may be washed in a solution of warm water and dishwashing detergent and then rinsed thoroughly with warm tap water and toweled dry. The filter should be

completely dry before it is reinstalled. The particle filter may also be cleaned daily by using a vacuum cleaner attachment without removing the filter from the concentrator. The filter must still be washed weekly.

3. If humidification has been prescribed:

a. Fill the humidifier reservoir with distilled water to the "fill" line and then thread the humidifier directly onto the fixed oxygen Diameter Index Safety System (DISS) outlet so that the humidifier is suspended.

b. Attach the desired length of oxygen delivery tubing (not to exceed 50 feet, or 15 meters) to the humidifier outlet. If condensation occurs when using longer lengths of oxygen tubing, condensation may be reduced by using a removable humidifier stand.

4. If humidification has not been prescribed:

a. Thread a green "Christmas Tree" fitting onto the fixed oxygen DISS outlet fitting and attach the desired length of oxygen delivery tubing (not to exceed 50 feet, or 15 meters).

5. Connect the cannula, transtracheal cannula, or mask to the oxygen delivery tubing.

6. Check to be certain that the power switch is in the "OFF" position. Select an electrical outlet (120 V, 60 Hz) that is not connected by a wall switch and is independent of other appliances.

7. Depress the power switch to the "ON" position.

8. Adjust the flowmeter to the prescribed oxygen setting by turning the flowmeter knob counterclockwise to increase the flow of oxygen. Verify oxygen flow through the cannula/delivery tubing and or the humidifier. An oxygen analyzer can be used to confirm that the concentration being delivered is correct.

Troubleshooting

Follow the suggested troubleshooting algorithm (ALG 1-2) to assist you in troubleshooting this concentrator.

1. If the unit fails to operate when turned on:

a. Check to be certain that the power cord is plugged into a 120 V, 60 Hz electrical outlet.

b. The electrical outlet may not have power. Test the outlet with a household lamp or radio. If the power is not on at the outlet, use another outlet.

c. The circuit breaker has tripped. Press the black reset button on the rear cover. If the breaker trips again, contact your dealer for service.

2. If the air intake or exhaust is blocked:

a. Check and service the gross particle filter if required.

b. Check for objects blocking discharge air from the bottom right side of the unit.

3. If the unit is operating but you are unable to obtain the desired flow of enriched gas, check the following:

a. Blocked oxygen delivery device or connecting tubing.

(1) Remove the delivery device (cannula, catheter, or transtracheal catheter) from the extension tubing. If flow is restored, clean or replace the delivery device.

(2) Disconnect the extension tubing from the humidifier. If flow is restored, check the tubing for kinks or obstructions, or replace the tubing as required.

b. Blocked or defective humidifier.

(1) Remove the humidifier from the outlet of the MC84. If flow is restored, clean or replace the humidifier.

c. Use of excessive length of connecting tubing. Use a maximum of 50 feet, or 15 meters, of tubing.

4. If the unit operates but you are unable to obtain the appropriate oxygen concentration:

a. Ensure the patient has an adequate supply of compressed oxygen or liquid oxygen.

b. Remove the unit from service and return it to an authorized service center.

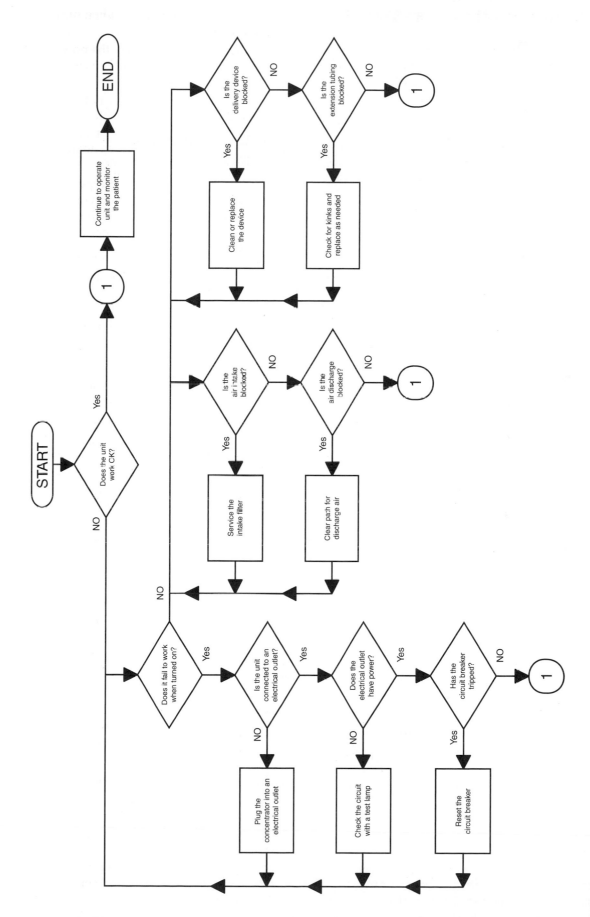

ALG 1-2 *An algorithm describing how to troubleshoot oxygen concentrators.*

LIQUID RESERVOIR SYSTEMS

Bulk Supply Systems

Bulk supply systems are used to supply large amounts of medical gas to a hospital or other institution. It is more economical to operate a bulk system than to use many small cylinders. The construction of a bulk liquid storage reservoir is very similar to an enlarged steel thermos. An outer steel shell encloses several layers of insulation in a near vacuum. The inner wall contains the liquid gas (Figure 1-19). Standards of bulk reservoir construction have been established by the American Society of Mechanical Engineers. Liquid oxygen is stored in the reservoir at a temperature of –183° Celsius. Liquid oxygen continuously vaporizes, creating pressure. Pressure relief valves are incorporated into the reservoir to release pressure. The release of pressure, as the gas expands, cools the reservoir (Gay-Lussac's law).

It is important to size the reservoir properly, so that the use of gas exceeds the rate of vaporization. If too much gas is lost to the atmosphere by vaporization, it may not be economical to operate the bulk system. An advantage of storing oxygen in liquid form is that one cubic foot of liquid oxygen expands to 861 heat exchanger cubic feet of gaseous oxygen (1:861 ratio). The liquid oxygen is fed

into a heat exchanger like a radiator; it warms the liquid to a gas (Figure 1-19). Once the liquid has vaporized to a gas, pressure will have increased. The pressure is reduced to 50 psi by passing through a reducing valve. After the pressure has been reduced to 50 psi, the gas is then fed into the piping system.

Portable Reservoirs

Smaller liquid reservoirs have been designed for home and ambulatory use (Figure 1-20). The principles of construction are similar to the large bulk systems described earlier, only smaller in scale.

The larger reservoirs designed for stationary use in the home vary in capacity from 20 to 43 liquid liters. Although the capacity may seem small, remember that one liquid liter of oxygen is equal to 861 gaseous liters. This makes the capacity in gaseous liters range from 16,400 to 35,200 liters. Physical size ranges of these reservoirs are diameters of 12–15 inches and heights of 27–38 inches and weights that vary, when full, between 84 and 160 lbs.

The smaller portable reservoirs are designed to be easily carried on the shoulder or placed into a small cart for ambulation. The liquid capacities of these portable units range from .6 liters to 1.23 liters, giving them a gaseous capacity of 500 to 1058 liters. Weights

Figure 1-19 *A bulk liquid oxygen storage and supply system. Note the insulated container, control valve, and heat exchanger. The heat exchanger converts the liquid to a gas by warming it.*

Figure 1-20 *A contemporary portable liquid home oxygen system. The larger reservoir is for use in the home. The smaller portable reservoir may be filled from the larger one for trips away from home lasting up to eight hours at flow rates less than 2 liters per minute. (Courtesy CAIRE, Inc., Bloomington, MN)*

Figure 1-21 *A photograph of the HELiOS® portable oxygen system.*

of these units when full vary from 5.3 to 9.0 lbs. Oxygen conservation devices such as pulse demand flow regulators (described later in this chapter), when used in conjunction with the liquid reservoirs, can dramatically extend the duration of oxygen supply. These devices, when coupled with liquid supply systems and cylinders, can result in oxygen savings of 3–7 times when compared to conventional continuous oxygen flow delivery.

Mallinckrodt Puritan Bennett® HELiOS® Portable Liquid Oxygen System

The HELiOS® portable oxygen system is a small lightweight liquid oxygen reservoir that incorporates a pneumatic oxygen conserving device (Figure 1-21). Patients requiring continuous oxygen may be independent and ambulatory with this unit for up to 8 to 10 hours at a setting of 2 on the conserving device. The weight of the unit when full is 3.6 pounds and only 2.7 pounds when empty. The unit must be used with the dual lumen nasal cannula

that allows the pneumatic system to sense the patient's inspiration, delivering oxygen during the inspiratory phase of ventilation. The rate of oxygen evaporative loss from the unit is between 1 to 1.5 pounds per day. The portable unit can be filled from a larger liquid reservoir in less than one minute (40 seconds).

Portable Oxygen Duration

It may be necessary to calculate the duration of oxygen flow from these portable liquid reservoirs. These calculations are all based upon the weight of the units. All portable systems incorporate some form of spring scale to estimate the contents remaining. Many are calibrated in fourths and some use LED displays to further subdivide the contents into smaller increments. However, these scales are only estimates and do not accurately reflect the contents remaining in the reservoirs.

Sometimes it may be necessary to accurately calculate the number of liters or duration in time remaining in a portable liquid system. These calculations are also based upon weight. However, since the accuracy of spring scales varies, all calculations shown incorporate a scale factor (.80) to allow for variation in scales. It is also required that you know the empty weight of the reservoir you are working with. This can be found in the owner's manual or service manual.

Derivation of the formula:

(1) Density of O_2 at its boiling point
    = 1141 kg/m³

(2) 1141.0 kg/m³ (2.2 lb/kg) = 2510.2 lb/m³

(3) 2510.2 lbs/m³ (.001 m³/L)
    = 2.5102 lbs/L

(4) 1 liter (liquid) = 860.6 liters (gaseous)

$$\frac{860.6 \text{ liters (gas)}}{2.5102 \text{ lbs/L (liquid)}} = \frac{324.8 \text{ L (gas)}}{\text{lbs (liquid)}}$$

RESULT: There are 342.8 L gaseous oxygen per lb of liquid oxygen.

For example:

You are working with a patient in her home who is using a large portable reservoir at 2 L/min. She wants to know how long her reservoir will last before it needs to be refilled. The indicator says it is ½ full, but she is still concerned. What is the duration of the reservoir?

Empty Weight = 60 lbs (from service manual)

Current Weight = 145 lbs

Scale Factor = .80

(145 lbs − 60 lbs [liquid]) = 342.8 L (gas)/lb (liquid) × .80 = 23,310 L (gas)

$$\frac{23,310 \text{ L (gas)}}{2 \text{ L min}} = 11,655 \text{ minutes}$$

$$\frac{11,655 \text{ minutes}}{60 \text{ minutes/hour}} = 194 \text{ hours, or 8 days}$$

Notice in the calculation that the capacity in liters was multiplied by .80. This scale factor gives you a reserve or cushion of 20% to allow for accuracy variation in the spring scale used to weigh the liquid reservoir.

ASSEMBLY AND TROUBLESHOOTING

Assembly—Portable Liquid Oxygen Systems

Little is required for proper assembly of portable liquid reservoirs. The following guide will help you in the assembly and preparation of the reservoir for use.

1. Ensure that the reservoir is filled by checking the weight gauge provided.
   a. Should the reservoir require filling, contact your local vendor.

2. Attach a flowmeter and humidifier to the threaded outlet of the reservoir.

3. Attach the oxygen therapy equipment to the outlet of the humidifier.

4. Turn on the flowmeter to the ordered setting and observe for proper flow. When transfilling the ambulatory reservoirs, follow the manufacturer's instructions carefully. Since connections and attachment vary, specific instructions are not included here. When transfilling the portable reservoir, exercise caution. The extreme cold temperatures of the fittings may result in cryogenic burns!

Troubleshooting

When troubleshooting this equipment, please follow the suggested troubleshooting algorithm (ALG 1-3).

1. If gas fails to flow from the oxygen therapy device:
   a. Check to ensure the reservoir is full, using the weight gauge or other gauge provided by the manufacturer.
   b. Check all connections for tightness. Check for leaks by feeling and by listening for escaping gas.
   c. Make certain that the humidifier is assembled correctly and that it is not obstructed. Check to ensure that all threaded connections are tight.
   d. Check oxygen tubing for kinks or obstruction.
   e. If (a) through (d) are satisfactory, contact your local vendor.

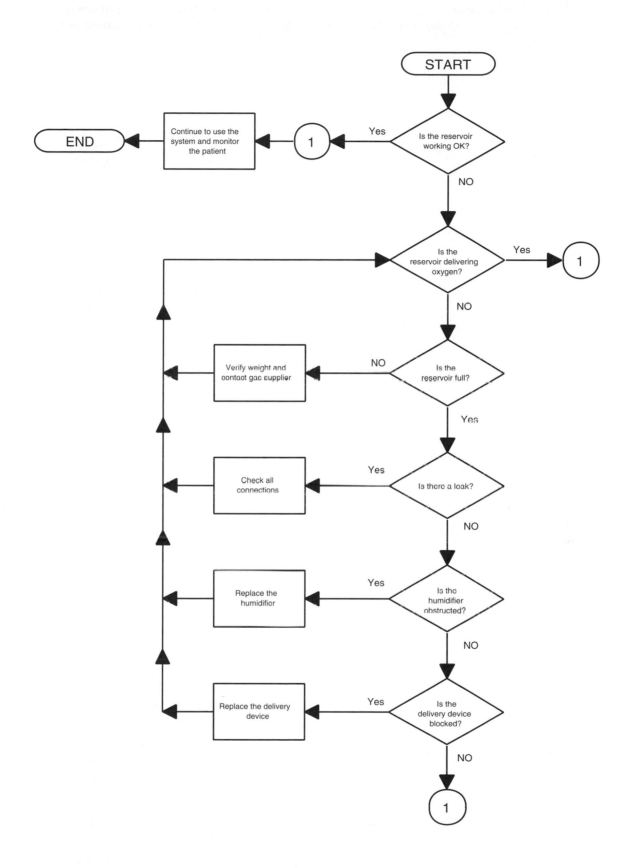

ALG 1-3 *An algorithm describing how to troubleshoot a portable liquid oxygen reservoir.*

PIPING SYSTEMS

Piping systems provide a safe, convenient way to distribute medical gases throughout an institution. The initial cost of these systems is quite high; however, over time they may be more cost effective than cylinders, depending on the quantity of medical gases used.

CONSTRUCTION OF PIPING SYSTEMS

The National Fire Protection Association has established standards for the construction and operation of medical gas piping systems.

Supply

Oxygen may be supplied from a **manifold** of two or more cylinders, a bulk liquid reservoir or both. A manifold consists of two or more cylinders connected together using high-pressure steel or copper tubing. When two or more cylinders are interconnected, the total volume of gas available is greater than a single cylinder alone. Part C of Figure 1-22 depicts a schematic of an oxygen supply system using two cylinder manifolds. Figure 1-22 illustrates the three primary types of supply systems. The supply system is designed to meet the

institution's needs, and requires periodic filling from an oxygen vendor. Liquid gas can be delivered whenever the reservoir requires filling, or on a regularly scheduled basis. It is transported to the institution by truck or by rail.

A reserve supply is required to provide up to 24 hours of oxygen in the event that the main supply becomes depleted. The reserve supply can consist of a smaller liquid reservoir or a manifold of cylinders. When pressure in the main supply drops, a valve automatically opens, activating the reserve supply.

The pressure is reduced by means of a regulator or reducing valve before the gas enters the piping system.

Piping System Construction

A piping system conducts the gas through copper pipes to points of use. This piping system is similar in design to the water system in your home or apartment; however, it must conform to stricter standards of construction. These systems are made from seamless K- or L-type copper tubing. The tubing must meet specific standards regarding its ability to withstand pressure without rupturing. All joints are sweat soldered using silver solder.

Sweat soldering is accomplished by applying heat to the joint using a torch. The solder is melted, flows into the joint, and seals it. Flux may be used to clean the joint and allow the solder to adhere to the metal better.

After soldering, joints are carefully checked for leaks. The pipes are independently supported to the building structure at specified intervals. This means that nothing else may be attached to the building's structure at the same point where the medical gas piping system is attached. Following construction, the system is cleaned of any flux or debris and pressure tested. The system is pressurized to 1.5 times its working pressure with dry, oil-free air or with nitrogen. Each joint is then checked for leaks. The system is allowed to stand for 24 hours at this pressure and must remain leak free during this time in order to pass final inspection.

Following the pressure test, both the oxygen and air supply lines are charged with gas. The oxygen piping system is supplied by a bulk oxygen system, while a medical air compressor supplies gas for the air piping system. The outlets are then tested for purity. Oxygen and air lines are checked with analyzers to ensure that they are delivering the correct gas.

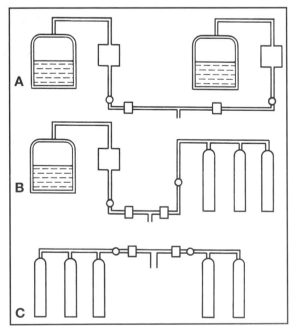

Figure 1-22 *Bulk oxygen supply systems that are typical for most medical care facilities. (A) Liquid primary and liquid reserve, (B) Liquid primary and cylinder reserve, and (C) Cylinder primary and cylinder reserve.*

Once the purity test has been completed, the system may be used for patient care.

Safety Features

Safety features in a medical gas piping system include alarms, zone valves, riser valves and pressure sensors.

Alarms are included in a piping system. These alert personnel to pressure drops in the system caused by leaks or depletion of the gas supply. The alarm must be placed in an area that is attended 24 hours a day. For this reason, the hospital telephone switchboard is a common location for medical gas alarm panels.

Zone valves are shutoff valves placed at strategic positions so that gas supply to different areas may be cut off in the event of a fire. Zone valves also are placed at the base of risers (pipes conducting gas from one floor to another), as shown in Figure 1-23. In some acute care facilities, Respiratory Care Practitioners (RCPs), are required to identify and turn off the appropriate zone valves in the

event of a fire. If a zone valve is turned off, the RCP is also responsible to ensure that patients requiring oxygen receive it from cylinders or another source during transport from the scene of a fire and also when returning the patients to their rooms.

Pressure sensors are placed throughout the piping system to monitor pressure. Line pressure in most hospital systems is 50 psi.

Station Outlets

Medical gas outlets, located at the points of desired use, are termed station outlets. Special fittings are incorporated into these outlets, preventing the connection of equipment designed for a different gas. Examples of these fittings include Diameter Indexed Safety Fittings and quick-connect fittings.

The Diameter Indexed Safety System (DISS) was designed by the Compressed Gas Association. This system utilizes differing thread pitch, connection diameter, and internal and external threading to prevent the

Figure 1-23 *Placement of safety shutoff valves in a piping system. Note the placement of the main supply shutoff, riser valves, and zone valves.*

Figure 1-24 *A photograph of a DISS oxygen fitting.*

valves, incorporated into station outlets, to prevent gas loss when not in use.

Quick-connect fittings vary from one manufacturer to another. These fittings are designed to be rapidly connected or disconnected without the use of threads. Figure 1-25 shows an example of common quick-connect outlets.

CYLINDERS

Oxygen cylinders provide a convenient method of providing oxygen delivery to a patient. The smaller cylinder sizes are portable, facilitating their use in an emergency, ambulatory, or transport setting. Oxygen cylinders are safe and effective when handled correctly.

Cylinder Construction

The construction of oxygen cylinders is strictly regulated by the Department of Transportation (DOT). Medical gas cylinders are seamless, either made from high strength chrome molybdenum steel or a high strength aluminum alloy. Steel cylinders are spun into shape while the steel is still hot. Following shaping, the steel is heat treated to retain its tensile strength. Recently, the aluminum alloy cylinders have gained popularity due to their lighter weight. High strength steel cylinders are stamped with the marking "DOT 3AA."

attachment of equipment designed for dissimilar gases or gas mixtures (Figure 1-24). It is designed for pressures less than 200 psi, which by definition is termed low pressure. Check

Figure 1-25 *Three quick-connect fittings. Left to right are oxygen, air, and vacuum.*

Figure 1-26 *A photograph of a carbon fiber-wrapped cylinder developed for ambulatory patient use.*

"DOT" refers to the Department of Transportation and "3AA" indicates heat treated high strength steel. The designation "3AL" denotes aluminum construction. Typically, cylinders are filled to a pressure 10% greater than the working pressure indicated on its shoulder, providing the cylinder has passed the required hydrostatic testing.

Light weight aluminum cylinders reinforced with carbon fiber wrap have been developed for ambulatory patient use (Figure 1-26). These cylinders incorporate an ultra-thin aluminum wall reinforced with helical and hoop wraps of carbon fiber impregnated with epoxy resin for reinforcement. The weight savings over steel cylinders of similar size is approximately 70%, and about a 30% weight savings is realized compared with conventional aluminum cylinder construction. The cylinders are designed to be filled to a service pressure of 3000 psi. When used with oxygen-conserving devices, these cylinders can provide a long duration with a very light-weight package for ambulatory use.

Cylinder Markings

The DOT requires that cylinder data be stamped on the shoulder of the cylinder (Figures 1-27 and 1-28).

Hydrostatic Testing

Every five years a cylinder is subjected to a hydrostatic test to measure its elasticity. The cylinder is filled to a pressure equal to 5/3 its working pressure and cylinder expansion is measured. If the expansion is within tolerance, the cylinder is returned to service. If the cylinder fails the test, it is removed from service and destroyed. The inspector's mark and the date of the test, followed by a "+" sign (steel cylinders only), are then stamped into the shoulder of the cylinder. If a star follows the inspection date, the cylinder may go for ten years before another hydrostatic test is performed (steel cylinders only).

Some communities may be limited in their ability to provide hydrostatic testing for fiber-wrapped cylinders since the designed service pressure is 3000 psi. The testing site would need equipment capable of exceeding 5000 psi pressure to hydrostatically test a fiber-wrapped cylinder.

Figure 1-27 *Cylinder markings indicate the cylinder has passed inspection. The inspection was performed in March 1982. The inspector's mark is between the month and year. The "+" sign indicates the cylinder complies with the hydrostatic test. The star marking indicates the cylinder may go ten years before being tested again.*

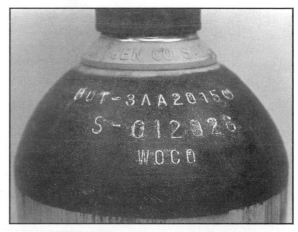

Figure 1-28 *Cylinder markings indicate that the cylinder is made from high tensile strength heat-treated steel (DOT 3AA) and has a service pressure of 2015 psi (2015). The serial number is below the DOT numbers and the owner's stamp is below the serial number.*

Cylinder Sizes

Medical gas cylinders are manufactured in many sizes (Figure 1-29). The most common sizes encountered in the hospital environment are the "H" and the "E" cylinders. The "H" cylinder contains 244 cubic feet of oxygen and weighs approximately 135 pounds. The "E" cylinder contains 22 cubic feet of oxygen and weighs approximately 16 pounds. Since the "E" cylinder is smaller and lighter, it is usually used for ambulation of patients (with a cart) and for transporting patients from one place to another within the hospital.

Color Coding

The Compressed Gas Association has developed a color code for the different medical gases and gas mixtures. This code was published by the Department of Commerce through the recommendation of the Bureau of Standards. An international color code also exists for medical gases. The only difference between the two color codes is the color for

COMMON METRIC EQUIVALENTS (APPROX.)
1 Cubic Foot....7.48   gallons....28.3   liters
1 Gallon.........3.785 liters.......0.132 cubic feet
1 Liter..........0.264 gallons....0.035 cubic feet

		B/BB	D/DD	E	M	G	H
CO_2	Liters	370	940	1590	7570	12300	15800
	Gals.	100	250	420	2000	3263	4180
	C.F.	13.37	33.2	56.1	267	436	558
	Wt.	1 lb. 8 oz.	3 lbs. 13 oz.	6 lbs. 7 oz.	30 lbs. 10 oz.	50 lbs. 0 oz.	64 lbs. 0 oz.
CO_2/O_2	Liters		400	660	3000	5330	6000
	Gals.		105	174	793	1408	1585
	C.F.		14.1	23.3	106	188	212
	Wt.		1 lb. 3 oz.	2 lbs. 0 oz.	8 lbs. 15 oz.	15 lbs. 14 oz.	17 lbs. 14 oz.
C_3H_6	Liters	378	871				
	Gals.	100	230				
	C.F.	13.37	30.75				
	Wt.	1 lb. 7.25 oz.	3 lbs. 5.5 oz.				
He	Liters		300	500	2260	4000	6000
	Gals.		79.2	132	597	1057	1585
	C.F.		10.6	17.6	79.8	141	213
	Wt.		0 lbs. 1.8 oz.	0 lbs. 2.9 oz.	0 lbs.13.2 oz.	1 lb. 7.5 oz.	2 lbs. 2.8 oz.
He/O_2	Liters			500	2260	4000	4500
	Gals.			132	597	1057	1189
	C.F.			17.6	79.8	141	159
	Wt.						
N_2O	Liters		940	1590	7570	13800	15800
	Gals.		249	420	2000	3657	4200
	C.F.		33.2	56.1	267	489	558
	Wt.		3 lbs. 13 oz.	6 lbs. 7 oz.	30 lbs. 10 oz.	56 lbs. 0 oz.	64 lbs. 0 oz.
O_2	Liters	200	400	660	3450	5300	6900
	Gals.	52.8	105	174	912	1400	1825
	C.F.	7	14.1	23.3	122	187	244
	Wt.	9.4 oz.	1 lb. 3 oz.	1 lb. 15 oz.	10 lbs. 1 oz.	15 lbs. 8 oz.	20 lbs. 3 oz.
Air	Liters		375	625	3275	5050	6550
	Gals.		99	165	865	1334	1730
	C.F.		13.2	22	116	178	232
	Wt.		1 lb. 0 oz.	1 lb. 10 oz.	8 lbs. 11 oz.	13 lbs. 5 oz.	17 lbs. 6 oz.
N_2	Liters			610			6400
	Gals.			161			1676
	C.F.			21.5			224
	Wt.			1 lb. 9 oz.			16 lbs. 6 oz.

Figure 1-29 *Cylinders are manufactured in different sizes. (Courtesy BOC Gases, formerly Airco, Murray Hill, NJ)*

TABLE 1-3 Cylinder Color Coding

Gas	Color Code	
	United States	International
Oxygen	Green	White
Carbon dioxide	Gray	Gray
Nitrous oxide	Light blue	Light blue
Cyclopropane	Orange	Orange
Helium	Brown	Brown
Carbon dioxide and oxygen	Gray and green	Gray and white
Helium and oxygen	Brown and green	Brown and white
Air	Yellow	White and black

cylinders containing oxygen (see Table 1-3). The international color is white, while the United States still uses green. In addition to the color code, each cylinder is required to have a label indicating the cylinder's contents.

Labeling of cylinder contents is required by the United States Pharmacopeia (USP), a division of the Food and Drug Administration (FDA). The USP controls the purity standards of compressed gases for medical use.

If the label and the color code do not match, the cylinder should not be used and should be returned to the vendor. The most reliable indicator of what is contained in the cylinder is the label.

SAFETY RULES FOR CYLINDER USE

Common sense and the practice of certain safety precautions will ensure safety for both you and your patient. Remember at all times that a medical gas cylinder contains gas pressurized up to 2200 psi. If the cylinder or cylinder valve were to rupture, disastrous consequences could result. Rules and precautions, recommended by the Compressed Gas Association and published in their pamphlet "Characteristics and Safe Handling of Medical Gases, 1971," are summarized in Table 1-4.

TABLE 1-4 Safety Rules for Cylinder Use

Moving Cylinders
1. Always leave protective valve caps in place when moving a cylinder.
2. Do not lift a cylinder by its cap.
3. Do not drop a cylinder, strike two cylinders against one another, or strike other surfaces.
4. Do not drag or slide cylinders; use a cart.
5. Use a cart whenever loading or unloading cylinders.

Storing Cylinders
1. Comply with local and state regulations for cylinder storage as well as with those established by the National Fire Protection Association.
2. Post the names of gases stored.
3. Keep full and empty cylinders separate. Place the full cylinders in a convenient spot to minimize handling of cylinders.
4. Keep storage areas dry, cool, and well ventilated. Storage rooms should be fire-resistant.
5. Do not store cylinders close to flammable substances such as gasoline, grease, or petroleum products.

(continues)

TABLE 1-4 *(continued)*

6. Protect the cylinders from being damaged by cuts or abrasions. Do not store them in areas where they may be damaged by moving or falling objects. Keep cylinder valve caps on at all times.

7. Cylinders may be stored in the open; however, keep them on a platform so they are above the ground.In some parts of the country, shading may be required due to high temperatures. If ice and snow accumulate, thaw at room temperature or use water cooler than 125° F.

8. Protect cylinders from potential tampering by untrained, unauthorized individuals.

Withdrawing Cylinder Contents
1. Allow cylinders to be handled by experienced, trained individuals only.

2. The user of the cylinder is responsible for verifying the cylinder contents before use. If the contents are in doubt, do not use the cylinder. Return it to the supplier.

3. Leave the protective valve cap in place until you are ready to attach a regulator or other equipment.

4. Follow safety precautions. Make sure the cylinder is well supported and protected from falling over.

5. Always crack the cylinder valve prior to attaching a regulator or reducing valve. (Refer to previous "Assembly and Troubleshooting" section.)

6. Use appropriate reducing valves or regulators when attaching equipment designed for lower operating pressures than those contained in the cylinder.

7. Do not force any threaded connections.Verify that the threads you are using are designed for the same gas or gas mixture in accordance with the American Standard Safety System.

8. Connect a cylinder to a manifold designed for high pressure cylinders only.

9. Use equipment only with cylinders containing the gases for which the equipment was designed.

10. Open cylinder valves slowly. Never use a wrench or hammer to force a cylinder valve open. Treat cylinders and cylinder valves with care.

11. Do not use compressed gases to dust off yourself or your clothing.

12. Keep all connections tight to prevent leakage.

13. Before removing a regulator, turn off the valve and bleed the pressure.

14. Never use a flame to detect leaks with flammable gases.

15. Do not store flammable gases with oxygen. Keep all flammable anesthetic gases stored in a separate area.

Reprinted with permission from Gary C.White, Basic Clinical Lab Competencies for Respiratory Care, *4th Edition, Thomson Delmar Learning, 2003.*

DURATION OF GAS FLOW

In order to calculate how long a cylinder will last at a given liter flow, it is important to remember four key facts:

1. When full, an "H" cylinder contains 244 cubic feet of oxygen.

2. When full, an "E" cylinder contains 22 cubic feet of oxygen.

3. Full cylinders contain 2200 psi pressure.

4. One cubic foot of oxygen equals 28.3 liters.

Once these facts have been committed to memory, the duration of any "H" or "E" cylinder may be calculated.

Tank Factors

It is common practice to use tank factors in the calculation of cylinder duration. By knowing the four key facts listed above, these factors may be derived. Table 1-5 illustrates how these factors are derived.

Once these factors have been derived, it is

TABLE 1-5 Tank Factor Calculation

$$\text{Tank Factor} = \frac{\text{Size (cu ft.)} \times 28.3 \text{ liters/cu ft}}{\text{Pressure when full}}$$

$$\text{"H" cylinder} = \frac{244 \text{ cu ft(28.3 liters/cu ft)}}{2200 \text{ psi}}$$

$$= 3.14 \text{ liters/psi}$$

$$\text{"E" cylinder} = \frac{22 \text{ cu ft(28.3 liters/cu ft)}}{2200 \text{ psi}}$$

$$= .28 \text{ liters/psi}$$

easy to convert from gauge pressure (psi) directly to liters. To accomplish this, multiply the gauge pressure by the tank factor for that cylinder. For example:

You are asked to help move a patient from the Emergency Room to the Intensive Care Unit, which usually takes about twenty minutes. You are manually ventilating the patient using a resuscitation bag at a liter flow of 15 liters per minute. Will the department's "E" cylinder containing 1000 psi have enough gas for the transport?

Step 1:
"E" tank factor

$$= \frac{22 \text{ cu ft(28.3 liters/cu ft}}{2200 \text{ psi}}$$

$$= 0.28 \text{ liters/psi}$$

Step 2:
Content of cylinder

$$= \text{tank factor} \times \text{gauge pressure}$$
$$= .28 \text{ liters/psi} \times 1000 \text{ psi}$$
$$= 280 \text{ liters}$$

Step 3:
Duration in minutes

$$= \frac{\text{cylinder contents}}{\text{liter flow}}$$

$$= \frac{280 \text{ L}}{15 \text{ L/min}}$$

$$= 18 \text{ minutes}$$

Answer: No, the cylinder will not last!

Note: It is common to arrive at an answer of hours expressed as a decimal form—for example, 6.3 hours. Each tenth of an hour is 6 minutes, so 6.3 hours equals 6 hours and 18 minutes.

It is common clinical practice to leave 500 psi remaining in the cylinder prior to changing it, providing that a maximum duration is not desired (airborne or ground transport). By leaving 500 psi in the cylinder, water, other gases and foreign material cannot enter the cylinder, helping to extend its useful life.

To calculate the cylinder duration, leaving 500 psi in a cylinder, follow the example outlined below.

You are asked to set a patient up on an oxygen mask at 12 L/min in the X-ray department. The facility is in an older part of the institution and does not have piped oxygen. You move an "H" cylinder to the area to supply oxygen for your patient. The cylinder gauge reads 1250 psi. How long will the cylinder last if you leave 500 psi remaining in the cylinder?

Step 1:
"H" tank factor

$$= \frac{244 \text{ cu ft(28.3 liter/cu ft)}}{2200 \text{ psi}}$$

$$= 3.14 \text{ L/psi}$$

Step 2:
Content of cylinder

$$= \text{tank factor} \times (\text{gauge pressure} - 500 \text{ psi})$$
$$= .28 \text{ L/psi (1250 psi} - 500 \text{ psi)}$$
$$= 2355 \text{ L}$$

Step 3:
Duration in minutes

$$= \frac{\text{cylinder contents}}{\text{liter flow}}$$

$$= \frac{2355 \text{ L}}{12 \text{ L/min}}$$

$$= 196 \text{ minutes}$$

$$= 3 \text{ hours 12 minutes}$$

This type of problem and others like it are very common in clinical practice. Your patient's safety may depend on your ability to remember how to perform these simple calculations.

ASSEMBLY AND TROUBLESHOOTING

Assembly—Oxygen Cylinders

To prepare a cylinder for use, complete the following instructions.

1. Transport the cylinder to the point of use by employing a cylinder cart. Be sure that the protective valve cap is in place when transporting the cylinder.

2. Position the cylinder upright and attach it using chains provided at the point of use, or use a cylinder stand to prevent it from tipping over.

3. Remove the protective cap ("H" cylinder). The smaller "E" cylinders have a piece of shrink-wrap plastic tape protecting the cylinder valve and outlet. Remove the protective tape prior to attaching a regulator or reducing valve.

4. Announce to personnel or patients in the area that a loud noise will occur.

5. Position the cylinder such that the cylinder valve opening is pointing away from any people in the room. "Crack" the cylinder by quickly opening and closing the valve to eliminate debris from the cylinder valve opening.

6. Attach an appropriate regulator to the cylinder and attach the oxygen therapy equipment to the regulator.

7. Slowly turn on the cylinder valve.

8. Read the pressure gauge and determine if the contents of the cylinder are adequate for the duration of therapy.

Troubleshooting

Troubleshooting a cylinder is quite simple since this oxygen supply system has so few moving parts. The following is a suggested troubleshooting algorithm (ALG 1-4).

1. Check for leaks at the connection between the cylinder and regulator. If leaks are present, tighten the connection.
   a. A leak can be detected by a hissing sound. The amplitude or volume of the sound indicates the severity of the leak.
   b. Subtle leaks may be detected by feeling for gas flow with your hands around the connections.
   c. If you suspect a leak but can't detect it:
      (1) Use a solution of mild detergent and water, and brush the solution around the fittings. Leaks will cause bubbles to form, indicating the presence of a leak.
   d. If a leak is detected, turn off the cylinder valve (bleeding all pressure from the regulator) and retighten all connections.

2. Check for leaks between the regulator and the oxygen therapy equipment and tighten as appropriate.
   a. A leak can be detected by a hissing sound. The amplitude or volume of the sound indicates the severity of the leak.
   b. Subtle leaks may be detected by feeling for gas flow with your hands around the connections.
   c. If you suspect a leak but can't detect it:
      (1) Use a solution of mild detergent and water, and brush the solution around the fittings. Leaks will cause bubbles to form, indicating the presence of a leak.
   d. If a leak is detected, turn off the cylinder valve (bleeding all pressure from the regulator) and retighten all connections.

3. If gas fails to flow from the cylinder, check the pressure gauge to ensure that the cylinder has pressure.
   a. If the cylinder contains pressure, check the regulator outlet for obstructions.
   b. If the above is satisfied, replace the regulator with another and try again.

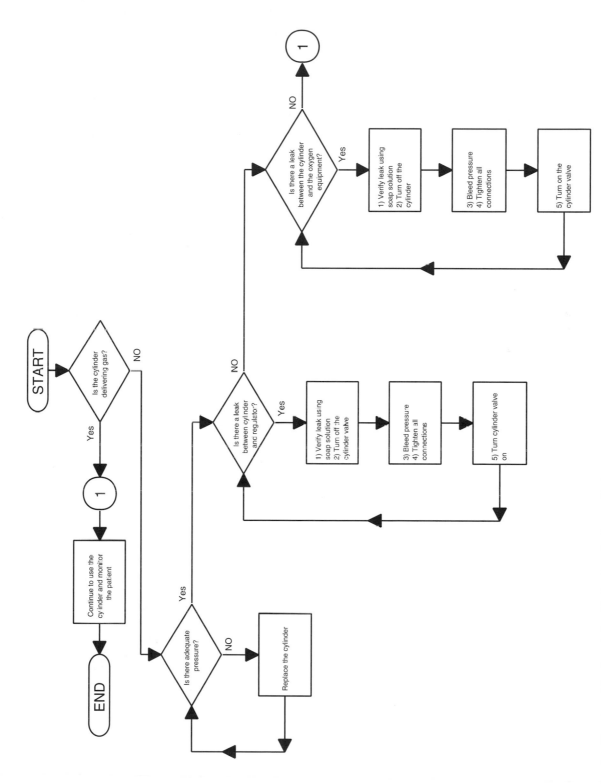

ALG 1-4 *An algorithm describing how to troubleshoot medical gas cylinders.*

OXYGEN REGULATION DEVICES

Cylinders that contain highly pressurized gas would be dangerous to use without specialized equipment to regulate gas flow and allow safe attachment of other equipment. It is important to understand the operation of cylinder valves and reducing valves to safely use cylinders.

Direct Acting Cylinder Valve

As its name implies, the **direct acting cylinder valve** operates by opening and closing the valve seat directly. As the valve stem or wheel is turned, the valve plunger moves up or down, acting directly on the valve seat. As the valve seat is opened, gas moves from the area of high pressure (within the cylinder) to the area of lower pressure (out of the cylinder). Figure 1-30 shows the component parts of the cylinder valve. The valve plunger is threaded, so as the stem is turned, it opens or closes. The direct acting cylinder valve is a type of needle valve.

Diaphragm Cylinder Valve

In this type of cylinder valve, a diaphragm opens or closes the valve seat. As the valve stem is turned, the threaded plunger moves up or down, allowing the diaphragm to open or close the valve seat. Gas pressure then displaces the diaphragm, allowing gas to flow out of the cylinder. These valves are usually employed with cylinders having a lower working pressure of 1500 psi or less (Figure 1-31).

Cylinder Valve Safety Features

Several safety features are incorporated into cylinder valves.

Since cylinders contain many different gases, the Compressed Gas Association (CGA) has designed a system to prevent the interchange of dissimilar gases. In other words, the safety system is designed to prevent the attachment of an oxygen regulator to a nitrous oxide medical gas cylinder. The two types of valve outlet safety systems are the American Standard and the Pin Index Safety System (PISS).

The American Standard Safety System (ASSS) is incorporated into the valves for the larger cylinders (sizes "M," "G," "H"). This system uses differing thread pitches, internal

Figure 1-30 *A full section of a direct acting cylinder valve. (Courtesy BOC Gases, formerly Airco, Murray Hill, NJ)*

Figure 1-31 *A functional diagram of an indirect acting cylinder valve.*

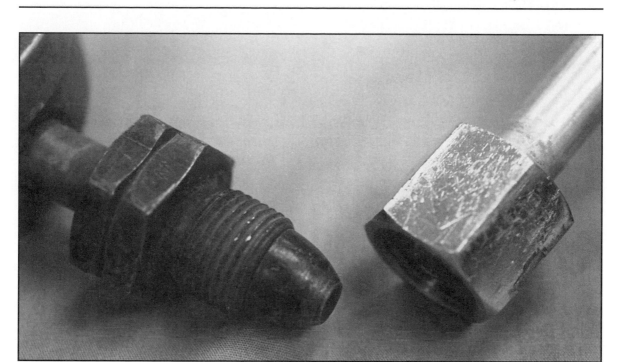

Figure 1-32 *Differing threads and pitches for cylinder valve connections. Note the threads on the left are external (acetylene), and the threads on the right are internal (oxygen).*

left- and right-hand threads, and external threading to prevent the attachment of equipment not designed for the gas contained in the cylinder. Figure 1-32 shows acetylene and oxygen American Standard fittings. Note how one is internally threaded and the other is externally threaded.

The smaller cylinder valves (sizes "AA"–"E") use a yoke type connection between the cylinder valve and the reducing valve. The Pin Index Safety System incorporates pins in the reducing valve yoke and holes on the cylinder valve at specified positions to prevent the attachment of equipment not designed for the gas contained in the cylinder. Figure 1-33 illustrates how this safety system works using the different pin positions.

In addition to the indexing safety systems, pressure release devices are built into the cylinder valves. These pressure relief devices will open if pressure or temperature rises beyond safe limits. The two types of pressure relief devices are the frangible disk and the fusible plug. These devices may be used singly or in combination with one another.

The frangible disk pressure relief consists of a thin metal disk that contains the pressure within the valve. If the pressure within the cylinder rises abnormally, the disk will burst or fracture, releasing pressure before the cylinder walls rupture.

The fusible plug pressure relief is made from an alloy that will melt when the ambient temperature exceeds 208–220° Fahrenheit. When the plug melts or distorts, pressure will be released, preventing rupture of the cylinder.

OXYGEN	2-5
AIR	1-5
He/O_2 (80% and under)	2-4
CO_2/O_2 (7% or under)	2-6
NITROUS OXIDE	3-5

Figure 1-33 *Pin index positions for medical gases.*

REDUCING VALVES

Single-Stage Reducing Valve

A single-stage **reducing valve** reduces the pressure from the cylinder to a working pressure in one step or stage. All reducing valves operate by using two opposing forces, spring tension and gas pressure separated by a flexible diaphragm. Figure 1-34 illustrates the component parts of a single-stage reducing valve and its operation. Gas pressure in the cylinder displaces the diaphragm upward. When gas pressure and spring tension are equal, the diaphragm is flat, closing the poppet valve. As the pressure within the chamber drops, spring tension forces the diaphragm down, opening the poppet valve. This cycle repeats itself with the diaphragm oscillating back and forth, opening and closing the poppet valve. Spring tension determines the outlet pressure from the reducing valve. The tension may be fixed or adjustable depending on the reducing valve's construction. If the tension is adjustable, there is usually a screw provided that will allow adjustment of the tension against the diaphragm.

Modified Single-Stage Reducing Valve

The modified single-stage reducing valve is similar to the single-stage reducing valve. The difference between the two is that the modified single stage reducing valve has a poppet closing spring in addition to the spring above the diaphragm. Figure 1-35 illustrates the component parts of this reducing valve. The poppet closing spring allows the poppet valve to open and close faster, providing greater flow rates.

Multistage Reducing Valves

Multistage reducing valves are simply two or more single-stage reducing valves in series with one another. Figure 1-36 shows the component parts of this reducing valve. The first stage reduces the cylinder to an intermediate pressure of approximately 200 psi. The second stage then reduces the pressure to the desired working pressure, usually 50 psi. Each stage operates independently from the other.

The addition of the additional stage allows more precise regulation of pressure and a greater flow rate than is possible with a single-stage reducing valve. Common applications of multistage reducing valves include powering of mechanical ventilators. These applications require high flows and a stable pressure source.

Reducing Valve Safety Features

Several safety features are incorporated into the design of reducing valves. These include pressure relief valves, or pop-off valves, and indexing of the inlet and outlet.

Each stage of a reducing valve is required to have a safety relief valve in the event that excess pressure develops within the stage. The safety relief will exhaust excessive pressure before the reducing valve housing bursts.

The inlet of the reducing valve is indexed with either American Standard indexing or the Pin Index Safety System indexing. Both of these systems were developed by the Compressed Gas Association and discussed earlier in this chapter.

The outlet of the reducing valve uses Diameter Indexed Safety System threads. This safety system was also discussed earlier in this chapter.

Figure 1-34 *Functional diagram of a single-stage reducing valve.*

Figure 1-35 *Functional diagram of a modified single-stage reducing valve. Note the addition of a poppet closing spring.*

Figure 1-36 *Functional diagram of a two-stage reducing valve. Note how two single-stage regulators are connected in series to form a two-stage regulator.*

REGULATORS

When a flowmeter and a reducing valve are joined together into a common unit, it is termed a **regulator**. Regulators are more convenient than separate reducing valves and flowmeters. Only one high pressure connection is required (between the cylinder and the regulator) and they are more compact in size. A regulator consists of a reducing valve with a Bourdon-type flowmeter, or a reducing valve with a Thorpe tube flowmeter. Both of these flowmeters are discussed later in this chapter.

ASSEMBLY AND TROUBLESHOOTING

Assembly—Oxygen Reducing Valves

Follow the suggested guidelines when assembling a reducing valve for use.

1. Select a reducing valve appropriate for the intended use. If high flow rates are desired (80–120 liters/min.), use a two-stage or modified single-stage reducing valve.

2. Remove the protective valve cap ("H" cylinder) or protective tape ("E" cylinder) and "crack" the tank by opening and closing the valve quickly to expel any foreign material. Perform this task with the valve pointing away from yourself and other people.

3. Attach the reducing valve to an appropriate cylinder valve (American Standard fitting or Pin Index fitting).

4. Attach the oxygen equipment to the reducing valve.

5. Turn on the cylinder valve.

Troubleshooting

Troubleshooting a cylinder and reducing valve primarily involves checking for leaks. The following is a suggested troubleshooting algorithm (ALG 1-5).

1. Check for leaks at the connection to the cylinder. If leaks are present, tighten the connection.

2. Check for leaks between the reducing valve and the oxygen therapy equipment and tighten as appropriate.

3. If gas fails to flow from the cylinder, check the pressure gauge to ensure that the cylinder has pressure.
   a. If the cylinder contains pressure, check the reducing valve outlet for obstructions.
   b. If the above is satisfied, replace the reducing valve with another and try again.

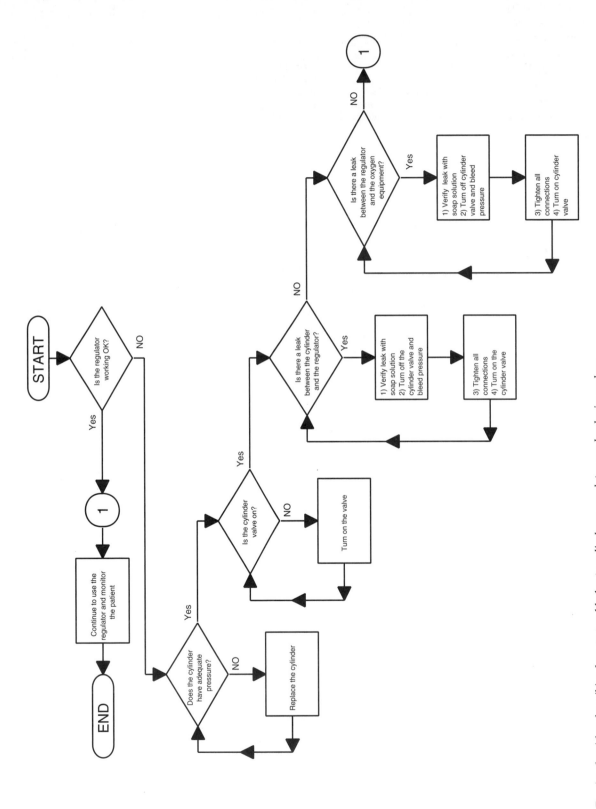

ALG 1-5 *An algorithm describing how to troubleshoot medical gas regulators and reducing valves.*

PROPORTIONERS (AIR-OXYGEN BLENDERS)

Blenders are devices that mix air and oxygen to precise concentrations. These devices provide a stable 50 psi source of mixed gas. Common applications of blenders include, but are not limited to, powering ventilators, Continuous Positive Airway Pressure (CPAP) systems, and controlled oxygen therapy. Blenders are very compact and convenient to use, requiring a 50 psi source of oxygen and air.

Principle of Operation

Air and oxygen entering the blender are first directed into two chambers on opposite sides of a diaphragm that balances the air and oxygen pressures (regulator section). If the incoming pressures are unequal, the regulator portion of the blender balances the pressures so that they are equal (Figure 1-37).

It is important that the pressures are equal, because if one gas entered the proportioning valve at a greater pressure, more of that gas would be delivered, altering the percentage from what is desired.

Gas exiting from the regulator section then passes through a proportioning valve. The oxygen percentage control adjusts the proportions of air and oxygen. If 80% oxygen is desired, turning the control opens the oxygen side more while proportionally closing the air side.

Most manufacturers incorporate a built-in alarm system into the blender. If gas pressure from the supply lines (air or oxygen) drops within the regulation section, an audible alarm will sound.

Figure 1-37 *A functional diagram of an oxygen blender.*

ASSEMBLY AND TROUBLESHOOTING

Assembly—Oxygen Blenders

To prepare a blender for use, follow the instructions listed below.

1. Ensure a supply of compressed oxygen and air at 50 psi. The supply devices may include an oxygen piping system or cylinders with appropriate regulators.

2. Connect a 50-psi hose to the air supply and to the air inlet fitting on the blender.

3. Connect a 50-psi hose to the oxygen supply and to the oxygen inlet on the blender.

4. Read the pressure gauges on the blender to verify line pressure (if provided).

5. Check the pressure alarm by disconnecting the air or oxygen source.

6. Adjust the blender to the desired F_IO_2 (fraction of inspired oxygen).

7. Attach the oxygen therapy device or other medical equipment to the outlet of the blender.
   a. If the outlet does not have a one-way check valve, attach the equipment to the blender before attaching the oxygen and air supply lines.

8. Verify oxygen concentration with an oxygen analyzer.

Troubleshooting

Troubleshooting a blender consists of checking for leaks and verifying oxygen concentration. The following is a suggested algorithm (ALG 1-6).

1. Sources of leaks:
   a. Between the gas source (piping system or regulator) and the high pressure hoses.
   b. Between the high pressure hoses and the blender.
   c. Between the blender and the oxygen equipment.

2. Verify the oxygen concentration using an oxygen analyzer. If there is a tremendous discrepancy (greater than ±2%), calibrate the analyzer and repeat verification. If the discrepancy still exists, replace the blender and have the defective unit repaired by your local vendor or authorized biomedical repair facility.

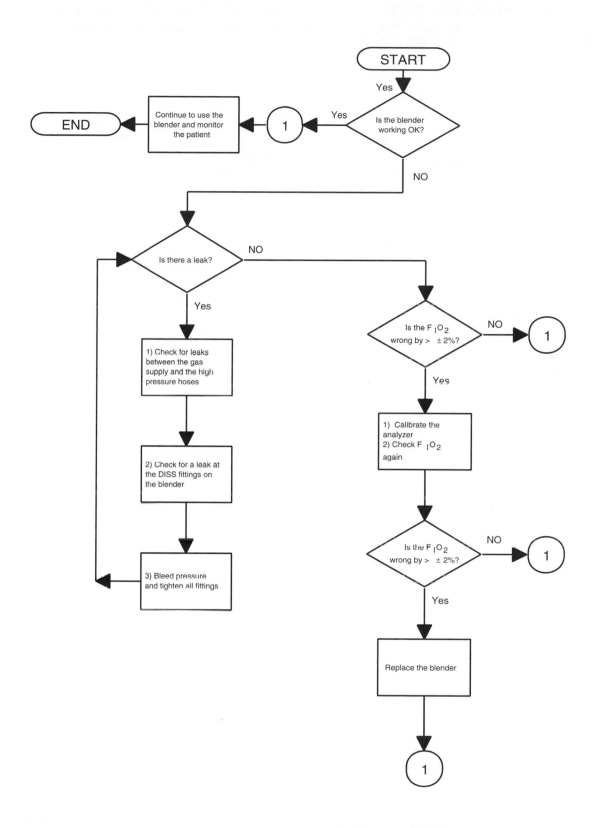

ALG 1-6 *An algorithm describing how to troubleshoot an oxygen blender.*

OXYGEN FLOWMETERS

Bourdon Gauge (Fixed Orifice Flowmeter)

A **Bourdon gauge flowmeter** consists of a Bourdon gauge and an adjustable reducing valve (Figure 1-38). Gas flows through the adjustable reducing valve, past the Bourdon gauge, and then passes through a fixed orifice distal to the Bourdon gauge. The adjustable reducing valve can vary the pressure between the reducing valve outlet and the fixed orifice. As pressure increases, flow out of the device also increases. The increase in pressure between the reducing valve outlet and the fixed orifice causes the coiled tube in the Bourdon gauge to straighten. The gauge, however, is recalibrated to indicate flow rather than pressure as the coiled tube straightens (employing Poiseuille's law).

This flowmeter is accurate as long as the outlet is at ambient pressure. Any increase in pressure distal to the fixed orifice will cause this flowmeter to read inaccurately. This can be caused by obstructions to flow or attachment of equipment that causes back pressure

to develop. It is possible to obstruct the outlet and the Bourdon gauge will indicate a flow higher than is being delivered.

The Bourdon gauge flowmeter is lightweight and very compact. Another advantage of this device is that it will operate in any position. The flowmeter will operate in unusual positions because none of the moving parts is gravity dependent. Therefore, it is popular in emergency and transport settings (ambulance, intra-hospital transport, airborne transport).

Any oxygen connecting tubing, or tubing to oxygen administration devices, must be carefully checked for kinks or obstructions. In a noisy, bumpy environment (ambulance or airborne transport), physically touch and follow the tubing with your hands to verify that the tubing has not been obstructed. Stretchers, equipment or other care providers' feet placed on the tubing could obstruct oxygen flow. You can't tell by monitoring the gauge if oxygen is flowing or not!

Fixed Orifice Flowmeters

Fixed orifice flowmeters are designed to provide specific flow rate settings by selecting

Figure 1-38 *A functional diagram of a Bourdon flowmeter. This is also known as a fixed orifice flowmeter.*

or adjusting an outlet orifice size. At a given inlet pressure, only so much flow can pass through a restricted orifice (choked flow principle). When a large orifice is selected, flow will be high. Conversely, a small orifice will provide a lower flow rate for a given inlet pressure. It is important to use these flowmeters with the correct inlet pressure the flowmeter is designed for (typically 50 psi). Figure 1-39 is an example of a fixed orifice regulator for an E cylinder. This unit incorporates a reducing valve and a fixed orifice flowmeter into a single compact unit.

Uncompensated Thorpe Tube Flowmeter

The components of an uncompensated **Thorpe tube flowmeter** include a "V"-shaped tapered tube (Thorpe tube), a float, and a needle valve (Figure 1-40). Note how the needle valve is positioned proximal to the Thorpe tube.

The Thorpe tube becomes a variable orifice. The Thorpe tube gradually increases in diameter from its base to the top of the tube. The flowmeter is calibrated with the pressure inside of the tube equal to ambient pressure.

Figure 1-40 *An uncompensated Thorpe tube flowmeter.*

The float provides a means of indicating the flow rate. As the needle valve is opened, gas pressure pushes the ball up in the Thorpe tube, overcoming gravity. At equilibrium, gas pressure equals gravitational attraction and the float is stable. As the float moves up in the Thorpe tube, the tube becomes larger and more and more gas flows around it.

The needle valve provides a means of adjusting gas flow into the Thorpe tube. As the needle valve is progressively opened, more gas flows into the tube. The term "uncompensated Thorpe tube flowmeter" refers to the fact that it is uncompensated for back pressure. If pressure is applied distally to the Thorpe tube, for example from a kinked connecting tube or other obstruction, the Thorpe tube becomes pressurized. As the pressure in the Thorpe tube increases, the pressure gradient between the bottom and the top of the float decreases, causing the float to fall. The flow indication may actually be lower than the delivered flow.

Compensated Thorpe Tube Flowmeter

A compensated Thorpe tube flowmeter is similar in design to an uncompensated one

Figure 1-39 *A photograph of a fixed orifice regulator for an E cylinder.*

with one exception. A compensated Thorpe tube's needle valve is distal to the Thorpe tube (Figure 1-41). Since the needle valve is placed distal to the Thorpe tube, pressure within the tube is equal to line pressure or 50 psi when connected to a gas source.

Back pressure applied distally to the needle valve has no effect on its performance. Additional pressure or restriction causes the flowmeter to behave as if the needle valve is closed further, restricting flow. If enough pressure is applied to stop the flow, eventually the pressure proximal and distal to the needle valve will equal 50 psi, the float will no longer be suspended, and gas flow will cease.

When working with Thorpe tube flowmeters, it is often necessary to know if it is compensated or uncompensated. There are three ways to identify a compensated flowmeter:

1. The label will state, "Calibrated at 760 mmHg, 70° F, 50 psig inlet and outlet pressure."

2. With the needle valve closed, the float will rapidly jump up the Thorpe tube when the flowmeter is connected to an oxygen source.

3. Check the position of the needle valve; if it is downstream from the Thorpe tube, it is compensated.

Ranges of Flowmeters

Several manufacturers offer flowmeters with expanded calibration scales that extend beyond the range of the typical 0- to 15-L/min flowmeter's calibrated range. A high-range flowmeter is calibrated from 0 to 75 L/min in 5-L/min units (Figure 1-42A). The high-range flowmeter is useful in Continuous Positive Airway Pressure (CPAP) and high-flow oxygen delivery systems with high-flow clinical applications. Low-range flowmeters have scales calibrated between 0 and 3 L/min in quarter-L/min intervals (Figure 1-42B) and are useful in pediatrics and chronic obstructive lung disease patients.

Figure 1-41 *A compensated Thorpe tube flowmeter.*

(A)   **(B)**

Figure 1-42 *(A) A photograph of a high-range flowmeter, calibrated from zero to seventy-five liters per minute. (B) A photograph of a low-range (pediatric) flowmeter, calibrated from zero to three liters per minute.*

ASSEMBLY AND TROUBLESHOOTING

Assembly—Oxygen Flowmeters

Flowmeters are very easy to assemble for use. Complete the following instructions to prepare a flowmeter.

1. Attach the flowmeter to an appropriate 50-psi gas source using DISS or quick-connect fittings.

2. Attach the appropriate therapy equipment to the DISS fitting on the flowmeter outlet.

3. When using a Bourdon flowmeter, carefully check all supply tubing for kinks or obstructions.

4. Adjust the flow to the desired setting.

5. A Thorpe tube flowmeter can be identified when it is connected to a 50-psi gas source. The float on a Thorpe tube flowmeter will quickly rise and fall when the tube is pressurized to the 50-psi line pressure.

Troubleshooting

Troubleshooting a flowmeter primarily consists of checking for leaks. Periodically, a flowmeter should be checked against a calibration standard for accuracy (calibration flowmeter or volume displacement spirometer). When troubleshooting this equipment, please follow the suggested troubleshooting algorithm (ALG 1-7).

1. Sources of leaks:
   a. Connection between flowmeter and 50-psi gas source.
   b. Connection between flowmeter and the therapy equipment.

2. If the flowmeter fails to deliver expected flow or behaves erratically, check it against a calibration standard and if necessary have it repaired.

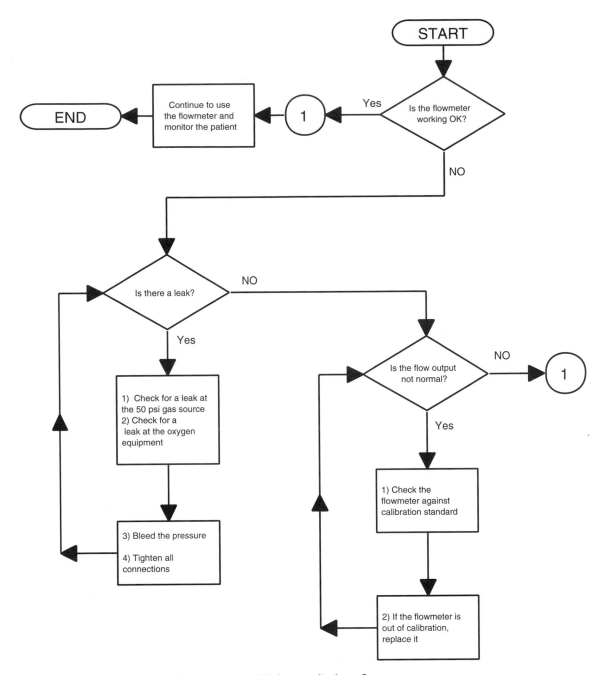

ALG 1-7 *An algorithm describing how to troubleshoot medical gas flowmeters.*

DEMAND PULSE FLOW OXYGEN DELIVERY DEVICES

Demand pulse flow oxygen delivery devices are oxygen delivery devices which are designed to deliver oxygen only during the inspiratory phase. A common name for these devices is an **oxygen conserving device (OCD)**. During a normal ventilatory cycle, when using continuous flow oxygen, oxygen delivered during the last part of inspiration (dead space volume) and the oxygen delivered during exhalation are not usable. Dead space volume is the portion of oxygen delivered which does not participate in gas exchange at the alveoli (Figure 1-43). Demand pulse flow oxygen delivery devices are able to sense the start of the inspiratory phase, and deliver oxygen only during inspiration (Figure 1-44). By delivering oxygen only during that part of the ventilatory cycle that is usable (oxygen

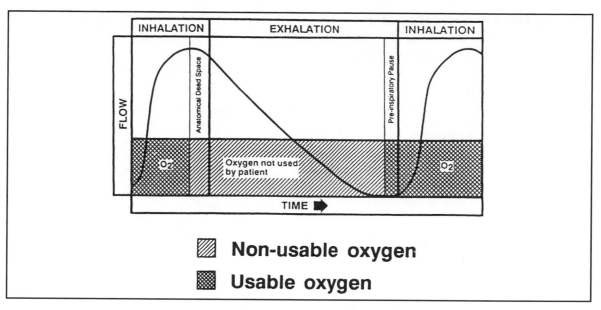

Figure 1-43 *A graph illustrating usable and nonusable oxygen during continuous flow delivery. (Courtesy Puritan Bennett Corporation, Lenexa, KS)*

that can participate in gas exchange), oxygen is conserved when these devices are compared to continuous flow oxygen delivery devices. Since these devices deliver a minimal flow of dry gas, humidification requirements are eliminated. These devices are most commonly used in the home setting, where oxygen conservation can result in substantial cost savings.

When initially setting up an oxygen system on ambulatory patients, it is helpful to perform an exercise oximetry study with both continuous flow and demand pulse flow oxygen systems to insure adequate oxygen saturation. Not all patients will be able to maintain adequate oxygen saturations during demand pulse flow delivery. Therefore, it is important to adjust the demand pulse oxygen delivery flow rate to meet the patient's needs during exercise, as documented by oximetry. Some patients with severe pulmonary disease may not tolerate demand pulse flow oxygen delivery systems at all. In these patients, continuous flow oxygen systems are required to maintain adequate oxygen saturations.

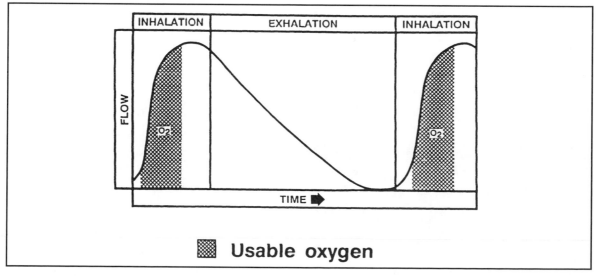

Figure 1-44 *A graph illustrating usable and nonusable oxygen during pulsed demand flow delivery. (Courtesy Puritan Bennett Corporation, Lenexa, KS)*

Transtracheal Systems DOC 2000 Demand Oxygen Controller

The Transtracheal Systems DOC 2000 demand oxygen controller is a pulse demand oxygen delivery device that conserves oxygen by delivering it only during inspiration (Figure 1-45). The unit is electronically controlled and may be powered by a rechargeable Ni-Cad battery or a 120 v, 60Hz power adapter, which also functions to recharge the Ni-Cad battery. When the Ni-Cad battery is fully charged, the DOC 2000 can operate between 8 and 10 hours before requiring a recharge.

Inspiratory Detection

The DOC 2000 detects inspiration using a sensitive pressure transducer. During inspiration, a sub-ambient pressure is created in the patient's nares as the lungs expand. When the pressure transducer senses the drop in pres-

sure, a valve opens, delivering oxygen to the patient.

Oxygen Flow Control

The operation of the DOC 2000 is based upon switching the patient between the oxygen source (valve 2) and the pressure sensor (valve 1). When valve 2 is not energized, oxygen flows from the source directly to the patient (Figure 1-46). Simultaneously, when valve 2 is not energized, valve 1 is energized, which connects the transducer (U11) to the normally closed atmospheric port. Each time the pressure transducer is referenced to ambient pressure, it recalibrates itself, which maintains a consistent sensitivity threshold.

During exhalation, valve 2 is energized, which closes it and stops the flow of oxygen. Valve 1 is not energized, which connects the pressure transducer to the patient through the normally open port of valve 1 (Figure 1-46). Once a pressure drop is detected, valve 2 opens and valve 1 closes, beginning the inspiratory cycle once again.

Monitoring System

The DOC 2000 uses a green light-emitting diode (LED) for two functions. When the unit is first turned on, the LED illuminates and stays on for approximately 1 second, indicating that power is on and that the unit is self-calibrating. Once the patient is connected to the DOC 2000, the green LED will illuminate during inspiration. This tells the operator/user that

Figure 1-45 *A photograph of the DOC 2000 demand oxygen controller. (Courtesy Transtracheal Systems, Englewood, CO)*

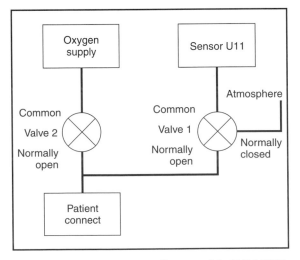

Figure 1-46 *A schematic diagram of the DOC 2000 demand oxygen controller. (Courtesy Transtracheal Systems, Englewood, CO)*

inspiration has been detected and that oxygen flow is initiated.

A yellow LED and audible alarm alerts the operator/user of a low battery level. In the event this alarm system is activated, discontinue battery operation and connect the unit to its AC power pack/charging unit. The Ni-Cad battery can be recharged in approximately 13 hours.

The DOC 2000 also incorporates a system default signal indicator/alarm detector. A red LED illuminates if the unit does not sense an inspiratory effort within approximately 45 seconds. When this occurs, the red LED illuminates and a continuous audible alarm sounds. If an inspiratory effort is detected within 8 to 10 seconds, the unit will reset itself. If no inspiratory effort is detected within approximately 50 seconds, valve 2 opens, delivering the prescribed oxygen flow continuously.

DeVilbiss OMS 20 and EX2000D

DeVilbiss Health Care, Inc., markets two electronically controlled demand pulse flow oxygen delivery devices (Figure 1-47A and B). The OMS 20 is designed to be used with 20 psi liquid oxygen systems. The OMS 20 may be operated from an internal battery for up to 23 hours or by an optional 115 V, 60 Hz power

adapter. The unit senses the patient's inspiratory efforts and delivers a pulse of oxygen during early inspiration. Pulsed oxygen delivery may be provided at flows of between 0.25 and 6 liters per minute.

The EX2000D is designed for use on small oxygen cylinders having a yoke type cylinder valve. The EX2000D is powered by a standard alkaline "C" cell battery. Once the battery is installed, the unit is slipped over the cylinder yoke, and the T-handle is hand-tightened until it seals against the cylinder valve, much like a standard regulator is secured. A selector switch on the right of the unit allows the operator to select between continuous flow and pulsed dose oxygen delivery.

Inspiratory Detection

The DeVilbiss units use a very sensitive pressure transducer to detect the patient's inspiration. As the patient inhales through his or her nasal cannula, the sub-ambient pressure created in the patient's lungs is transmitted to the DeVilbiss unit through the cannula. A sub-ambient pressure (Trigger Level—0.02 cm H_2O) causes an electrical signal to be sent from the pressure transducer (sensor) to the solenoid valve. Once inspiration is detected by the transducer, an electrical signal opens the solenoid valve, delivering a pulse of oxygen.

(A)

(B)

Figure 1-47 *(A) A photograph of the DeVilbiss OMS 20. (B) A photograph of the DeVilbiss EX2000D pulse flow oxygen system. (Courtesy DeVilbiss Health Care, Inc. Somerset, PA)*

Oxygen Flow Control

Oxygen flow (OMS 20) is determined by the setting on the Pulse Dosage switch. The Pulse Dosage switch is a rotary switch which determines how long the solenoid valve remains open. As the flow rate setting is increased by turning the Pulse Dosage switch, the time the solenoid valve remains open is also increased. This is a time-based variable circuit with a constant flow rate. The volume of oxygen delivered to the patient is solely determined by the amount of time the solenoid valve remains open. Therefore, when the respiratory rate increases, the patient actually receives more oxygen. This would be referred to as a "rate response" type of oxygen delivery.

Liter flow on the EX2000D is adjusted by connecting the unit to a cylinder and by attaching a short length of tubing between the EX2000D and an external flowmeter used for calibration purposes. An Allen wrench is inserted into the fitting on the bottom of the EX2000D, and flow is adjusted until the desired flow is displayed on the external flowmeter. Once the desired flow is set, the wrench is removed, along with the calibration flowmeter and connecting tubing.

Monitoring Systems

The DeVilbiss OMS 20 and EX2000D have several monitoring features built into the units. These features include low battery detection, pulse delivery indication and a detection delay indicator.

The low battery indicator will light and an audible alarm will sound when the battery power becomes low. When this condition is detected, it is important to recharge the internal battery using the 120 V, 60 Hz adapter supplied with the unit.

During inspiration, a green LED will illuminate when a pulse is delivered. The sensor circuit sends an electrical signal to illuminate the LED simultaneously with the signal sent to the solenoid valve. Whenever the solenoid valve is opened, the green Pulse Dose LED is also illuminated for the duration of the valve's open time.

A detection delay system is also incorporated into the design of the DeVilbiss units. If an inspiratory effort is not detected within a specified time interval (the time interval is adjustable from 6 to 60 seconds), a red LED will illuminate and a continuous audible alarm will sound. This feature may be turned "ON" or "OFF" by using the two-position Delay Detector switch.

Chad Therapeutics Oxymatic 301 and Oxymatic 2400

Chad Therapeutics, Inc. has designed and is marketing two electronic demand flow pulse delivery oxygen conserving devices (Figure 1-48). The model 301 is designed for portable operation (intermittent), and the model 2400 is designed for continuous use, although it may also be used with portable

Figure 1-48 *Photographs of (A) the Chad Therapeutics Oxymatic 301 and (B) Oxymatic 2400 pulse flow oxygen delivery systems. (Courtesy Chad Therapeutics, Inc., Chatsworth, CA)*

oxygen systems. Both units electronically sense the end of expiration and the beginning of inspiration and deliver a pulse of oxygen within .2 seconds following the start of inspiration. Both units are powered by common alkaline "C" size batteries. The battery life averages 3 to 4 weeks of use.

Inspiratory Detection

During inspiration, a sub-ambient pressure is created in the lungs as the lungs expand. During exhalation, chest wall recoil creates a pressure in the lungs that is greater than ambient pressure. These very small pressure changes are communicated to the Oxymatic units through the patient's nasal cannula.

The Oxymatic units have an internal flexible diaphragm that changes position in response to the pressure changes in the patient's lungs. The neutral position (position between exhalation and inspiration) is electronically detected. When diaphragm motion away from the neutral position is detected, inspiration is detected. An electronic signal is transmitted to the solenoid valve, opening it and delivering a 35-mL pulse of oxygen within 0.2 seconds of the start of inspiration.

Oxygen Flow Control

The Oxymatic units deliver a constant 35-mL pulse of oxygen when the solenoid valve opens. The units control oxygen flow delivery by altering how frequently these constant volume pulses are delivered.

Clinical trials have shown that when the Oxymatic units deliver 35-mL pulse of oxygen every breath, this is equivalent to a continuous oxygen flow of 4 L/min (determined by oxygen saturation). When a pulse is delivered three out of every four breaths (75% of the time), this is equivalent to a continuous flow of 3 L/min. When a pulse is delivered every other breath (50% of the time), this is equivalent to 2 L/min continuous flow. When oxygen is delivered one out of every four breaths (25% of the time), this is equivalent to 1 L/min continuous flow.

Because of the unique pulse delivery (alternate breath delivery below 4 L/min), some patients may be uncomfortable initially when using these units. It is important to explain how these units work and that even though the patient may not feel oxygen flow on each breath, it is equivalent to what they have been receiving. As noted earlier in this section, it is important to conduct an oximetry trial to determine the oxygen needs of a patient who is using a conserving device.

Monitoring Systems: Oxymatic 301

The monitor on the Oxymatic 301 is a battery test indicator. To use the battery tester, move the thumbwheel selector on the top of the unit to the "Battery Test" position. Observe the indicator to assess the battery's condition. If the indicator is red, replace the battery before use. If the indicator is amber, you should have a replacement battery available to use. If the indicator is green, the battery has sufficient electrical energy to operate the unit. The Oxymatic 301 uses a common alkaline "C" size battery.

Monitoring Systems: Oxymatic 2400

The Oxymatic 2400 has a battery test feature, a low battery warning indicator and an apnea alarm. All of these conditions can be monitored on the top of the unit. The battery test can be performed by moving the black rocker switch to the "ON/BATT" position while the unit is on. The "BATT TEST" display will indicate the battery's condition. If the display is dark green, the battery is in good condition. With use, the color of the green indicator becomes progressively lighter. When the display is amber in color, approximately 48 hours of battery life remains. If the indicator is red, 24 hours of life remains and the battery should be changed.

The low battery warning is a blinking LED display in the Indicator Setting window that resembles a battery. When the battery life falls to around 24 hours of continuous use, the low battery warning will flash intermittently. When this condition is observed, the battery should be changed as soon as possible.

Apnea detection is built into the Oxymatic 2400. If the unit fails to sense inspiration over a period of 40 seconds, the alarm system is activated. An audible and visual alarm will alert the user to this condition. A flashing red light labeled "ALARM" on the top of the unit will flash intermittently along with the audible alarm. Besides apnea, kinks in the patient's tubing or patient disconnects can also cause this alarm.

ASSEMBLY AND TROUBLESHOOTING

Assembly—Oxygen Conserving Devices

1. Connect the conserving device to an oxygen source (cylinder or liquid system).
   a. An oxygen cylinder requires the use of a regulator to reduce the cylinder pressure and to set the oxygen delivery to the prescribed flow. The conserving device is attached to the outlet of the regulator.
   b. A liquid system requires the use of a flowmeter, which is used to set the desired flow rate. The conserving device is attached to the outlet of the flowmeter.
   c. A portable liquid reservoir may also be used by threading a barbed hose-fitting adapter into the inlet port of the conserving device and attaching the other end to the outlet of the portable reservoir set at the appropriate flow rate.

2. Connect the delivery tubing of the nasal cannula or transtracheal catheter to the barbed outlet of the conserving device. Delivery tubing should never exceed 35 feet in length.

3. Depress the "On/Off" button on the top of the unit to turn the unit on. The unit will perform a self-calibration (about 1 second) and then will operate normally.

Troubleshooting

When troubleshooting oxygen conserving devices, please follow the suggested troubleshooting algorithm (ALG 1-8).

1. If the unit fails to deliver oxygen flow:
   a. Check tubing and cannula or transtracheal catheter for obstructions or kinks.
   b. Make certain that the oxygen flowmeter is on and that there is a sufficient quantity of oxygen (pressure for cylinders or weight for liquid systems).
   c. The patient may not be generating a sufficient inspiratory effort to activate the inspiratory detection circuit. Patients with advanced lung disease may not be candidates for pulsed oxygen delivery and may require continuous flow.
   d. Verify that the batteries are in good condition and are in place if the unit is battery powered.

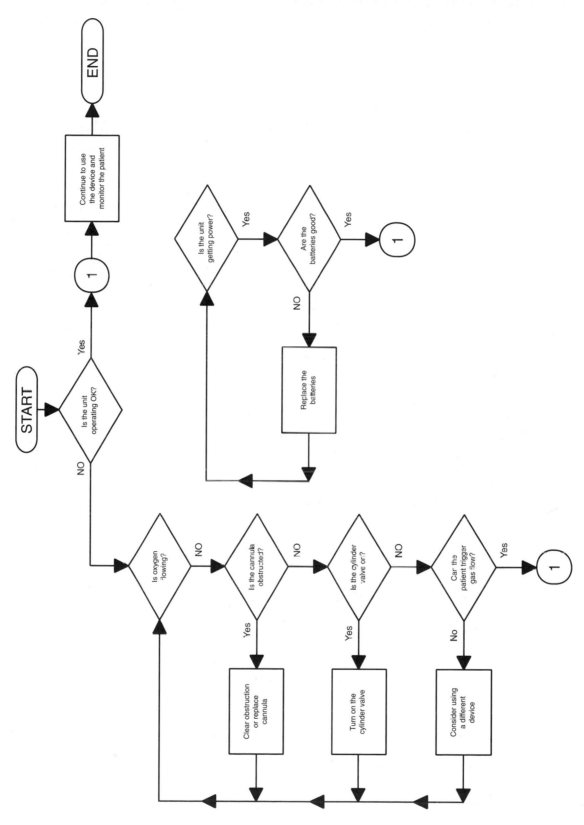

ALG 1-8 *An algorithm describing how to troubleshoot an oxygen conserving device.*

CLINICAL CORNER

Medical Gas Supply Equipment

1. You are on-call for a home care company that employs you as a respiratory care practitioner. A patient who was just set up at home on a liquid oxygen system calls with a complaint. Over the phone, Mr. Smith says: "My new oxygen bottle is hissing. I am worried it might explode." What should you tell your new client, and what would you recommend that he do?

2. You are preparing to transport a patient from the intensive care unit (ICU) to the floor. In order to do so, you set up an "E" cylinder to provide oxygen to his cannula. When you turn on the cylinder valve, you hear a leak. Describe the steps you would take to correct the problem.

3. You are setting up a new patient at home with an oxygen concentrator. The patient requests that she be allowed enough freedom of movement to reach the bathroom, the kitchen, and her bedroom (the location of the concentrator). Describe how you would evaluate the concentrator's placement and any limitations you might impose regarding maximum lengths of extension tubing.

4. Describe a clinical situation in which you might select a single-stage reducing valve and another in which you might select a two-stage reducing valve.

5. You are evaluating a patient for a pulsed demand regulator for his portable oxygen system. Describe how you would appropriately evaluate him, state which of the devices discussed in the text is best for a given patient, and explain why.

6. You are using a Bourdon gauge flowmeter for a helicopter transport. What safety precautions should you be aware of when using this type of regulator?

Self-Assessment Quiz

1. "Gases being composed of discrete molecules in random motion" best describes:
   a. the ideal gas law.
   b. the kinetic theory of gases.
   c. Dalton's law.
   d. Charles' law.

2. The kinetic activity of gases is largely dependent upon:
   a. their concentration.
   b. the pressure.
   c. the temperature.
   d. the type of gas.

3. Chambers A and B are connected by high-pressure tubing and separated by a valve. If chamber A contains 500 psi of gas and chamber B contains 50 psi of gas, what will occur when the valve is opened?
   a. The pressures in the chambers will remain equal.
   b. Chamber A will be pressurized by chamber B.
   c. Gas will flow from chamber A to chamber B until pressures equalize.
   d. The pressure in chamber B will increase to a level greater than in chamber A.

4. Pascal's law best describes:
   a. the relationship between volume and pressure of a gas.
   b. the relationship between pressure and temperature of a gas.
   c. the relationship between temperature and volume of a gas.
   d. the equal distribution of pressure transmitted by a fluid.

5. A device used clinically to measure small pressures is termed a:
   a. mercury barometer.
   b. aneroid barometer.
   c. manometer.
   d. reducing valve.

6. A Bourdon gauge:
   I. uses a coiled tube.
   II. uses a sealed diaphragm.
   III. measures pressure.
   IV. measures flow.
   a. I and II
   b. I and IV
   c. II and III
   d. II and IV

7. The statement, "As temperature increases, pressure also increases," best describes:
   a. Gay-Lussac's law.
   b. Dalton's law.
   c. Henry's law.
   d. Charles' law.

8. Bernoulli's theorem best describes:
   a. the relationship between temperature and pressure of a gas.
   b. the relationship between volume and pressure of a gas.
   c. an energy balance or conservation between velocity and pressure.
   d. the relationship between pressure of a gas and its ability to dissolve into a liquid.

9. An air entrainment mask operates by mixing source gas (oxygen) and room air. This device operates using:
   a. viscous shearing and vorticity.
   b. Bernoulli's theorem.
   c. Venturi's principle.
   d. Poiseuille's law.

10. You are analyzing the F_IO_2 of a patient's HAFOE device, which reads 0.85. The entrainment port is set at 40%. Why would the analyzed oxygen concentration differ so much from the setting?
    a. The analyzer is malfunctioning.
    b. The patient's respiratory rate is affecting oxygen delivery.
    c. More room air is being entrained.
    d. There may be an obstruction distal to the entrainment port.

11. A gas's velocity is said to be choked when:
    a. velocity can no longer increase.
    b. a maximum temperature is reached.
    c. pressure is at a maximum.
    d. the concentration is at a maximum.

12. A patient with reactive airway disease is experiencing bronchospasm. The patient's work of breathing has dramatically increased in the last few minutes. This is an example of:
    I. Poiseuille's law.
    II. the Bernoulli theorem.
    III. increased airway resistance.
    IV. decreased lateral pressure.
    a. I and III
    b. I and IV
    c. II and III
    d. II and IV

13. You measure the volume of gas exiting a delivery device at 22 degrees Celsius to be 1.50 liters. The gas passes through a heater, warming it to 37 degrees Celsius. What is the actual volume delivered to the patient?
    a. 1.56 liters
    b. 2.00 liters
    c. 2.50 liters
    d. 3.12 liters

14. "The rate of gas diffusion into or out of a liquid is directly proportional to the partial pressure of the gas" best describes:
    a. Charles' law.
    b. Fick's law.
    c. Henry's law.
    d. Gay-Lussac's law.

15. Given the following gas mixture:
    Gas A = 20%
    Gas B = 50%
    Gas C = 30%
    Total pressure equals 600 mmHg.
    Find the partial pressure of Gas A.
    a. 10 mmHg
    b. 20 mmHg
    c. 80 mmHg
    d. 60 mmHg

16. Which of the following is constructed in a similar way to a thermos bottle?
    a. oxygen cylinder
    b. oxygen concentrator
    c. liquid oxygen reservoir
    d. oxygen piping system

17. Safety features incorporated into regulators or reducing valves include:
    I. DISS outlet.
    II. PISS inlet.
    III. American Standard inlet.
    IV. pressure relief valve(s).
    a. I only
    b. I and II only
    c. I, II, and III only
    d. I, II, III, and IV

18. Which of the following is (are) true for an "H" size oxygen cylinder?
    I. When full, it contains 2,200 psi.
    II. It contains 22 cubic feet of gas.
    III. It will have "3AA" stamped on the shoulder.
    IV. It contains 244 cubic feet of gas.
    a. I and II only
    b. I and III only
    c. I, III, and IV only
    d. I, II, and III only

19. The marking "3AA" indicates:
    a. the cylinder type.
    b. the contents of the cylinder.
    c. the cylinder serial number.
    d. the cylinder size.

20. The lightest compressed gas cylinder for ambulatory use is:
    a. a 3AA steel cylinder.
    b. an aluminum (3AL) cylinder.
    c. a fiber wrapped cylinder.
    d. a portable liquid reservoir.

21. A device that mixes air and oxygen is termed a (an):
    a. concentrator.
    b. oxygen enricher.
    c. oxygen proportioner.
    d. reducing valve.

22. When troubleshooting an oxygen concentrator, you find that the device is operating yet you are unable to obtain the desired flow of oxygen-enriched gas. Possible problems include:
    I. a tripped circuit breaker.
    II. obstructed delivery tubing.
    III. obstructed humidifier.
    IV. a dirty filter.
    a. I
    b. I and II
    c. II and III
    d. I and IV

23. Advantages of transfilling portable cylinders from a home oxygen concentrator include:
    I. convenience.
    II. cost savings
    III. speed of filling the cylinder.
    a. I only
    b. I and II
    c. I and III
    d. I, II, and III

24. When making a call on a home care patient, you weigh her liquid reservoir, which registers 80 lbs. You know the manufacturer's weight to be 60 lbs, and that your patient uses 3 L/min oxygen. How much gas does her reservoir contain, and can she wait for 5 hours before your company's delivery truck arrives?
    I. 12,340 L oxygen remaining
    II. 5,484 L oxygen remaining
    III. 30 hours' duration remaining
    IV. 84 hours' duration remaining
    a. I and III
    b. I and IV
    c. II and III
    d. II and IV

25. An advantage of using a demand pulse flow oxygen delivery system in the home care environment is that:
    I. less oxygen is used.
    II. it is less expensive for the patient.
    III. a humidifier is not required.
    a. I
    b. II
    c. I and II
    d. I, II, and III

26. When selecting an oxygen conserving device for ambulatory use, it is important to:
    a. select the unit based upon overall cost.
    b. perform an ambulatory oxygen saturation trial using the unit.
    c. draw arterial blood gases before and after ambulation.
    d. none of the above.

27. A potential disadvantage to the Mallinckrodt Puritan Bennett® HELiOS® system is:
    a. it is heavier than other portable liquid reservoirs.
    b. it has a smaller capacity than competing units.
    c. it must be used with the HELiOS7 dual lumen cannula.
    d. it can only provide flow rates of up to 2 L/min.

28. Back pressure will affect the accuracy of which of the following flowmeters?
    I. Compensated Thorpe tube
    II. Uncompensated Thorpe tube
    III. Bourdon flowmeter
    a. I and II only
    b. II and III only
    c. I and III only
    d. III only

29. A back pressure compensated flowmeter:
    I. reads correctly if back pressure is applied.
    II. reads lower than the actual flow when back pressure is applied.
    III. has the needle valve downstream from the Thorpe tube.
    IV. has the needle valve upstream from the Thorpe tube.
    a. I and III
    b. I and IV
    c. II and III
    d. II and IV

30. When using a fixed orifice flowmeter, it is important to:
    a. calibrate it using a calibration flowmeter.
    b. use the correct inlet pressure.
    c. ensure that there isn't a restriction in the inlet tubing.
    d. adjust the regulator to the pressure on the label.

Selected Bibliography

Chad Therapeutics. (1993). *Product information and instructions for use, Model 301 Oxymatic electronic oxygen conserver.* Chatsworth, CA: Author.

Chad Therapeutics. (1993). *Product information and instructions for use, Model 2400 Oxymatic, electronic oxygen conserver system.* Chatsworth, CA: Author.

Chigier, N. (1981). *Energy, combustion, and environment.* McGraw-Hill.

Compressed Gas Association. (1981). *Handbook of compressed gases.* Van Nostrand Reinhold Company.

Contemporary Products, Inc. (2003). *Composite fiber wrapped cylinder owners manual.* Portland, ME: Author.

DeVilbiss Health Care. (1988). *DeVO/MC29 and DeVO/MC44 patient guide.* Somerset, PA: Author.

DeVilbiss Health Care. (1987). *DeVilbiss DeVO/MC44-90 oxygen concentrator service manual.* Somerset, PA: Author

Grenard, S. (1973). *The hazards of respiratory therapy equipment.* Lenn Educational Medical Services.

Gonzales, S. C. (1986). Efficacy of the oxymizer pendant in reducing oxygen requirements of hypoxemic patients. *Respiratory Care, 31*(8), 681–688.

Kerby, G. R., et al. (1990). Clinical efficacy and cost benefit of pulse flow oxygen in hospitalized patients. *Chest, 97*(2), 369–372.

Invacare Corporation. (2003). *IRC5LX 5-liter concentrator owners manual.* Elyria, OH: Author.

Invacare Corporation. (2003). *Venture® HomeFill™ oxygen filling system, owners manual.* Elyria, OH: Author.

Pierson, D. J., et al. (1992). *Foundations of respiratory care.* Churchill Livingstone, Inc.

Pulsair. (1990). *Oxygen management systems 20/50 liquid oxygen and high pressure oxygen, service and repair manual.* Ft. Pierce, FL: Author.

Puritan Bennett Corporation. (2003). *HELiOS® portable liquid oxygen unit, operating instructions.* Pleasanton, CA: Author.

Puritan Bennett Corporation. (1989). *Companion 5 oxygen saver operating instructions.* Lenexa, KS: Author.

Puritan Bennett Corporation. (1989). *Puritan Bennett Companion 5 oxygen saver, service manual.* Lenexa, KS: Author.

Sacci, R. (1979). Air entrainment masks: Jet mixing is how they work; The Bernoulli and Venturi principles are how they don't. *Respiratory Care, 24*(10), 928–931.

Tiep, B. L., et al. (1990). Pulsed nasal and transtracheal oxygen delivery. *Chest, 97*(2), 364–368.

Ward, J. J. (1988). Equipment for mixed gas and oxygen therapy. In T. A. Barnes, et al. (eds.), *Respiratory care practice.* Year Book Medical.

CHAPTER 2

MEDICAL GAS THERAPY EQUIPMENT

INTRODUCTION

Administration of oxygen and other therapeutic gases is an important aspect of the practice of respiratory care. The profession of respiratory care began when early practitioners delivered and set up oxygen cylinders at the bedside. Administration of medical gases today not only includes oxygen administration, but hyperbaric oxygen therapy, helium/oxygen therapy, carbon dioxide/oxygen therapy, and nitric oxide therapy.

As a respiratory care practitioner, it is important for you to understand the indications for therapeutic gas administration. You must also understand what equipment is required for administration of specific gases, and how to assemble, troubleshoot, and monitor the patient during medical gas administration.

OBJECTIVES

After completing this chapter, the student will accomplish the following objectives:

- List the indications for oxygen therapy in the acute, sub-acute, and home settings.
- Differentiate between high-flow and low-flow oxygen devices.
- List three characteristics common to oxygen enclosures or environmental devices.
- Differentiate between the following oxygen delivery devices, classify each as a high flow or low-flow delivery device, and discuss its principle of operation.
  — nasal cannula
  — reservoir and pendant cannula
  — simple mask
  — partial rebreathing mask (reservoir mask)
  — non-rebreathing mask (reservoir mask)
  — HiOx^{80} disposable high F_IO_2 mask
  — transtracheal catheter

- Describe the operation of high-flow air entrainment devices.
  — Vapotherm 2000i high flow gas therapy system
- Describe the contraindications for oxygen therapy in the acute, sub-acute, and home settings.
- Differentiate between the following enclosures or environmental devices:
  — isolette
  — head box
  — mist tent (croupette)
- Explain the principle behind hyperbaric oxygen therapy and the equipment utilized for this therapy.
- Differentiate between the equipment utilized for mixed-gas therapy (O_2/He and O_2/CO_2) and that used for oxygen administration.
  — Describe the use of nitric oxide and the equipment required for its administration.

KEY TERMS

Anatomic reservoir	Hypoxemia	Non-rebreathing	Simple oxygen mask
F_IO_2	Incubator	mask	Transtracheal
Head box	Low-flow oxygen	Oxyhood	catheter
High-flow oxygen	delivery devices	Partial rebreathing	Venturi or HAFOE
delivery system	Mist tents	mask	mask
Hyperbaric oxygen	Nasal cannula	Pendant cannula	
therapy	Nasal catheter	Reservoir cannula	

INDICATIONS FOR OXYGEN THERAPY

The indications for oxygen therapy have been well described and defined by the American Association for Respiratory Care's Clinical Practice Guidelines (CPGs). These guidelines provide a research based framework for the administration of oxygen and other therapeutic procedures in the practice of respiratory care.

Oxygen is indicated for the treatment and prevention of hypoxemia. **Hypoxemia** is defined in the CPGs as a $PaO_2 \leq 60$ mmHg or an $SaO_2 \leq 90\%$ for patients in the acute care setting. In the sub-acute or home care settings, hypoxemia is defined as a $PaO_2 \leq 55$ mmHg

or $SaO_2 \leq 88\%$ in subjects breathing room air. Additionally, oxygen may be prescribed in the sub-acute or home care setting when the PaO_2 is 56–59 mmHg or the SaO_2 or $SpO_2 \leq$ 89% in association with specific clinical conditions (e.g., cor pulmonale, congestive heart failure, or erythro-cythemia with hematocrit > 56). Medicare also includes pulmonary hypertension as a qualifier for home oxygen if a patient does not meet the PaO2 or SaO2 criteria breathing room air. Oxygen may also be used for patients who desaturate during ambulation, or sleep in the sub-acute and home care settings. The clinical practice guidelines should be used as resource when assessing, initiating treatment, and monitoring patients receiving oxygen therapy (Figures 2-1 and 2-2).

AARC CLINICAL PRACTICE GUIDELINE
Oxygen Therapy for Adults in the Acute Care Facility
2002 Revision & Update

OT-AC 1.0 PROCEDURE:
The procedure addressed is the administration of oxygen therapy in the acute care facility other than with mechanical ventilators and hyperbaric chambers.

OT-AC 2.0 DEFINITION/DESCRIPTION:
Oxygen therapy is the administration of oxygen at concentrations greater than that in ambient air with the intent of treating or preventing the symptoms and manifestations of hypoxia.

OT-AC 3.0 SETTING:
This Guideline is confined to oxygen administration in the acute care facility.

OT-AC 4.0 INDICATIONS:
4.1 Documented hypoxemia. Defined as a decreased PaO_2 in the blood below normal range.(2) PaO_2 of < 60 torr or SaO_2 of < 90% in subjects breathing room air or with PaO_2 and/or SaO_2 below desirable range for specific clinical situation.
4.2 An acute care situation in which hypoxemia is suspected substantiation of hypoxemia is required within an appropriate period of time following initiation of therapy.
4.3 Severe trauma
4.4 Acute myocardial infarction
4.5 Short-term therapy or surgical intervention (e.g., post-anesthesia recovery, hip surgery)

Figure 2-1 *American Association for Respiratory Care, Clinical Practice Guideline: Oxygen Therapy for Adults in the Acute Care Facility—2002 Revision & Update.* **(continues)**

OT-AC 5.0 CONTRAINDICATIONS:

No specific contraindications to oxygen therapy exist when indications are judged to be present.

OT-AC 6.0 PRECAUTIONS AND/OR POSSIBLE COMPLICATIONS:

6.1 With PaO_2 > or = 60 torr, ventilatory depression may occur in spontaneously breathing patients with elevated $PaCO_2$.

6.2 With F_IO_2 > or = 0.5, absorption atelectasis, oxygen toxicity, and/or depression of ciliary and/or leukocytic function may occur.

6.3 Supplemental oxygen should be administered with caution to patients suffering from paraquat poisoning and to patients receiving bleomycin.

6.4 During laser bronchoscopy, minimal levels of supplemental oxygen should be used to avoid intratracheal ignition.

6.5 Fire hazard is increased in the presence of increased oxygen concentrations.

6.6 Bacterial contamination associated with certain nebulization and humidification systems is a possible hazard.

OT-AC 7.0 LIMITATIONS OF PROCEDURE:

Oxygen therapy has only limited benefit for the treatment of hypoxia due to anemia, and benefit may be limited with circulatory disturbances. Oxygen therapy should not be used in lieu of but in addition to mechanical ventilation when ventilatory support is indicated.

OT-AC 8.0 ASSESSMENT OF NEED:

Need is determined by measurement of inadequate oxygen tensions and/or saturations, by invasive or noninvasive methods, and/or the presence of clinical indicators as previously described.

OT-AC 9.0 ASSESSMENT OF OUTCOME:

Outcome is determined by clinical and physiologic assessment to establish adequacy of patient response to therapy.

OT-AC 10.0 RESOURCES:

For other types of oxygen delivery devices used outside of the acute care facility, reference the AARC Clinical Practice Guideline: Oxygen Therapy in the Home or Extended Care Facility for further description. *Respiratory Care* 1992; 37(8): 918–922.

10.1 Equipment

10.1.1 Low-flow systems deliver 100% (i.e., $F_DO_2 = 1.0$) oxygen at flows that are less than the patient's inspiratory flowrate (i.e., the delivered oxygen is diluted with room air) and, thus, the oxygen concentration inhaled (F_IO_2) may be low or high, depending on the specific device and the patient's inspiratory flowrate.

10.1.1.1 Nasal cannulas can provide 24%–40% oxygen with flowrates up to 6 L/min in adults (depending on ventilatory pattern). Oxygen supplied via nasal cannula at flowrates < or = 4 L/min need not be humidified. Care must be taken when assigning an estimated F_IO_2 to patients as this low-flow system can have great fluctuations.

10.1.1.2 Simple oxygen masks can provide 35%–50% F_IO_2, depending on fit, at flowrates from 5–10 L/min. Flowrates should be maintained at 5 L/min or more in order to avoid rebreathing exhaled CO_2 that can be retained in the mask. Caution should be taken when using a simple mask where accurate delivery of low concentrations of oxygen is required. Long-term use of simple mask can lead to skin irritation and pressure sores.

10.1.1.3 Partial rebreathing mask is a simple mask with a reservoir bag. Oxygen flow should always be supplied to maintain the reservoir bag at least one third to one half full on inspiration. At a flow of 6–10 L/min the system can provide 40%–70% oxygen. It is considered a low-flow system. The non-rebreathing mask is similar to the partial rebreathing mask except it has a series of one-way valves. One valve is placed between the bag and the mask to prevent exhaled air from returning to the bag. There should be a minimum flow of 10 L/min. The delivered F_IO_2 of this system is 60%–80%.

10.1.1.4 Patients who have been receiving transtracheal oxygen at home may continue to receive oxygen by this method in the acute care facility setting provided no problems present. If difficulties related to the transtracheal route of administration appear, oxygenation should be assured by other means.

10.1.2 High-flow systems deliver a prescribed gas mixture—either high or low F_DO_2 at flowrates that exceed patient demand.

10.1.2.1 Currently available air-entrainment masks can accurately deliver predetermined oxygen concentration to the trachea up to 40%. Jet-mixing masks rated at 35% or higher usually do not deliver flowrates adequate to meet the inspiratory flowrates of adults in respiratory distress.

Figure 2-1 *(continues)*

10.1.2.2 Aerosol masks, tracheostomy collars, T-tube adapters, and face tents can be used with high-flow supplemental oxygen systems. A continuous aerosol generator or large-volume reservoir humidifier can humidify the gas flow. Some aerosol generators cannot provide adequate flows at high oxygen concentrations.

10.2 Personnel

10.2.1 Level I personnel—i.e., any person who has adequately demonstrated the ability to perform the task—may check and document that a device is being used appropriately and the flow is as prescribed.

10.2.2 Level II personnel—licensed or credentialed respiratory care practitioners or persons with equivalent training and documented ability to perform the tasks—may assess patients, initiate and monitor oxygen delivery systems, and recommend changes in therapy.

OT-AC 11.0 MONITORING:

11.1 Patient

11.1.1 clinical assessment including but not limited to cardiac, pulmonary, and neurologic status

11.1.2 assessment of physiologic parameters: measurement of PaO_2s or saturation in any patient treated with oxygen. An appropriate oxygen therapy utilization protocol is suggested as a method to decrease waste and to realize increased cost savings. Consider need/indication to adjust F_DO_2 for increased levels of activity and exercise.

11.1.2.1 in conjunction with the initiation of therapy; or

11.1.2.2 within 12 hours of initiation with $F_IO_2 < 0.40$

11.1.2.3 within 8 hours, with $F_IO_2 >$ or $=$ 0.40 (including postanesthesia recovery)

11.1.2.4 within 72 hours in acute myocardial infarction

11.1.2.5 within 2 hours for any patient with the principal diagnosis of COPD

11.2 Equipment

11.2.1 All oxygen delivery systems should be checked at least once per day.

11.2.2 More frequent checks by calibrated analyzer are necessary in systems

11.2.2.1 susceptible to variation in oxygen concentration (e.g., high-flow blending systems)

11.2.2.2 applied to patients with artificial airways

11.2.2.3 delivering a heated gas mixture

11.2.2.4 applied to patients who are clinically unstable or who require an F_IO_2 of 0.50 or higher.

11.2.3 Care should be taken to avoid interruption of oxygen therapy in situations including ambulation or transport for procedures.

OT-AC 12.0 FREQUENCY:

Oxygen therapy should be administered continuously unless the need has been shown to be associated only with specific situations (e.g., exercise and sleep).

OT-AC 13.0 INFECTION CONTROL:

Under normal circumstances, low-flow oxygen systems (including cannulas and simple masks) do not present clinically important risk of infection and need not be routinely replaced. High-flow systems that employ heated humidifiers and aerosol generators, particularly when applied to patients with artificial airways, can pose important risk of infection. In the absence of definitive studies to support change-out intervals, results of institution-specific and patient-specific surveillance measures should dictate the frequency with which such equipment is replaced.

Reprinted with permission from *Respiratory Care* 2002; 47(6): 717–720. The complete AARC Clinical Practice Guidelines are available from the AARC Web site (*http://www.aarc.org*), or from the AARC Executive Office, or from *Respiratory Care* journal.

Figure 2-1 *(continued)*

AARC CLINICAL PRACTICE GUIDELINE
Oxygen Therapy in the Home or Extended Care Facility

OT-CC 1.0 PROCEDURE:
The procedure addressed is the administration of oxygen therapy in the home or in the extended care facility other than by mechanical ventilator.

OT-CC 2.0 DESCRIPTION/DEFINITION:
Oxygen therapy is the administration of oxygen at concentrations greater than that in ambient air with the intent of treating or preventing the symptoms and manifestations of hypoxia.

OT-CC 3.0 SETTING:
This Guideline is confined to oxygen administration in the home or extended care facility.

OT-CC 4.0 INDICATIONS:
Documented hypoxemia: In adults, children and infants older than 28 days: (1) PaO_2 < or = 55 torr or SaO_2 < or = 88% in subjects breathing room air,1,2 or (2) PaO_2 of 56–59 torr or SaO_2 or SpO_2 < or = 89% in association with specific clinical conditions (e.g., cor pulmonale, congestive heart failure, or erythrocythemia with hematocrit > 56).

Some patients may not qualify for oxygen therapy at rest but will qualify for oxygen during ambulation, sleep, or exercise. Oxygen therapy is indicated during these specific activities when SaO_2 is demonstrated to fall to < or = 88%.

OT-CC 5.0 CONTRAINDICATIONS:
No absolute contraindications to oxygen therapy exist when indications are present.

OT-CC 6.0 PRECAUTIONS AND/OR POSSIBLE COMPLICATIONS:
6.1 In spontaneously breathing hypoxemic patients with chronic obstructive pulmonary disease, oxygen administration may lead to an increase in $PaCO_2$.
6.2 Undesirable results or events may result from noncompliance with physician's orders or inadequate instruction in home oxygen therapy.
6.3 Complications may result from use of nasal cannulae or transtracheal catheters.
6.4 Fire hazard is increased in the presence of increased oxygen concentrations.
6.5 Bacterial contamination associated with certain nebulizers and humidification systems is a possible hazard.

6.6 Possible physical hazards can be posed by unsecured cylinders, ungrounded equipment, or mishandling of liquid oxygen (resulting in burns). Power or equipment failure can lead to an inadequate oxygen supply.

OT-CC 7.0 LIMITATIONS OF PROCEDURE:
Oxygen therapy has only limited benefit for the treatment of hypoxia due to anemia and benefit may be limited when circulatory disturbances are present.

OT-CC 8.0 ASSESSMENT OF NEED:
8.1 Initial assessment: Need is determined by the presence of clinical indicators as previously described and the presence of inadequate oxygen tension and/or saturation as demonstrated by the analysis of arterial blood. Concurrent pulse oximetry values must be documented and reconciled with the results of the baseline blood gas analysis if future assessment is to involve pulse oximetry.
8.2 Ongoing evaluation or reassessment: Additional arterial blood gas analysis is indicated whenever there is a major change in clinical status that may be cardiopulmonary related. Arterial blood gas measurements should be repeated in 1–3 months when oxygen therapy is begun in the hospital in a clinically unstable patient to determine the need for long-term oxygen therapy (LTOT). Once the need for LTOT has been documented, repeat arterial blood gas analysis or oxygen saturation measurements are unnecessary other than to follow the course of the disease, to assess changes in clinical status, or to facilitate changes in the oxygen prescription.

OT-CC 9.0 ASSESSMENT OF OUTCOME:
Outcome is determined by clinical and physiologic assessment to establish adequacy of patient response to therapy.

OT-CC 10.0 RESOURCES:
10.1 Equipment
10.1.1 Low-flow oxygen systems: Such devices supply oxygen at flows that are less than the patient's inspiratory demand (i.e., the delivered oxygen is diluted with room air). These devices may supply either a low

Figure 2-2 *American Association for Respiratory Care, Clinical Practice Guideline: Oxygen Therapy in the Home or Extended Care Facility. (Courtesy of American Association for Respiratory Care, Irving, TX)* ***(continues)***

or high F_IO_2 depending upon the specific design. Reservoir masks or other devices designed to provide for a high F_IO_2 are usually not appropriate for long-term oxygen therapy outside of the hospital.

10.1.1.1 Nasal cannulae can provide 24–40% oxygen (depending on patient's inspiratory flowrate) with flowrates up to 6 L/min in adults; infant flows should be limited to a maximum of 2 L/min. Oxygen supplied to adults by nasal cannulae at flows < or = to 4 L/min need not be humidified.

10.1.1.2 Transtracheal oxygen catheters can provide continuous oxygen therapy with oxygen consumption compared to nasal cannulas of only about one-half of that used at rest and two-thirds of that used with exercise. Transtracheal catheters may require greater patient supervision and have an increased risk for complication.

10.1.1.3 Oxygen-conserving devices: Oxygen reservoir cannulae (nasal or pendant), demand oxygen delivery devices, and transtracheal catheters are currently being utilized for oxygen conservation. Each of these devices may have advantages or disadvantages that are related to specific design.

10.1.2 High-flow oxygen delivery systems: Such devices can provide a prescribed gas mixture of high or low oxygen concentration at flows that exceed patient demand; however, they are impractical for home use except for humidifying devices that are compressor-driven with supplemental oxygen bled in at low flows. Tracheostomy collars and T-tube adapters may be used with high-flow supplemental oxygen systems. The gas should be humidified by a continuous aerosol generator or a heated humidifier. The humidifier is preferable because of the greater likelihood for the transmission of contagion via nebulizer.

10.1.3 Oxygen supply systems

10.1.3.1 Oxygen concentrators: Concentrators extract oxygen from ambient air and should deliver oxygen at concentrations of 85% or greater at up to 4 L/min. Membrane oxygen concentrators typically provide oxygen at a lower F_DO_2, and higher flows are required to 'compensate' for the reduced F_DO_2.

10.1.3.2 Liquid oxygen systems: Liquid oxygen is provided in large reservoir canisters with smaller portable units that can be transfilled by the patient. There is evaporation loss from the canisters when they are not in use. Many of the portable liquid oxygen units are appropriate for ambulatory therapy and can be utilized with oxygen-conserving devices to extend their functional time.

10.1.3.3 Compressed gas cylinders: Oxygen may be supplied in large cylinders (e.g., G or H cylinders) as stationary units for home oxygen therapy. Smaller cylinders (e.g., D and E cylinders) may be equipped with wheels and used as portable oxygen units (strollers). E cylinders may also be used as a backup for oxygen concentrators in the event of a power or equipment failure. Smaller cylinders coupled with oxygen conserving devices may be used as ambulatory units.

10.2 Personnel: Credentialed respiratory care practitioners (RRT or CRTT) or other credentialed persons with equivalent training and documented ability to perform the tasks may assess patients, initiate and monitor oxygen delivery systems, recommend changes in therapy, and instruct caregivers. Caregivers may operate and maintain oxygen delivery devices and assess a specific patient after they have been instructed by credentialed practitioners and have demonstrated the appropriate level of skill.

OT-CC 11.0 MONITORING:

11.1 Patient

11.1.1 Clinical assessment should routinely be performed by the patient and/or the caregiver to determine changes in clinical status (e.g., use of dyspnea scales and diary cards). Patients should be visited/monitored at least once a month by credentialed personnel unless conditions warrant more frequent visits.

11.1.2 Measurement of baseline oxygen tension and saturation is essential before oxygen therapy is begun. These measurements should be repeated when clinically indicated or to follow the course of the disease. Measurements of SO_2 also may be made to determine appropriate oxygen flow for ambulation, exercise, or sleep.

11.2 Equipment Maintenance and Supervision: All oxygen delivery equipment should be checked at least once daily by the patient or caregiver. Facets to be assessed include proper function of the equipment, prescribed flowrates, F_DO_2, remaining liquid or compressed gas content, and backup supply. A respiratory care practitioner or

Figure 2-2 *(continues)*

equivalent should during monthly visits reinforce appropriate practices and performance by the patient and caregivers and assure that the oxygen equipment is being maintained in accordance with manufacturers' recommendations. Liquid systems need to be checked to assure adequate delivery. Oxygen concentrators should be checked regularly to assure that they are delivering 85% oxygen or greater at 4 L/min.

OT-CC 12.0 FREQUENCY:

Oxygen therapy should be administered continuously unless the need has been shown to be associated only with specific situations (e.g., exercise and sleep).

OT-CC 13.0 INFECTION CONTROL:

Under normal circumstances low-flow oxygen systems without humidifiers do not present a

clinically important risk of infection and need not be routinely replaced. High-flow systems that employ heated humidifiers or aerosol generators, particularly when applied to subjects with artificial airways, can be important sources of infection and should be cleaned and disinfected on a regular basis. (Although studies have suggested that tubing should be changed every 48 hours in the hospital, there are no definitive studies regarding the frequency of tube changes at home or in long-term care facilities.)

Reprinted with permission from *Respiratory Care* 1992; 37: 918–922. The complete AARC Clinical Practice Guidelines are available from the AARC Web site (*http://www.aarc.org*), from the AARC Executive Office, or from *Respiratory Care* journal.

Figure 2-2 *(continued)*

HIGH- AND LOW-FLOW OXYGEN DELIVERY SYSTEMS

The term **high-flow oxygen delivery system** does not refer to the liter flow of oxygen powering the device. Rather it refers to the fact that the device delivers all of the patient's inspiratory flow needs. With a high-flow system, all of the inspired gas the patient breathes is delivered by the oxygen device, and none is provided from the ambient air.

These oxygen delivery systems most commonly employ viscous shearing or vorticity to mix ambient air with oxygen. (Viscous shearing was discussed earlier in Chapter 1.) Oxygen powering the device mixes with room air delivering a high flow of mixed gas at a precise **F_IO_2** (fraction of inspired oxygen, expressed as a decimal). The total flow delivered to the patient is greater than the flow set on the oxygen flowmeter due to the additional gas drawn into the device by viscous shearing and vorticity. Total flows and air/oxygen entrainment ratios will be discussed later in this chapter.

Low-flow oxygen delivery devices provide part of a patient's inspiratory gas flow needs. The remainder of the gas the patient inhales comes from room air. Since the gas

delivered from the oxygen device mixes with unknown and varying amounts of room air, the amount of F_IO_2 delivered varies.

The variation in the F_IO_2 is dependent upon the patient's tidal volume (depth of breathing) and respiratory rate. If the tidal volume is large, more room air will be inspired in proportion to the oxygen delivered from the device. As the respiratory rate increases, room air entrainment also increases. If the proportion of room air increases, the delivered F_IO_2 will decrease.

HIGH-FLOW OXYGEN DELIVERY SYSTEMS

Venturi Masks/High Air Flow with Oxygen Entrainment (HAFOE)

The **venturi or HAFOE mask** utilizes the viscous shearing effect mixing two different gases (oxygen and air), increasing total flow for precise oxygen concentration delivery (Figure 2-3). The term "venturi" is really incorrectly applied to describe the operation of these devices. The high-flow gas from the jet forms a boundary layer, cleaving the relatively stationary room air. This viscous shearing effect entrains the room air, mixing the oxygen with it. By varying the size of the oxygen jet and the entrainment ports, differing oxygen

Figure 2-3 *A pictorial representation of a venturi mask. Note the room air entrainment lateral to the oxygen jet. (A) High-velocity jet. (B) Region of viscous shearing. (C) Room air entrainment.*

concentrations may be obtained. The ratio of air entrainment to oxygen flow may be calculated using the following formula:

$$\frac{\text{Liters of Air Entrained}}{\text{Liters of Oxygen}} = \frac{1.0 - F_IO_2}{F_IO_2 - 0.21}$$

F_IO_2 = Desired Oxygen Concentration

It is important to remember that F_IO_2 is expressed as a decimal and not as a percentage when solving this equation.

For example:

You are using an entrainment device set at an F_IO_2 of .40. What is the air-to-oxygen entrainment ratio?

$$\frac{\text{Liters of Air Entrained}}{\text{Liters of Oxygen}} = \frac{1.0 - F_IO_2}{0.40 - 0.21}$$

$$\frac{\text{Liters of Air Entrained}}{\text{Liters of Oxygen}} = \frac{1.0 - 0.40}{0.40 - 0.21}$$

$$\frac{\text{Liters of Air Entrained}}{\text{Liters of Oxygen}} = \frac{0.6}{0.19}$$

$$\frac{\text{Liters of Air Entrained}}{\text{Liters of Oxygen}} = \frac{3}{1}$$

Often you will be required to calculate the total flow rate from an entrainment device. To calculate the total flow (air and oxygen) being delivered to the patient, you must know (1) the air-to-oxygen entrainment ratio, and (2) the liter flow of oxygen entering the device.

Total Flow =
    Liters of Air Entrained + Liters of Oxygen

For example:

An entrainment mask is set at 24%. The oxygen flow to the mask is 3 L/min. What is the total flow (air and oxygen) to the patient?

Step 1: What is the air-to-oxygen entrainment ratio?

$$\frac{\text{Liters of Air Entrained}}{\text{Liters of Oxygen}} = \frac{1.0 - F_IO_2}{F_IO_2 - 0.21}$$

$$\frac{\text{Liters of Air Entrained}}{\text{Liters of Oxygen}} = \frac{1.0 - 0.24}{0.24 - 0.21}$$

$$\frac{\text{Liters of Air Entrained}}{\text{Liters of Oxygen}} = \frac{25}{1}$$

This means that for every liter of oxygen entering the mask, there are 25 liters of air being entrained.

Step 2: What is the total flow?

Total Flow =
    Liters of Air + Liters of Oxygen

Total Flow = (3 × 25) + 3

Total Flow = 78 Liters per Minute

Manufacturers have developed specific combinations of entrainment ports and jet sizes to deliver precise F_IO_2 levels. These combinations depend on the ratio of air entrainment in proportion to oxygen flow to determine the oxygen concentration. These ratios are summarized in Table 2-1.

High-flow systems are designed to flood the patient's face with a high flow of gas con-

TABLE 2-1 Air to Oxygen Entrainment Ratios

Room Air-to-Oxygen Ratio	Concentration
25:1	24%
10:1	28%
8:1	30%
5:1	35%
3:1	40%
1.7:1	50%
1:1	60%
0:1	100%

Reprinted with permission from Gary C. White, Basic Clinical Lab Competencies for Respiratory Care, 4th Ed., Thomson Delmar Learning, 2003.

taining a constant F_IO_2. The theory behind the use of this system is that if enough flow is provided, the patient will not entrain any room air. The success of the concept depends on the oxygen percentage (air-to-oxygen entrainment ratio) and the patient's inspiratory flow demands. If the patient's inspiratory flow demands exceed the flow from the mask, room air will be entrained and the F_IO_2 will become variable and not fixed.

For example:

A patient is ordered a 35% venturi mask. He is breathing at a rate of 20 breaths per minute with a minute volume of 8 liters at an Inspiratory-to-Expiratory ratio (I:E) of 1:2. Is the device providing adequate flow if the flowmeter is set at 6 liters per minute?

1. Calculate the patient's inspiratory flow demands.

    Tidal volume

    = minute volume/frequency

    = 8 liters/20 breaths per minute

    = .4L (400 mL)

    Total ventilatory cycle

    = 60 seconds/20 bpm

    = 3 seconds

    Inspiratory time is 1 second at an I:E ratio of 1:2.

    Inspiratory flow demand

    = .4 liters/second

    = .4 liters/second × 60 seconds/minute

    = 24 liters/minute

2. Calculate flow through the device and compare. Air-to-oxygen entrainment ratio at 35% = 5:1.

    Total flow at 6 liters/min

    = 30 liters air + 6 liters oxygen

    = 36 liters per minute

3. Conclusion: The device exceeds the patient's inspiratory flow needs by 12 liters/minute.

Anesthesia Bag-Mask Systems

Anesthesia bags can be combined with ventilation masks and valves to construct a true non-rebreathing system (Figure 2-4). One one-way valve prevents exhaled gas from mixing with the oxygen delivered to the bag and the other one-way valve prevents the entrainment of room air during inspiration. If the fit is tight and the flow is adequate, this device

Figure 2-4 *An anesthesia bag-mask system. Note the one-way valves and their flow direction.*

can provide up to 100% oxygen delivery. The oxygen flow is adjusted so that the reservoir bag never collapses during inspiration. This device also may be used to administer mixed gas therapy such as He/O_2 or O_2/CO_2.

LOW-FLOW OXYGEN DELIVERY DEVICES

Nasal Cannula and Catheter

The **nasal cannula** is an example of a low-flow oxygen delivery device. The cannula rests on the patient's upper lip, with the curve of the prongs directed posteriorly into the nasal passages. Oxygen at a flow between 1 to 6 liters per minute enters the patient's nose, filling the anatomic reservoir (Figures 2-5 and 2-6).

The **anatomic reservoir** consists of the nasopharynx and oropharynx (Figure 2-7). In the adult its volume is approximately 50 milliliters. As a patient breathes, there is a slight pause in time between exhalation and inspiration. During this pause, the anatomic reservoir

Figure 2-5 *A typical nasal cannula.*

Figure 2-6 *A patient wearing a nasal cannula.*

TABLE 2-2	Nasal Cannula Oxygen Concentrations
100% O² Flow in Liters	**Approximate F_IO_2**
1 L	0.24
2 L	0.28
3 L	0.32
4 L	0.36
5 L	0.40
6 L	0.44

Adapted from Gary C. White, Basic Clinical Lab Competencies for Respiratory Care, 4th Ed., Thomson Delmar Learning, 2003.

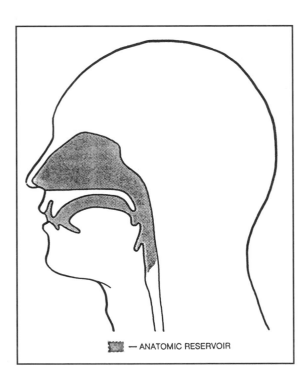

— ANATOMIC RESERVOIR

Figure 2-7 *The anatomic reservoir.*

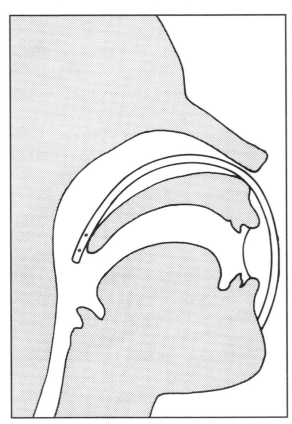

Figure 2-8 *A pictorial representation indicating the correct placement of the nasal catheter. Note that the tip of the catheter is immediately posterior to the uvula and has not been advanced past it.*

fills with oxygen. Therefore, the first 50 milliliters of each breath is pure oxygen, and the remainder consists of oxygen mixed with room air. As discussed earlier, the F_IO_2 varies depending on the patient's tidal volume and respiratory rate. Table 2-2 indicates the approximate F_IO_2 delivery with these devices.

The **nasal catheter** operates on a similar principle to that of the nasal cannula. The catheter is positioned by passing it through the nose and the turbinates with the tip resting at the level of the uvula in the oropharynx (Figure 2-8). Oxygen entering the device flows directly into the oropharynx. The F_IO_2 delivery is similar to that of the nasal cannula.

ASSEMBLY AND TROUBLESHOOTING

Assembly—High-Flow Oxygen Delivery Devices

Correct assembly and troubleshooting of high-flow oxygen delivery systems is important for correct operation and patient safety. The following is a suggested assembly guide.

1. Obtain an appropriate oxygen source (cylinder, piping system, liquid reservoir, or concentrator) with a flowmeter calibrated for an appropriate flow range.

2. Attach the flowmeter to the 50 psi oxygen source.

3. Attach a humidifier to the flowmeter. *Note:* If you are using a venturi mask, do not use a humidifier. Water droplets and particles may alter the performance from the desired F_IO_2.

4. Attach the oxygen connecting tube to the humidifier.

5. Adjust the flow so that the entrainment device exceeds the patient's inspiratory needs or, when using an anesthesia bag-mask, adjust the flow so the reservoir bag does not deflate during inspiration.

6. Placement of the oxygen therapy device:
   a. Place the mask on the bridge of the patient's nose, adjusting the strap so it is snug but not tight.
   b. If the mask is a reservoir type, ensure that the reservoir is free to expand without pressure from bed covers or other objects.
   c. When using an anesthesia bag-mask, check for proper operation of the one-way valves and for correct assembly.
   d. Adjust the head strap so it is snug but not too tight.
   e. Verify oxygen concentration of the venturi mask system.

Troubleshooting

Troubleshooting high-flow oxygen masks consists of checking for leaks and proper flow from the mask. The following is a suggested algorithm (ALG 2-1).

1. Check the following sources for leaks:
   a. Check the connection between the flowmeter and the 50-psi gas source.
   b. Check the connection between the flowmeter and the humidifier.
   c. Check the connection between the connecting tube and the humidifier.

2. If gas fails to flow from the mask:
   a. Verify that the oxygen flowmeter is turned on and an adequate supply of gas exists.
   b. Check the oxygen connecting tube for kinks or obstructions.
   c. Verify that the humidifier is operating properly.

ALG 2-1 *An algorithm describing how to troubleshoot high-flow oxygen systems.*

ASSEMBLY AND TROUBLESHOOTING

Assembly—Nasal Cannula

Nasal cannulas are one of the most common oxygen administration devices. Although a nasal catheter is used less frequently, it is also important to understand its use. It is essential to understand how to assemble and troubleshoot these devices. The following is a suggested assembly guide.

1. Obtain an appropriate oxygen source (cylinder, piping system, liquid reservoir, or concentrator) with a flowmeter calibrated for an appropriate flow range.

2. Attach the flowmeter to the 50-psi oxygen source.

3. Attach a humidifier to the flowmeter.

4. Attach the oxygen connecting tube to the flowmeter.

5. Adjust the flow to the ordered level prior to placing the device on the patient.

6. Placement of the oxygen therapy device:

   a. Nasal catheter
      (1) Lubricate the catheter with sterile water-soluble lubricant.
      (2) Estimate the length of the catheter by measuring from the pinna of the ear to the tip of the nose.
      (3) Pass the catheter gently down one nare until the tip is visible behind the uvula.
      (4) If the patient gags following placement of the nasal catheter, it has been placed too far down the airway. Withdraw the catheter a centimeter or two.
      (5) You may find that it is helpful to use a tongue depressor to depress the tongue and a flashlight, or otoscope, to visualize the nasal catheter and its placement.

   b. Nasal cannula
      (1) Place the cannula resting on the upper lip with the prongs pointed down into the nasal passages.
      (2) Secure the strap around the head so it is snug but not tight, or adjust the lariat strap beneath the chin as shown in Figure 2-6.

   c. Reservoir cannula
      (1) Place the reservoir so it rests on the upper lip and adjust the strap so it is comfortable.

   d. Pendant cannula
      (1) Place the pendant reservoir on the patient's chest. Rest the prongs of the cannula on the upper lip and direct them into the nasal passages.
      (2) Adjust the strap so the cannula is comfortable.

Troubleshooting

Troubleshooting cannulas and catheters primarily consists of checking for flow from the device and checking for leaks. The following is a suggested troubleshooting algorithm (ALG 2-2).

1. Check the following sources for leaks:
   a. The connection between the flowmeter and the 50-psi gas source may not be tight.
   b. The connection between the flowmeter and the humidifier may be loose.
   c. The connection between the cannula and the humidifier may not be snug.

2. If gas fails to flow from the cannula or catheter:
   a. Verify that the oxygen flowmeter is turned on and an adequate supply of gas exists.
   b. Check the oxygen connecting tube for kinks or obstructions.
   c. Verify that the humidifier is operating correctly.
   d. Check the cannula or catheter for obstruction caused by dried secretions. If obstructed, replace the cannula or catheter.

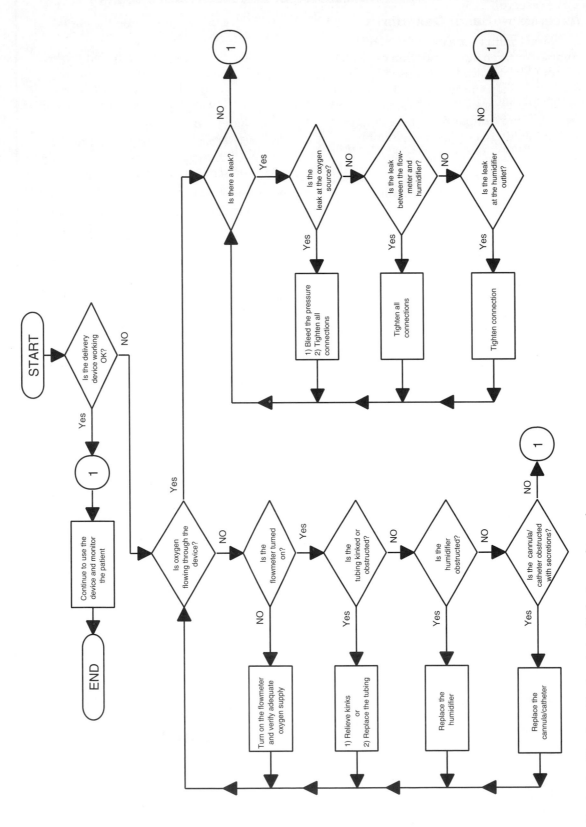

ALG 2-2 *An algorithm describing how to troubleshoot a nasal cannula.*

Reservoir and Pendant Cannulas

The **reservoir cannula** and the **pendant cannula** are two contemporary devices designed to maintain FIO2 levels at lower flow rates. By providing a small reservoir, oxygen flow may be reduced without affecting the oxygen delivery. This is a particular advantage during ambulation or exercise. The performance of these devices, however, is variable. Figure 2-9 shows a pendant cannula (A) and a reservoir cannula (B) and their application.

Transtracheal Catheter

A **transtracheal catheter** is a small catheter surgically inserted into the trachea at the second cartilage ring. By supplying oxygen flow directly into the trachea, this device can maintain F_IO_2 levels at a lower oxygen flow than with a nasal cannula. These devices are used primarily for patients who require continuous long-term oxygen therapy. The transtracheal catheter may use up to 59% less oxygen than conventional oxygen cannulas. This is because adequate PaO_2 levels (arterial oxygen tensions) may be achieved at oxygen flows as low as ¼ liter per minute. Figure 2-10 shows a transtracheal oxygen catheter and its placement.

Hazards involving the use of these devices include infection, subcutaneous emphysema, and hemoptysis. Lower costs and cosmetic advantages must be carefully weighed against these potential hazards.

Simple Oxygen Mask

A **simple oxygen mask** is a lightweight mask applied to a patient's face. Figures 2-11 and 2-12 show a typical simple mask and how it is applied. The principle behind a simple mask is to add reservoir space (the mask) in addition to the anatomic reservoir. During the pause between exhalation and inspiration, the mask and anatomic reservoir fill with pure oxygen. During the first part of inspiration, pure oxygen is inhaled. During the latter part, oxygen and room air are mixed in the mask and inhaled. As with nasal cannula use, F_IO_2 delivery varies depending upon tidal volume and respiratory rate. Typical oxygen delivery is between 35% and 50% oxygen at 5–12 L/min.

(A)

(B)

Figure 2-9   *(A) A pendant oxygen cannula applied to a patient. (B) A reservoir oxygen cannula applied to a patient.*

Figure 2-12 *A patient correctly wearing a simple oxygen mask.*

Figure 2-10 *A transtracheal catheter and a pictorial representation showing its correct placement.*

Figure 2-11 *A simple oxygen mask.*

The minimum liter flow a simple mask should be set is 5 L/min.

Since the patient also exhales into the mask, the mask may collect exhaled carbon dioxide. This is not desired. Therefore, it is important to maintain enough oxygen flow into the mask to flush the exhaled carbon dioxide, usually 6–12 liters per minute or greater, and monitor the patient.

Partial Rebreathing and Non-Rebreathing Masks

The partial rebreathing and non-rebreathing masks are sometimes referred to as reservoir masks. A reservoir bag is added to the mask to provide an additional reservoir for oxygen.

The **partial rebreathing mask** (Figure 2-13) has a reservoir bag attached that is open to the mask. As the name implies, the patient rebreathes part of his exhaled gas. When the patient exhales, approximately the first third of expiration is from the anatomic dead space that has not participated in gas exchange and is rich in oxygen. It is this portion that fills the reservoir bag. The remaining exhaled gas exits through the exhalation ports. As the patient pauses between expiration and inspiration, additional oxygen flows into the mask and reservoir bag. When the patient inhales, a mixture of oxygen and air is inhaled. The oxygen

Figure 2-13 *A disposable partial rebreathing mask.*

delivered by this mask typically contains up to 70% oxygen. Oxygen flow is adjusted so that the reservoir bag is not allowed to fully collapse during inspiration.

The **non-rebreathing mask** is similar to the partial rebreathing mask except that one-way valves have been added to the mask's exhalation port(s) and between the mask and the reservoir bag (Figure 2-14). The one-way valve between the mask and reservoir helps to prevent exhaled gas from mixing with the oxygen in the reservoir bag. The one-way valve on the

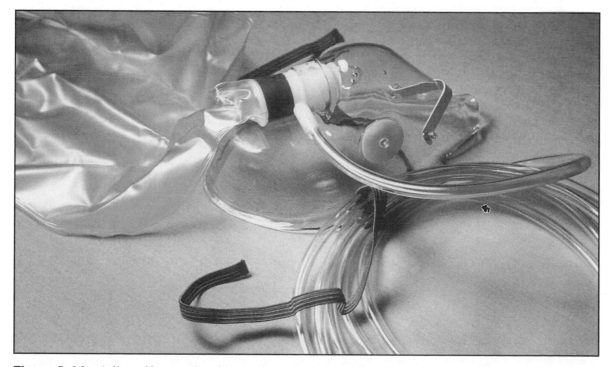

Figure 2-14 *A disposable non-rebreathing mask.*

exhalation port(s) closes during inspiration to prevent room air from entering the mask. Many manufacturers include only a single one-way valve on the side of the mask. In the event oxygen flow were to be interrupted, the patient may still inhale through the side port without the one-way valve.

The performance of the disposable non-rebreathing mask can vary considerably. The fit of the mask, operation of one-way valves, and oxygen flow may all contribute to decrease the F_IO_2 delivery. The disposable non-rebreathing masks can typically deliver oxygen concentrations of up to 80%. Liter flow into the mask should be set at a minimum flow rate of 10 liters per minute.

HIOX[80] DISPOSABLE HIGH F_IO_2 OXYGEN MASK

The HiOx[80] is a disposable high F_IO_2 delivery mask that was developed to deliver high oxygen concentrations (80 %) consistently with less room air entrainment (Figure 2-15). The HiOx[80] mask has a molded vinyl facemask without air entrainment ports or one-way valves covering exhalation holes. The bridge of the mask is also fitted with a moldable foam cushion to better seal the fit of the mask to the patient's nose. Two straps are provided (one above the ears and one below) to better secure the mask to the patient's face.

The base of the mask is fitted with a manifold consisting of three one-way valves. Two of the one-way valves fitted to a wye at the base of the mask direct inspiratory flow from the reservoir and ensure that exhaled air is exhausted into the room (Figure 2-16). A 750-mL reservoir attached to the inspiratory limb of the wye provides a source of pure

Figure 2-15 *A photograph of the HiOx[80] high F_IO_2 mask. (Courtesy of American Association for Respiratory Care, Irving, TX)*

oxygen during inspiration. All one-way valves are of a large diameter low resistance design (< 1.5 cmH$_2$O). In the event the patient's inspiratory demand exceeds the 750-mL reservoir capacity, a one-way valve in the inspiratory limb opens, admitting room air.

Oxygen concentrations of 80 % can be achieved at oxygen flow rates of 8 L/min. The lower oxygen consumption can be advantageous during patient transport or other applications where the oxygen supply from cylinders or liquid reservoirs is limited.

Figure 2-16 *A diagram illustrating gas flows during inhalation (with and without room air entrainment) and exhalation. (Courtesy of Viasys Healthcare, Yorba Linda, CA)*

VAPOTHERM 2000*i*

The Vapotherm 2000*i* is a high-flow oxygen therapy system that is capable of delivering oxygen flows from 5 to 40 L/min at a humidity content of 55 mg/liter at a temperature of 41 degrees Celsius (Figure 2-17). This equates to a relative humidity delivery of greater than 95%.

Humidification is accomplished using membrane technology, where the water source is routed through a membrane (vapor transfer cartridge) and passes into the gas stream as water vapor. The membrane only passes particles smaller than 0.01 microns, effectively eliminating bacteria and other microorganisms (Figure 2-18). Operational range for temperature may be adjusted between 35 and 43 degrees Celsius.

Since the gas delivered to the patient is both warmed and humidified, higher flow rates at higher F_IO_2 levels may be tolerated through delivery devices such as nasal cannulas. Oxygen flow through a nasal cannula can

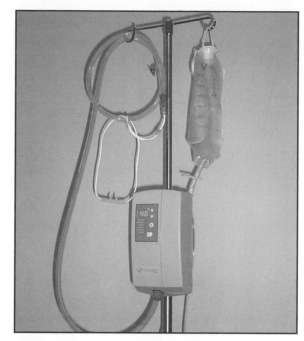

Figure 2-17 *A photograph of the Vapotherm 2000i oxygen delivery system. (Courtesy of Vapotherm, Inc., Annapolis, MD)*

ASSEMBLY AND TROUBLESHOOTING

Assembly—Oxygen Masks

Oxygen masks are quite common in clinical practice. Therefore, it is important to understand how to assemble and troubleshoot these oxygen administration devices correctly. The following is a suggested assembly guide.

1. Obtain an appropriate oxygen source (cylinder, piping system, liquid reservoir, or concentrator) with a flowmeter calibrated for an appropriate flow range.

2. Attach the flowmeter to the 50-psi oxygen source.

3. Adjust the flow to the ordered level or, when using a partial rebreathing or non-rebreathing mask, adjust the flow so the reservoir bag does not deflate during inspiration.

4. Placement of the oxygen therapy device:
   a. Place the mask on the bridge of the patient's nose first, adjusting the strap so it is snug but not too tight.
   b. If the mask is a reservoir type, ensure that the reservoir is free to expand without pressure from bed covers or other objects.
   c. When using a non-rebreathing mask, check for proper operation of the one-way valves.

Troubleshooting

Troubleshooting oxygen masks consists of checking for leaks and proper flow from the mask. The following is a suggested troubleshooting algorithm (ALG 2-3).

1. Check the following sources for leaks:
   a. Check the connection between the flowmeter and the 50-psi gas source.
   b. Check the connection between the flowmeter and the humidifier.
   c. Check the connection between the connecting tube and the humidifier.

2. If gas fails to flow from the mask:
   a. Verify that the oxygen flowmeter is turned on and an adequate supply of gas exists.
   b. Check the oxygen connecting tube for kinks or obstructions.

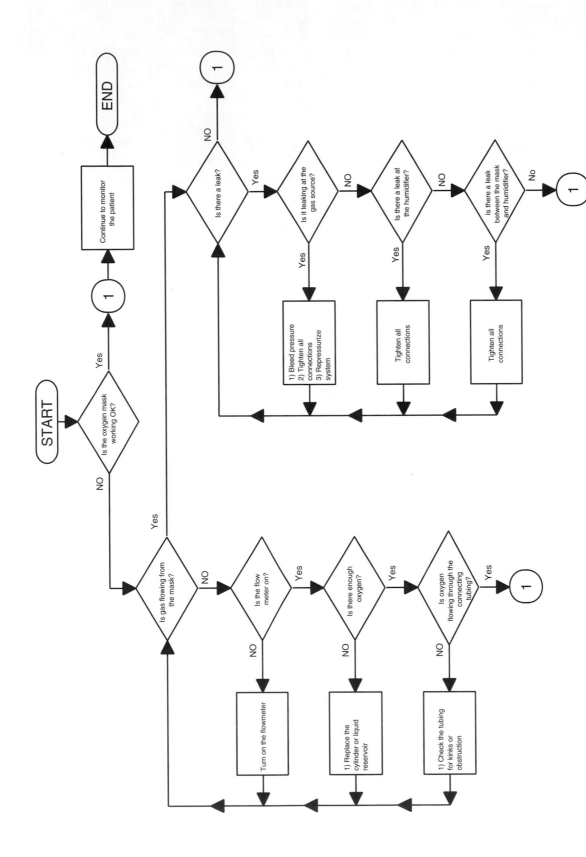

ALG 2-3 *An algorithm describing how to troubleshoot an oxygen mask.*

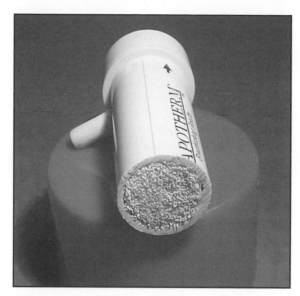

Figure 2-18 *A photograph of the Vapor Transfer Cartridge. (Courtesy of Vapotherm, Inc., Annapolis, MD)*

be delivered up to 40 liters per minute without significant patient discomfort and flows of up to 20 liters per minute may be delivered via transtracheal catheter.

OXYGEN ENCLOSURES OR ENVIRONMENTAL DEVICES

Incubators

The **incubator** is a transparent box used to regulate an infant's environmental temperature. It also may be used to control the F_IO_2 (Figure 2-19). Due to the large volume of the incubator and the frequent nursing care an infant requires, it is difficult to maintain a consistent oxygen concentration. Therefore, these devices are rarely used for oxygen regulation, but rather are used to control the thermal environment.

Head Box

The **head box** or **oxyhood** is a transparent box designed to enclose an infant's head (Figure 2-20). Frequently, head boxes are used inside an isolette, with the isolette controlling the thermal environment and the head box providing the consistent F_IO_2. Flow is adjusted into the head box so that the infant will not entrain any room air around its neck. The gas entering the head box is premixed (usually using a blender) and then humidified and

Figure 2-19 *A photograph of a contemporary incubator.*

Figure 2-20 *A photograph of a head box.*

heated. Nebulizers are not recommended since noise levels may become excessive. Since the head box encloses the infant's head, the isolette may be opened for nursing care to other portions of the body without affecting the F_IO_2.

When delivering oxygen to an infant in a head box, it is important to analyze the F_IO_2. Using a calibrated oxygen analyzer (refer to Chapter 6 for the assembly, calibration, and troubleshooting of oxygen analyzers), measure the oxygen concentration at the infant's face near the bottom of the head box. A variation of oxygen concentrations can occur between the bottom and top of the head box. If a variation is found, repeated measurements at various locations can determine how that particular hood "mixes" gases and what settings work best. Pulse oximetry and trans-cutaneous monitoring are also helpful to ensure that the F_IO_2 delivered is adequate to maintain the patient's oxygen requirements.

ASSEMBLY AND TROUBLESHOOTING

Assembly—Oxygen Hood/Head Box

Infants requiring a hood need close supervision and attention. Careful assembly and troubleshooting is important for optimal therapy. The following is a suggested assembly guide.

1. Choose a proper sized hood for the infant. Select one that covers the head without being too large.

2. Ensure a proper gas source for the blender or mixing device. Attach a flowmeter calibrated in the appropriate flow range.

3. Confirm correct blender assembly and operation as discussed earlier in the chapter.

4. Select an appropriate heated humidifier to meet inspiratory flow needs. Examples may include the Bear VH-820, Bird Humidifier, Conchapack, Fisher and Paykel MR730 or equivalent.

5. Connect large bore tubing to the outlet of the humidifier and to the head box.

6. Provide a means of temperature monitoring at the inlet of the head box.

7. Verify oxygen concentration and flow using an oxygen analyzer and observing for flow.

Troubleshooting

Troubleshooting oxygen hoods primarily involves checking for leaks, ensuring flow, and monitoring temperature. When troubleshooting this equipment, please follow the suggested troubleshooting algorithm (ALG 2-4).

1. Sources for leaks:
   a. Between the gas source (piping system or regulator) and the high pressure hoses.
   b. Between the high pressure hoses and the blender.
   c. The connection between the blender and the humidifier.

2. Verify the oxygen concentration using an oxygen analyzer. If there is a tremendous discrepancy, calibrate the analyzer and repeat verification. If the discrepancy still exists, replace the blender and have the defective unit repaired by your local vendor or authorized biomedical repair facility.

3. Temperature monitoring:
   a. Many of the new humidifiers have provisions for servo control. A sensor automatically adjusts the temperature to the desired level. Even with servo control, it is important to monitor inlet temperatures.

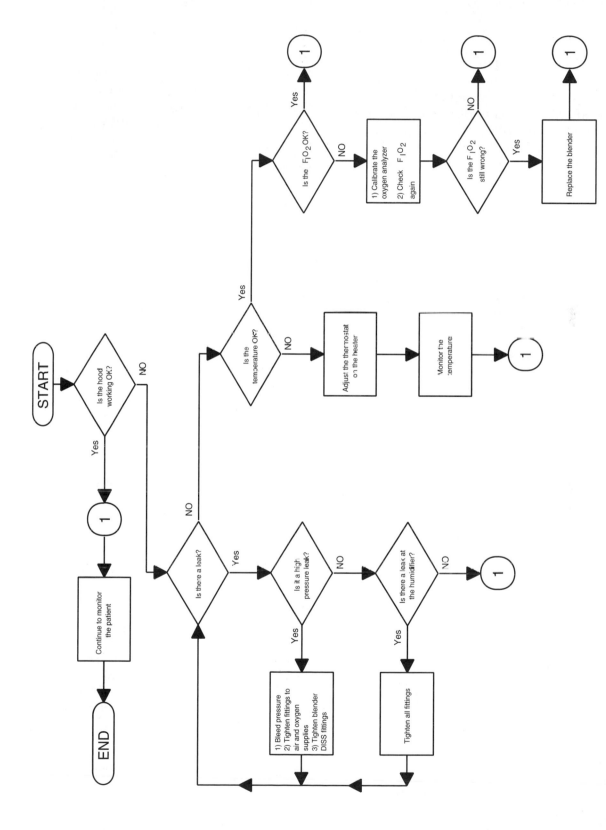

ALG 2-4 *An algorithm describing how to troubleshoot a head box or oxyhood.*

MIST TENTS

Mist tents (croupettes) are plastic tents that are large enough to enclose a small child (Figure 2-21). The primary application of these tents is for aerosol therapy. However, the oxygen environment also may be controlled using these devices. The child's activity, opening and closing the tent for nursing care, and difficulty in sealing the tent all contribute to variations in the F_IO_2. These tents are usually powered by a high-output aerosol device. If additional oxygen is required, the oxygen may be bled in from a flowmeter or another nebulizer.

Figure 2-21 *A photograph of a croupette.*

ASSEMBLY AND TROUBLESHOOTING

Assembly—Croupette

Assembly of croupettes and mist tents will vary with manufacturers. The following is a suggested assembly guide.

1. Ensure a source of 50-psi gas to power the unit and an oxygen flowmeter.

2. Attach the canopy frame to the bed per manufacturer's instructions.

3. Attach the canopy to the frame following the manufacturer's instructions.

4. Fill the nebulizer with sterile distilled water.

5. Add ice to the reservoir as required or connect the cooling unit to an appropriately rated 110-volt electrical outlet.

6. Adjust the oxygen flow to between 12 and 15 liters per minute.

7. Place the infant into the canopy and tuck the edges under the mattress.

8. After 20 to 30 minutes, verify oxygen concentration and adjust as appropriate.

Troubleshooting

Troubleshooting croupettes consists of checking for leaks and verifying oxygen concentrations. When troubleshooting this equipment, please follow the suggested troubleshooting algorithm (ALG 2-5).

1. Sources for leaks:
   a. Check the connection between the flowmeter and oxygen connecting tube.
   b. Check the canopy seal between the mattress and the canopy.
   c. See if the canopy zippers are open.

2. Factors that affect oxygen concentration:
   a. Opening and closing the canopy frequently.
   b. Child's toys obstructing inlets or circulation outlets.

3. Fire hazards:
   a. Croupette canopies contain a large volume of oxygen. Therefore children's toys should be limited to non-battery operated toys and ones that do not generate sparks!

ALG 2-5 *An algorithm describing how to troubleshoot a croupette.*

HYPERBARIC OXYGEN THERAPY

Hyperbaric oxygen therapy, as defined by the Undersea Hyperbaric Medical Society (UHMS), is the exposure of a patient or patients to a pressure greater than one atmosphere absolute while breathing 100% oxygen either continuously or intermittently. This therapy was once confined to decompression sickness (caisson disease), but now has been utilized in the treatment of other disorders. The physiological effects of hyperbaric oxygen therapy include the mechanical effects as well as the oxygenation effects.

Physiological Effects of Hyperbaric Oxygen Therapy

The mechanical effects of hyperbaric oxygen therapy are related to the increased pressures. Any trapped gas bubbles, when exposed to the increased pressure during hyperbaric treatment, will decrease in size (Boyle's law). At a constant temperature (body temperature), the increased pressure causes the volume of the trapped gas bubbles to decrease. This effect is utilized in the treatment of decompression sickness and gas embolisms.

The oxygenation effects of hyperbaric oxygen therapy include the supersaturation of plasma, vasoconstriction, gas washout (gases other than oxygen), increased effectiveness of white blood cells, and neovascularization of tissue by improved collagen synthesis.

The supersaturation of the plasma occurs due to the increased partial pressure of oxygen under the hyperbaric conditions. PaO_2 levels can reach 1500 mmHg during therapy. This increase in plasma saturation improves oxygen transport even to areas with minimal perfusion.

Vasoconstriction during hyperbaric oxygen therapy has also been documented. It is not known how this occurs, but it is important in the management of localized "compartmented" disorders.

Increased elimination of other gases during hyperbaric treatment is possible due to the high driving force (partial pressure) of oxygen. Other gases, such as nitrogen and carbon monoxide, can be more quickly eliminated from the body by use of hyperbaric therapy than is possible at ambient pressures.

White blood cells have an increased ability to fight infections when exposed to hyperbaric oxygen therapy. It is thought that the increase in available oxygen results in increased oxidative mechanisms, which help the cells to perform their function better. Additionally, hyperbaric oxygen therapy is lethal to anaerobic microorganisms.

Neovascularization to poorly perfused tissues occurs as a result of hyperbaric oxygen therapy. The periodic increased oxygenation promotes the formation of fibroblasts, osteoblasts, and granulocytes, and collagen formation. This promotes capillary budding into areas that were previously not perfused, improving circulation. This effect has been helpful in the management of radiation necrosis of bone tissue, necrotizing fasciitis, gas gangrene and other difficult-to-manage wounds and disorders.

The accepted conditions that may benefit from hyperbaric oxygen therapy include:

- Gas gangrene
- Radiation necrosis
- Carbon monoxide/cyanide poisoning
- Ischemic tissue transplants
- Necrotizing soft tissue infections
- Decompression sickness
- Refractory osteomyelitis
- Refractory anaerobic infections
- Severe acute anemia or hemorrhage (blood loss anemia)
- Crush injury/Traumatic ischemia
- Ischemic tissue transplants
- Enhanced healing of problematic wounds

Equipment for Hyperbaric Oxygen Therapy

To deliver hyperbaric oxygen therapy, a specialized chamber is required. The two types of chambers are the multiplace and the monoplace chambers.

The multiplace chamber is a large vessel that can accommodate more than one patient at a time. The chamber is pressurized with room air, and the patient breathes oxygen via a non-rebreathing mask or other device. Additionally, these chambers allow for a health care provider to be with the patient during the therapy. The advantages of the multiplace chamber are that more than one patient can be treated simultaneously, and the health care provider can treat any emergent conditions that may arise during treatment. The disadvantages of the multiplace chambers are that they are very large, and very expensive to purchase and maintain.

The monoplace chamber is a small chamber capable of treating only one patient at a time (Figure 2-22). Typically, these chambers are pressurized with oxygen, although air may also be used. They are much smaller and can be placed more conveniently than the multiplace chambers. The disadvantage of the monoplace chambers is that the health care provider must depressurize the chamber to treat any emergent problems that may arise during therapy.

Contraindications/Hazards

The only absolute contraindication for hyperbaric oxygen therapy is an untreated pneumothorax that occurred during therapy. During decompression, the gas in the pneumothorax will greatly expand (Boyle's law). It is important to provide a path for the gas to escape by the placement of a chest tube or needle thoracentesis.

Patients with upper respiratory infections may have difficulty clearing their ears during pressurization and decompression. Decongestants may help alleviate the problem. It may be required in some cases to delay treatment (if not emergent), until the upper respiratory infection subsides.

Patients with predisposed pulmonary disease, who air trap, may have difficulty with hyperbaric treatment. A slower decompression rate may assist these patients in eliminating gas as it expands due to decreased pressures.

Some patients may be unable to equalize pressures in their middle ears. Tympanic membrane rupture is possible during hyperbaric oxygen therapy. Some patients may require the placement of bilateral tympanotomy tubes for this type of therapy.

MIXED GAS THERAPY

He/O_2 Therapy

Helium/oxygen mixtures have been administered for some time in the treatment of obstructive airway diseases. The rationale is that a gas of lesser density can more easily bypass the obstruction and therefore be inspired with less effort and resistance. Gas mixtures are available in 20/80% and 30/70% oxygen-to-helium mixtures. The densities of the mixtures compared to oxygen are 1.8

Figure 2-22 *A photograph of a monoplace hyperbaric chamber.*

(20/80%) and 1.6 (30/70%) times less dense, respectively.

A tight-fitting anesthesia bag-mask system is usually employed for therapy (see Figure 2-4). Gas flow is adjusted so that the reservoir bag never collapses. Typically, precise gas flow is not required. The purpose of the tight-fitting mask is to ensure that the lighter gas will not escape from the mask and avoid being inhaled.

If accurate flows are ordered, one can use the density difference to calculate what an oxygen flowmeter should read. The oxygen flowmeter setting is equal to the desired flow (ordered flow) divided by the density difference from oxygen (1.8 or 1.6). Alternatively, specially calibrated flowmeters can be purchased to be used with the specific gas mixtures.

CARBON DIOXIDE/OXYGEN THERAPY

CO_2/O_2 therapy has been used for many years for treatment of various disorders. The scientific rationale for such therapy, however, is questionable. This therapy is typically administered using a disposable, non-rebreathing mask. Gas mixtures are available in 5/95% and 7/93% carbon dioxide–to-oxygen mixtures. Therapy should be limited to between five and fifteen minutes at a time.

When administering this gas mixture, it is important to monitor the patient's heart rate, respiratory rate, and blood pressure carefully. Alterations in these readings or a change in mental state would warrant discontinuation of therapy.

NITRIC OXIDE (NO) THERAPY

Inhaled nitric oxide therapy is used to treat persistent pulmonary hypertension of the newborn, having been approved by the

Figure 2-23 *A photograph of the Ohmeda I-NOvent.*

United States Food and Drug Administration for this application. Nitric oxide is supplied in aluminum cylinders at a 99% purity (combined with nitrogen) level. Nitric oxide is highly reactive and can combine with oxygen or water to form nitrogen dioxide (NO_2) or nitric acid (HNO_3) respectively. Therapeutic levels of nitric oxide range from 2 to 80 parts per million (ppm). Nitric oxide is delivered via the I-NOvent (Figure 2-23). The I-NOvent interfaces with critical care ventilators to deliver the desired nitric oxide concentration to the inspiratory limb of the ventilator circuit.

CLINICAL CORNER

1. Describe two clinical situations, one in which you would select a low-flow device and another in which you would select a high-flow device. Be specific regarding pathology, blood gases, and respiratory assessment.
2. You adjust a patient's venturi mask from 40% to 50%. However, you observe that the patient is still desaturating, despite the higher oxygen concentration. Describe what you should evaluate to determine whether the mask is meeting the patient's needs.
3. You are called to set up a head box in the nursery for a newborn who is desaturating. What equipment should you take with you (assume that the unit has piped oxygen and air), and how would you set up the system?

Self-Assessment Quiz

1. Which of the following are criteria for oxygen therapy according to the American Association for Respiratory Care's Clinical Practice Guideline for acute care patients?
   I. $PaO_2 \leq 75$ mmHg breathing room air
   II. $PaO_2 \leq 60$ mmHg breathing room air
   III. $SaO_2 \leq 95$ % breathing room air
   IV. $SaO_2 \leq 90$ % breathing room air
   a. I and III
   b. I and IV
   c. II and III
   d. II and IV

2. Which of the following are criteria for oxygen therapy according to the American Association for Respiratory Care's Clinical Practice Guideline for sub-acute and homecare patients?
   I. $PaO_2 \leq 55$ mmHg breathing room air
   II. $PaO_2 \leq 60$ mmHg breathing room air
   III. $SaO_2 \leq 88$ % breathing room air
   IV. $SaO_2 \leq 90$ % breathing room air
   a. I and III
   b. I and IV
   c. II and III
   d. II and IV

3. Which of the following disease states may qualify a patient for home oxygen therapy if they don't meet the PaO_2 or SaO_2 criteria?
   I. cor pulmonale
   II. congestive heart failure
   III. erythro-cythemia with hematocrit > 56
   IV. pulmonary hypertension
   a. I only
   b. I and II only
   c. I, II, and III only
   d. I, II, III, and IV

4. You have set a patient up on a venturi mask at 50%. The oxygen flowmeter is set at 15 liters per minute. What is the total flow to the patient?
   a. 15 liters per minute
   b. 25 liters per minute
   c. 41 liters per minute
   d. 50 liters per minute

5. A partial rebreathing mask, when properly fitted and when the bag remains inflated, can deliver up to:
   a. 35% oxygen.
   b. 50% oxygen.
   c. 70% oxygen.
   d. 80% oxygen.

6. A non-rebreathing mask, when properly fitted and when the bag remains inflated, can deliver up to:
   a. 35% oxygen.
   b. 50% oxygen.
   c. 70% oxygen.
   d. 80% oxygen.

7. A simple oxygen mask, when properly fitted and when the bag remains inflated, can deliver up to:
   a. 35% oxygen.
   b. 50% oxygen.
   c. 70% oxygen.
   d. 80% oxygen.

8. A patient is on a venturi mask at 35%. The patient wishes to eat. What flowmeter setting on a nasal cannula would be sufficient to meet the patient's needs during meals?
   a. 3 liters per minute
   b. 4 liters per minute
   c. 5 liters per minute
   d. 6 liters per minute

9. A 65-year-old male patient arrives via ambulance in the emergency department. The patient weighs 64 Kg and is somewhat thin. The patient is on a nasal cannula at 3 L/min. You note the following vital signs:
   respiratory rate: 28–35 / min
   tidal volume: 200–240 mL
   SpO_2:   85% on 3 L/min nasal cannula
   ventilatory pattern: Irregular
   The emergency room physician asks for your recommendation. What would you suggest?
   a. nasal cannula at 3 L/min
   b. venturi mask at 40%
   c. non-rebreathing mask at 12 liters per minute
   d. nasal cannula at 5 liters per minute

10. Which of the following are low-flow oxygen delivery devices?
    I. venturi mask
    II. nasal cannula
    III. anesthesia bag-mask
    IV. disposable non-rebreathing mask
    a. I and II only
    b. II and III only
    c. II and IV only
    d. I and IV only

11. You are assessing a patient on a nasal cannula at 3 L/min. His SpO_2 is only 88% when just an hour ago it was 93%. What might you check when troubleshooting the oxygen delivery system?
    I. Make sure both prongs are in the nares.
    II. Check the tubing connections.
    III. Verify the liter flow at the flowmeter.
    IV. Determine if the patient has removed the cannula for any length of time.
    a. I only
    b. I and II only
    c. I, II, and III only
    d. I, II, III, and IV

12. Which of the following is a low-flow oxygen delivery device that provides therapeutic F_IO_2 levels at liter flows of less than 1 liter per minute?
    a. partial rebreathing mask
    b. nasal catheter
    c. nasal cannula
    d. transtracheal catheter

13. The simple mask, partial rebreathing mask, and non-rebreathing mask increase the F_IO_2 delivery compared with a nasal cannula by:
    a. adding a reservoir.
    b. increasing liter flow.
    c. viscous shearing and vorticity.
    d. entraining room air.

14. A venturi mask set at 24% oxygen with an oxygen flow of 4 L/min provides a total flow of:
    a. 40 L/min.
    b. 55 L/min.
    c. 95 L/min.
    d. 104 L/min.

15. When checking on a patient wearing a partial rebreathing mask, you note that the bag deflates markedly during inspiration. You should:
    a. not be concerned.
    b. increase the oxygen flow.
    c. leave the oxygen flow the same.
    d. change the patient to a simple oxygen mask.

16. A patient is wearing a venturi mask set at 40%. The patient is cold and pulls up the bed linen to cover his shoulders, covering the entrainment ports to the mask. What would you expect might occur?
    I. The F_1O_2 will increase.
    II. Total flow will remain unchanged.
    III. More air will enter the mask through the exhalation ports.
    IV. More oxygen will flow through the system in relation to air.
    a. I and III
    b. I and IV
    c. II only
    d. IV only

17. What device is able to achieve high F_1O_2 levels at lower liter-flow settings when compared with a disposable non-rebreathing mask?
    a. a venturi mask
    b. a HiOx^{80} mask
    c. the Vapotherm oxygen therapy system
    d. a partial rebreathing mask

18. What device is able to deliver humidified oxygen at high flow rates?
    a. a venturi mask
    b. a HiOx^{80} mask
    c. the Vapotherm oxygen therapy system
    d. a partial rebreathing mask

19. You must set up a patient in the emergency room on an oxygen delivery device administering a high F_1O_2 as quickly as possible. The best oxygen delivery device to use would be:
    a. a simple mask.
    b. a partial rebreathing mask.
    c. a disposable non-rebreathing mask.
    d. a venturi mask.

20. You must select an oxygen delivery device for a patient who is sensitive to small changes in F_1O_2. The patient requires moderate oxygen concentrations. However, if the patient's oxygen concentration varies much, she might rapidly desaturate. The best delivery device for this patient would be:
    a. a simple mask.
    b. a partial rebreathing mask.
    c. a disposable non-rebreathing mask.
    d. a venturi mask.

21. A patient is on a 40% venturi mask set at 10 L/min. What is the total flow of gas through the mask?
    a. 10 L/min
    b. 20 L/min
    c. 30 L/min
    d. 40 L/min

22. You must provide humidified oxygen for a newborn that has an SpO$_2$ of 68% on room air. What device would provide the most consistent F$_I$O$_2$ delivery while allowing good access for nursing care?
    a. nasal cannula
    b. head box or hood
    c. isolette
    d. croupette

23. When setting up a head box or hood, what is required to adequately monitor the infant's environment in the hood?
    I. oxygen analyzer
    II. thermometer
    III. oxygen saturation monitor
    a. I only
    b. I and II only
    c. I and III only
    d. I, II, and III

24. What is the minimum flow a simple oxygen mask should be set at?
    a. 3 liters per minute
    b. 5 liters per minute
    c. 8 liters per minute
    d. 10 liters per minute

25. You must set a patient up on a mixture of 30% oxygen and 70% helium. You know the density difference is 1.6 times less than oxygen alone. The doctor orders a specific liter flow of 15 liters per minute. With only an oxygen flowmeter available, what would you set the flow at?
    a. 9 liters per minute
    b. 12 liters per minute
    c. 15 liters per minute
    d. 24 liters per minute

26. A hazard of administering F$_I$O$_2$ levels greater than 0.50 for extended periods of time is:
    a. ventilatory depression.
    b. oxygen toxicity.
    c. absorption atelectasis.
    d. oxygen emboli.

27. You must set a patient up on a mixture of 20% oxygen and 80% helium. You know the density difference is 1.8 times less than oxygen alone. The doctor orders a specific liter flow of 10 liters per minute. With only an oxygen flowmeter available, what would you set the flow at?
    a. 6 liters per minute
    b. 10 liters per minute
    c. 18 liters per minute
    d. none of the above

28. A physician presents with an arterial blood gas, and she is questioning the PaO$_2$, which is 1000 mmHg. What is a possible explanation for this?
    a. It is an instrumentation error.
    b. Air bubbles affected the sample.
    c. The patient is on 100% oxygen.
    d. The patient is in a hyperbaric chamber.

29. Hyperbaric oxygen therapy utilizes which gas law to achieve its effect?
    a. Boyle's law
    b. Charles' law
    c. Henry's law
    d. Dalton's law

30. Which of the following conditions are accepted for treatment using hyperbaric oxygen therapy?
    I. gas gangrene
    II. carbon monoxide poisoning
    III. radiation necrosis
    IV. necrotizing soft tissue infections
    a. I only
    b. I and II only
    c. I, II, and III only
    d. I, II, III, and IV

Selected Bibliography

American Association for Respiratory Care. (2002). Clinical practice guildeline: Oxygen therapy for adults in the acute care facility—2002 revision and update. *Respiratory Care, 47*(6), 717–720.

American Association for Respiratory Care. (1992). Clinical practice guildeline: Oxygen therapy in the home or extended care facility. *Respiratory Care, 37*(8), 918–922.

Aranda, M., et al. (1999). The biology of nitric oxide. *Respiratory Care, 44*(2), 156–168.

Branson, R. D. (1999). Inhaled nitric oxide: Delivery systems and monitoring. *Respiratory Care, 44*(3), 281–307.

Fussell, K. M. (2003). Assessing need for long-term oxygen therapy: A comparison of conventional evaluation and measures of ambulatory oximetry monitoring. *Respiratory Care, 48*(2), 115–119.

Hess, D. R. (2003). Detection and monitoring of hypoxemia and oxygen therapy. *Respiratory Care, 45*(1), 65–83.

McCoy, R. M. (2003). Oxygen-conserving techniques and devices. *Respiratory Care, 45*(1), 95–104.

Robinson, T. D. (2000). The role of hypoventilation and ventilation-perfusion redistribution in oxygen-induced hypercapnia during acute exacerbations of chronic obstructive pulmonary disease. *American Journal of Respiratory and Critical Care Medicine, 56*, 314–332.

Sacci, R. (1989). Air entrainment masks; jet mixing is how they work; the Bernoulli and Venturi principles are how they don't. *Respiratory Care, 24*(10), 928–931.

CHAPTER 3

HUMIDITY AND AEROSOL THERAPY EQUIPMENT

INTRODUCTION

Many respiratory care procedures involve the administration of humidity or aerosol. Normally, humidification of inspired gases is physiologically accomplished in our upper airways. Medical gases are anhydrous (free of water) and must be humidified to prevent undesirable pathological consequences such as retained secretions, mucous plugging, and irritation.

Many pieces of equipment are used in respiratory care to humidify gases and produce aerosols. Each operates using several fundamental principles. In this chapter you will learn the physics of humidity, the principles of humidification and aerosol generation, and the equipment used to humidify gases and aerosolize liquids.

OBJECTIVES

After completing this chapter, the student will accomplish the following objective: be able to achieve a score of 80% or better on a written self-assessment quiz.

PHYSICS OF HUMIDITY AND AEROSOL THERAPY

- Define and differentiate between humidity and aerosol.
- Explain how humidity is measured.
- Define the term *evaporation*.
- Explain how a temperature increase can increase a gas's capacity for humidity.
- Define the term *humidity deficit*, and explain how humidity therapy may reduce it.
- Describe the physical characteristics of aerosols.
- Describe four factors that influence an aerosol particle's deposition in the pulmonary system.
- Explain how choked flow is applied to generate an aerosol.
- Discuss the clinical application of humidity therapy.

HUMIDITY THERAPY EQUIPMENT

- Explain three ways a humidifier can be designed to increase its efficiency.
- Explain the principles of operation of the following types of humidifiers:
  - Pass-Over
  - Misty Ox Laminar Diffuser Humidifier
  - Wick
  - Diffusion Grid (Cascade Type)
  - Heat and Moisture Exchangers
- Discuss the clinical application of aerosol therapy.

AEROSOL THERAPY EQUIPMENT

- Differentiate between a mainstream and a sidestream nebulizer.
- Explain the principles of operation of small volume nebulizers, their assembly, and how to troubleshoot them.
- Explain the principle of operation, assembly, and troubleshooting of large volume jet nebulizers.
- Explain the operation and application of metered dose inhalers (MDIs) and holding chamber devices.

- Explain the functional characteristics and application of the following aerosol delivery devices:
  — Aerosol mask
  — Trach mask
  — Face tent
  — Brigg's adapter
  — Drainage bag
- Explain the principle of operation of an ultrasonic nebulizer.

- Explain the assembly and troubleshooting of the following ultrasonic nebulizers.
  — DeVilbiss Ultra-Neb 99
  — Timeter Compu-neb
  — Small volume ultrasonic nebulizers for medication delivery
- Describe the characteristics of a pediatric mist tent and its assembly and troubleshooting.

KEY TERMS

Aerosol	Evaporation	Humidity deficit	Metered dose
Amplitude	Frequency	Hygroscopic	inhalers
Anhydrous	Heat and moisture	Hypertonic	Nebulizer
Babbington principle	exchanger	Hypotonic	Piezoelectric crystal
Baffle	Hertz	Inertial impaction	Relative humidity
Body humidity	Holding chamber	Isotonic	Tonicity
Capacity	Humidifier	Maximum absolute	
Carrier gas	Humidity	humidity	

PHYSICS OF HUMIDITY AND AEROSOL THERAPY

HUMIDITY AND AEROSOLS

Humidity

Humidity is water that is in the gaseous state. Water vapor is composed of individual water molecules contained in a gas. Water vapor or humidity behaves in a similar way to gas molecules—it exerts a pressure and is in constant random motion. In order to calculate the partial pressure of a gas containing humidity, the partial pressure of water vapor must be accounted for when adding the partial pressures. For example, when calculating the partial pressures of ambient air that is fully saturated with water vapor, the partial pressure of the water vapor must be accounted for (Dalton's law of partial pressures).

Barometric pressure
$$= 760 \text{ mmHg}$$

Partial pressure of H_2O at 24° Celsius
$$= 23.8 \text{ mmHg}$$

$$760 \text{ mmHg} - 23.8 \text{ mmHg}$$
$$= 736.2 \text{ mmHg}$$
(partial pressure of gases)

Partial pres. of O_2
$$= 736.2 \times .2095 = 154.23$$

Partial pres. of N_2
$$= 736.2 \times .7808 = 574.83$$

Partial pres. of Ar
$$= 736.2 \times .0093 = 6.85$$

Partial pres. of CO_2
$$= 736.2 \times .0003 = .22$$

Inert gases
$$= 736.2 \times .0001 = .07$$

Aerosols

An **aerosol** by definition is particulate matter suspended in a gas. The particulate matter can be liquid or solid. An example of an aerosolized solid is Cromolyn sodium, a medication that can be delivered in powdered form and inhaled while suspended. Liquids are aerosolized in clinical practice both for bland aerosol therapy (primarily for the hydration of the pulmonary tract) and for administration of medications directly to the pulmonary system.

MEASUREMENT OF HUMIDITY

Humidity can be quantified several ways, including actual content in grams or milligrams of water, partial pressure of water vapor, and relative humidity.

Water Content or Absolute Humidity

Desiccants are compounds that absorb water. By drying a desiccant so that it is **anhydrous** (without any water content) and weighing it, then passing a gas through it so that the water is removed from the gas, one can determine the actual water content of the gas. The difference in weight before and after passing the gas through the desiccant would equal the water content of the gas. As you recall from basic physics or chemistry classes, one gram of water equals one milliliter of water. The process of measuring water content has been done for gases at various temperatures, a sample of which is shown in Table 3-1. Notice that as temperature increases, the ability of a gas to hold water also increases. The actual water content when a gas is fully saturated is termed **maximum absolute humidity** or **capacity**.

Partial Pressure

Water vapor behaves like a gas. The random motion of water molecules exerts a pressure in a way similar to gas exerting pressure (see Chapter 1, Dalton's law). Therefore, it is possible to measure the partial pressure water vapor exerts at various contents and pressures (Table 3-1). As the temperature of a gas increases, kinetic activity increases, so the pressure also increases.

The magnitude of the pressure exerted by water vapor is independent of the barometric pressure. Its magnitude is solely dependent upon temperature and relative humidity. Therefore, at a given temperature and relative humidity, the partial pressure of water vapor is a constant regardless of the barometric pressure. The partial pressure of water vapor must always be accounted for (subtracted) when calculating the partial pressures of other gases in a mixture.

Relative Humidity

Relative humidity is humidity expressed as a percentage of a gas's capacity (water content when fully saturated). The capacity may be determined by using tables such as Table 3-1. Relative humidity is derived by dividing the actual water content of a gas by its capacity at that temperature, as shown in the following equation.

$$\text{Relative humidity} = \frac{\text{Actual Humidity}}{\text{Capacity}}$$

Example: You are administering a humidified gas containing 23 mg/L water. The temperature of the gas is 30° Celsius. What

---

TABLE 3-1 Water Content and Pressures at Different Temperatures

Temperature (° Celsius)	Water Content (mg/L) Capacity	Partial Pressure (torr)
0	4.85	4.58
5	6.80	6.54
10	9.40	9.20
15	12.83	12.79
20	17.30	17.51
25	23.04	23.69
30	30.35	31.71
35	39.60	42.02
37	43.90	47.00
40	51.10	55.13
45	65.60	71.66
50	83.20	92.30

Adapted from Table 17-2, Burton, Hodgkin, and Gee, Respiratory Care: A Guide to Clinical Practice, J. B. Lippincott, 1984. Reprinted with permission.

is the relative humidity of the gas you are administering?

$$\text{Relative humidity} = \frac{\text{Actual Humidity}}{\text{Capacity}}$$

$$= \frac{23 \text{ mg/L}}{30.35 \text{ mg/L}}$$

$$= .757 \text{ or } 75.7\%$$

Example: The local radio announcer states that it is 30° Celsius and the relative humidity is 45%. What is the actual humidity? Relative humidity

$$\text{Relative humidity} = \frac{\text{Actual Humidity}}{\text{Capacity}}$$

$$\text{Actual humidity} = \text{Relative humidity} \times \text{Capacity}$$

$$= .45 \times 30.35 \text{ mg/L}$$

$$= 13.66 \text{ mg/L}$$

Note: 30.35 mg is the capacity at 30° C (from Table 3-1).

EVAPORATION

Evaporation is the process of water moving from a liquid to a gaseous state. Molecules in a liquid, like those in a gas, are in random motion. The kinetic energy of molecules in a liquid, however, is less than the kinetic energy of molecules in a gas. There are also variations in the energy levels of molecules within a liquid. Those molecules with sufficient kinetic energy will overcome the attractive forces between molecules in the liquid and escape as vapor. When those molecules with sufficient energy escape from the liquid, the overall energy level of the liquid declines, and the temperature decreases (evaporative heat loss). When this occurs at room temperature, heat from the ambient air transfers to the liquid, restoring the energy level, and the process is repeated until the liquid is gone.

As the temperature of a liquid is increased, the kinetic activity of its molecules is also increased. Therefore, more molecules will have sufficient energy to escape as vapor.

HUMIDITY DEFICIT

Humidity deficit is a physiological term that refers to the difference between the inspired gas's water content and the water content of a gas at body temperature and pres-

sure. At body temperature and pressure saturated (BTPS), inspired gas is at 37° Celsius, contains 43.9 mg/L of water, exerts a partial pressure of 47 mmHg, and is fully saturated. These conditions at BTPS are termed **body humidity**. Humidity deficit then is the difference between body humidity and the actual humidity of the inspired gas as illustrated in the following formula.

Humidity deficit
= Body humidity − Actual humidity

Example: You are administering a gas at 25° Celsius with a relative humidity of 50%. What is the humidity deficit?

(a) Fully saturated, a gas at 25° C contains 23.04 mg/L.

Relative humidity × Capacity
= Actual humidity

.50 × 23.04 mg/L = 11.52 mg/L

(b) Humidity deficit
= Body humidity − Actual humidity

= 43.9 mg/L − 11.52 mg/L

= 32.38 mg/L

Humidity deficit becomes clinically significant when it is large and is sustained for a prolonged period of time. Pathological changes occur in the pulmonary system causing retention of secretions, airway plugging, or obstruction and infection with pathogenic bacteria.

Since medical gases are anhydrous, it is important to humidify the gases before they are administered. Proper humidification of inspired gases will reduce the humidity deficit and prevent any adverse pathological changes from occurring.

PHYSICAL CHARACTERISTICS OF AEROSOLS

As discussed earlier, aerosols are particles suspended in a gas. Clinically liquids are aerosolized more frequently than solids. Therefore, the majority of this discussion will focus on the aerosolization of liquids.

Particle Size and Mass

As the size of an aerosol particle increases, so does its mass. If the radius of a sphere doubles, the volume will increase approximately eight times ($V = 4 \times k \times r^3$). As volume increases, mass will increase proportionally. Therefore, an increase or reduction in the size of a particle will dramatically change its mass. As the mass of the aerosol particle decreases, gravity will have less effect on it and it will remain suspended longer.

PHYSICAL NATURE OF PARTICLES

A discussion of the physical nature of aerosol particles is important in understanding how they behave clinically. Physical factors include its tonicity, its electric charge, and whether a particle is hygroscopic. As you will learn later, physical features influence a particle's ability to remain suspended and how deeply it penetrates the pulmonary system.

Hygroscopic

If an aerosol is **hygroscopic**, it has a tendency to absorb water. As the particle absorbs water, it increases in size and mass. When inhaled, hygroscopic aerosols will deposit in the pulmonary system sooner than non-hygroscopic aerosols. This is because the particles will coalesce or combine, forming larger particles with greater mass, which will no longer remain in suspension.

Tonicity

Tonicity refers to the concentration of solutes in a solution relative to their concentration in body fluids. A hypertonic solution will gain water from body fluids, due to its greater concentration of solutes. An isotonic solution will remain stable (neutral toward water absorption), since solute concentrations are similar to body fluids. A hypotonic solution will lose water, since its solute concentrations are less than that of body fluids.

Hypertonic solutions (>.9% NaCl) absorb water. When aerosolized they become hygroscopic, increasing in size as discussed earlier.

Isotonic solutions (.9% NaCl), when aerosolized, are neutral in their affinity to water. Therefore, particle sizes tend to remain stable.

Hypotonic solutions (<.9% NaCl) release water and, when aerosolized, decrease in size. As their size decreases, so does their mass.

Electrical Charge

Due to the methods employed to aerosolize liquids, the aerosol particles become electrically charged. Electrical charge seems to have little effect physiologically; however, it may have significant effect on the function of surrounding electrical equipment. Sensitive amplification instrumentation (e.g., ECG monitors) have been affected by the static charge that can build up in plastic 22-mm diameter corrugated tubing carrying aerosol at high flow rates.

FACTORS INFLUENCING AEROSOL DEPOSITION IN THE AIRWAYS

Many factors influence an aerosol's ability to deposit into the pulmonary system. These factors include (1) particle size and gravitational effects, (2) inertia, (3) temperature and humidity, and (4) the patient's respiratory pattern (Table 3-2).

Particle Size and Gravity

As particle size and mass increase, gravitational forces act on the particle to a greater degree, tending to remove it from suspension. Ideally, all particles should be small enough that effects of gravity are minimal. However, when particles become too small, they remain suspended and never deposit in the pulmonary system. Particle sizes between 1 and 5 microns are clinically optimal for peripheral deposition in the respiratory bronchioles.

Inertia

Inertia is also related to particle size and mass. As Newton stated, kinetic energy equals ½ times the mass times velocity squared. A particle with greater mass, when placed in motion, will have a greater inertia than a particle with a smaller mass. Newton also stated that once an object is placed in motion, it tends to stay in motion unless acted upon by an outside force. An aerosol particle with a large

---

TABLE 3-2 Factors that Influence Aerosol Stability and Penetration into the Airways

---

Particle size

Hygroscpoic properties

Tonicity

Inertia

Temperature and humidity of the delivery gas

Patient's respiratory pattern

---

mass will tend to travel in a straight line even if the gas suspending it changes direction. Larger particles will be removed from suspension in the upper airways, and not penetrate further into the pulmonary system. Smaller particles with less mass will travel further into the lungs.

Temperature and Humidity

As the temperature of the **carrier gas** (the gas conducting the suspended aerosol particles) increases with humidity held constant, the aerosol particles will have a tendency to evaporate into the carrier gas. If the aerosol is introduced into a humid carrier gas, the particles will coalesce (combine), forming larger particles.

Respiratory Pattern

A significant factor influencing pulmonary deposition of aerosols is the patient's respiratory pattern. A slow, deep inspiration followed by a brief pause before exhalation will increase aerosol deposition into the lungs. An example of this desired effect can be illustrated by the administration of bronchodilators. Maximal penetration and deposition is desired to reduce bronchospasm. Good patient instruction and monitoring can influence the effectiveness of aerosol therapy to a large degree. If a patient is properly instructed, the patient can inhale slowly to a larger than normal tidal volume, and hold his or her breath at end inspiration. By modifying the breathing pattern in this way, aerosol penetration and deposition can be maximized.

APPLICATION OF CHOKED FLOW

Choked flow is applied in many aerosol generators to produce an aerosol. As described in Chapter 1, choked flow occurs when a gas's velocity through a nozzle can no longer be increased by increasing the head pressure. When the flow is choked, the flow at the nozzle exit is sonic, or greater than the speed of sound (343 m/second at standard conditions). Liquids may be entrained into the gas flow by placing a capillary tube into the boundary layer near the nozzle exit.

Liquid is drawn from the reservoir, up the capillary tube and into the gas stream by a combination of shear forces, vorticity, and a pressure differential (Figure 3-1). The shear forces are the greatest within a distance of three

Figure 3-1 *A functional diagram of a pneumatic nebulizer. (1) The high pressure nozzle. (2) Area of maximum shear force. (3) Capillary tube. (4) Baffle. (5) Area of vorticity (approximately three nozzle diameters from the nozzle exit). (6) Reservoir.*

times the diameter of the nozzle's opening. The effect of vorticity is most pronounced once the boundary layer becomes turbulent and vortices form. The pressure differential is created by the removal of fluid from the capillary tube at the top by shear forces and vorticity. Since the base of the tube is occluded (immersed in water), the removal of fluid (mass) at the top results in a region of low pressure within the capillary tube. The greater pressure at the base of the capillary tube (atmospheric pressure) forces water up the tube, filling the void (conservation of mass). Once the liquid reaches the top of the capillary tube, it is continuously entrained into the high velocity gas by shear forces and vorticity. Once entrained, the liquid is instantly broken up into an aerosol with a wide range of particle sizes.

The baffle distal to the jet and capillary tube stabilizes the aerosol particle size by **inertial impaction**. A **baffle** may consist of a ball or a wall downstream from the nozzle exit. As discussed earlier, the aerosol particles with a large volume have a large mass. As the gas flow changes direction around the baffle, the large particles resist changes in direction and impact against the baffle. Only smaller particles with small masses are able to follow the gas flow around the baffle and remain suspended. The difference between an atomizer and a nebulizer is that an atomizer does not have a baffle to stabilize particle size. A nebulizer has a baffle and is therefore able to better control the particle size.

HUMIDITY THERAPY EQUIPMENT

FACTORS INFLUENCING HUMIDIFIER EFFICIENCY

A **humidifier** is a device that adds water vapor (water in its molecular or gaseous state) to a gas. Humidifier efficiency can be increased by controlling the temperature, the surface area for gas-to-liquid contact, and the time that the gas is exposed to the liquid. Manufacturers utilize these three factors to improve the clinical efficiency of their humidifiers.

Temperature

By increasing the temperature of the liquid, the molecules' kinetic activity increases. As the molecules gain energy, more of them will have enough energy to escape as a vapor, increasing the humidity output.

Furthermore, as the temperature of the solution is increased, the temperature of the gas is also increased as it passes over the solution. A warm gas has a greater capacity for water vapor than a cold gas.

Surface Area

Surface area for gas-to-water contact is also an important factor in determining humidity. Increasing the surface area for contact will increase the humidity.

Time for Contact

The time that the gas is allowed to interface with the solution also influences humidity. If the time for contact can be increased, humidity also will be increased. Slowing the flow of gas may not be desired since many clinical applications require high flows, in excess of 50 liters per minute.

CLINICAL APPLICATIONS OF HUMIDITY THERAPY

The American Association for Respiratory Care Clinical Practice Guideline: Humidification during Mechanical Ventilation is included in Figure 3-2.

When an artificial airway is placed, by-passing the upper airway, humidification is necessary to prevent hypothermia, inspissation of airway secretions, destruction of airway epithelium, and atelectasis (due to mucous plugging). A heated humidifier or a heat and moisture exchanger (HME) can be used to help prevent these problems. The humidifier should provide a minimum of 30 mg H_2O/L of delivered gas at 30°C. When using a heated humidifier, appropriate monitoring should include temperature probe(s) at the humidifier and the airway to monitor heat output so as not to damage the airway epithelium.

Humidity may also be used when administering low-flow oxygen therapy. Medical gases are anhydrous and contain no water vapor. By using simple bubble humidifiers, water vapor is added to the inspired gas, reducing the humidity deficit. Often, use of bubble humidifiers is determined by patient comfort.

Humidity is also applied when delivering oxygen to neonates in a hood or isolette. A newborn's hypothalamus is not fully developed and thus is unable to adequately regulate his body temperature. Therefore, warm humidified gas is delivered to assist in adequate thermal regulation of the neonate's temperature. A thermometer or thermister probe (servo-controlled humidifier) should be placed proximal to the patient to ensure that excessive heat is not being administered to the patient.

HUMIDIFIERS

Room Humidifier

Contemporary room humidifiers employed in clinical practice are, in reality, aerosol generators. The majority of these devices operate using centrifugal force. The aerosol exiting the device evaporates in the ambient air, increasing the humidity of the room.

Centrifugal force is applied using a spinning disk (Figure 3-3). As an electric motor spins the disk, water is drawn up through the hollow shaft by capillary action. When the water encounters the spinning disk, it is thrown outward by centrifugal force. The breaker combs surrounding the spinning disk shatter the water particles, producing an aerosol. The evaporating aerosol causes the humidity of the room to increase.

Large amounts of air pass through this type of humidifier, making it a potential

AARC CLINICAL PRACTICE GUIDELINE
Humidification during Mechanical Ventilation

HMV 1.0 PROCEDURE:
The addition of heat and moisture to inspired gases delivered to the patient during mechanical ventilatory support via an artificial airway

HMV 2.0 DESCRIPTION/DEFINITION:
When the upper airway is bypassed, humidification during mechanical ventilation is necessary to prevent hypothermia, inspissation of airway secretions, destruction of airway epithelium, and atelectasis. This may be accomplished using either a heated humidifier or a heat and moisture exchanger (HME). (HMEs are also known as hygroscopic condenser humidifiers, or artificial noses). The chosen device should provide a minimum of 30 mg H_2O/L of delivered gas at 30°C. Heated humidifiers operate actively to increase the heat and water vapor content of inspired gas. HMEs operate passively by storing heat and moisture from the patient's exhaled gas and releasing it to the inhaled gas.

HMV 3.0 SETTINGS:
3.1 Critical care
3.2 Acute care inpatient
3.3 Extended care and skilled nursing facility
3.4 Home care
3.5 Prolonged transport

HMV 4.0 INDICATIONS:
Humidification of inspired gas during mechanical ventilation is mandatory when an endotracheal or tracheostomy tube is present.

HMV 5.0 CONTRAINDICATIONS:
There are no contraindications to providing physiologic conditioning of inspired gas during mechanical ventilation. An HME is contraindicated under some circumstances.
5.1 Use of an HME is contraindicated for patients with thick, copious, or bloody secretions.
5.2 Use of an HME is contraindicated for patients with an expired tidal volume less than 70% of the delivered tidal volume (eg, those with large bronchopleurocutaneous fistulas or incompetent or absent endotracheal tube cuffs).
5.3 Use of an HME is contraindicated for patients with body temperatures less than 32°C.

5.4 Use of an HME may be contraindicated for patients with high spontaneous minute volumes (> 10L/min).
5.5 An HME must be removed from the patient circuit during aerosol treatments when the nebulizer is placed in the patient circuit.

HMV 6.0 HAZARDS/COMPLICATIONS:
Hazards and complications associated with the use of humidification devices include
6.1 potential for electrical shock—heated humidifiers;
6.2 hypothermia—HME or heated humidifiers; hyperthermia—heated humidifiers;
6.3 thermal injury to the airway from heated humidifiers; burns to the patient and tubing meltdown if heated-wire circuits are covered or circuits and humidifiers are incompatible;
6.4 underhydration and impaction of mucus secretions—HME or heated humidifiers;
6.5 hypoventilation and/or alveolar gas trapping due to mucus plugging of airways—HME or heated humidifier;
6.6 possible increased resistive work of breathing due to mucus plugging of airways—HME or heated humidifiers;
6.7 possible increased resistive work of breathing through the humidifier—HME or heated humidifiers;
6.8 possible hypoventilation due to increased dead space—HME;
6.9 inadvertent overfilling resulting in unintentional tracheal lavage—heated reservoir humidifiers;
6.10 the tact that when disconnected from the patient, some ventilators generate a high flow through the patient circuit that may aerosolize contaminated condensate, putting both the patient and clinician at risk for nosocomial infection—heated humidifiers;
6.11 potential for burns to caregivers from hot metal—heated humidifiers;
6.12 inadvertent tracheal lavage from pooled condensate in patient circuit—heated humidifiers;
6.13 elevated airway pressures due to pooled condensation—heated humidifiers;
6.14 patient-ventilator dysynchrony and improper ventilator performance due to

Figure 3-2 *AARC Clinical Practice Guideline: Humidification During Mechanical Ventilation. (Courtesy American Association of Respiratory Care, Irving, TX)* **(continues)**

pooled condensation in the circuit—heated humidifiers;

6.15 ineffective low-pressure alarm during disconnection due to resistance through HME.

HMV 7.0 LIMITATIONS OF METHODS:

7.1 Insufficient heat and humidification can occur with some HME devices, resulting in complications noted in HMV 6.0.

7.2 Insufficient heat and humidification can occur with heated humidifiers and result in complications noted in HMV 6.0 when

7.2.1 improper temperature settings are selected.

7.2.2 water level in the humidifier falls below manufacturer's suggested level.

7.3 The HME selected should be appropriate to the patient's size and tidal volume.

HMV 8.0 ASSESSMENT OF NEED:

Humidification is needed by all patients requiring mechanical ventilation via an artificial airway. Conditioning of inspired gases should be instituted using either an HME or a heated humidifier.

8.1 HMEs are better suited for short-term use (< or = 96 hours) and during transport.

8.2 Heated humidifiers should be used for patients requiring longterm mechanical ventilation (> 96 hours) or for patients who exhibit contraindications for HME use.

HMV 9.0 ASSESSMENT OF OUTCOME:

Humidification is assumed to be appropriate if, on regular careful inspection, the patient exhibits none of the hazards or complications listed in HMV 6.0.

HMV 10.0 RESOURCES:

10.1 Equipment: Appropriate equipment should be available to provide for adequate humidification of the inspired gas. Such equipment may include but is not limited to

10.1.1 humidification device;

10.1.2 a system to monitor inspired gas temperature and to alarm when the temperature falls outside a preset range (for heated humidifier);

10.1.3 sterile water for heated humidifiers;

10.1.4 equipment necessary to comply with Universal Precautions.

10.2 Humidifier performance specifications should be checked to assure adequate heating and humidification during expected peak inspiratory flowrate and minute ventilation delivered by the mechanical ventilator. Heated humidifiers selected for use should meet specifications of the American National Standards Institute.

10.3 Personnel:

10.3.1 Level-I personnel should possess

10.3.1.1 a complete understanding of the operation, maintenance, and troubleshooting of the ventilator, circuit, and humidifying device;

10.3.1.2 knowledge of and ability to implement Universal Precautions.

10.3.2 Level-II personnel should possess the abilities described in 10.3.1.1 and 10.3.1.2 and should also have

10.3.2.1 the ability to assess patient response to humidification;

10.3.2.2 the ability to recognize an adverse response to humidification;

10.3.2.3 the ability to appropriately respond to adverse events;

10.3.2.4 the ability to recommend modifications in humidification techniques as

HMV 11.0 MONITORING:

The humidification device should be inspected visually during the patient-ventilator system check and condensate should be removed from the patient circuit as necessary. HMEs should be inspected and replaced if secretions have contaminated the insert or filter. The following variables should be recorded during equipment inspection:

11.1 Humidifier setting (temperature setting or numeric dial setting or both). During routine use on an intubated patient, a heated humidifier should be set to deliver an inspired gas temperature of 33 ± 2°C and should provide a minimum of 30 mg/L of water vapor.

11.2 Inspired gas temperature. Temperature should be monitored as near the patient's airway opening as possible, if a heated humidifier is used.

11.2.1 Specific temperatures may vary with patient condition, but the inspiratory gas should not exceed 37°C at the airway threshold.

11.2.2 When a heated-wire patient circuit is used (to prevent condensation) on an infant, the temperature probe should be located outside of the incubator or away from the direct heat of the radiant warmer.

11.3 Alarm settings (if applicable). High temperature alarm should be set no higher than 37°C, and the low temperature alarm should be set no lower than 30°C.

Figure 3-2 *(continues)*

11.4 Water level and function of automatic feed system (if applicable).

11.5 Quantity and consistency of secretions. Characteristics should be noted and recorded. When using an HME, if secretions become copious or appear increasingly tenacious, a heated humidifier should replace the HME.

HMV 12.0 FREQUENCY:

All patients with an artificial airway requiring mechanical ventilation should receive continuous humidification of inspired gases.

HMV 13.0 INFECTION CONTROL:

13.1 Reusable heated humidifiers should be subjected to high-level disinfection between patients. Clean technique should be observed when manually filling the water reservoir. Sterile water should be used.

13.2 When using a closed, automatic feed system, the unused portion of water in the water feed reservoir remains sterile and need not be discarded when the patient circuit is changed. However, the water feed system should be designated for single patient use only.

13.3 Condensation from the patient circuit should be considered infectious waste and disposed of according to hospital policy using strict Universal Precautions.

13.4 Because condensate is infectious waste, it should never be drained back into the humidifier reservoir.

_____

Reprinted with permission from *Respiratory Care* 1992; 37: 887–890. The complete AARC Clinical Practice Guidelines are available from the AARC Web site (*http://www.aarc.org*), from the AARC Executive Office, or from *Respiratory Care* journal.

Figure 3-2 *(continued)*

Figure 3-3 *A photograph and a functional diagram of a centrifugal room humidifier.*

source of nosocomial infections. The large water reservoir is also a source for bacterial growth or contamination. When these devices are used, it is important to keep them clean and change the water in the reservoir frequently.

ASSEMBLY AND TROUBLESHOOTING

Assembly—Room Humidifiers

Room humidifiers are quite simple and have few moving parts. The following is a suggested assembly guide.

1. Remove the motor housing from the humidifier and fill the reservoir with water to the correct level indicated on the side of the unit.

2. Replace the motor housing with the hollow shaft immersed in the water reservoir.

3. Connect the power cord to a suitable 110-volt outlet and turn on the humidifier.

4. Observe for aerosol output.

Troubleshooting

Since these humidifiers are simple in their operation, troubleshooting them is quite easy. However, if the unit fails to operate, little can be done by the respiratory care practitioner to correct malfunctions. When troubleshooting this equipment, please follow the suggested troubleshooting algorithm (ALG 3-1).

1. If the humidifier fails to produce adequate aerosol and the motor functions properly:
   a. First, disconnect the power.
   b. Check the outlet for obstructions.
   c. Be certain the reservoir is filled properly.
   d. Check the breaker combs for integrity. If the breaker combs are broken or absent, replace the unit or take it to an authorized repair center.

2. If the motor fails to operate:
   a. Check the integrity of the electrical outlet by using another electrical device to test it.
   b. If the electrical outlet is good and the motor still fails to operate, replace the unit or take it to an authorized repair center.

3. Clean the humidifier daily and change the water at least twice each day.

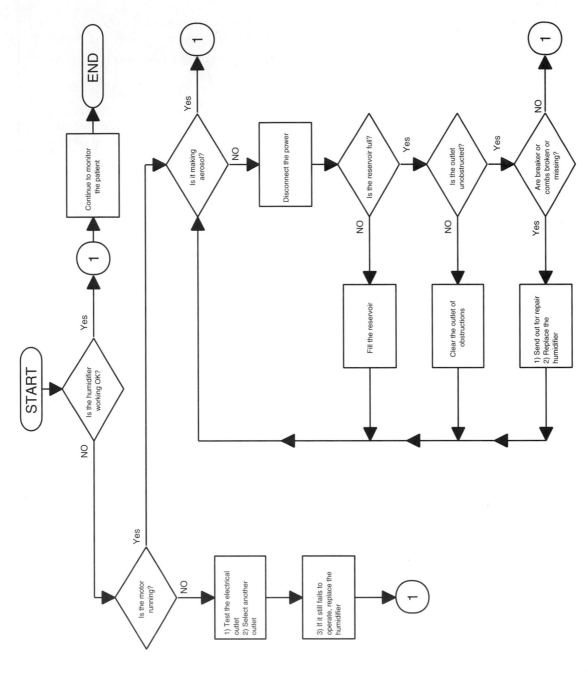

ALG 3-1 *An algorithm describing how to troubleshoot a centrifugal room humidifier.*

Pass-Over Humidifier

The pass-over humidifier is the simplest of all the humidifiers. Gas flow passes over a reservoir of water. Water evaporates into the gas, increasing the humidity of the gas. Efficiency of these humidifiers can be increased by heating the water, thereby increasing the rate of evaporation. Figure 3-4 shows this type of humidifier, which is used in the Emerson 3-PV adult ventilator.

Bubble Humidifier

The majority of the disposable humidifiers used for oxygen therapy are bubble humidifiers. Efficiency and output vary, depending on many factors. These factors include liter flow through the humidifier, ambient temperature, and time of operation. The output of these devices may vary from 33% to 40% relative humidity at 37° Celsius.

These humidifiers operate by bubbling gas up through a reservoir of water (Figure 3-5). Gas enters the humidifier through the DISS fitting on the top of the unit. Gas flows down through a hollow tube to a diffusing element. The diffuser breaks the gas flow up into small bubbles. As the gas bubbles float to the surface, the water evaporates into them. The efficiency of these humidifiers is improved by the diffuser, which increases surface area and the

Figure 3-4   *A pass-over humidifier used in the Emerson 3-PV ventilator.*

time the gas is allowed to interface with the water.

A safety relief valve is incorporated into the upper housing of the humidifier to relieve pressure in the event the gas path becomes obstructed. Most of these relief valves operate at 2 psi. Many manufacturers incorporate an audible whistle alarm to alert practitioners when the relief is activated.

Figure 3-5   *A photograph and a functional diagram of a bubble humidifier.*

ASSEMBLY AND TROUBLESHOOTING

Assembly—Bubble Humidifiers

Bubble humidifiers are the most common humidifiers utilized in respiratory care. There are numerous models and manufacturers producing these devices. Disposable humidifiers are available, both prefilled with sterile water and unfilled. Construction of these humidifiers varies, as does their assembly. Follow the manufacturer's instructions when assembling these units for clinical use. The following assembly guide will apply to the majority of the humidifiers in use today.

1. Disposable humidifiers are packaged aseptically in a plastic wrap. Open the package and remove the parts, maintaining aseptic technique.

2. Most humidifiers come in two parts (see Figure 3-6). The top portion consists of the DISS oxygen fitting, pressure relief, and oxygen nipple outlet. The bottom part is the water reservoir.

Prefilled:

   a. Attach the top portion to the bottom following the manufacturer's recommendations.
   b. When the parts are attached, gently squeeze the sides of the reservoir, listening for gas escaping through the outlet. By doing this you can be assured that the reservoir has been properly pierced by the top part of the humidifier.
   c. Attach the humidifier to the DISS fitting on a flowmeter.
   d. Attach the oxygen therapy equipment to the outlet of the humidifier.
   e. Adjust the flowmeter to the desired oxygen flow rate.
   f. Check for oxygen flow and bubbles in the reservoir.

   g. Check the safety relief valve by obstructing the oxygen connecting tube. Pinch it or aseptically obstruct the humidifier outlet.

Non-prefilled:

   a. Aseptically fill the reservoir to the indicated level, using sterile distilled water.
   b. Attach the top portion to the reservoir, following the manufacturer's instructions.
   c. Attach the humidifier to the DISS fitting on a flowmeter.
   d. Attach the oxygen therapy equipment to the nipple outlet of the humidifier.
   e. Adjust the flowmeter to the desired oxygen flow rate.
   f. Check the safety relief valve by obstructing the oxygen connecting tube. Pinch it or aseptically obstruct the humidifier outlet.

Troubleshooting

When troubleshooting this equipment, please follow the suggested troubleshooting algorithm (ALG 3-2). If oxygen fails to flow from the humidifier:

1. Check to ensure that the flowmeter is turned on.

2. If the humidifier is prefilled, ensure that the reservoir has been pierced and that gas can flow through it.

3. Check the outlet for obstructions.

4. Check the oxygen containing tubing for obstructions or kinks.

5. If (1) through (4) are satisfactory, replace the humidifier.

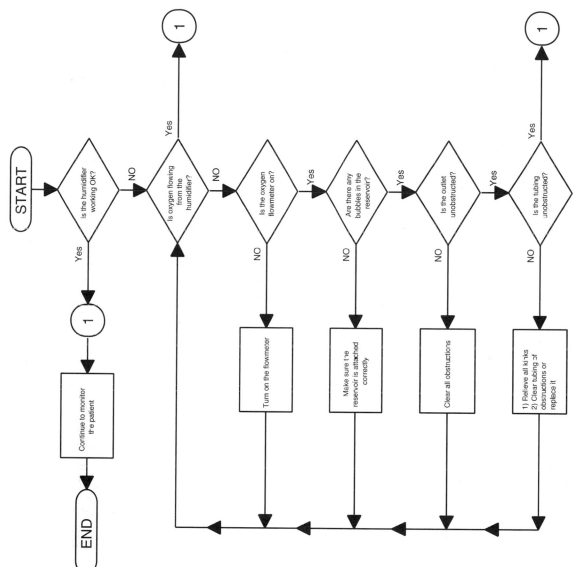

ALG 3-2 *An algorithm describing how to troubleshoot a bubble humidifier.*

Misty Ox Laminar Diffuser Humidifier

Vital Signs is marketing and distributing a disposable humidifier which incorporates some unique features. This humidifier is unique in that aerosol produced by a high output nebulizer is evaporated into the gas flowing through the device, producing high humidity outputs at high flow rates. When combined with the TurboHeater, the Laminar

Diffuser Humidifier (LDH) is capable of producing heated molecular high humidity (HMHH) at flows of up to 80 L/min.

The design of the humidifier incorporates the Misty Ox Gas Injection Nebulizer (GIN) head (discussed later in this chapter) to produce a dense aerosol at high flow rates. The aerosol output from the nebulizer is directed downward into two perforated disks (Figure 3-6), which form an evaporation chamber. The perforated disks increase the turbulence of the gas/aerosol mixture flowing through them, while the large surface areas presented by the square-shaped perforations in the disks cause the suspended aerosol to deposit onto the disks, forming a thin film of water. Turbulent gas flowing through the disks, and the chamber created between them, evaporates the thin film of water, increasing the relative humidity of the gas. Gas flow is directed down through a converging duct into a conical-shaped mixing chamber. The shape of this chamber causes the gas to flow through it in a swirling pattern. Positioned along the outer wall of this mixing chamber are radially spaced baffles. The baffles further remove aerosol particles from the flowing gas by inertial impaction. The gas is then discharged through a short piece of tubing into the accumulator chamber where the gas comes into contact with the heater platen

Figure 3-6 *A functional diagram (left) and a detailed diagram (right) of the Vital Signs, Inc. Misty Ox Laminar Diffuser Humidifier (LDH).*

ASSEMBLY AND TROUBLESHOOTING

Assembly—Misty Ox LDH Humidifier

1. Remove the cap from the sterile distilled water bottle you wish to use as a reservoir.

2. Aseptically remove the Laminar Diffuser Humidifier (LDH) from its package. Use caution not to contaminate the long capillary tube that will be immersed into the sterile reservoir.

3. Insert the capillary tube into the bottle and screw the nebulizer into place using the 38-mm threaded fitting. Make sure that the nebulizer is on tight and is not cross threaded.

4. Connect the primary gas source (DISS fitting on the top of the LDH) to a flowmeter (air or oxygen) or an oxygen blender. Be certain that you have screwed the DISS fittings together tightly to preserve flow to the patient.

   a. If oxygen and air flowmeters are used for the primary and secondary gas sources, high-range flowmeters (0–74 L/min) are recommended.

   b. In lieu of a high-range flowmeter, a standard 0–15 L/min flowmeter may be substituted for the primary gas source. When adjusting the flow, open the needle valve to its maximum open position (beyond flush). When opened this far, most standard flowmeters will deliver between 60–90 L/min. The nozzle in the GIN nebulizer head will limit flow through it to 40 L/min.

5. Attach large-bore (22 mm) aerosol tubing to the outlet of the LDH. Use of a drainage bag is recommended due to the high water vapor output of this humidifier.

6. Connect the desired delivery device to the aerosol tubing.

7. Adjust the flowmeters to the desired setting (Table 3-5 and Table 3-6, p. 157), or adjust the blender to the desired F_IO_2. Set the flow to maintain adequate flows to meet the patient's inspiratory demands.

8. Check the F_IO_2 level using a calibrated oxygen analyzer.

9. If using the TurboHeater, place an in-line thermometer near the patient to monitor the temperature of the delivered gas.

10. Replace the solution reservoir when the fluid level is ¼ inch from the bottom of the container.

Troubleshooting

When troubleshooting this equipment, please follow the suggested troubleshooting algorithm (ALG 3-3).

No flow from the humidifier:

1. Check to ensure that there is an adequate oxygen supply when using cylinders.

2. Verify that the flowmeter is correctly connected to the 50-psi oxygen or air source.

3. Check the connection between the humidifier and the flowmeter.

   a. Make sure it is securely attached.

   b. Check for any obstruction where the nebulizer attaches to the flowmeter.

   c. Verify that the secondary gas inlet tube is free of obstruction or kinks.

Little or no humidity output:

1. Check to ensure that the reservoir bottle contains fluid.

2. Check the capillary tube to ensure it is immersed into the solution in the reservoir bottle.

3. Check the capillary tube for obstructions.

4. Check the large bore aerosol delivery tubing for kinks or obstructions.

5. If using a standard flowmeter (0–15 L/min), verify that the needle valve has been opened to its maximum setting (beyond flush).

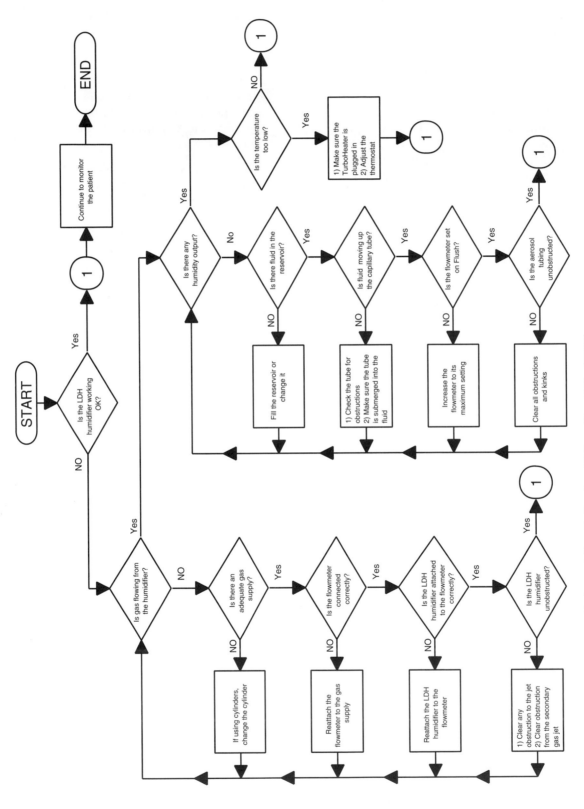

ALG 3-3 *An algorithm describing how to troubleshoot a Misty Ox Laminar Diffuser Humidifier (LDH).*

of the TurboHeater. Increased pressure in the center of the humidifier and gravity cause the aerosol particles, which coalesce following removal from suspension, to flow down through the precipitate chamber (center of the humidifier) and to drain radially outward onto the heater platen. The hot platen causes the water to be vaporized, further increasing the relative humidity of the gas while also warming it. The heated, humidified gas flows radially through the accumulator chamber to the outlet where it then flows to the patient. It is important to note that the output from the humidifier is molecular water, or water vapor, which contains very few suspended aerosol particles.

The Gas Injection Nebulizer (GIN) head also provides greater flexibility in delivery of variable F_IO_2 levels and flow rates using a closed system. The nebulizer may be powered by oxygen or air (primary gas), while the injected gas (air or oxygen) provides additional flow. To determine the desired F_IO_2 and flow rates refer to Table 3-4 and Table 3-5 later in this chapter (pp. 153 and 157). The LDH humidifier, being a closed system, gives this humidifier further flexibility in that it may be used for positive pressure applications, such as CPAP, since oxygen dilution is not accomplished using jet mixing or air entrainment.

Cascade and Cascade II Humidifiers

The Puritan Bennett Cascade and Cascade II humidifiers are very efficient diffuser type humidifiers, capable of producing body humidity (BTPS) even with high flows of gas. This makes this humidifier suitable for adult mechanical ventilation or other high flow applications.

The efficiency of the Cascade humidifiers is accomplished by increasing surface area and incorporating a heating element. The Cascade II can deliver 100% relative humidity at body temperature at minute volumes of up to 10 liters per minute. Gas entering the humidifier is directed down through the tower and passes through a one-way valve below the diffusion grid (Figure 3-7). The one-way valve prevents the gas from flowing back up the tower into the equipment attached to it. The bolus of gas entering below the diffusion grid causes the water to be displaced, increasing the water level and allowing some water to enter the diffusion grid. Water then enters a

Figure 3-7 *A functional diagram of a Cascade humidifier.*

port above the grid, forming a thin sheet. The gas forms a froth, which creates a large air-water surface area.

A small port located above the water level on the tower acts as a sensing port. Pressure changes created by the patient's inspiratory efforts can be conveyed to the equipment attached. Without the sensing port, the patient would need to generate a force equal to the depth of water in the reservoir.

A heating element increases the temperature of the reservoir, thereby increasing the rate of evaporation. The electrical heating element is not in direct contact with the water in the reservoir. Rather it is inserted into a well, which is a part of the reservoir assembly in contact with the water. A switch located on the heater assembly must close by contacting a raised part of the jar lid casting located in the depression. The switch closes when the jar assembly is attached to the heater. Failure to assemble the unit correctly will result in the heater not operating.

The Cascade II is similar to the Cascade humidifier except that it incorporates a servo-controller that controls the temperature. The respiratory care practitioner adjusts the desired temperature level with the temperature control knob. A proximal sensor is placed near the patient's airway to measure the temperature there. Its signal is sent to the heater, which adjusts the output to maintain the temperature level established by the practitioner. This function is an example of servo feedback control.

ASSEMBLY AND TROUBLESHOOTING

Assembly—Cascade Humidifier

1. Be certain that the two red "O" rings are in place on the well where it attaches to the lid. Attach the heater well to the lid of the Cascade using the two small screws.

2. Attach the tower to the lid by inserting the top of the tower into the inlet on the lid. Secure it to the lid using the plastic stud. Verify that the one-way valve is installed correctly at this time.

3. Check to be sure the large "O" ring is in place on the lid where it attaches to the reservoir jar.

4. Aseptically fill the reservoir with sterile distilled water.

5. Screw the lid to the reservoir jar.

6. Attach the Cascade to its heater using the two twist tabs on the top surface of the lid.

7. Attach large-bore aerosol tubing to the inlet and outlet of the humidifier.

Troubleshooting

When troubleshooting this equipment, please follow the suggested troubleshooting algorithm (ALG 3-4).

If the Cascade fails to generate adequate foam or bubbles:

1. Check the water level in the reservoir.

2. Check to ensure that the tower is attached properly.

3. Check the tower for the one-way valve.

4. Check the inlet and outlet for obstruction to gas flow.

Leaks may be a problem when troubleshooting these humidifiers. Common sources include:

1. The large "O" ring in the lid.

2. The red "O" rings on the heater well. Presence of water in the lid's depression will alert you to a leak in this area.

3. Failure to tighten the lid sufficiently or cross threading the lid.

If the Cascade fails to heat properly:

1. Tighten the studs holding the locking tabs on top of the lid by gently tapping them farther down into their seats. If these become loose, the lid may fail to activate a switch on the bottom of the heater assembly. Lift up on the reservoir and listen for the faint "click" of the switch closing.

2. If the switch is closed and the heater still fails to operate, replace the heater and take the potentially bad one to an authorized biomedical repair facility.

3. Check to see if a circuit breaker has tripped, and reset it if required.

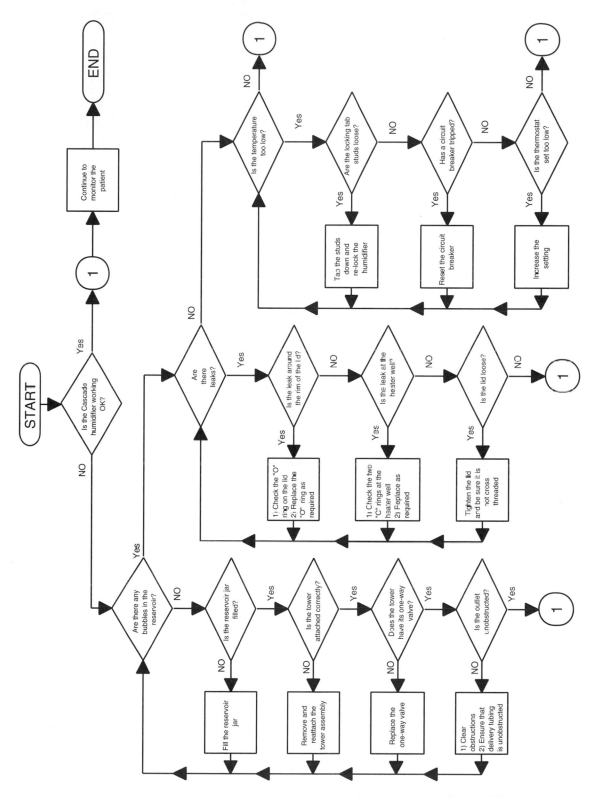

ALG 3-4 *An algorithm describing how to troubleshoot a Cascade humidifier.*

Hudson RCI ConchaTherm®
IV Humidifier

The Hudson RCI ConchaTherm® IV humidifier is a microprocessor-controlled, wick-type humidifier that incorporates provisions for a heated wire circuit (Figure 3-8). The ConchaTherm® IV humidifier incorporates the same Concha-Column and feeds system employed on the earlier Conchapack and Conchatherm III designs, in which the wick assembly increases the surface area, thus improving output and performance. The wick assemblies are disposable and may be changed as frequently as required to maintain adequate asepsis.

The wick assembly consists of the wick, heating element, gas inlet and outlet, and water feed system fittings. Gas flowing into the unit flows down past the wick. The heating element surrounds the wick and increases the rate of evaporation.

The wick assembly mates to the Concha-Therm® IV heater control assembly. The heater/control assembly servo controls the airway temperature, servo controls the heated wire circuit, and provides alarm functions to alert the clinician of potentially dangerous

Figure 3-8 *The Conchatherm IV made by Hudson RCI, Inc.*

events. The alarms incorporated into the ConchaTherm® IV humidifier are summarized in Table 3-3.

ASSEMBLY AND TROUBLESHOOTING

Assembly—Hudson RCI ConchaTherm® IV Humidifier

1. Mate a wick Concha-Column to the heater/control assembly by slipping it in from the top, ensuring that the plastic clamps on the feed tubes are closed.

2. Attach the disposable reservoir to the side of the heater assembly.

3. Connect the feed lines to the top and bottom positions on the reservoir by piercing them using a twisting motion. Open the clamps on the feed lines.

4. Attach the power cord to a suitable AC power source.

5. Connect the proximal airway probe to the patient circuit and, if you are using a heated wire circuit, connect the heated wire cables to the appropriate cables on the humidifier.

6. Select the correct mode (infant/adult), set the airway temperature, and set the column-to-patient temperature gradient.

Troubleshooting

1. Feed system problems:
   a. Check the water level in the reservoir.
   b. Check for correct installation of the feed probes into the water reservoir.
   c. Check to be sure the clamps are in the open position.

2. Probe/Heated wire problems:
   a. Check connections at the humidifier and patient circuit.
   b. Check for breaks or faults in the cables and wires.

TABLE 3-3 Hudson RCI ConchaTherm®
IV Alarms

Emergency Alarms (Red)

    High temperature

    Check probe

    Bad probe

    Adult

    Inspiratory wire and disconnect

    Service

Cautionary Alarms (Yellow)

    Adult/Infant

    Low temperature

    Expiratory wire and disconnect

Figure 3-9 *The Fisher and Paykel MR 730 humidifier.*

Fisher and Paykel Healthcare MR 730 Humidifier

The Fisher and Paykel MR 730 humidifier is a servo-controlled wick humidifier (Figure 3-9). This humidifier is capable of delivering heated humidified gas between 29° and 40° Celsius. These humidifiers may be used with heated wire circuits, which reduce condensate due to a more constant temperature distribution from the humidifier to the patient through the circuit.

Disposable and reusable chambers are available which slide into and lock into the computer controlled heater assembly. The

---

ASSEMBLY AND TROUBLESHOOTING

Assembly—Fisher and Paykel

1. Slide the module onto the heater and lock into place with the locking tab.

2. Attach the water feed tubing from a disposable fill set to the center pole on the module.

3. Attach appropriate large-bore aerosol tubing to the inlet and outlet of the humidifier. Alternatively, a heated wire circuit may be used, in which case the appropriate electrical connections must be made at the servo controller, the chamber, and proximal to the patient's airway.

4. Place the proximal airway probe near the patient's airway.

5. Initiate gas flow through the unit, and adjust the temperature control to the desired temperature.

Troubleshooting

Troubleshooting primarily relates to breaks occurring in the cable from the temperature probe. Periodically these require replacement. Leaks are not a problem since it is a sealed unit.

chamber assemblies consist of the inlet, outlet, wick, and heating platen.

Alarms include high and low chamber temperature, high and low airway temperature, probe disconnection and or heater wire disconnection, and microprocessor failure.

Bear VH-820 Humidifier

The Bear VH-820 humidifier is another example of a heated wick humidifier. This humidifier may be used for both infants and adults.

Gas entering the center of the humidifier passes by the heater rod (Figure 3-10). The gas is then channeled through a spiral-shaped chamber that contains the wick. The spiral shape ensures a large surface area and a longer time for gas to interface with water.

The humidifier is servo controlled with three temperature probe positions: proximal airway, heater rod, and humidifier outlet. All three temperatures are monitored, and the operation of the humidifier is regulated by a microprocessor.

The feed system is automatic and operates by a sensing system controlling a pinch valve. When the water level drops about 1 milliliter,

Figure 3-10 *A functional diagram of the Bear VH-820 humidifier.*

the valve opens, admitting water to the humidity chamber. Gravity causes the water to flow from a reservoir bag (bottle) to the chamber. The volume within the chamber varies between 5 and 10 milliliters.

ASSEMBLY AND TROUBLESHOOTING

Refer to Figure 3-11 when following the assembly procedure.

Assembly—Bear VH-820

1. Attach the "O" ring to the chamber jar by seating it into the groove provided.

2. Mate the cover assembly and the jar together by twisting them. The outlet should be on the same side as the water feed port.

3. Insert the heater into the jar, ensuring that the heater is perpendicular to the feed tubing.

4. Insert the humidification chamber into the heater/control chamber.

5. Insert the water feed tubing into the pinch valve assembly.

6. Attach large-bore aerosol tubing to the inlet and outlet fittings.

7. Plug in the proximal airway probe and place it near the patient's airway.

Troubleshooting

Troubleshooting this humidifier relates primarily to alarm conditions and problems with the temperature probe cable.

CHAMBER TOP

O-RING

CHAMBER BASE

WATER INLET
TUBING

PINCH VALVE
ASSEMBLY

HEATER/CONTROL
CHAMBER

HUMIDIFIER

Figure 3-11 *An assembly drawing of the Bear VH-820 humidifier.*

DHD Healthcare Thera-Mist P35000 Humidifier

The Thera-Mist P35000 is a wick type heated humidifier (Figure 3-12). It is capable of producing body humidity up to minute volumes of 20 L/min. The design is unique, in that neither the water or gas stream comes into contact with the heater element. (Figure 3-12).

By keeping both the inhaled gas and water in isolation from the heating element, cross contamination and routine sterilization are eliminated.

The Thera-Mist P35000 consists of an adjustable heater, wick humidifier and heating platen, and a water reservoir bottle. The heater is adjustable via a knob that can be rotated to increase the heater's output. Temperature varies depending upon gas flow through the circuit. As gas flow increases, the temperature delivered decreases. The use of a temperature probe proximal to the patient's airway is important in patient monitoring.

Figure 3-12 *A photograph of the DHD Healthcare Thera-Mist P35000 humidifier.*

The humidifier's wick passes through the heater and into the reservoir bottle below it. Water is transported to the humidifier's platen via capillary action. The humidifier/platen assembly attaches to the heater via a threaded base assembly. This assembly is totally isolated from the heater because it is a separate sealed unit. This minimizes the potential for cross contamination by direct contact.

The reservoir bottle has a standardized 38-mm diameter top. This top facilitates the use of the majority of prefilled sterile solution bottles. The reservoir mates to the heater base via the 38-mm threaded top. Once the Thera-Mist system is assembled, it is important to squeeze the reservoir bottle or invert the system to prime the wick and transport at least 30 mL of water to the humidifier/platen surface. This priming action will assure that the wick will continue to transport water to the heater unit.

The system remains connected in the ventilator circuit and is only changed when the ventilator circuit is changed. Additional water reservoirs may be added at any time without breaking the patient/ventilator circuit when needed.

ASSEMBLY AND TROUBLESHOOTING

Assembly—Thera-Mist P35000 Humidifier

1. Visually inspect the heater to ascertain whether it is clean and the power cord and plug are intact and free of any visible wear.

2. Turn the heater "OFF."

3. Turn the heater thermostat control fully counterclockwise.

4. Attach a humidifier top by screwing it firmly into the top of the Thera-Mist P3500 heater by turning it clockwise.

5. Attach a water reservoir by screwing it onto the threads beneath the heater assembly.

6. Thoroughly wet the wick in the humidifier top by briefly inverting the assembly to wet the wick and then by squeezing the bottle slightly to force water into the upper chamber.

7. Turn the power switch "ON" and adjust the temperature to the desired range (verify the temperature using an inline thermometer proximal to the patient's connection).

8. Attach large-bore aerosol tubing to the inlet and outlet of the humidifier. Make certain that a thermometer is placed proximal to the patient to monitor the temperature output of the heater.

9. Connect the outlet tubing to the patient using an appropriate interface.

Troubleshooting

Troubleshooting primarily consists of ensuring that the tubing is free from obstruction due to condensation and verifying that the water reservoir is adequately filled. Malfunction of the heater can be assessed by verifying electrical connections and ensuring that the switch light is illuminated, indicating its proper operation.

Heat and Moisture Exchangers (Artificial Nose)

Heat and moisture exchangers are simple devices whose function can replace that of a humidifier. The **heat and moisture exchanger** consists of a honeycomblike-tubular structure made of aluminum or hygroscipic materials (Figure 3-13).

Moisture and heat from the patient's exhaled gas is absorbed into the tubular structure of the exchanger. The inspired gas is warmed and humidified by evaporation as it passes through the exchanger. The efficiency of these devices varies between manufacturers from 70% to 90 % relative humidity between 30° and 31° Celsius.

The heat and moisture exchanger should be placed between the patient's artificial airway and the ventilator circuit or oxygen therapy equipment. Minimizing resistance, dead space, and compliance are critical factors in a

Figure 3-13 *A photograph and a functional diagram of a heat and moisture exchanger (HME).*

good design. Should these devices become obstructed with mucous, resistance can increase dramatically.

The placement and adjustment of external pressure disconnect alarms is also important for patient safety. The alarm should be set near the peak airway pressure and, if the sensor placement can be moved, it should be between the patient's airway and the moisture exchanger. This is due to the increased resist-ance that a moisture exchanger may develop, even if disconnected from the patient.

These devices are effective for short-term usage (less than 96 hours). For long-term use, a humidifier is recommended. Bronchial cast formation due to secretion retention from long-term use has been reported. This is caused by the comparatively low relative humidity and the fact that artificial airways bypass the upper airway.

ASSEMBLY AND TROUBLESHOOTING

Assembly—HME

1. Aseptically open the package containing the heat and moisture exchanger.

2. Using the adapters provided, match the 15 mm artificial airway connection on the patient side of the exchanger and the ventilator tubing or oxygen therapy equipment on the other.

3. Place the heat and moisture exchanger on the airway and attach the circuit to the other side.

4. If required, provide additional support to the artificial airway to prevent the weight of the heat and moisture exchanger from producing adverse traction on the airway.

5. Carefully monitor peak pressures (if mechanically ventilating the patient) before and after installation. If the patient is spontaneously ventilating, monitor respiratory effort and minute ventilation for adverse changes.

Troubleshooting

Troubleshooting primarily consists of monitoring the device for obstruction. Signs of obstruction would include increased peak airway pressures and increased work of breathing.

The heat and moisture exchanger should be replaced at the intervals recommended by the manufacturer. By replacing the device, problems with obstruction and bacterial contamination can be minimized.

CLINICAL APPLICATIONS OF AEROSOL THERAPY

INDICATIONS FOR AEROSOL THERAPY

The administration of aerosols include the use of bland agents (sterile water, hypotonic, isotonic, or hypertonic saline), various classifications of drugs (beta adrenergics, anticholinergics, anti-inflammatory agents, etc.), antimicrobial agents, surfactants, and enzymes. The American Association for Respiratory Care has published several Clinical Practice Guidelines specific to the administration of aerosol therapy (Figures 3–14 through 3-17). The clinical practice guidelines focus on the delivery of bland aerosols, delivery of aerosols to the upper airway, and delivery of aerosols to the lung parenchyma.

Bland aerosol therapy is indicated to treat airway edema, provide heated aerosol in the presence of a bypassed upper airway, and aid in sputum induction or mobilization. Cool aerosols are indicated to reduce airway edema. The upper airway is the region most often treated by the use of cool aerosols. The cool aerosol can result in vasoconstriction, reducing airway edema. Common situations in which cool aerosol is utilized include post-extubation, post-operative management of the upper airway, subglottic edema, and laryngotracheobronchitis.

Heated bland aerosol is indicated if the aerosol is applied to an artificial airway that bypasses the upper airway. The function of the upper airway is to warm, filter, and humidify inspired gas. Heated aerosol helps to make up for the temperature and humidity deficit resulting from the bypassed upper airway.

Delivery of medications to the upper and lower airway for systemic absorption is commonly performed via the aerosol route. Often, the lung parenchyma is the desired site of medication activity. Selecting the aerosol route and inhaling the medication results in rapid onset, with fewer systemic side effects at lower doses when compared with other routes of administration. The upper airway may be selected as a site of medication action when topical anesthesia is required, or control of rhinitis or upper airway edema is needed. Depending upon the desired site of action, the selection of the delivery device is important due to differences in particle size and output.

AARC CLINICAL PRACTICE GUIDELINE
Bland Aerosol Administration
2003 Revision & Update

BAA 1.0 PROCEDURE:
Bland aerosol administration

BAA 2.0 DESCRIPTION/DEFINITION:
For purposes of this guideline, bland aerosol administration includes the delivery of sterile water or hypotonic, isotonic, or hypertonic saline in aerosol form. Bland aerosol administration may or may not be accompanied by oxygen administration.

   2.1 The use of cool, bland aerosol therapy is primarily indicated for upper airway administration; therefore, a mass median aerodynamic diameter (MMAD) micron is desirable.

   2.2 The use of hypo- and hypertonic saline is primarily indicated for inducing sputum specimens; therefore, a MMAD of 1–5 microns is desirable.

   2.3 The use of heated bland aerosol is indicated primarily for minimizing humidity deficit when the upper airway has been bypassed; therefore, a MMAD of 2–10 microns is desirable.

BAA 3.0 SETTINGS:
Bland aerosol therapy can be administered in settings that include hospital, clinic, extended care facility, and home.

BAA 4.0 INDICATIONS:
   4.1 The presence of upper airway edema—coolbland aerosol
   4.1.1 Laryngotracheobronchitis (LTB)
   4.1.2 Subglottic edema
   4.1.3 Post-extubation edema
   4.1.4 Postoperative management of the upper airway

Figure 3-14 *The American Association for Respiratory Care Clinical Practice Guideline: Bland Aerosol Administration—2003 Revision & Update. (Courtesy American Association of Respiratory Care, Irving, TX)* **(continues)**

4.2 The presence of a bypassed upper airway

4.3 The need for sputum specimens or mobilization of secretions

BAA 5.0 CONTRAINDICATIONS:

5.1 Bronchoconstriction

5.2 History of airway hyperresponsiveness

BAA 6.0 HAZARDS/COMPLICATIONS:

6.1 Wheezing or bronchospasm

6.2 Bronchoconstriction when artificial airway is employed

6.3 Infection

6.4 Overhydration

6.5 Patient discomfort

6.6 Caregiver exposure to droplet nuclei of *Mycobacterium tuberculosis* or other airborne contagious microorganism produced as a consequence of coughing, particularly during sputum induction

6.7 Edema of the airway wall

6.8 Edema associated with decreased compliance and gas exchange and with increased airway resistance

6.9 Sputum induction by hypertonic saline inhalation can cause bronchoconstriction with patients who have COPD, asthma, cystic fibrosis, or other pulmonary diseases.

BAA 7.0 LIMITATIONS OF METHOD:

7.1 The efficacy of intermittent or continuous use of bland aerosol as a means of reducing mucus has not been established. Bland aerosol is not a substitute for systemic hydration.

7.2 The physical properties of mucus are only minimally affected by the addition of water aerosol

7.3 Bland aerosol for humidification when the upper airway has been bypassed is not as efficient or effective as are heated water humidifiers or adequately designed heat moisture exchangers (HME) because of the

7.3.1 Difficulties in maintaining temperature at patient airway

7.3.2 Possible irritation to the airway

7.3.3 Infection risk

BAA 8.0 ASSESSMENT OF NEED:

8.1 The presence of one or more of the following may be an indication for administration of sterile water or isotonic or hypotonic saline aerosol:

8.1.1 Stridor

8.1.2 Brassy, croup-like cough

8.1.3 Hoarseness following extubation

8.1.4 Diagnosis of LTB or croup

8.1.5 Clinical history suggesting upper airway irritation and increased work of breathing (e.g., smoke inhalation)

8.1.6 Patient discomfort associated with airway instrumentation or insult

8.1.7 Bypassed upper airway

8.2 The presence of the need for sputum induction (e.g., for diagnosis of Pneumocystis carinii, pneumonia, tuberculosis) is an indication for administration of hypertonic saline aerosol.

BAA 9.0 ASSESSMENT OF OUTCOME:

9.1 With administration of sterile water or hypotonic or isotonic saline, the desired outcome is the presence of one or more of the following:

9.1.1 Decreased work of breathing

9.1.2 Improved vital signs

9.1.3 Decreased stridor

9.1.4 Decreased dyspnea

9.1.5 Improved arterial blood gas values

9.1.6 Improved oxygen saturation as indicated by pulse oximetry (SpO_2)

9.2 With administration of hypertonic saline, the desired outcome is a sputum sample adequate for analysis.

BAA 10.0 RESOURCES:

10.1 Equipment—Depending upon the specific application, components may include:

10.1.1 Aerosol generator

10.1.1.1 Large-volume nebulizer

10.1.1.2 Ultrasonic nebulizer

10.1.1.3 Small-volume nebulizer

10.1.2 Heater or cooling device

10.1.3 Patient application device

10.1.3.1 Mist tent

10.1.3.2 Hood

10.1.3.3 Mouthpiece

10.1.3.4 Mask

10.1.3.5 T-piece

10.1.3.6 Face tent

10.1.3.7 Tracheostomy collar

10.1.4 Corrugated aerosol tubing and water trapp

10.1.5 Tissues and emesis basin or container for collecting or disposing of expectorated sputum

10.1.6 Gloves, goggles, gown, and mask

10.1.7 Suction device and catheters

10.1.8 Oxygen analyzer

10.1.9 Device for filtering exhaled gas during sputum induction, with scavenger or filter system

10.1.10 Thermometer

10.2 Resources—Personnel

Figure 3-14 *(continues)*

10.2.1 Level I caregiver may be the provider of service after Level II personnel have established need for a specific device by patient assessment and the first administration has been completed. Level I personnel must demonstrate:

10.2.1.1 Proper preparation, measurement, and mixing of solution

10.2.1.2 Proper technique for administration of solution to be aerosolized

10.2.1.3 Proper use of equipment

10.2.1.4 Effective cleaning of equipment

10.2.1.5 Appropriate disposal of wastes

10.2.1.6 Ability to encourage effective breathing patterns and coughing techniques

10.2.1.7 Ability to modify techniques in response to adverse reactions as instructed and to appropriately communicate with physician, detailing the severity of symptoms

10.2.1.8 Compliance with Standard Precautions and proper infection control procedures

10.2.2 Level II personnel supervise Level I personnel, are responsible for initial assessments and care of the unstable patient, and must demonstrate knowledge and skill related to:

10.2.2.1 Indications and limitations for aerosol devices and associated equipment

10.2.2.2 Proper use, maintenance, and cleaning of equipment, including filter and scavenging systems

10.2.2.3 Risks inherent to the aerosolized solution and specific devices

10.2.2.4 Procedures for safely disposing of hazardous wastes

10.2.2.5 Breathing patterns and coughing techniques

10.2.2.6 Modification of technique in response to adverse reactions

10.2.2.7 Modification of flowrates and temperature as prescribed, in response to severity of symptoms

10.2.2.8 Assessment of patient condition and response to therapy

10.2.2.9 Auscultation, inspection, and monitoring of vital signs

10.2.2.10 Determination of peak expiratory flowrate, spirometry, and ventilatory mechanics

10.2.2.11 Recognition and response to adverse reactions and complications of procedure

10.2.2.12 Understanding of and compliance with Standard Precautions

10.2.2.13 Proper disposition of medical waste

BAA 11.0 MONITORING:

The extent of patient monitoring should be determined on the basis of the stability and severity of the patient's condition.

11.1 Patient subjective response—pain, discomfort, dyspnea, restlessness

11.2 Heart rate and rhythm, blood pressure

11.3 Respiratory rate, pattern, mechanics, accessory muscle use

11.4 Sputum production: quantity, color, consistency

11.5 Skin color

11.6 Breath sounds

11.7 Pulse oximetry

11.8 Spirometry equipment (if concern of adverse reaction)

BAA 12.0 FREQUENCY:

12.1 Critical care or emergency room settings that require continuous administration of bland aerosol necessitate close monitoring.

12.1.1 Short duration: 4–8 hours following extubation

12.1.2 Subglottic edema: until clinical evidence of edema has subsided

12.1.3 Long duration: artificial airways

12.1.4 Re-evaluation every 8 hours or with change in clinical condition

12.2 Acute care patients should be evaluated for response to therapy of continuous administration of bland cool aerosol for LTB and reevaluated at least every 48–72 hours or with change in clinical response.

12.3 Home care patients should be re-evaluated periodically for response to therapy or with change in status.

12.4 Sputum induction should be performed as often as necessary to yield appropriate specimen for desired examination (e.g., each morning for 3 days for acid-fast bacillus).

BAA 13.0 INFECTION CONTROL:

13.1 Standard Precautions for body fluid isolation are to be implemented.

13.2 Centers for Disease Control and Prevention recommendations for control of exposure to tuberculosis and droplet nuclei are to be implemented when patient is known or suspected to be immunosuppressed, is known to have tuberculosis, or has other risk factors for the disease.

13.2.1 To reduce aerosol contamination of room air

13.2.1.1 Enclose and contain aerosol administration.

Figure 3-14 *(continues)*

13.2.1.2 Filter aerosols that bypass or are exhaled by patient.

13.2.1.3 When aerosol release to the atmosphere cannot be routed through a filter:

13.2.1.3.1 Use filtered scavenger systems to remove aerosols that cannot be contained.

13.2.1.3.2 Provide local exhaust ventilation to remove aerosols that are released into room air.

13.2.1.3.3 Provide frequent air exchange to dilute concentration of aerosol in room.

13.2.1.3.4 Allow exchange of gas in the room to eliminate 99% of aerosol before next patient enters or receives treatment in that area.

13.2.1.3.5 Provide booths or stalls for sputum induction in areas in which multiple patients are treated. Booths or stalls should be designed to provide adequate airflow to draw aerosol and droplet nuclei from the patient and into an appropriate filtration system with exhaust directed to an appropriate outside vent. Booths should be adequately cleaned between patients.

13.2.2 Filters, nebulizers, and other contaminated disposable components of the aerosol delivery system should be treated as hazardous waste.

13.2.3 Personal protection devices should be used to reduce exposure when engineer-ing alternatives are not adequate or in place.

13.2.3.1 Use properly fitted respirator with adequate filtration when flow exhaust cannot control removal of aerosols.

13.2.3.2 Goggles, gloves, masks, and gowns should be used to serve as splatter shields and to reduce exposure to body substances.

13.2.4 Personnel should safely dispose of hazardous wastes.

13.2.5 Personnel who are at high risk for adverse effects from exposure should be given alternative assignments.

13.3 Nebulizers should not be reused between patients without disinfection.

13.4 Nebulizers should be sterilized, changed, or cleaned according to institutional infection control policy or at conclusion of a procedure that is not to be repeated.

13.5 Solutions should be handled aseptically.

13.6 Solutions from multidose sources must be handled aseptically and discarded after 24 hours.

Reprinted with permission from *Respiratory Care* 2003;48: 529–533. The complete AARC Clinical Practice Guidelines are available from the AARC Web site (http://www.aarc.org), from the AARC Executive Office, or from *Respiratory Care* journal.

Figure 3-14 *(continued)*

AARC CLINICAL PRACTICE GUIDELINE
Selection of Aerosol Delivery Device

AD 1.0 PROCEDURE:
Selection of a device for delivery of aerosol to the lower airways

AD 2.0 DESCRIPTION:
The selection of a device for administration of pharmacologically active aerosol to the lower airway. The device selected should produce particles with a mass median aerodynamic diameter (MMAD) of 2-5 microns.
These devices include
Metered dose inhalers (MDI)
MDIs with accessory device (e.g., spacer)
Dry powder inhalers (DPI)
Small volume nebulizers (SVN)
Large volume nebulizers (LVN)

Ultrasonic nebulizers (USN)
This guideline does not address bland aerosol administration and sputum induction.

AD 3.0 SETTING:
Aerosol therapy can be administered in a number of settings including hospital, clinic, extended care facility, and home.

AD 4.0 INDICATIONS:
The need to deliver—as an aerosol to the lower airways—a medication from one of the following drug classifications:
Beta adrenergic agents
Anticholinergic agents (antimuscarinics)
Anti-inflammatory agents
(e.g., corticosteroids)

Figure 3-15 *The American Association for Respiratory Care Clinical Practice Guideline: Selection of Aerosol Delivery Device. (Courtesy American Association of Respiratory Care, Irving, TX)* *(continues)*

Mediator-modifying compounds
(e.g., cromolyn sodium)
Mucokinetics

The selection of a device for delivery of aerosol for parenchymal deposition (e.g., antibiotics) will be addressed in another Guideline.

AD 5.0 CONTRAINDICATIONS:

5.1 No contraindications exist to the administration of aerosols by inhalation.

5.2 Contraindications related to the substances being delivered may exist. Consult the package insert for product-specific contraindications.

AD 6.0 HAZARDS/COMPLICATIONS:

6.1 Malfunction of device and/or improper technique may result in underdosing.

6.2 The potential exists for malfunction of device and/or improper technique (inappropriate patient use) to result in overdosing.

6.3 Complications of specific pharmacologic agent may occur.

6.4 Cardiotoxic effects of Freon have been reported as an idiosyncratic response that may be a problem with excessive use of MDI.

6.5 Freon may affect the environment by its effect on the ozone layer.

6.6 Repeated exposure to aerosols has been reported to produce asthmatic symptoms in some caregivers.

AD 7.0 LIMITATIONS OF PROCEDURE OR DEVICE:

7.1 Only a small percent of output deposits in the airway (< or = 10%).

7.2 Efficacy of the device is technique dependent (e.g., coordination, breathing pattern, inspiratory hold). The reader is referred to *Kacmarek RM, Hess D. The interface between patient and aerosol generator. Respir Care 1991;36:952–976* for detailed descriptions of optimal technique.

7.3 Efficacy of the device is design dependent (i.e., output and particle size).

7.4 Reduced deposition of aerosol to the lower airways is associated with the following and may require consideration of increased dose:

7.4.1 mechanical ventilation;

7.4.2 artificial airways;

7.4.3 airway caliber (e.g., infants and children);

7.4.4 severity of obstruction.

7.5 Patient compliance

7.6 Limitations of specific devices

7.6.1 Metered Dose Inhaler:

7.6.1.1 Environmental concerns (CFC)

7.6.1.2 Inadequate technique

7.6.1.3 Inadequate instruction

7.6.2 MDI accessory device (spacer or holding chamber):

7.6.2.1 Adds to cost over MDI alone

7.6.2.2 More bulky than MDI alone

7.6.3 Dry powder inhaler:

7.6.3.1 At the present time, patients must load each dose for most medications.

7.6.3.2 Reduced inspiratory flow (< 60 L/min) can lead to reduced deposition.

7.6.3.3 Irritation to airway

7.6.3.4 Humidity may cause clumping of particles.

7.6.4 Small-Volume Nebulizer:

7.6.4.1 Time- and labor-intensive

7.6.4.2 Less portable

7.6.4.3 Requires compressed-gas source or electricity

7.6.4.4 Vulnerable to contamination

7.6.4.5 Lack of convenience may affect patient compliance

7.6.5 Large-Volume Nebulizer:

7.6.5.1 Limited to acute and critical care setting

7.6.5.2 Requires close monitoring

7.6.5.3 Time- and cost-intensive

7.6.5.4 Vulnerable to contamination

7.6.5.5 Reconcentration of solution may occur over long period of time due to evaporation by dry gas.

7.6.6 Ultrasonic Nebulizer:

7.6.6.1 Cost of device

7.6.6.2 Mechanical reliability

7.6.6.3 Requires electrical power source

7.6.6.4 Vulnerable to contamination

AD 8.0 ASSESSMENT OF NEED:

8.1 Based on proven therapeutic efficacy, variety of available medications, and cost-effectiveness the MDI with accessory device should be the first method to consider for administration of aerosol to the airway.

8.2 Lack of availability of prescribed drug in MDI, dry powder, or solution form.

8.3 Inability of the patient to use device properly with coaching and instruction should lead to consideration of other devices.

8.4 Patient preference for a given device that meets therapeutic objectives should be honored.

8.5 When there is need for large doses, MDI, SVN, or LVN may be used. Clear superiority of any one method has not been established. Convenience and patient tolerance of procedure should be considered.

8.6 When spontaneous ventilation is inadequate (e.g., as in kyphoscoliosis or neuromuscular disorders, exacerbation of severe bronchospasm with impending respiratory failure that does not respond to other forms of therapy), delivery by a positive pressure breathing device (IPPB) should be considered.

AD 9.0 ASSESSMENT OF OUTCOME:

9.1 Proper technique applying device

Figure 3-15 *(continues)*

9.2 Patient response to or compliance with procedure

9.3 Objectively measured improvement (e.g., increased FEV_1 or peak flow)

AD 10.0 RESOURCES:

10.1 Equipment:

10.1.1 MDI-canister with actuator supplied by manufacturer; MDI accessory device that properly fits MDI mouthpiece or mask; adapters for specific circumstances (e.g., tracheostomy)

10.1.2 Small volume nebulizer—gas source, tubing, flowmeter, and mouthpiece or mask

10.1.3 Large volume nebulizer—gas source, flowmeter, connecting tubing, and mouthpiece or mask

10.1.4 Mechanical ventilator—SVN or MDI, adapter in inspiratory line of circuit

10.1.5 IPPB machine (i.e., pressure-limited ventilator)-nebulizer, gas source, connecting tubing, and mouthpiece or mask

10.1.6 Manual resuscitator—for 'bagging in' aerosol from MDI or SVN

10.2 Personnel:

10.2.1 Knowledge and skills at several levels are required to fully utilize and apply these devices.

10.2.1.1 Level II personnel provide initial assessments and care of the unstable patient:

10.2.1.1.1 utilizing proper technique for administration of MDI, accessory device, dry powder inhaler, SVN, LVN, USN; and SVN via IPPB;

10.2.1.1.2 practicing proper use, maintenance, and cleaning of equipment;

10.2.1.1.3 encouraging effective breathing patterns and coughing techniques;

10.2.1.1.4 modifying technique in response to adverse reactions;

10.2.1.1.5 modifying dosages and/or frequency as prescribed in response to severity of symptoms;

10.2.1.1.6 assessing patient condition and response to therapy;

10.2.1.1.7 performing auscultation and inspection and taking vital signs;

10.2.1.1.8 performing peak expiratory flowrate, spirometry, or ventilatory mechanics;

10.2.1.1.9 recognizing and responding to therapeutic and adverse responses and complications of medication and/or procedure;

10.2.1.1.10 understanding and complying with Universal Precautions.

10.2.1.2 The patient, family, or home caregiver; Level-I hospital personnel provide routine care of the patient:

10.2.1.2.1 preparing, measuring, and mixing medication;

10.2.1.2.2 demonstrating proper technique for administration of medication;

10.2.1.2.3 using equipment properly;

10.2.1.2.4 cleaning equipment;

10.2.1.2.5 encouraging effective breathing patterns and coughing techniques;

10.2.1.2.6 modifying technique in response to adverse reactions as instructed, with appropriate communication with physician or Level-II care provider;

10.2.1.2.7 modifying dosages and/or frequency as prescribed, with appropriate communication with physician, in response to severity of symptoms;

10.2.1.2.8 using the peak flowmeter properly and documenting results.

AD 11.0 MONITORING:

11.1 Performance of the device

11.2 Technique of device application

11.3 Assessment of patient response including changes in vital signs

AD 12.0 FREQUENCY:

12.1 Initiation of therapy after careful assessment of need (as outlined above)

12.2 The change from one type of device to another is based on a change in patient's condition or ability to use the specific device.

AD 13.0 INFECTION CONTROL:

13.1 Universal Precautions must be exercised for body substance isolation.

13.2 SVN and LVN are for single patient use or should be subjected to high-level disinfection between patients.

13.3 Published data establishing a safe use-period for SVN and LVN are lacking; however they probably should be changed or subjected to high-level disinfection at approximately 24-hour intervals.

13.4 Medications:

13.4.1 Medications should be handled aseptically.

13.4.2 Tap water should not be used as the diluent.

13.4.3 Medications from multidose sources in acute care facilities must be handled aseptically and discarded after 24 hours, unless manufacturer's recommendations specifically state that medications may be stored longer than 24 hours.

13.5 MDI accessory devices are for single patient use only. Cleaning of accessory devices is based on aesthetic criteria.

13.6 There are no documented concerns with contamination of medication in MDI canisters.

Reprinted with permission from *Respiratory Care* 1992; 37: 891–897. The complete AARC Clinical Practice Guidelines are available from the AARC Web site (*http://www.aarc.org*), from the AARC Executive Office, or from *Respiratory Care* journal.

Figure 3-15 *(continued)*

AARC CLINICAL PRACTICE GUIDELINE
Delivery of Aerosols to the Upper Airway

AUA 1.0 PROCEDURE:
Administration of aerosols to the upper airway

AUA 2.0 DESCRIPTION:
Delivery of therapeutic aerosols to the upper airway including the nose, pharynx, and larynx—therapeutic aerosols are indicated for upper airway inflammation, anesthesia, rhinitis, and administration of medications for systemic effect.

Devices for upper airway delivery include metered dose inhalers (MDI), metered spray pumps (MSP), hand-bulb atomizers (HBA), and small-volume (SVN), large-volume (LVN), and ultrasonic nebulizers (USN).

Nasopharyngeal deposition is greatest for particles in the range of 5–20 microns.

AUA 3.0 SETTING:
Bland or pharmacologically active aerosol therapy can be administered in a number of settings, including hospital, clinic, diagnostic laboratory, extended care facility, and home.

AUA 4.0 INDICATIONS:
4.1 Upper airway inflammation (e.g., to relieve inflammation due to laryngotracheobronchitis)
4.2 Anesthesia (e.g., to control pain and gagging during endoscopic procedures)
4.3 Rhinitis (e.g., to relieve inflammation and vascular congestion)
4.4 Systemic disease (e.g., to deliver peptides such as insulin)

AUA 5.0 CONTRAINDICATIONS:
Known hypersensitivity to the medication being delivered

AUA 6.0 HAZARDS/COMPLICATIONS:
6.1 Administration of medications for upper airway inflammation may result in
6.1.1 bronchospasm,
6.1.2 rebound of symptoms,
6.1.3 systemic side effects.
6.2 Administration of medications for anesthesia may result in
6.2.1 inhibition of gag reflex,
6.2.2 choking,
6.2.3 dehydration of epithelium,
6.2.4 allergic reactions,
6.2.5 excessive systemic effect,
6.2.6 bronchospasm,
6.2.7 nosocomial infection from contaminated delivery device or medication (See AARC CPG on Selection of Aerosol Delivery Device).
6.3 Administration of medications for rhinitis may result in
6.3.1 nasal rebound (including rhinitis medicamentosa) after extended use of alpha adrenergic decongestants;
6.3.2 delayed effect (e.g., effects of steroids are not immediate);
6.3.3 sensation of irritation and burning in the nose;
6.3.4 sneezing attacks (immediately following administration);
6.3.5 mucosal ulceration and bleeding;
6.3.6 postnasal drip.
6.4 Systemic disease—medication may cause nasal irritation or toxic effects.

AUA 7.0 LIMITATIONS OF PROCEDURE:
7.1 Upper airway inflammation—patient cooperation is not essential but may be desirable for effective administration in some applications.
7.2 Anesthesia—direct local application of anesthetic agents may require direct visualization.
7.3 Rhinitis
7.3.1 In the presence of excessive nasal mucus secretion or edema of the nasal mucosa, the drug may fail to reach the site of intended action. Deposition may be compromised by the presence of nasal polyps or a deviated septum.
7.3.2 Response may not be readily observable for drugs such as cromolyn sodium and steroids.
7.4 Systemic disease
7.4.1 In the presence of excessive nasal mucus secretion or edema of the nasal mucosa, the drug may fail to reach the site of intended action. Deposition may also be compromised by the presence of nasal polyps or a deviated septum.
7.4.2 Response may not be immediately apparent.

AUA 8.0 ASSESSMENT OF NEED:
The presence of one or more of the following may suggest the need for aerosol application.
8.1 In upper airway inflammation—

Figure 3-16 *The American Association for Respiratory Care Clinical Practice Guideline: Delivery of Aerosols to the Upper Airway. (Courtesy American Association of Respiratory Care, Irving, TX)* **(continues)**

8.1.1 stridor

8.1.2 brassy croup-like cough

8.1.3 hoarseness following extubation

8.1.4 diagnosis of laryngeotracheobronchitis or croup

8.1.5 recent extubation

8.1.6 evidence of inflamed upper airway

8.1.7 soft-tissue radiograph suggesting edema

8.1.8 increased work of breathing

8.2 For anesthesia—

8.2.1 severe localized pain in upper airway

8.2.2 impending invasive instrumentation of the upper airway

8.3 In rhinitis—

8.3.1 diagnosis of allergic, non-allergic, or infectious rhinitis

8.3.2 symptomatic need:

8.3.2.1 nasal congestion

8.3.2.2 rhinorrhea

8.3.2.3 sneezing

8.3.2.4 itching of nose, eyes, or palate

8.4 In systemic disease—presence of a systemic disease that warrants intranasal delivery of a therapeutic agent

AUA 9.0 ASSESSMENT OF OUTCOME:

9.1 In upper airway inflammation, effectiveness of administration may be indicated by

9.1.1 reduced stridor,

9.1.2 reduced hoarseness,

9.1.3 improvement in soft-tissue radiograph,

9.1.4 decreased work of breathing, as evidenced by decreased use of accessory muscles.

9.2 For anesthesia, effectiveness of administration is marked by reduced discomfort in the patient.

9.3 In rhinitis, effectiveness of administration may be indicated by

9.3.1 reduced nasal congestion,

9.3.2 improved airflow through nose,

9.3.3 reduced rhinorrhea,

9.3.4 reduced sneezing,

9.3.5 reduced itching of nose, eyes, or palate.

9.4 Systemic disease—effectiveness of administration of agent is marked by the presence of the appropriate systemic therapeutic response.

AUA 10.0 RESOURCES:

10.1 Equipment:

10.1.1 metered dose inhaler, or MDI, with nasal adapter

10.1.2 metered spray pump, or MSP

10.1.3 hand-bulb atomizer, or HBA

10.1.4 small volume nebulizer, or SVN, (use requires gas source, flowmeter, connecting tubing, and mask or mouthpiece)

10.1.5 large volume nebulizer, or LVN, (use requires gas source, flowmeter, large-bore tubing, and mask or mouthpiece)

10.1.6 ultrasonic nebulizer, or USN, (use requires electrical source, large-bore tubing and mouthpiece, mask, or nasal adapter)

10.2 Personnel:

10.2.1 A Level I caregiver may be the provider of service after Level II personnel have established need for a specific device by patient assessment, initial administration(s) has been completed, and patient is considered stable. Level I personnel (typically CRTT or RRT) must demonstrate appropriate technique for

10.2.1.1 preparing and measuring medications;

10.2.1.2 administering medication;

10.2.1.3 equipment use;

10.2.1.4 cleaning equipment;

10.2.1.5 disposal of wastes;

10.2.1.6 encouraging effective breathing patterns;

10.2.1.7 modifying treatment in response to adverse reactions as instructed, with appropriate communication with physician and Level II caregiver, in response to severity of symptoms;

10.2.1.8 Universal Precautions and proper infection control

10.2.2 Level II personnel should perform initial assessments of all patients and care for the unstable patient. The Level II caregiver should be an RRT or have equivalent training in patient assessment, aerosol administration, pulmonary function, and lung mechanics and should have demonstrated his/her knowledge and ability to perform related to the following:

10.2.2.1 indications and limitations for MDI, MSP, MBA, SVN, LVN, and USN;

10.2.2.2 proper use, maintenance, and cleaning of equipment, including filter and scavenging systems;

10.2.2.3 risks inherent in the medications and specific devices;

10.2.2.4 procedures for safely disposing of medical wastes;

10.2.2.5 breathing patterns and coughing techniques;

10.2.2.6 technique modification in response to adverse reactions;

Figure 3-16 *(continues)*

10.2.2.7 dose and/or frequency modification in response to severity of symptoms, as prescribed;

10.2.2.8 assessment of patient condition and response to therapy;

10.2.2.9 auscultation, inspection, and vital-signs determination;

10.2.2.10 measurement of peak expiratory flowrate, flow-volumes, timed volumes, and ventilatory mechanics;

10.2.2.11 recognition and response to adverse reactions to and complications of medication and/or procedure;

10.2.2.12 instructing patients and families.

AUA 11.0 MONITORING:

The extent of patient monitoring should be determined on the basis of the stability and severity of the patient's condition:

11.1 patient compliance and increase or decrease in symptoms, signs, and patient subjective response as specified in Section 8;

11.2 heart rate and rhythm, blood pressure;

11.3 change in indicators of therapeutic effect (e.g., blood-glucose level with insulin).

AUA 12.0 FREQUENCY:

Frequency of administration is specific for purpose of administration and medication used.

AUA 13.0 INFECTION CONTROL:

13.1 Universal Precautions for body fluid isolation are to be implemented.

13.2 Centers for Disease Control and Prevention recommendations for control of exposure to tuberculosis and droplet nuclei are to be implemented when patient is known to have tuberculosis or has other risk factors for the disease.

13.2.1 To reduce aerosol contamination of room air,

13.2.1.1 enclose and contain aerosol administration;

13.2.1.2 filter aerosols that bypass or are exhaled by patient;

13.2.2 When aerosol release to the atmosphere cannot be routed through a filter,

13.2.2.1 use filtered scavenger systems to remove aerosols that cannot be contained;

13.2.2.2 provide local exhaust ventilation to remove aerosols that are released into room air;

13.2.2.3 provide frequent air exchange to dilute concentration of aerosol in room;

13.2.2.4 allow exchange of gas in the room to eliminate 99% of aerosol before next patient enters or receives treatment in that area.

13.2.3 It remains unclear whether high efficiency particulate air (HEPA) filters completely remove infectious particles from the air.

13.2.4 Filters, nebulizers, and other contaminated disposable components of the aerosol delivery system should be treated as medical waste. Applicator nozzles for multi-dose atomizers should be changed between patients.

13.2.5 Personal protection devices should be used to reduce exposure when engineering alternatives are not adequate or in place.

13.2.5.1 Use properly fitted respirator with adequate filtration when flow exhaust cannot control removal of aerosols.

13.2.5.2 Goggles, gloves, masks, and gowns should be used to serve as splatter shields and to reduce exposure to body substances.

13.2.6 Personnel should safely dispose of hazardous wastes.

13.2.7 Personnel who are at high risk for adverse effects from exposure should be offered an opportunity for alternative assignments.

13.3 Nebulizers should not be reused between patients without disinfection.

13.4 Nebulizers should be changed or sterilized

13.4.1 at conclusion of a procedure that is not to be repeated;

13.4.2 every 24 hours with repeated or continuous administration or more often when visibly soiled;

13.5 Nebulizers *should not* be rinsed with tap water between treatments.

13.6 Solutions should be handled aseptically.

13.7 Diluent solutions from multidose vials (e.g., distilled water and normal saline) must be handled aseptically and should be discarded after 24 hours.

Reprinted with permission from *Respiratory Care* 1994; 39:803–807. The complete AARC Clinical Practice Guidelines are available from the AARC Web site (*http://www.aarc.org*), from the AARC Executive Office, or from *Respiratory Care* journal.

Figure 3-16 *(continued)*

AARC CLINICAL PRACTICE GUIDELINE
Selection of a Device for Delivery of Aerosol to the Lung Parenchyma

DALP 1.0 PROCEDURE:

Selection of a device for delivery of aerosol to the lung parenchyma

DALP 2.0 DESCRIPTION:

A device selected for administration of pharmacologically active aerosol to the lung parenchyma should produce particle sizes with a mass median aerodynamic diameter (MMAD) of 1–3 microns.

Such devices include ultrasonic nebulizers (USNs, including the Porta-Sonic), some large volume nebulizers (LVNs, such as the Small Particle Aerosol Generator™, or SPAG, which is intended only for ribavirin delivery), some small volume nebulizers (such as the Circulaire, RespirGard II, and Pari IS 2,) Other devices including metered dose inhalers (MDIs) may be developed for parenchymal deposition. Although some parenchymal deposition of particles < 1 micron probably does occur, selection of a specific device should be based on its ability to produce particles within MMAD of 1–3 microns.

DALP 3.0 SETTING:

Aerosol therapy can be administered in a number of settings including but not limited to hospital, clinic, extended care facility, or home.

DALP 4.0 INDICATIONS:

The indication for selecting a suitable device is the need to deliver a topical medication (in aerosol form) that has its site of action in the lung parenchyma or is intended for systemic absorption. Such medications may possibly include antibiotics, antivirals, antifungals, surfactants, and enzymes.

DALP 5.0 CONTRAINDICATIONS:

5.1 No contraindications exist to choosing an appropriate device for parenchymal deposition.

5.2 Contraindications related to the substances being delivered may exist. Consult the package insert for product-specific contraindications to medication delivery.

DALP 6.0 HAZARDS/COMPLICATIONS:

6.1 Malfunction of device and/or improper technique may result in underdosing or overdosing.

6.2 In mechanically ventilated patients, the nebulizer design and characteristics of the medication may affect ventilator function (e.g., filter obstruction, altered tidal volume, decreased trigger sensitivity) and medication deposition.

6.3 Complications related to specific pharmacologic agents can occur.

6.4 Aerosols may cause bronchospasm or irritation of the airway.

6.5 Exposure to medications and patient-generated droplet nuclei may be hazardous to clinicians.

6.5.1 Exposure to medication should be limited to the patient for whom it has been ordered. Nebulized medication that is released into the atmosphere from the nebulizer or exhaled by the patient becomes a form of "secondhand" exposure that may affect health-care providers and others in the vicinity of the treatment.

There has been increased awareness of possible health effects of aerosols, such as ribavirin and pentamidine. Anecdotal reports associate symptoms such as conjunctivitis, decreased tolerance to presence of contact lenses, headaches, bronchospasm, shortness of breath, and rashes in health-care workers exposed to secondhand aerosols. Similar concerns have been expressed concerning health-care workers who are pregnant or are planning to be pregnant within 8 weeks of administration. Less often discussed are the potential exposure effects of aerosolized antibiotics (which may contribute to the development of resistant organisms), steroids, and bronchodilators.

Because the data regarding adverse health effects on the health-care worker and on those casually exposed are incomplete, the prudent course is to minimize exposure in all situations.

6.5.2 The Centers for Disease Control and Prevention recommend addressing exposure control issues by (1) administrative policy, (2) engineering controls, and (3) personal protective equipment, in that order.

6.5.2.1 Administrative controls: Should include warning signs to apprise all who enter a treatment area of potential hazards of

Figure 3-17 *The American Association for Respiratory Care Clinical Practice Guideline: Selection of a Device for Delivery of Aerosol to the Lung Parenchyma. (Courtesy American Association of Respiratory Care, Irving, TX)*
(continues)

exposure. Accidental exposures should be documented and reported according to accepted standards.

Measures to reduce aerosol contamination of room air include:

6.5.2.1.1 discontinuing nebulization of medication while patient is not breathing the aerosol;

6.5.2.1.2 ensuring that staff who administer medications understand risks inherent with the medication and procedures for safely disposing of hazardous wastes;

6.5.2.1.3 screening of staff for adverse effects of exposure to aerosol medication;

6.5.2.1.4 providing alternative assignments for those staff who are at high risk of adverse effects from exposure (e.g., pregnant women or those with demonstrated sensitivity to the specific agent).

6.5.2.2 Engineering controls:

6.5.2.2.1 Filters or filtered scavenger systems to remove aerosols that cannot be contained.

6.5.2.2.2 Frequent air exchanges to dilute concentration of aerosol in room to eliminate 99% of aerosol before the next patient enters and receives treatment in the area.

6.5.2.2.3 Booths or stalls for sputum induction and aerosolized medication administration in areas in which multiple patients are treated. Booths or stalls should be designed to provide adequate air flow to draw aerosol and droplet nuclei from the patient and into an appropriate filtration system, with exhaust directed to an appropriate outside vent.

6.5.2.2.4 Handling of filters, nebulizers, and other contaminated components of the aerosol delivery system used with suspect agents (such as pentamidine and ribavirin) as hazardous waste.

6.5.2.3 Personal protection devices:

6.5.2.3.1 Personal protection devices should be used to reduce exposure when engineering alternatives are not in place or are not adequate. Use properly fitted respirators with adequate filtration when exhaust flow cannot adequately remove aerosol particles.

6.5.2.3.2 Goggles, gloves, and gowns should be used as splatter shields and to reduce exposure to medication residues and body substances.

DALP 7.0 LIMITATIONS OF PROCEDURE OR DEVICE:

7.1 A relatively small fraction of nebulizer output deposits in the lung parenchyma.

7.2 Efficacy of the device is technique dependent (e.g., coordination, ability to follow instructions, and breathing pattern including inspiratory flow and inspiratory hold).

7.3 Efficacy of the device is design dependent (i.e., output and particle size).

7.4 The following clinical situations are associated with reduced deposition of aerosol to the lung parenchyma and may require consideration of increased dose:

7.4.1 Mechanical ventilation

7.4.2 Artificial airways

7.4.3 Reduced airway caliber (e.g., infants and pediatrics)

7.4.4 Severity of obstruction

7.4.5 Hydrophilic formulations

7.4.6 Failure of patient to comply with procedure.

7.5 Limitation of specific devices:

7.5.1 MDI:

7.5.1.1 Particle size varies with drug formulation, propellants, evaporation rate, and humidity.

7.5.1.2 Accessory device is recommended with MDI use

7.5.1.2.1 assure optimal deposition

7.5.1.2.2 reduce oropharyngeal deposition

7.5.1.2.3 decrease caregiver exposure.

7.5.1.3 Relatively few formulations are targeted to the lung parenchyma.

7.5.2 SPAG™40 (intended only for ribavirin delivery)

7.5.2.1 Limited to acute and critical care setting

7.5.2.2 Requires close monitoring

7.5.2.3 Requires compressed gas source

7.5.2.4 Vulnerable to contamination

7.5.2.5 Reconcentration of solution may occur over a long period of time due to evaporation by dry gas source.

7.5.3 SVN:

7.5.3.1 Few devices produce particles with MMAD of 1–3 microns.

7.5.3.2 MMAD may vary with nebulizer model, medication, gas flow, and gas pressure.

7.5.3.3 Requires compressed gas source.

7.5.3.4 Vulnerable to contamination.

7.5.3.5 Reconcentration may occur.

7.5.4 LVN:

7.5.4.1 Generally limited to acute and critical care setting although anecdote suggest some home use.

7.5.4.2 Requires close monitoring.

Figure 3-17 *(continues)*

7.5.4.3 Few devices produce particles with MMAD of 1–3 microns.

7.5.4.4 Vulnerable to contamination.

7.5.5 USN:

7.5.5.1 Cost may be a factor.

7.5.5.2 May be mechanically unreliable.

7.5.5.3 Requires electrical power source.

7.5.5.4 Some units do not reliably produce MMAD of ; microns.

7.5.5.5 Reconcentration of solution may occur over long period of time due to evaporation by heat generated by piezoelectric cell. The ultrasonic device may denature the medication.

DALP 8.0 ASSESSMENT OF NEED (SELECTION CRITERIA FOR DEVICE):

8.1 Availability of prescribed drug in solution or MDI formulation.

8.2 Availability of appropriate scavenging or filtration equipment.

8.3 Patient preference for a given device that meets therapeutic objectives.

8.4 Although specific devices may give known ranges of particle size and output, clear superiority of any one method or device for achieving specific clinical outcomes has not been established. Cost, convenience, effectiveness, and patient tolerance of procedure should be considered.

8.5 When spontaneous ventilation is inadequate (e.g., kyphoscoliosis, neuromuscular disorders, or respiratory failure) consider augmentation with mechanical ventilation.

DALP 9.0 ASSESSMENT OF OUTCOME

Appropriate device selection is reflected by evidence of

9.1 use of proper technique in applying device;

9.2 patient compliance with procedure;

9.3 a positive clinical outcome. (However, appropriate device selection and application does not guarantee a positive outcome.)

DALP 10.0 RESOURCES

10.1 Equipment:

10.1.1 MDI and accessory device (holding chamber or spacer).

10.1.2 SPAG (nebulizer with drying chamber supplied by manufacturer); gas source; tent, hood or ventilator; scavenger or filter system to prevent aerosol from being released outside immediate treatment area.

10.1.3 SVN, gas source, tubing, one-way valves, mouthpiece or mask, scavenger or filter system to prevent aerosol from being released outside immediate treatment area.

10.1.4 LVN, gas source, flowmeter, connecting tubing, mouthpiece or mask scavenger or filter system to prevent aerosol from being released outside immediate treatment area.

10.1.5 Mechanical ventilator with SPAG unit, adapter in inspiratory line of circuit, filter system in expiratory line to prevent obstruction of expiratory valves, scavenger or filter system to prevent aerosol from being released outside immediate treatment area.

10.1.6 IPPB machine (i.e., pressure-cycled ventilator), nebulizer gas source, connecting tubing, mouthpiece or mask, scavenger or filter system to prevent aerosol from being released outside immediate treatment area.

10.2 Personnel

10.2.1 Level-II personnel should establish the need for a specific device by patient assessment and complete the first administration of the medication. Level-II personnel should continue to care for the unstable patient. We recommend that the Level-II caregiver be credentialed (e.g., RRT, CRTT, RN). Level-II personnel must have documented knowledge of and demonstrated ability to perform regarding:

10.2.1.1 Indications and limitations for SPAG, MDI with accessory devices, SVN, LVN, and USN.

10.2.1.2 Proper use, maintenance and cleaning of equipment, including filter and scavenging systems.

10.2.1.3 Risks inherent to the medications and specific devices.

10.2.1.4 Safe disposal of hazardous wastes and medical waste.

10.2.1.5 Optimal breathing patterns and coughing techniques.

10.2.1.6 Technique modification in response to adverse reactions.

10.2.1.7 Dosages and/or frequency modification as prescribed, in response to severity of symptoms.

10.2.1.8 Assessment of patient condition and response to therapy.

10.2.1.9 Performance of auscultation, inspection, and monitoring of vital signs.

10.2.1.10 Performance of peak expiratory flowrate, spirometry, and ventilatory mechanics.

10.2.1.11 Recognition and response to therapeutic or adverse response and complications of medication administration and/or the procedure.

Figure 3-17 *(continues)*

10.2.1.12 Understanding and compliance with Universal Precautions and guidelines for prevention of the spread of tuberculosis and other infection control measures.

10.2.2 Level-I caregiver may be the provider of service to the stable patient after Level-II personnel have established need for a specific device by patient assessment and the first administration has been completed. We recommend that Level-I personnel be credentialed (e.g., RRT, CRTT, RN). They must have documented knowledge and demonstrated ability to perform related to:

10.2.2.1 preparing, measuring, and mixing medication;

10.2.2.2 demonstrating proper technique for administration of medication;

10.2.2.3 using equipment properly;

10.2.2.4 cleaning equipment;

10.2.2.5 properly disposing of wastes;

10.2.2.6 encouraging effective breathing patterns and coughing techniques;

10.2.2.7 modifying technique in response to adverse reactions as instructed, with appropriate communication with physician, in response to severity of symptoms;

10.2.2.8 implementing and observing Universal Precautions and guidelines to avoid transmission of tuberculosis and proper infection control.

DALP 11.0 MONITORING:

11.1 Performance of the device and scavenging system

11.2 Technique of device application

11.3 Assessment of patient response

DALP 12.0 FREQUENCY:

A device for delivery of aerosolized medication to the lung parenchyma is selected

12.1 on initiation of therapy, after careful assessment of need (as outlined);

12.2 when the decision is made to change the device because of a change in patient condition or because the patient is unable to use the specific device.

DALP 13.0 INFECTION CONTROL:

13.1 Caregiver should exercise Universal Precautions for body substance isolation and follow CDC recommendations for control of exposure to tuberculosis and droplet nuclei.

13.2 Nebulizers should not be used between patients without disinfection.

13.3 Nebulizers should be changed or sterilized:

13.3.1 at conclusion of dose administration or at least every 24 hours;

13.3.2 at 24-hour intervals with continuous administration;

13.3.3 when visibly soiled.

13.4 Nebulizers should not be rinsed with tap water between treatments but may be rinsed with sterile water. CDC Guidelines recommend sterile water rinsing and air drying.

13.5 All medications should be handled aseptically.

13.6 CDC guidelines suggest that if multi-dose medications containers are dated upon opening and handled aseptically, medication may be used until exhausted or until the manufacturer's expiration date unless visible or suspected contamination occurs. However, it is not clear whether this applies only to solutions containing a bacteriostatic agent. Caution is advised particularly for reconstituted solutions.

Reprinted with permission from *Respiratory Care* 1996; 41: 647–653. The complete AARC Clinical Practice Guidelines are available from the AARC Web site (*http://www.aarc.org*), from the AARC Executive Office, or from *Respiratory Care* journal.

Figure 3-17 *(continued)*

AEROSOL THERAPY EQUIPMENT

NEBULIZER

A **nebulizer** is a device that produces particulate matter that is delivered into a gas stream. The particles may be liquids or solids. The particles are suspended in the gas stream provided that they are small enough so that gravity, inertial impaction and other forces discussed earlier in this chapter do not remove them from suspension.

Mainstream and Sidestream Nebulizers

Mainstream and sidestream are two classifications of nebulizers based upon the nebulizer's placement in relation to the flow of

Figure 3-18 *A diagram of a mainstream (A) and sidestream (B) small volume nebulizer.*

carrier gas. The carrier gas is the main gas flow that carries the aerosol particles to the patient.

With a mainstream nebulizer, the nebulizer is placed directly in the path of the carrier gas (Figure 3-18). The aerosol produced by the nebulizer is conducted out of the device by the main flow of carrier gas. Particle sizes from this type of nebulizer tend to be larger since the aerosol flows in a relatively straight path.

Sidestream nebulizers have a nebulizer that is placed adjacent to the flow of carrier gas (Figure 3-18). The aerosol output must change direction before merging with the carrier gas. Due to this direction change, particle sizes are smaller in these nebulizers than in the mainstream type.

Small-Volume Nebulizers

Pneumatic nebulizers may be further classified by the volume of the reservoirs that they possess. A small-volume nebulizer is one with a volume of less than 30 milliliters and is primarily utilized for short-term medication delivery. These devices produce aerosol particles that range from 1.5 to 7 microns in diameter.

Bulb-Type Handheld Nebulizers

Bulb-type nebulizers are commonly used by outpatients receiving home therapy. These devices are small handheld nebulizers that are powered by squeezing a rubber bulb (Figure 3-19).

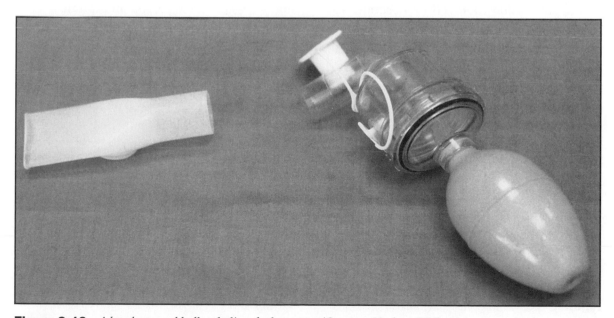

Figure 3-19 *A hand-powered bulb nebulizer for home use. (Courtesy Hudson RCI)*

Squeezing the bulb forces gas through the jet, creating a reduction in pressure and nebulization of the liquid in the reservoir (Bernoulli's principle). Each time the bulb is squeezed, a small amount of medication is delivered.

Patient instruction is critical with this type of nebulizer. Coordination of inspiration with the squeezing of the bulb sometimes becomes difficult. If the coordination is off, medication delivery is compromised.

ASSEMBLY AND TROUBLESHOOTING

Assembly—Bulb Nebulizer

1. Fill the reservoir with the ordered amount and dilution of medication.

2. Attach the bulb to the distal end of the nebulizer.

3. Insert the proximal end into the mouth.

4. Squeeze the bulb during a deep inspiration. Holding the breath at the end of inspiration for approximately

10 seconds helps to improve aerosol deposition.

Troubleshooting

Troubleshooting primarily consists of coordinating inspiration with squeezing the bulb. The nebulizer should be thoroughly cleaned after use to prevent the jet from becoming obstructed. Proper disinfection of home therapy equipment is also important to minimize infection.

Disposable Gas-Powered Small-Volume Nebulizers

In the clinical setting, disposable gas-powered small-volume nebulizers are very common. They are used to administer bronchodilators and other topical agents to the respiratory tract. The variety of styles and manufacturers are numerous. Most operate using similar principles.

Most small-volume nebulizers are updraft (draw medication up vertically) nebulizers that operate using choked flow, described earlier in this chapter. The liquid medication is

atomized and entrained into the gas flow by a combination of shear forces and vorticity (Figures 3-20 and 3-21). The aerosolized medication is then directed into a baffle, stabilizing the particle size before the aerosol exits the nebulizer.

Respigard II Small-Volume Nebulizer

The Respigard II small-volume nebulizer is a unique nebulizer which incorporates two one-way valves, a wye, and an expiratory filter (Figure 3-22). These nebulizers are capa-

Figure 3-20 *A functional diagram of a small-volume nebulizer.*

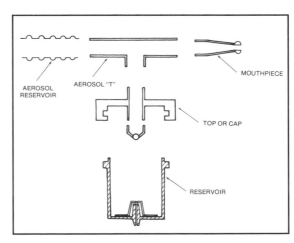

Figure 3-21 *An assembly drawing of a small-volume nebulizer.*

Filter   One-way valve

Mouthpiece

Nebulizer

One-way valve

Reservoir

(A)

Figure 3-23   *A photograph of the Salter Labs Medical Products NebuTech™ HDN™ small-volume nebulizer.*

(B)

Figure 3-22   *(A) An assembly drawing and (B) a photograph of the Respigard II small volume nebulizer.*

Figure 3-24   *An illustration showing inspiratory and expiratory gas flow through the Salter Labs Medical Products NebuTech™ HDN™ small-volume nebulizer.*

ble of producing particle sizes of less than 2 microns. The Respigard II is commonly used in the administration of Pentamidine, an antimicrobial drug used to treat Pneumocystis carinii pneumonia (PCP).

Salter Labs Medical Products NebuTech™ HDN™ Small-Volume Nebulizer

The Salter Labs Medical Products Nebu-Tech™ HDN™ small-volume nebulizer is a breath enhanced nebulizer that utilizes inspiratory and expiratory one-way valves to enhance aerosol delivery during inspiration (Figures 3-23 and 3-24). During exhalation, the exhaled gas is directed into the ambient room. Also, aerosolized medication is collected in the upper chamber, ready for delivery on the next breath. Up to 50 mL of dense aerosol is held in the upper chamber ready for delivery during the next inspiration. The convoluted gas path flow also helps to stabilize particle size, enhancing small particle output. Approximately 80% of the delivered aerosol from the nebulizer is less than 5 microns in diameter.

Monaghan Medical Corporation AeroEclipse® Breath-Actuated Nebulizer

The Monaghan Medical Corporation Aero-Eclipse® breath-actuated nebulizer is a nebulizer that incorporates a unique diaphragm/spring assembly and a sliding actuator piston that results in aerosol delivery only during inspiration (Figures 3-25 and 3-26).

During inspiration, the sub-ambient pressure causes a diaphragm to compress a spring moving an actuator piston closer to the high pressure gas jet. Once the actuator piston is in position, nebulization begins. At the end of inspiration, sub-ambient pressure diminishes, and the spring moves the actuator piston away from the high pressure gas jet, ending nebulization. In the event the patient fails to generate sufficient inspiratory sub-ambient pressure to activate the nebulizer, a green button on the top of the nebulizer may be depressed to activate nebulization by compressing the spring manually.

Breath activation during inspiration

Figure 3-25 *A photograph of the Monaghan Medical Corporation AeroEclipse® breath-actuated nebulizer.*

reduces medication waste, since no aerosol is delivered during the expiratory phase. Also, clinical trials have shown that smaller doses may be given for the same clinical efficacy in shorter therapy times.

Figure 3-26 *A line drawing showing inspiratory and expiratory gas flow through the Monaghan Medical Corporation AeroEclipse® breath-actuated nebulizer.*

ASSEMBLY AND TROUBLESHOOTING

Refer to ALG 3-5 and Figure 3-21 when following the assembly and troubleshooting procedures.

Assembly—Small-Volume Nebulizer

1. Aseptically remove the component parts from the package.

2. Add the ordered volume and dilution of medication to the reservoir.

3. Attach the reservoir to the nebulizer top, screwing them together or pushing them together, depending upon the design.

4. Attach the aerosol T to the outlet of the nebulizer.

5. Attach the aerosol tubing reservoir to one end of the aerosol T and the mouthpiece to the other.

6. Attach the oxygen connecting tube to the nipple on the bottom of the nebulizer.

7. Attach the distal end of the oxygen connecting tube to a flowmeter. Adjust the flow to between 5 and 7 liters per minute.

Troubleshooting

When troubleshooting this equipment, please follow the suggested troubleshooting algorithm (ALG 3-5).

If aerosol output is absent or low:

1. Check to be sure the oxygen connecting tube is attached to the flowmeter and nebulizer.

2. Check the flowmeter to ensure the flow is properly set.

3. Check the jet for obstruction.

4. If (1) through (3) are satisfactory, replace the unit with a new one.

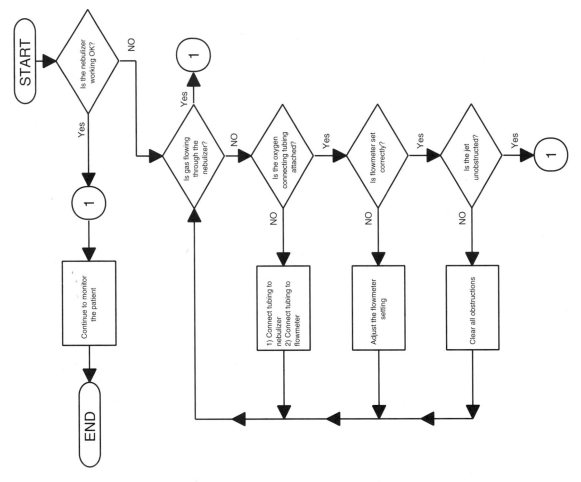

ALG 3-5 *An algorithm describing how to troubleshoot a small-volume nebulizer.*

METERED DOSE INHALERS

Metered dose inhalers (MDIs) are small self-contained nebulizers designed for administration of medications (Figure 3-27A). Many bronchodilators and steroids can be administered using MDIs. MDIs are advantageous in that they are very small and are easy to use.

How MDIs Operate

Contained in the MDI canister is the medication to be delivered (solution or powder) mixed with an inert liquified gas under pressure (Figure 3-27B). The majority of MDIs use fluorocarbons as the propellant. When the patient depresses the mouthpiece toward the canister using a squeezing action, a valve opens, discharging a premeasured dose of medication along with the propellant. The propellant rapidly evaporates, leaving the medication in suspension as an aerosol. These devices operate in a way that is similar to an aerosol paint can.

There have been some reports of patient sensitivity to the propellant, causing bronchospasm and other unwanted side effects. More studies are currently being conducted regarding how safe and non-reactive these agents are in the population. These devices are very popular and can be very cost-effective.

By United States law, fluorocarbons will be eliminated as a propellant from MDIs. HFA and other propellants may be used as a substitute for the fluorocarbons in MDIs. More medications will likely become available as dry powder preparations for use in dry powder inhalers.

MDI HOLDING CHAMBERS

The use of a holding chamber (Figure 3-28), enhances the effectiveness of aerosol deposition and improves delivery for patients who have problems coordinating the sequencing of squeezing the MDI and inspiration. A **holding chamber** is a valved reservoir that helps to slow the delivery of medication and act as a temporary reservoir for containing the medication

(A)

(B)

Figure 3-27 *(A) A photograph and (B) a functional diagram of a metered dose inhaler (MDI).*

Figure 3-28 *A drawing showing several different types of spacers.*

before inhalation. The MDI is inserted into the holding chamber at the opposite end from the mouthpiece (Figure 3-29). When the patient squeezes the MDI, the medication is discharged into the holding chamber, which acts as a reservoir and baffle device. The larger particles impact the walls of the holding chamber, removing them from suspension. The larger size of the holding chamber (reservoir) facilitates the further evaporation of the propellant. The net result is that smaller particles are inspired by the patient. If a patient has difficulty timing the release of medication with his or her ventilatory cycle, the holding chamber may improve medication delivery.

Figure 3-29 *A drawing illustrating how the MDI and spacer are assembled together.*

Patient Instructions for Use

The assembly and troubleshooting of the MDI device itself is relatively easy. The most difficult part of MDI use is educating the patient on how to correctly use it. The effectiveness of MDI administration is highly technique dependent. Therefore, it is important that you thoroughly instruct your patient on its proper use.

Use without a Holding Chamber

Have the patient sitting or standing comfortably. It is important that the patient be upright to allow for good chest expansion to facilitate a deep breath. Make certain that the patient is not wearing restrictive clothing that may hamper his or her ability to take a deep breath.

Have the patient hold the MDI a few centimeters away from his or her open mouth. Have the patient exhale, then slowly inhale deeply a few times. Once the patient is cognizant of his or her breathing pattern, instruct the patient to squeeze the MDI just after beginning a breath and to continue slowly inhaling deeply to a maximal inspiration. Have the patient hold his or her breath a few seconds (5 to 10 seconds) at the end of inspiration. Have the patient slowly exhale after MDI administration. Repeat the procedure as many times as ordered by the patient's physician, waiting between puffs.

Use with a Holding Chamber

As discussed above, thorough patient instruction is important. Position the patient as described earlier. Connect the MDI to the holding chamber as shown in Figure 3-29. Have the patient insert the mouthpiece into his or her mouth. Instruct the patient to exhale and to take a slow deep breath. Just after the patient begins a breath, have him or her squeeze the MDI delivering the medication. Have the patient continue his or her inhalation, performing a breath hold at the end of inspiration (5 to 10 seconds). Have the patient remove the holding chamber /MDI and slowly exhale following medication administration. Repeat the procedure as many times as ordered by the patient's physician, waiting between puffs.

ASSEMBLY AND TROUBLESHOOTING

Assembly—MDI

1. Remove the MDI from its box and assemble the mouthpiece by placing it on top of the canister.

2. Thoroughly shake the MDI vigorously for a few seconds.

3. If using a spacer, connect the MDI to the spacer as shown in Figure 2-23.

4. Instruct the patient on the use of MDIs.

Troubleshooting

When troubleshooting this equipment, please follow the suggested troubleshooting algorithm (ALG 3-6).

If the MDI fails to activate when the valve is depressed:

1. Check for correct assembly of the mouthpiece and how it mates to the propellant canister.

2. The MDI may be exhausted of propellant and medication. To check the contents of the MDI, float it in water in a small bowl or basin.

   a. If the MDI sinks to the bottom it is full.

   b. If the MDI floats upright it is partially full.

   c. If the MDI floats horizontally, it is empty.

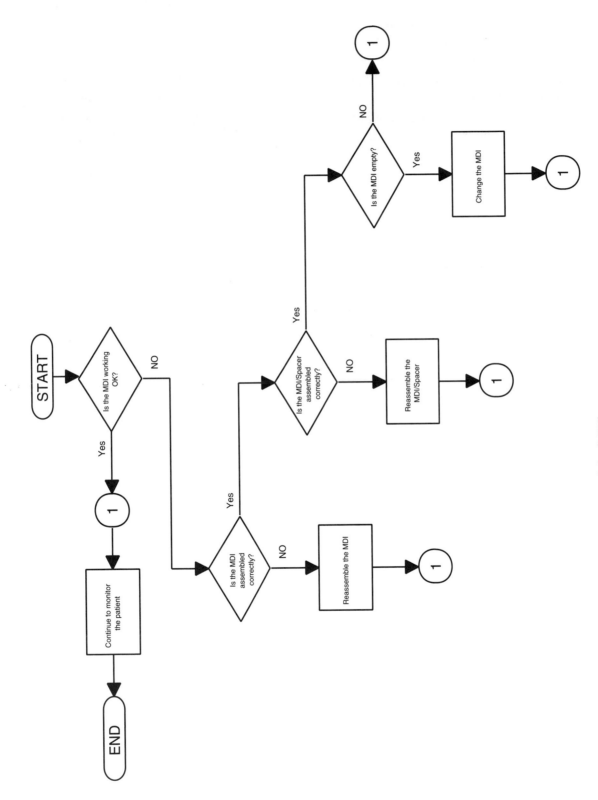

ALG 3-6 *An algorithm describing how to troubleshoot a Metered Dose Inhaler (MDI).*

DRY POWDER INHALERS (DPIs)

A dry powder inhaler (DPI) is an aerosol delivery device that administers aerosols in a dry powder form. A DPI creates an aerosol by drawing ambient air through a small dose of dry powdered medication. As the air passes through the powdered medication, it is aerosolized into suspension in the carrier gas (ambient air). If the particles are fine enough, they will be carried into the airway and deposited into the lung parenchyma.

Unlike MDIs, DPIs do not require a propellant for their operation. The patient, however, must have strong enough inspiratory muscle strength to produce an inspiratory flow sufficient to aerosolize the medication. DPIs do not require the same coordination, or a breath hold like MDIs.

There are several different types of DPIs available (Figures 3-30 through 3-32), including the Diskhaler, Discus and Turbuhaler. Depending upon the type of DPI, the way it is assembled and how it is used varies. Most manufacturers provide a placebo inhaler for practice and demonstration purposes. You should practice with the placebo inhaler until you are proficient in its use before instructing a patient on how to use the device.

Diskhaler

The Diskhaler is shown in Figure 3-30. To use the diskhaler, begin by removing the mouthpiece cover by sliding it off. Pull the tray out from the Diskhaler and place a disk containing medication onto the tray with the numbers facing up. Slide the tray into Diskhaler, which rotates the tray, making the medication dose available for use. Lift the back of the lid upright; this punctures the medication blister, opening it to the inspired gas flow for aerosolization. Keeping the Diskhaler level, insert the open mouthpiece into the mouth, and take a slow deep breath. The inspired air will aerosolize the medication for delivery into the lungs. Once inspiration is complete, remove the device from the mouth and exhale. Replace the cover to protect the mouthpiece from contamination or foreign material.

Diskus

The Diskus is shown in Figure 3-31. To use the Diskus, open it by rotating the cover away from the mouthpiece. Cock the lever on the side of the Diskus; this action peels a foil cover off of the medication blister, exposing it for aerosolization. Keeping it level, insert it into the mouth and take a slow deep breath. Once inspiration is complete, remove it from the mouth and exhale. A counter on the Diskus records the number of doses available for use. With each use the number decreases by one. Replace the cover by rotating it back into position and closing the mouthpiece.

Turbuhaler

The Turbuhaler is shown in Figure 3-32. To use the Tubuhaler, remove the cover from the mouthpiece by sliding it off. Holding the Turbuhaler upright, grasp the mouthpiece

Figure 3-30 *A photograph of the Diskhaler dry powder inhaler.*

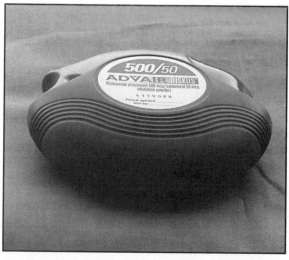

Figure 3-31 *A photograph of the Diskus dry powder inhaler.*

Figure 3-32 *A photograph of the Turbuhaler dry powder inhaler.*

assembly in one hand and the bottom grip in the other. Rotate the bottom grip first right then left; a distinct "click" can be heard when the action is performed correctly. Rotate the Turbuhaler carefully to the horizontal position and place the mouthpiece into the mouth. Take a slow deep breath, inhaling deeply. Following inspiration, remove the Turbuhaler from the mouth and exhale. Replace the mouthpiece cover to protect it from any contamination or foreign material.

ASSEMBLY AND TROUBLESHOOTING

Assembly – Dry Powder Inhalers (DPIs)

1. If assembly is required, correctly insert the foil-faced disk with medication blisters into the unit.

2. Once the DPI is assembled, correctly charge the unit with medication by twisting it or cocking a lever.

3. Position the DPI horizontally and instruct the patient to inhale deeply.

Troubleshooting

Incorrect assembly and failure to charge the unit with medication are the two most common causes of malfunctions. If the unit has a built-in counter, make certain that the number of doses has not been exceeded.

LARGE-VOLUME NEBULIZERS

Large-volume nebulizers are used to provide continuous aerosol therapy. They are designed with large reservoirs that may require filling every four or eight hours, depending upon the flow through the nebulizer. All of these devices are designed to use large-bore aerosol tubing to maximize gas and aerosol delivery.

Allegiance Healthcare Corporation Large-Volume Nebulizer

Allegiance Healthcare Corporation manufactures a prefilled large-volume nebulizer (Figure 3-33). The unit is capable of providing cool or heated aerosol (with the optional slip-on heater) at oxygen percentages varying from 28% to 100 %.

The nebulizer operates using the viscous shearing and vorticity principles to aerosolize liquid from the reservoir and to mix ambient air with oxygen to attain precise dilution ratios. Source gas (oxygen) is conducted down to the nebulizer jet where its velocity is increased. Water is drawn up a capillary tube where it encounters the high velocity gas stream. The water is aerosolized into fine particles, which are then baffled to further reduce particle size. The nebulizer is designed to use a 38-mm threaded fitting that matches the majority of brands of sterile solution 500-mL and 1000-mL bottles.

To deliver heated aerosol, an optional heater is inserted over the top of the nebulizer unit that surrounds the aluminum collar at the nebulizer top. The aluminum collar facilitates heat transfer to the aerosol as it passes through the unit. Some heater units are adjustable for temperature output, while others are not.

(A)   (B)

Figure 3-33 *A photograph (A) of the Allegiance Healthcare Corporation Large Volume Nebulizer and (B) a photograph showing it's assembly.*

ASSEMBLY AND TROUBLESHOOTING

Assembly – Large-Volume Nebulizers

1. Connect the reservoir bottle to the nebulizer top by screwing the top onto the bottle by turning it clockwise.

2. If heated aerosol is desired, place a heater over the top of the nebulizer top, ensuring that the heating element comes into contact with the aluminum surface above the entrainment ports. Adjust the heater thermostat to the desired temperature range and monitor the temperature using a thermometer proximal to the patient.

3. Connect the DISS inlet fitting to an oxygen or air flowmeter, adjust the flow to the desired range, and set the air entrainment port to desired F_IO_2.

4. Connect large-bore aerosol tubing to the humidifier's outlet and connect an appropriate patient interface to the distal end of the tubing. Use of a drainage bag or trap will help to prevent blockage of the delivery tubing with condensate.

Troubleshooting

1. If aerosol output is absent or inadequate:
   a. Ensure that the flowmeter is set at the correct setting.
   b. Check the water level in the reservoir bottle.
   c. Check the tubing for obstruction by condensate.

2. If the heater is not operating properly:
   a. Ensure that the electrical outlet is working, using a test lamp or other electrical device.
   b. Check the power cord for breaks or shorts.

3. If the oxygen concentration varies from the setting on the entrainment port:
   a. Verify that the entrainment port is set properly
   b. If the F_IO_2 is higher than was set, check for tubing obstructions.
   c. If the F_IO_2 is lower than was set, check for correct assembly and loose fittings.

Misty Ox Hi-Fi Nebulizer

Vital Signs, Inc. markets a nebulizer that can provide F_IO_2 levels from .60 to .96 at flow rates between 42 and 77 liters per minute (Figure 3-34). The Hi-Fi nebulizer is similar in appearance to the MultiFit nebulizer, also marketed by the same company. The major difference is that the MultiFit has a maximum flow restriction through the nozzle of 14 L/min, while the Hi-Fi has a maximum flow restriction through the nozzle of 40 L/min. This design allows for sufficient total flows to meet or exceed the patient's inspiratory demand

(43 L/min at F_IO_2 of .96, 77 L/min at F_IO_2 of .60). Without sufficient total flow to meet the patient's demand, you cannot achieve accurate oxygen concentration delivery to the patient.

The nebulizer operates using viscous shearing and jet mixing to nebulize water and entrain room air. Oxygen is conducted down through a small orifice jet, increasing the gas's velocity (Figure 3-35). Air is entrained at this point by viscous shearing, as described in Chapter 1. A capillary tube fitting, in close proximity to the jet, injects water into the high velocity gas stream by shear forces as described earlier in this chapter. The gas mixture and aerosol particles are directed through a converging duct downward and laterally form a swirling flow pattern in the mixing chamber. The swirling gas flow encounters baffles positioned radially along the edges of the mixing chamber which remove the larger aerosol particles from suspension. Careful design of the jet and mixing chamber allows the use of a 40-L/min jet (nozzle) to maintain higher total flow rates at higher F_IO_2 levels than other similar devices (Table 3-4). A Turbo-Heater is also available if heated aerosol is required.

The nebulizer is designed with a 38-mm threaded fitting to be used to attach the nebulizer to a reservoir bottle. The 38-mm fitting is a standard size fitting incorporated by many suppliers of sterile solutions. This is advantageous in that cost savings may be realized by using these solutions rather than purchasing prefilled nebulizers.

Figure 3-34 *A functional diagram of the Misty Ox Hi-Fi nebulizer.*

Figure 3-35 *A detailed diagram of the Misty Ox Hi-Fi nebulizer.*

ASSEMBLY AND TROUBLESHOOTING

Assembly—Misty Ox Hi-Fi Nebulizer

1. Remove the cap from the sterile distilled water bottle you wish to use as a reservoir.

2. Aseptically remove the nebulizer from its package. Use caution so that you do not contaminate the long capillary tube, which will be immersed into the reservoir bottle.

3. Insert the capillary tube into the bottle and screw the nebulizer into place using the 38-mm threaded fitting. Make sure that the nebulizer is on tight and is not cross threaded.

4. Attach the nebulizer to a high range flowmeter (0–75 L/min). Connect the flowmeter to a 50-psi oxygen source.
   a. Alternatively, a standard flowmeter (0–15 L/min) may be substituted. Open the needle valve to its maximum position (beyond flush). Most standard flowmeters will deliver between 60–90 L/min at this setting. The nozzle design in the Hi-Fi nebulizer will limit flow through it to 40 L/min even if the flowmeter exceeds this setting.

5. Attach large-bore aerosol tubing to the nebulizer outlet. Secure a drainage bag to collect any condensate at the midpoint of the tubing.

6. Attach the delivery device to the aerosol tubing (aerosol mask, face tent, aerosol T, trach mask).

7. Set the entrainment control to the desired F_IO_2 (.60, .65, .75, .85, .96), and adjust the flowmeter to the desired setting. Reduction in the entrainment settings from .96 to .60 will increase total flow through the Hi-Fi nebulizer. Maximum achievable flow is 77 L/min.
   a. If you are using a standard flowmeter set on its maximum position, the nozzle in the Hi-Fi will limit flow to 40 L/min.
   b. Verify the oxygen concentration using a calibrated oxygen analyzer (refer to Chapter 1).

8. Replace the reservoir bottle when the solution level is ¼ inch from the bottom of the container.

Troubleshooting

When troubleshooting this equipment, please follow the suggested troubleshooting algorithm (ALG 3-7).

No flow from the nebulizer:
1. Check to ensure that there is an adequate oxygen supply when using cylinders.
2. Verify that the flowmeter is correctly connected to the 50 psi oxygen source.
3. Check the connection between the nebulizer and the flowmeter.
   a. Make sure it is securely attached.
   b. Check for any obstruction where the nebulizer attaches to the flowmeter.

Little or no aerosol being generated:
1. Check to ensure that the reservoir bottle contains fluid.
2. Check the capillary tube to ensure it is immersed into the solution in the bottle.
3. Check the capillary tube for obstructions.
4. Check the large-bore aerosol delivery tubing for kinks or obstructions.
5. If using a standard 0-15 L/min flowmeter, make sure the flowmeter needle valve is opened to its maximum setting.

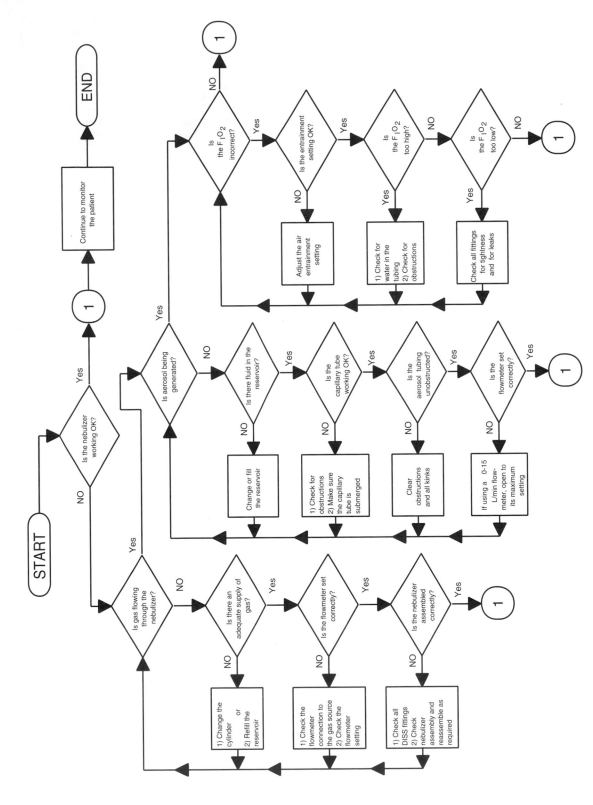

ALG 3-7 *An algorithm describing how to troubleshoot the Misty Ox Hi-Fi nebulizer.*

TABLE 3-4 Total Flow Rates Provided by Misty Ox Hi-Fi Nebulizer

Entrainment Setting	Oxygen Flow (L/min)	Total Flow (L/min)
60%	20–30	40–61
65%	30–40	54–72
75%	30–40	44–58
85%	30–40	37–49
96%	40	42

Misty Ox Gas Injection Nebulizer (GIN)

Vital Signs, Inc. is marketing a nebulizer that can provide high F_IO_2 levels (.21–1.0) and at high flow rates (over 100 L/min). Unlike other nebulizers available, the Gas Injection Nebulizer (GIN) is not an entrainment device. It is a closed system device which requires two gas sources (oxygen and air). The second gas is injected via an attached titration tube to achieve any FIO2 at any total flow. Being a closed system, the nebulizer can provide a positive pressure (CPAP), as well as hydration and variable oxygen concentrations.

To achieve oxygen concentrations from .21 to .50, the device should be connected to an air flowmeter (driving primary jet) and titrate oxygen to blend specific concentrations. To achieve oxygen concentrations between .50 and 1.0, the device should be connected to an oxygen flowmeter (driving the primary jet) and titrate air to blend specific concentrations.

In either configuration, the titration tube is connected to a "nipple adapter" or "Christmas tree" adapter on a flowmeter to provide the secondary injected gas flow. While the GIN part # 441G has a 40-L/min nozzle (same as the Hi-Fi) suited for adult applications, Medical Molding Corporation also produces another model (part # 441GB), the GIN Baby, for pediatric and infant applications. The GIN Baby's nozzle restricts flow to a maximum of 14 L/min.

The nebulizer operates using viscous shearing and jet mixing to nebulize water and mix room air. Oxygen is conducted down through a small orifice jet, increasing the gas's velocity (Figure 3-36). Another gas is injected at perpendicular to the primary jet (through the titration tube). The injected gas is directed against a curved baffle, causing a swirling flow pattern in the mixing chamber. The two gases mix together by vorticity and turbulent flow.

A capillary tube fitting, in close proximity to the jet, injects water into the high velocity primary gas stream by shear forces as described earlier in this chapter. The gas mixture and aerosol particles are directed through a converging duct downward and laterally forming a swirling flow pattern in the mixing chamber. The swirling gas flow encounters baffles positioned radially along the edges of the mixing chamber which remove the larger aerosol particles from suspension.

The nebulizer is designed with a 38-mm threaded fitting to be used to attach the nebulizer to a reservoir bottle. The 38-mm fitting is a standard-size fitting incorporated by many suppliers of sterile solutions. This is advantageous in that cost savings may be realized by using these solutions rather than purchasing prefilled nebulizers.

The total flow from the nebulizer and the F_IO_2 level is dependent upon what gas (oxygen or air) is the primary source and its flow rate, and what gas (oxygen or air) is the secondary gas (injected) and its flow rate. The oxygen concentrations and total flow rates are outlined in Tables 3-5 and 3-6 on page 157.

One investigator was able to achieve an F_IO_2 of 1.0, with a total flow of 91.2 liters per minute, when running the GIN nebulizer using oxygen as a secondary source at a maximum flow setting with the primary air source turned off.

Figure 3-36 *(A) A functional diagram and (B) a detailed diagram of the Misty Ox Gas Injection Nebulizer (GIN).*

ASSEMBLY AND TROUBLESHOOTING

Assembly—Misty Ox GIN Nebulizer

1. Remove the cap from the sterile distilled water bottle you wish to use as a reservoir.

2. Aseptically remove the nebulizer from its package. Use caution so that you do not contaminate the long capillary tube which will be immersed into the reservoir bottle.

3. Insert the capillary tube into the bottle and screw the nebulizer into place using the 38-mm threaded fitting. Make sure that the nebulizer is on tight and is not cross threaded.

4. Attach the nebulizer to a high range flowmeter (0–75 L/min). Connect the flowmeter to a 50-psi oxygen or air source, depending upon the total flow and F_IO_2 desired.

   a. Alternatively, a standard flowmeter (0–15 L/min) may be substituted. Turn the needle valve to its maximum setting (beyond flush). Most flowmeters will produce a flow of between 60 and 90 L/min at this setting. The GIN nebulizer will limit flow through its nozzle to 40 L/min at this setting.

5. Attach the secondary gas inlet tube to a second flowmeter powered by the desired secondary gas (air or oxygen). Use of a high-range flowmeter is also recommended for the secondary gas source.

6. Attach large-bore aerosol tubing to the nebulizer outlet. Secure a drainage bag, to collect any condensate, at the midpoint of the tubing.

7. Attach the delivery device to the aerosol tubing (aerosol mask, face tent, aerosol T, trach mask).

8. Adjust the primary and secondary gas flows to achieve your desired F_IO_2 and total flow rate.

   a. Verify the oxygen concentration using a calibrated oxygen analyzer (refer to Chapter 1).

9. Replace the reservoir bottle when the solution level is ¼ inch from the bottom of the container.

Troubleshooting

When troubleshooting this equipment, please follow the suggested troubleshooting algorithm (ALG 3-8).

No flow from the nebulizer:

1. Check to ensure that there is an adequate oxygen supply when using cylinders.

2. Verify that the flowmeter is correctly connected to the 50-psi oxygen or air source.

3. Check the connection between the nebulizer and the flowmeter.

   a. Make sure it is securely attached.

   b. Check for any obstruction where the nebulizer attaches to the flowmeter.

   c. Verify that the secondary gas inlet tube is free of obstruction or kinks.

Little or no aerosol being generated:

1. Check to ensure that the reservoir bottle contains fluid.

2. Check the capillary tube to ensure it is immersed into the solution in the bottle.

3. Check the capillary tube for obstructions.

4. Check the large-bore aerosol delivery tubing for kinks or obstructions.

5. If using a standard flowmeter (0–15 L/min), verify that the needle valve has been opened to its maximum setting (beyond flush).

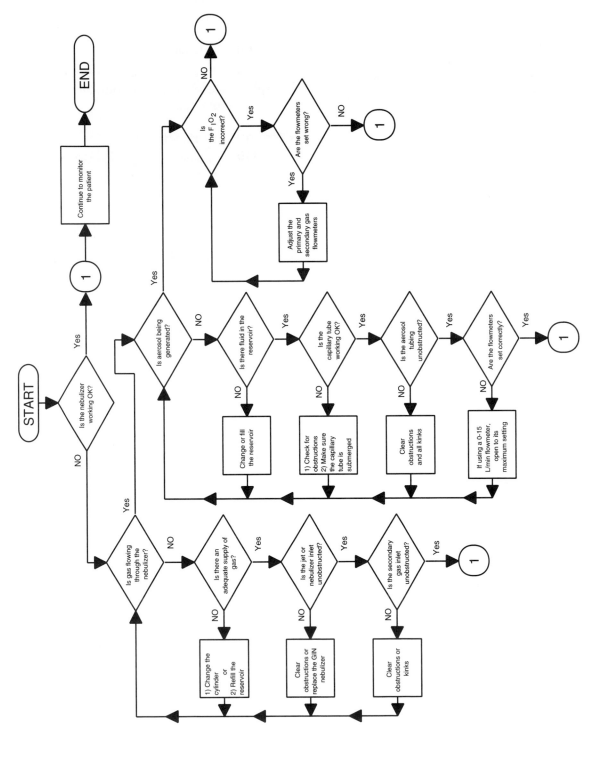

ALG 3-8 *An algorithm describing how to troubleshoot the Misty Ox Gas Injection Nebulizer (GIN).*

TABLE 3-5 Oxygen Concentration and Total Flow from the Misty Ox GIN Nebulizer

Oxygen (L/min)		Air (L/min)	
Primary Gas	Secondary Gas	Total Flow	Concentration
40	0	40	100%
40	10	50	84.2%
40	20	60	73.6%
40	30	70	66.1%
40	40	80	60.5%
40	50	90	56.1%
40	60	100	52.6%
40	70	110	49.7%

TABLE 3-6 Oxygen Concentration and Total Flow from the Misty Ox GIN Nebulizer

Air (L/min)		Oxygen (L/min)	
Primary Gas	Secondary Gas	Total Flow	Concentration
40	0	40	20.9%
40	10	50	36.8%
40	20	60	47.3%
40	30	70	54.9%
40	40	80	60.5%
40	50	90	64.9%
40	60	100	68.4%
40	70	110	71.3%

Vortan HEART Nebulizer

The Vortan HEART (High Output Extended Aerosol Respiratory Therapy) nebulizer is intended for continuous administration of aerosolized medication (Figure 3-37). In some patients, frequent administration of small-volume nebulizer treatments becomes ineffective, and continuous nebulization of bronchoactive agents is then warranted. The nebulizer has a 240-ml reservoir and obtains a particle size of between 3.5 and 2.2 microns in diameter.

Figure 3-37 *A photograph of the HEART nebulizer.*

Mistogen HV-12

The Mistogen HV-12 is a high-volume nebulizer intended for use with the Mistogen CAM 3 tent. It can also be used for room humidity by placing it on a stand designed for this use (Figure 3-38). It is a pneumatic nebulizer that uses choked flow to create a dense aerosol.

Figure 3-38 *The Mistogen HV-12 nebulizer.*

ASSEMBLY AND TROUBLESHOOTING

Assembly—Mistogen HV-12

1. Push the inlet filter into the air dilution control fitting and secure the dilution control assembly to the lid of the nebulizer.

2. Attach the feed/filter assembly tube to the jet/baffle assembly by pressing the feed tube onto the jet.

3. Screw the jet/baffle assembly into place on the gas inlet elbow.

4. Fill the reservoir with sterile distilled water.

5. Mate the lid to the reservoir, using the two slide clips on the lid to attach them.

6. Connect the nebulizer to a 50-psi gas source set for between 12 and 15 liters per minute.

Troubleshooting

When troubleshooting this equipment, please follow the suggested troubleshooting algorithm (ALG 3-9)

If aerosol production is inadequate or absent:

1. Check the water level in the reservoir.

2. Ensure the feed tube is attached properly and not obstructed and that the jet/baffle assembly is attached securely.

3. Ensure that the gas source is adequate.

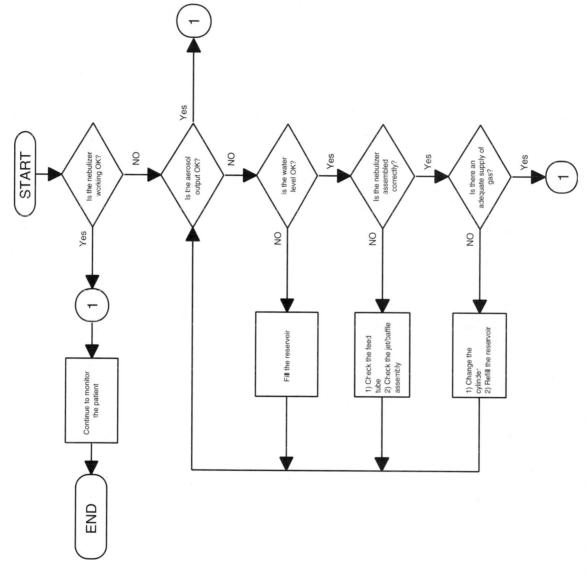

ALG 3-9 *An algorithm describing how to troubleshoot the Mistogen HV-12 nebulizer.*

BABBINGTON NEBULIZERS

Babbington nebulizers are pneumatically powered nebulizers that use the **Babbington principle** in their operation. The Babbington nebulizers have the brand names Solosphere, Hydrosphere, and Maxi-Cool. These are very efficient high output nebulizers that produce particle sizes ranging from 3 to 5 microns in diameter.

Gas entering the nebulizer is separated into two channels (Figure 3-39). One pressurizes a glass sphere and the other forms small bubbles that are pushed up a capillary tube to a reservoir above the glass sphere.

The bubbles carry small amounts of water up the tube to the reservoir, gradually filling it. The reservoir drains by gravity, and the water drips onto the glass sphere forming a very thin sheet.

Gas pressure exits the sphere through a very small hole, creating near supersonic velocities. The high velocity gas ruptures the thin sheet of water, producing a fine aerosol.

A baffle placed in the path of the gas flow further reduces the particle size.

Figure 3-39 *A functional diagram of a Babbington nebulizer.*

Solosphere

The Solosphere nebulizer is intended for long-term aerosol therapy and may be used interchangeably with the other large-volume nebulizers discussed earlier. Figure 3-40 shows a photograph and an assembly drawing of the Solosphere nebulizer.

The Solosphere nebulizer also incorporates an adjustable air entrainment port. When the nebulizer is powered with oxygen, the air entrainment ports allow F_IO_2 adjustments of .40, .50, .60, .80, and 1.00. Air is entrained into the nebulizer by jet mixing. As the air entrain-

Figure 3-40 *A photograph and an assembly drawing of the Solosphere nebulizer.*

ment is decreased, total flow through the nebulizer also decreases.

As with any entrainment device, downstream resistance in the tubing distal to the nebulizer will alter the room air entrainment characteristics of the device such that less air is entrained, increasing the delivered F_IO_2 and decreasing the total flow.

ASSEMBLY AND TROUBLESHOOTING

Assembly—Solosphere Nebulizer

1. Plug the bottom of the pick up tube (capillary tube) with the plug provided.

2. Push the bubble pump plug into place with the flat side facing the ball.

3. Be certain that the large "O" ring is in place on the lid assembly.

4. Insert the manifold assembly into the jar of the nebulizer and secure it in place using the two provided screws.

5. Fill the reservoir with sterile distilled water.

6. Screw the reservoir to the lid of the nebulizer.

7. Attach the nebulizer to a flowmeter and adjust to the ordered flow and F_IO_2.

Troubleshooting

When troubleshooting this equipment, please follow the suggested troubleshooting algorithm (ALG 3-10).

If aerosol production is inadequate:

1. Check the fluid level in the reservoir.

2. Check that the bottom and bubble pump plugs are in place.

3. Make certain the ball is in place and not damaged.

4. Check the DISS fitting for tightness.

5. Check the outlet and aerosol tubing for obstructions.

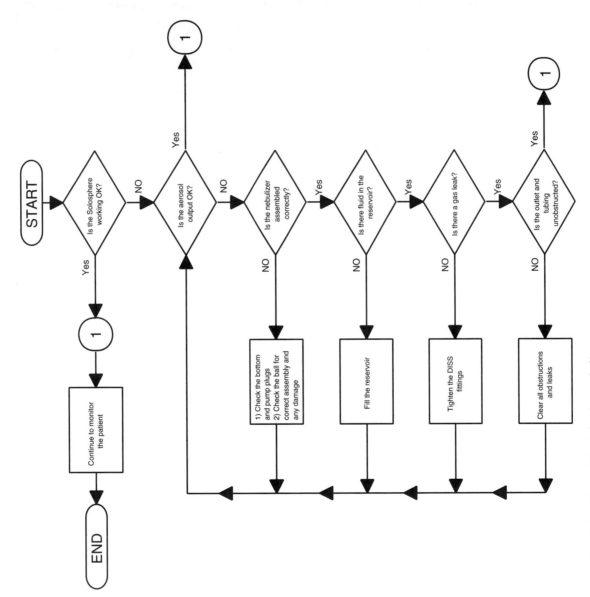

ALG 3-10   *An algorithm describing how to troubleshoot the Solosphere nebulizer.*

Maxi-Cool Nebulizer

The Maxi-Cool nebulizer is a dual ball Babbington nebulizer designed to be used with the Maxi-Cool aerosol tent. It operates using two Babbington nebulizers to produce a very fine dense aerosol (Figure 3-41).

An air entrainment fitting is provided to adjust the F_IO_2 to between .28 and .98 when powered by oxygen. Adjustment of the F_IO_2 control varies the air entrainment through the nebulizer. Total flows can vary from between 30 to 285 liters per minute, depending on the entrainment adjustment. If aerosol therapy without oxygen administration is the desired goal, the Maxi-Cool may be operated using compressed air.

ASSEMBLY AND TROUBLESHOOTING

Refer to ALG 3-11 and Figure 3-41 when following the assembly and trouble-shooting procedures.

Assembly—Maxi-Cool Nebulizer

1. Install the pump plug onto the base of the manifold by pressing it into place.

2. Install the two ball/baffle assemblies, checking the integrity of the "O" rings on their seats. Lock the assemblies into place with the tabs on the manifold.

3. Ensure that the large "O" ring is in place on the top of the nebulizer lid.

4. Press the manifold and the lid together, mating the two pieces.

5. Fill the reservoir with sterile distilled water.

6. Attach the lid to the reservoir by twisting the two components together.

7. Place the reservoir/nebulizer assembly into the housing base and press the cover into position, locking the reservoir/nebulizer assembly.

8. Attach the air entrainment fitting to the inlet opening and attach the large-bore delivery tubing to the other.

9. Connect the nebulizer to a 50-psi compressed gas source using a high pressure hose.

Troubleshooting

When troubleshooting this equipment, please follow the suggested troubleshooting algorithm (ALG 3-11).

If aerosol production is inadequate:

1. Check the fluid level in the reservoir.

2. Check that the bubble pump plug is in place.

3. Make certain the ball/baffle assemblies are in place and not damaged.

4. Check the DISS fitting for tightness.

5. Check the outlet and aerosol tubing for obstructions.

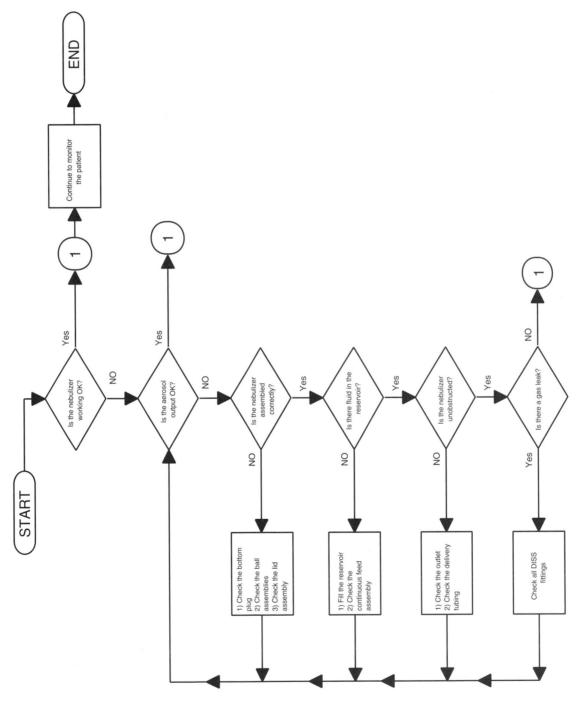

ALG 3-11 *An algorithm describing how to troubleshoot the Maxi-Cool nebulizer.*

Figure 3-41 *An assembly drawing of the Maxi-Cool nebulizer.*

SMALL-PARTICLE AEROSOL GENERATOR

ICN Pharmaceuticals, Inc., SPAG-2

The Small Particle Aerosol Generator-2 (SPAG-2) (Figure 3-42), manufactured by ICN Pharmaceuticals, Inc., is a pneumatically powered nebulizer designed specifically for the administration of ribaviran (Virazole®). Ribavirin is a medication that is specific for the treatment of respiratory syncytial virus (RSV), a common illness in infants and small children.

Ribaviran is a powder which is reconstituted by the addition of 300 ml of sterile water in the nebulizer flask or reservoir. Once the drug has been mixed, the nebulizer breaks the liquid into fine aerosol particles with a mean diameter of 1.3 microns. The SPAG-2 is unique when compared to other nebulizers, in that it has its own regulated gas supply (26 psi) and a secondary gas supply for drying the aerosol particles. The secondary gas supply has a flow adjustment of 2 to 9 L/min. The secondary gas supply is directed through a drying chamber where the aerosol particles evaporate, further reducing the diameter of the particles.

Precautions

Since infants and young children are unable to cooperate using small-volume nebulizers, the SPAG-2 has been designed to administer ribaviran to a tent or hood. When administered in this way, aerosolized ribaviran may be released into the patient's room.

Ribaviran has caused toxicity effects in some caregivers including conjunctivitis, rash, and bronchospasm. Additionally, women who are pregnant or nursing should not be exposed to ribaviran. Because these effects have been reported, environmental and personal protective equipment precautions should be taken when administering this drug.

Environmental precautions should include a private room with negative-pressure ventilation of at least six air changes per hour. When the patient requires routine types of care, the aerosol therapy should be interrupted, and sufficient time allowed for the aerosol particles to clear. Personal protective equipment should include a HEPA mask, gloves, gown, and goggles.

Figure 3-42 *A photograph of the ICN Pharmaceuticals, Inc., SPAG-2 nebulizer for the administration of ribaviran. (Courtesy ICN Pharmaceuticals, Inc., Costa Mesa, CA)*

ASSEMBLY AND TROUBLESHOOTING

Assembly—SPAG-2 Nebulizer

1. Reconstitute the ribaviran in the reservoir flask by mixing one vial (6 grams) of lyophilized ribaviran into 300 mL of sterile water using aseptic technique.

2. Insert the nebulizer stem into the reservoir cap and place the cap onto the reservoir flask.

3. Insert the reservoir assembly into the nebulizer housing and snap it into place in the bracket.

4. Insert the drying chamber through the wall of the SPAG-2 housing, pressing it into the "O" ring of the cap assembly.

5. Connect the two gas supplies, one to the nebulizer air fitting and the other to the drying air fitting.

6. Connect the gas source (40–60 psi regulated range) to the regulator inlet and adjust the pressure to 26 psi.

7. Open the nebulizer flowmeter completely. The nebulizer flowmeter should indicate 6½ to 8½ L/min. Readjust the regulator to 26 psi, if required.

8. Turn on the drying air flowmeter and readjust the reducing valve to 26 psi, as required. Adjust the drying air flowmeter to 3½ to 6½ L/min. Total flow (nebulizer + drying air) should be 15 L/min. Verify that there are three spray spots with a pattern of approximately 2.5-cm diameter.

Troubleshooting

When troubleshooting this equipment, please follow the suggested troubleshooting algorithm (ALG 3-12).

Little or no aerosol output:

1. Check to be sure that there is reconstituted ribaviran in the reservoir assembly.

2. Check the nebulizer stem for correct assembly. Check for obstruction in the nebulizer orifices.

3. Check the nebulizer drive line for correct attachment.

4. Make sure that the regulator is set for 26 psi.

5. Verify both the nebulizer and air flowmeter settings (total flow should equal 15 L/min).

6. Check all connectors for leaks.

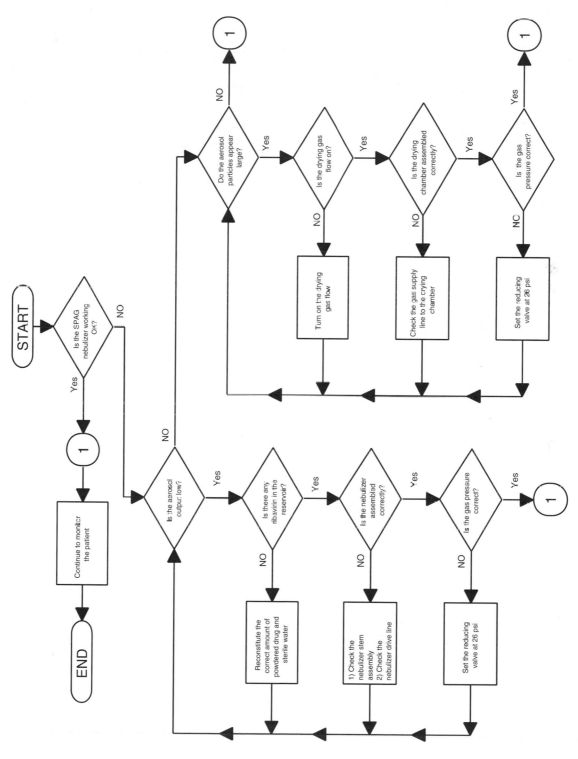

ALG 3-12 *An algorithm describing how to troubleshoot the SPAG-2 nebulizer.*

ULTRASONIC NEBULIZERS

Ultrasonic nebulizers operate by using high-frequency sound waves to produce a fine aerosol. The components of an ultrasonic nebulizer include a radio frequency generator, shielded cable, piezoelectric crystal or transducer, reservoir chamber, and a fan. Before discussing the operating principles of an ultrasonic nebulizer, it is important to understand the difference between frequency and amplitude of a wave form. **Frequency** refers to the number of wave forms per second, or **Hertz** (Hz). The term **amplitude** refers to the height of the wave form from the crest to the trough. In an ultrasonic nebulizer, increasing the frequency causes a decrease in particle size because more waves impact the surface of the water. By increasing amplitude without altering frequency, aerosol output or quantity is increased. This is because each wave has more energy (amplitude). Figure 3-43 illustrates two waveforms with differing amplitudes and frequencies.

The radio frequency (RF) generator produces electromagnetic energy or waves at approximately 1.35 MHz (million cycles per second). The RF generator is an electrically powered electronically controlled RF oscillator (Figure 3-44). The frequency (1.35 MHz) is fixed, while the amplitude is usually variable.

The RF energy from the radio frequency generator is conducted to the transducer via a shielded cable. The term "shielded" means that the core of the cable conducting the RF energy is completely surrounded by a braided wire that is connected to an electrical ground. This prevents RF energy from being radiated and causing interference to other electrical equipment close by.

The transducer contains the **piezoelectric crystal**. The piezoelectric crystal has the ability to change shape as an electrical current is applied to it. Thus, electrical energy (RF energy) is converted to mechanical energy (sound waves). The piezoelectric crystal oscillates at the same frequency as the RF energy applied to it.

The sound waves are directed and focused against the surface of the water in the reservoir. The high-frequency sound waves break the water up into a fine aerosol with particle sizes ranging from 1 to 10 microns.

The fan evacuates the aerosol from the reservoir chamber. The aerosol is then conducted to the patient using large-bore aerosol

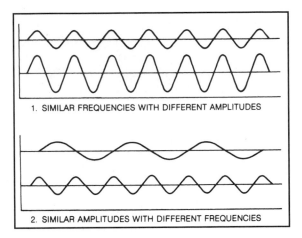

Figure 3-43 *A comparison between frequency and amplitude.*

Figure 3-44 *A functional diagram of an ultrasonic nebulizer.*

tubing. Without the fan, the aerosol would be produced but would lack clinically significant flow.

Hazards of ultrasonic nebulizers include nosocomial infections and electrical shock hazards. Nosocomial infection transmission is a problem due to the large, stagnant reservoir. Furthermore, many nebulizers are taken from one room to another and used with different patients. Frequent reservoir changes and cleaning or the use of disposable reservoirs will reduce infection complications. Electrical shock may be prevented by ensuring that the surrounding floor is kept free of water spills and condensation from the nebulizer. A wet floor serves as an excellent ground pathway.

Ultra-Neb 99

The DeVilbiss Ultra-Neb 99 is an ultrasonic nebulizer capable of producing a minimum of 6 ml per minute of aerosol at the maximum setting (Figure 3-45). These nebulizers are commonly employed in the clinical setting both for direct aerosol application (aerosol mask or face tent) and at the bedside. A reservoir holds up to 200 ml of solution for nebulization.

Timeter Compu-Neb

The Timeter Compu-Neb is an ultrasonic nebulizer commonly used in the clinical environment (Figure 3-46). It operates using the principles discussed in this chapter.

Figure 3-46 *The Timeter Model MP-500 Compu-Neb ultrasonic nebulizer. (Courtesy Allied Healthcare Products, Inc.–Timeter Instrument Corporation. Timeter Instrument Corporation is a division of Allied Healthcare Products, Inc., St. Louis, MO)*

Figure 3-45 *The DeVilbiss Ultra-Neb 99. (Courtesy DeVilbiss Health Care, Inc., Somerset, PA)*

ASSEMBLY AND TROUBLESHOOTING

Assembly— Ultrasonic Nebulizers

1. Connect the nebulizer to a 120 volt, 60 Hz power source.

2. Insert the nebulization chamber into the cylindrical receptacle at the front of the nebulizer. Align the nebulization chamber such that the slot matches the raised rib at the front of the receptacle.

3. Place the lid on the top of the nebulization chamber.

4. Attach the feed system to the reservoir bottle and clamp the feed tube. Invert the bottle and hang it from the bottle support arm.

5. Connect the feed system to the nebulization chamber by attaching the tubing to the nipple on the nebulizer lid. Unclamp the feed tubing, and the nebulizer will automatically fill.

6. Connect a short length of 22-mm diameter aerosol tubing between the nebulization chamber and the fan on the rear of the nebulizer. This will evacuate the aerosol from the nebulization chamber.

7. Connect a 60-inch length of 22-mm diameter aerosol tubing from the nebulization chamber to the patient.

8. If a disposable prefilled couplant chamber is to be used:
   a. Install the nebulization chamber as described in (2) above.
   b. Install the RF shield into the bottom of the nebulization chamber, aligning the notch on the circumference with the float assembly.
   c. Fill the chamber with sterile water to the fill line on the side of the chamber.
   d. Place the adapter ring onto the nebulizer chamber. Insert the disposable couplant into the nebulization chamber, seating it.
   e. Connect aerosol tubing to the prefilled chamber as described in (6) and (7).

Troubleshooting

When troubleshooting this equipment, please follow the suggested troubleshooting algorithm (ALG 3-13).

1. If the unit fails to operate and, when turned on, the "On/Off" switch does not illuminate:
   a. Ensure that the power cord is connected to a 120 v, 60 Hz outlet.
   b. Check the fuse at the rear of the nebulizer, and if necessary, replace it.

2. If aerosol output is diminished or absent:
   a. Check the "Check Chamber" indicator light. If the light is illuminated, the water level in the nebulization chamber is low.
   b. Check the delivery tubing for obstructions or accumulated condensate.
   c. Ensure that the tubing from the fan is attached to the chamber and that the fan is working.
   d. Check the float to ensure that it is free to travel up and down on its attachment rod.
   e. The chamber may have become contaminated. Wash the nebulizer chamber with alcohol or 2% acetic acid.

SMALL-VOLUME ULTRASONIC NEBULIZERS FOR MEDICATION DELIVERY

Small-volume (less than 10 ml) nebulizers have been developed for medication delivery. These devices use ultrasonic transducers to break liquid medication into fine aerosol particles for inhalation. Since these are ultrasonic nebulizers, more aerosol particles fall into the small particle size ranges, which improves aerosol penetration. Unlike the larger, continuous ultrasonic nebulizers, these smaller versions are very lightweight and portable. All of the units can be operated on internal battery packs, a 12 V DC power source or from a

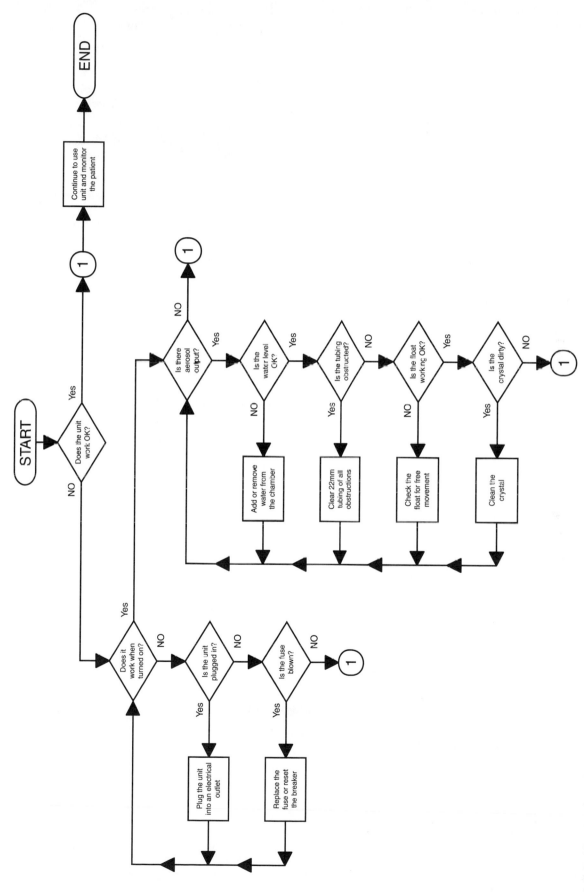

ALG 3-13 *An algorithm describing how to troubleshoot ultrasonic nebulizers.*

120 volt, 60 Hz adapter. The portability of these nebulizers makes them very convenient for patient use in the home or other settings away from acute care facilities.

DeVilbiss Pulmosonic 5500 Nebulizer

The DeVilbiss Health Care, Inc. Pulmosonic 5500 ultrasonic nebulizer is a small, portable ultrasonic nebulizer designed for medication administration (Figure 3-47). Being truly portable (10.3 ounces, or 292 grams), it can operate from an internal battery pack, 12 V DC power or via a 120 v, 60 Hz power adapter.

Theory of Operation

When the patient depresses a switch plate on the front of the unit, ultrasonic energy is directed into the medication dome, breaking the liquid medication into a fine aerosol. Aerosol will only be produced as long as the switch plate is depressed. The patient is encouraged to release the switch plate during exhalation, conserving medication. A one-way valve on the mouthpiece assembly allows the patient to exhale through the mouthpiece without removing it from the mouth.

Flow through the unit may be adjusted by rotating the flow cap on the back of the nebulizer. Rotating the flow cap adjusts the amount of ambient air entering the dome. By increas-

Figure 3-47 *A photograph of the DeVilbiss Pulmosonic 5500 ultrasonic nebulizer. (Courtesy Sunrise Medical)*

ing ambient air entrainment, flow is increased through the medication dome.

Microstat (CAIRE, Inc.)

The CAIRE, Inc., Microstat is a small, portable ultrasonic nebulizer designed for medication delivery (Figure 3-48). It weighs under 2 pounds, including the battery pack. The unit may also be powered by a 12 V DC power source or from a 115 v, 60 Hz electrical

Figure 3-48 *A photograph of the Microstat ultrasonic nebulizer. (Courtesy CAIRE, Inc., Bloomington, MN)*

outlet, using the adapter provided by the manufacturer.

Theory of Operation

The Microstat uses ultrasonic energy to break the liquid medication into a fine aerosol. The aerosol particles range between 3 and 5 microns. As the aerosol rises toward the outlet of the medicine chamber, it passes through a spiral-shaped set of baffles, which removes larger particles from suspension. The larger particles fall to the base of the medicine chamber, where they will be nebulized again. The baffling system ensures delivery of a uniform, stable particle size.

ASSEMBLY AND TROUBLESHOOTING

Assembly—Small-Volume Ultrasonic Nebulizers

1. Detach the nebulizer head cover assembly from the nebulizer head (Figure 3-48).

2. Fill the medicine chamber using the medication and dilution prescribed by the physician.

3. Attach the nebulizer head cover assembly to the nebulizer head.

4. Attach a mouthpiece to the nebulizer head cover assembly.

5. Depress the "On" button on the front of the unit. Aerosolized medication will appear in the nebulizer head cover within 10 seconds.

6. Instruct the patient to take slow, deep breaths. A one-way valve allows medication delivery only during inspiration. To exhale, have the patient remove the mouthpiece from his or her mouth and exhale passively or exhale through his or her nose.

   a. During therapy keep the nebulizer upright (vertical). If it is tipped, medication may be lost.

Cleaning

After each use it is recommended that the unit be cleaned.

1. Disconnect the nebulizer head and nebulizer head cover from the nebulizer control unit by unplugging the end plug.

2. Remove the nebulizer head cover from the nebulizer head and disassemble it.

3. Gently wash the parts in a mild detergent and water. Never immerse the end plug in water or any solution.

4. Rinse the parts in clean water and allow them to air dry.

5. Weekly, soak all parts (except the end plug) in a solution of white vinegar and water or cold disinfecting agent (Control III, Cidex, etc.).

Troubleshooting

When troubleshooting this equipment, please follow the suggested troubleshooting algorithm (ALG 3-14).

The nebulizer is operating but a light is rapidly flashing:

1. The battery level is low. Recharge the battery for 24 hours using the supplied AC power adapter.

The nebulizer will not work and a light is slowly flashing:

1. There is insufficient power in the internal battery pack to power the nebulizer. Recharge the battery as described above.

The nebulizer will not operate. The "ON" light illuminates for a few seconds, then turns off.

1. The nebulizer is not connected properly to the control unit. Reattach the end plug to the nebulizer control unit.

The nebulizer will not operate:

1. Check to ensure that the battery is properly installed.

2. Check to ensure the external power source and adapters are installed correctly.

3. The unit has malfunctioned. Contact your service representative.

4. The unit has overheated. Wait several minutes and restart the nebulizer.

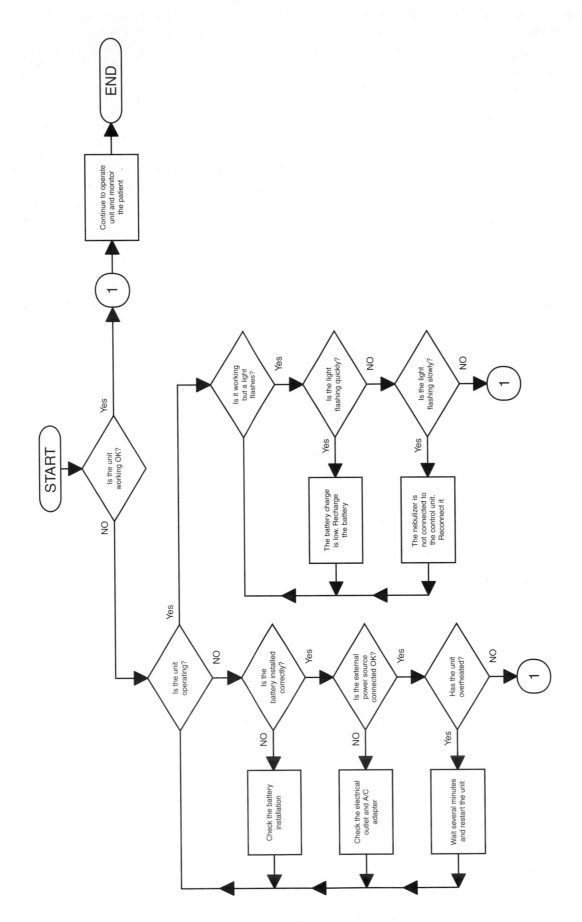

ALG 3-14 *An algorithm describing how to troubleshoot small-volume ultrasonic nebulizers.*

AEROSOL ADMINISTRATION DEVICES

Aerosol produced by a nebulizer must be safely and effectively conducted to the patient. Various devices have been designed to improve aerosol delivery for a variety of clinical applications. These devices include the aerosol mask, trach mask, face tent, and Brigg's adapter or aerosol T.

The aerosol mask (Figure 3-49) is similar to the simple oxygen mask. The inlet, however, is designed for large-bore tubing. The two outlet ports are also large to facilitate evacuation of any exhaled aerosol.

The trach mask is designed to fit over a tracheostomy tube (Figure 3-50). It is secured by an elastic strap that surrounds the neck. A 22-mm large-bore inlet fitting accommodates the aerosol tubing and a single large outlet port evacuates exhaled aerosol.

The face tent is designed to be strapped under the chin, enclosing the lower part of a patient's face (Figure 3-51). This device is commonly used in the recovery room following general anesthesia or for patients with facial burns.

Figure 3-50 *A tracheostomy aerosol mask.*

The Brigg's adapter is designed to be used with an artificial airway. It is also commonly referred to as an aerosol T. The Brigg's adapter has two 22-mm ports opposite one another

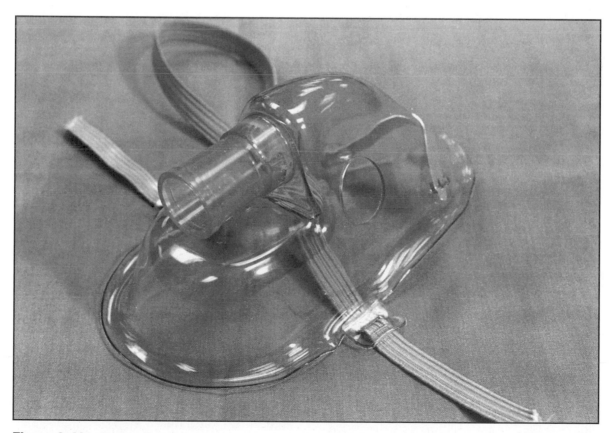

Figure 3-49 *An aerosol mask.*

Figure 3-51 *A patient wearing a face tent.*

and a 15-mm port at right angles to them, forming a T (Figure 3-52).

When using the Brigg's adapter with an artificial airway, it is important to install a short (approximately 6 inches) piece of aerosol tubing on the outlet of the adapter. This tubing serves as a reservoir, and prevents the patient from entraining room air during early inspiration. Adequate flow can be assured by observing the mist output through the reservoir. The flow of mist should never cease during the inspiratory phase; only then can you be sure that no air entrainment is occurring.

Although not technically an aerosol deliv-

Figure 3-52 *An aerosol T. This is also known as a Brigg's adapter.*

ery device, drainage bags are an important part of an aerosol therapy circuit (Figure 3-53). The drainage bag is placed at a low point in the tubing between the aerosol generator and the patient. Its purpose is to collect water condensation, thus preventing contamination of the reservoir and the patient. With air entrainment devices, the drainage bag also prevents water accumulation, created by condensation, from causing an increase in F_IO_2 due to back pressure.

PEDIATRIC AEROSOL TENTS

Pediatric aerosol tents are environmental devices frequently used in the treatment of croup, epiglottitis, and other pediatric upper airway disorders. They are designed to enclose the child in an atmosphere of cool aerosol. Oxygen may be administered, as well as aerosol, to correct hypoxemia, as required.

CROUPETTE

The croupette is commonly used for pediatric aerosol therapy. The croupette was discussed in Chapter 1, in the section on enclosures. Refer to Chapter 1 for its assembly and troubleshooting.

Figure 3-53 *A drainage bag. This bag is placed between the aerosol generator and the patient to collect condensate.*

OHMEDA PEDIATRIC AEROSOL TENT

The Ohmeda Pediatric Aerosol tent is a self-contained refrigerated aerosol generator (Figure 3-54). The tent provides both aerosol generation and refrigeration to keep the atmosphere inside the tent cool.

Figure 3-54 *The Ohmeda pediatric tent without a canopy attached.*

ASSEMBLY AND TROUBLESHOOTING

Assembly—Ohmeda Pediatric Aerosol Tent

1. Assemble the condensation bottle by screwing the cap on and attaching the condensate tube.

2. Place the condensation bottle into its bracket on the side of the main housing.

3. Assemble the cooling fan unit:
   a. Attach the radial finned plate to the evaporator bracket using the screws provided.
   b. Attach the blower wheel with the nut that secures it.
   c. Connect the condensation tube to the evaporator bracket.
   d. Attach the evaporator shroud by twisting it into place.

4. Attach the nebulizer to its bracket.

5. Erect the canopy support rod assembly over the bed or crib and secure it into place.

6. Attach the canopy to the frame, stretching the large opening over the rim of the evaporator shroud. Tuck the edges under the mattress for a tight seal.

7. Attach the large supply tubes to the two small holes in the canopy at the head of the bed.

8. Connect the nebulizer with high pressure hose to a flowmeter and set the flow between 12 and 15 liters per minute.

9. Fill the reservoir with sterile distilled water.

10. Connect the power cord to a 110-volt source.

11. Turn on the refrigeration unit.

Troubleshooting

When troubleshooting this equipment, please follow the suggested troubleshooting algorithm (ALG 3-15).

If aerosol output is low or absent:

1. Check to see if the reservoir is filled to the correct level.

2. Check the flowmeter setting and the high pressure hose connections.

3. Check the inlet tubing for obstructions.

4. Check the nebulizer jet for obstructions.

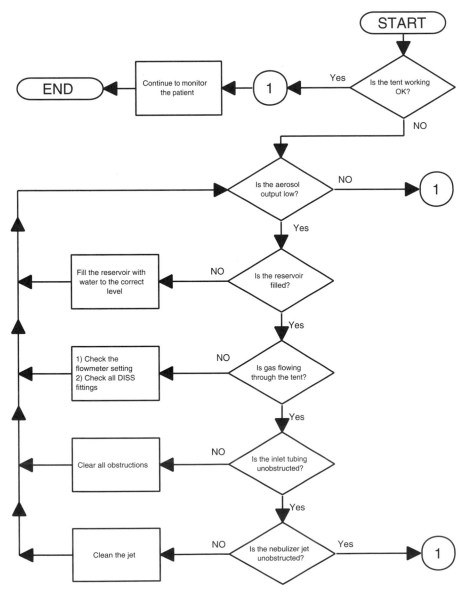

ALG 3-15 *An algorithm describing how to troubleshoot the Ohmeda pediatric aerosol tent.*

Mistogen Child Adult Mist (CAM) Tent

The Mistogen Child Adult Mist (CAM) tent (Figure 3-55) is designed to incorporate the Mistogen HV-12 nebulizer (discussed earlier) as its aerosol generator. In addition, the tent uses a refrigeration unit that chills and circulates water to cool the air inside the canopy.

Figure 3-55 *The Mistogen CAM tent. (Courtesy Allied Healthcare Products, Inc.—Timeter Instrument Corporation. Timeter Instrument Corporation is a division of Allied Healthcare Products, Inc., St. Louis, MO.)*

ASSEMBLY AND TROUBLESHOOTING

Assembly—Mistogen CAM Tent

1. Assemble the tent frame and position it at the head of the bed with the lower assembly under the mattress.

2. Connect the cooling panel by latching it and connecting the lower portion to its support blocks.

3. Attach the canopy to the canopy frame.

4. Fill the cooler reservoir with distilled water to the indicated level.

5. Install the coolant tubing between the cooling panel and the control unit.

6. Connect the drain tubing to the condensation trap on the control unit.

7. Assemble the HV-12 nebulizer as discussed earlier in this chapter and place it onto the cover of the control unit.

8. Connect the nebulizer tubing to the opening in the tent.

9. Plug the power cord into a 110-volt source and turn on the power.

Troubleshooting

When troubleshooting this equipment, please follow the suggested troubleshooting algorithm (ALG 3-16).

If aerosol production is inadequate or absent:

1. Check the water level in the reservoir.

2. Ensure the feed tube is attached properly and not obstructed and that the jet/baffle assembly is attached securely.

3. Ensure that the nebulizer is connected to a high-pressure gas source and that the flowmeter is on.

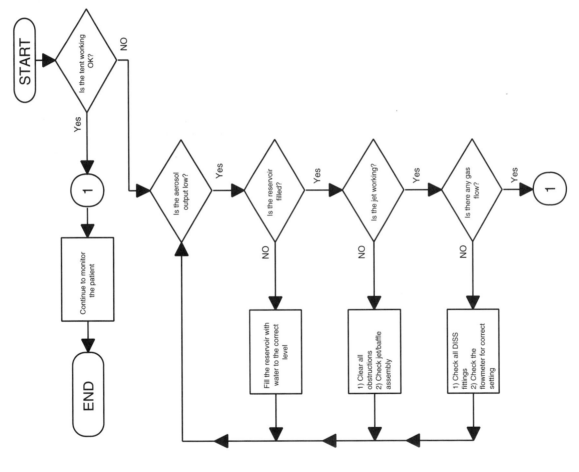

ALG 3-16 *An algorithm describing how to troubleshoot the Mistogen CAM tent.*

CLINICAL CORNER

Aerosol Therapy Equipment

1. You are taking care of a patient in an acute care setting and have just assembled a disposable, up-draft, small-volume nebulizer. When you turn on the flowmeter, the liquid medication simply bubbles and does not aerosolize. Describe the steps you would take to correct the situation.

2. You are taking care of a patient in the intensive care unit (ICU) who is on a 65% heated aerosol, and the flowmeter is set for 12 L/min. The patient is desaturating. Describe how you would assess the situation in the case where the flow from the nebulizer is adequate for the patient's inspiratory needs.

3. In a role-play situation, teach your instructor how to take a Metered Dose Inhaler treatment using a spacer.

4. You are expecting a new admission from surgery. The new patient is postoperative, having just had a tracheostomy tube placed. What equipment should you gather and how would you set it up to deliver 35% oxygen?

5. You are called to the medical floor to evaluate a patient on low-flow oxygen. A care assistant has called to alert you that the patient seems short of breath. Upon your arrival, you note the patient to be tachypneic and dyspneic. When you glance at the oxygen flowmeter, you notice that the disposable bubble humidifier is bulging and no bubbles can be observed. Describe the steps you would take in troubleshooting this situation.

6. You are setting up an ultrasonic nebulizer in preparation for a 20-minute treatment. When you turn the nebulizer on, the fan runs and the water in the reservoir is agitated, but no aerosol is produced. Describe how you would troubleshoot the situation.

Self-Assessment Quiz

1. Humidity is measured by:
   I. particle size.
   II. partial pressure.
   III. percentage.
   IV. water content.
   a. I and II only
   b. II and III only
   c. III and IV only
   d. III and IV only

2. An aerosol is defined as:
   a. water contained in a gas as vapor.
   b. particulate matter suspended in a gas.
   c. the maximum amount of water content a gas can contain at a given temperature.
   d. the actual water content of a gas at a given temperature.

3. The definition of capacity is:
   a. water contained in a gas as vapor.
   b. particulate matter suspended in a gas.
   c. the maximum amount of water content a gas can contain at a given temperature.
   d. the actual water content of a gas at a given temperature.

4. You must deliver a maximal amount of humidity to a patient's airway; how could this be accomplished using a diffusion grid humidifier?
   I. Increase the setting on the thermostat to a maximum of 37 degrees Celsius.
   II. Keep the water in the reservoir at the correct level.
   III. Ensure that the total flow through the humidifier exceeds the patient's requirements.
   IV. Use water traps or a drainage bag in the circuit.

a. I
b. I and II
c. I, II, and III
d. I, II, III, and IV

5. You are administering oxygen to a patient via a bubble-type humidifier. You know the humidity output is 14.5 mg/L (from a study published in *Respiratory Care*). What is the humidity deficit?
a. 14.5 mg/L
b. 29.4 mg/L
c. 43.9 mg/L
d. 47.0 mg/L

6. An advantage of the Misty Ox Laminar Diffuser Humidifier, when compared to a bubble jet humidifier, is:
a. High-flow outputs at high humidity are possible.
b. It is designed for low-flow oxygen delivery systems.
c. It only delivers cool aerosol.
d. None of the above are correct.

7. The majority of humidifiers operate using the phenomenon of:
a. Bernoulli's principle.
b. ultrasonic waves.
c. evaporation.
d. Venturi's principle.

8. Ways to improve a humidifier's efficiency include:
I. increase the temperature.
II. increase the jet's lateral pressure.
III. increase the surface area.
IV. increase the gas velocity through the device.
a. I and II only
b. III and IV only
c. II and III only
d. II and IV only

9. The magnitude of the pressure exerted by water vapor is dependent upon:
I. temperature.
II. relative humidity.
III. barometric pressure.
a. I
b. I and II
c. I and III
d. II and III

10. Factors that influence an aerosol's deposition in the lungs include:
I. particle size.
II. gravity.
III. inertia.
a. I only
b. II only
c. I and II only
d. I, II, and III only

11. The piezoelectric crystal in an ultrasonic nebulizer:
a. converts electrical energy to mechanical energy.
b. converts water to vapor.
c. vibrates at a low frequency causing hydrolysis.
d. cools the aerosol when operated with the fan.

12. Which of the following humidifiers would be suitable for use for a patient requiring a simple oxygen mask?
    I. bubble humidifier
    II. wick humidifier
    III. bubble jet humidifier
    IV. Misty Ox LDH humidifier
    a. I and II
    b. I and III
    c. II and III
    d. II and IV

13. You must provide humidified gas for a patient who is intubated; which of the following devices would be the most appropriate?
    I. bubble humidifier
    II. wick humidifier
    III. bubble jet humidifier
    IV. Misty Ox LDH humidifier
    a. I and II
    b. I and III
    c. II and III
    d. II and IV

14. When checking oxygen in a patient's room, you hear an audible chirping or whistling sound. The most likely cause is:
    a. the patient's inspiratory stridor.
    b. the nurse's call button.
    c. the humidifier pop-off.
    d. flow through the patient's venturi mask.

15. Contemporary high output humidifiers employ which of the following in their operation?
    I. Bernoulli's principle
    II. a wick
    III. a piezoelectric crystal
    IV. a heater
    a. I and II only
    b. I and III only
    c. II and III only
    d. II and IV only

16. The most common type of humidifier in clinical practice is:
    a. the bubble humidifier.
    b. the room humidifier.
    c. the wick humidifier.
    d. the pass-over humidifier.

17. An indication that a heat and moisture exchanger is becoming obstructed would be:
    a. The patient's work of breathing is increased.
    b. The water reservoir rarely needs filling anymore.
    c. The resistance to gas flow decreases.
    d. Pressure decreases distal to the exchanger.

18. A heat and moisture exchanger should be:
    I. placed between the ventilator circuit, or oxygen therapy equipment, and the patient's airway.
    II. utilized for short term applications (less than 24 hours).
    III. monitored for obstruction.
    a. I
    b. I and II
    c. II and III
    d. I, II, and III

19. Which of the following humidifiers would be suitable for use with a mechanical ventilator?
    I. Fisher and Paykel MR 730
    II. Ohmeda Ohio Bubble Jet humidifier
    III. Hudson RCI Conchapack
    IV. room humidifier
    a. I and II only
    b. I and III only
    c. III and IV only
    d. II and IV only

20. Advantages of metered dose inhalers (MDIs) include:
    I. small size.
    II. ease of use.
    III. inert nature of the propellants.
    a. I
    b. I and II
    c. II and III
    d. I, II, and III

21. A spacer device may be helpful:
    I. to improve the patient's coordination and timing.
    II. to improve the particle size inhaled by the patient.
    III. in that it acts as a baffle and reservoir.
    a. I
    b. I and II
    c. II and III
    d. I, II, and III

22. When using an MDI, the patient should be instructed to:
    I. take a slow deep breath.
    II. squeeze the MDI shortly after inspiration has begun.
    III. hold his or her breath following inspiration.
    IV. exhale passively.
    a. I
    b. I and II
    c. I, II, and III
    d. I, II, III, and IV

23. The most important aspect of using MDIs is:
    a. equipment care and cleaning.
    b. patient instruction.
    c. use of a spacer.
    d. infection control.

24. You are using a large-volume nebulizer to deliver aerosol and an F_IO_2 of 0.40 to a patient who is intubated. You measure the oxygen concentration and your analyzer reads 89%. The entrainment and flowmeter settings are correct. How might you troubleshoot this problem?
    I. check for water in the tubing
    II. check for kinks or obstructions
    III. check for loose fittings
    IV. make sure the nebulizer is assembled correctly and is not leaking
    a. I and II
    b. I and III
    c. II and III
    d. III and IV

25. An advantage of the Misty Ox Gas Injection Nebulizer (GIN) is that:
    I. high flow rates are possible.
    II. it may be heated.
    III. it is permanent and may be reused.
    IV. only one gas source is required.

a. I and II
b. I and III
c. II and III
d. III and IV

26. Entrainment of a liquid into a near sonic stream of gas by shear forces and vorticity is an application of:
    a. evaporation.
    b. Henry's law.
    c. choked flow.
    d. thermodynamics.

27. A patient may have difficulty using a bulb nebulizer:
    a. because the volume is so large.
    b. because the particle size is too large.
    c. because it produces body humidity.
    d. because of coordination.

28. Which of the following nebulizers employs choked flow in its operation?
    I. Bear VH-12
    II. Solosphere
    III. Mistogen HV-12
    IV. DeVilbiss Model 65
    a. I only
    b. II only
    c. III only
    d. IV only

29. Increasing the amplitude of an ultrasonic nebulizer:
    a. increases the water temperature.
    b. increases the rate of evaporation.
    c. increases the amount of aerosol output.
    d. decreases the particle size.

30. Which of the following mist tents incorporate(s) refrigeration units into their design?
    I. Croupette
    II. Ohio Pediatric Mist Tent
    III. Mistogen CAM tent
    a. I only
    b. I and II only
    c. II and III only
    d. I and III only

Selected Bibliography

American Association for Respiratory Care. (2003 rev.). Clinical practice guideline: Bland aerosol administration. *Respiratory Care, 48*(2), 529–533.

American Association for Respiratory Care. (1994). Clinical practice guideline: Delivery of aerosols to the upper airway. *Respiratory Care, 39*(8), 803–807.

American Association for Respiratory Care. (1996). Clinical practice guideline: Selection of a device for delivery of aerosol to the lung parenchyma. *Respiratory Care, 41*(7), 647–653.

American Association for Respiratory Care. (1992). Clinical practice guideline: Selection of aerosol delivery device. *Respiratory Care, 37*(8), 891–897.

American Association for Respiratory Care. Clinical practice guideline: Humidification during mechanical ventilation. *Respiratory Care, 37*(8), 887–890.

Bagwell, T. (1986). United States Patent Number, 4,767,576. Costa Mesa, CA: Medical Molding Corporation of America.

Bagwell, T. (1986). United States Patent Number, 4,629,590. Costa Mesa, CA: Medical Molding Corporation of America.

Branson, R. D., et al. Laboratory evaluation of moisture output of seven airway heat and moisture exchangers. *Respiratory Care, 32*(8), 741–747.

CAIRE, Inc. (1990). *Microstat user's guide.* Littleton, CO.

Darin, J. (1982). An evaluation of water-vapor output from four brands of unheated, prefilled bubble humidifiers. *Respiratory Care, 27*(1), 41–50.

Des Jardins, T. R. (2002). *Cardiopulmonary anatomy and physiology* (4th ed.). Clifton Park, NY: Thomson Delmar Learning.

DeVilbiss Health Care, Inc. (1993). *DeVilbiss AeroSonic Ultrasonic Nebulizer instruction guide.* Somerset, PA: Author.

Gagliardini, F. J. (1984). Ultrasonic nebulizers as room humidifiers (abstract). *Respiratory Care, 29*(10), 1025.

Greenway, L., et al. (1985). Static electricity generated by nebulizers (abstract). *Respiratory Care, 30*(10), 871.

ICN Pharmaceuticals, Inc. (1986). *Small Particle Aerosol Generator SPAG-2.* Costa Mesa, CA: Author.

Klopf, S., et al. (2000). Clinical evaluation of a breath actuated small volume nebulizer (BA-SVN). *Respiratory Care, 45*(8), 979.

Lewis, M. A., et al. (2000). Improving resource utilization with new technologies. *Respiratory Care, 45*(8), 981.

Op't Holt, T. (1988). Aerosol generators and humidifiers. In T. A. Barnes, et al. (Eds.), *Respiratory care practice.* Year Book Medical.

Perch, S. A., Jr., et al. (1984). Effectiveness of the Servo SH 150 artificial nose humidifier: A case report. *Respiratory Care, 29*(10), 1009–1012.

Rau, J. L. (2002). *Respiratory therapy pharmacology* (6th ed.). Year Book Medical.

Waskin, H. (1991). Toxicology of antimicrobial aerosols: A review of aerosolized ribaviran and pentamidine. *Respiratory Care, 36*(9), 1026–1036.

CHAPTER 4

HYPERINFLATION THERAPY EQUIPMENT

INTRODUCTION

Incentive spirometry is a mode of therapy commonly used to promote deep breathing and coughing. Both disposable and permanent equipment are available for this therapeutic modality. In this chapter you will learn about the equipment, how to operate it, and how to correctly assemble and troubleshoot it.

Positive-Expiratory-Pressure (PEP) mask therapy uses the application of positive end expiratory pressure with the patient exhaling actively to FRC, ending the breath at ambient pressure level. This application of expiratory pressure splints the airways open, facilitating secretion clearance.

Oscillating PEP therapy is similar to PEP therapy alone except that the device excites pressure vibrations throughout the lung parenchyma. The oscillating PEP therapy device incorporates a weighted ball valve that opens and closes at a high frequency, or a counterweighted lever and magnet that open and close a valve causing the vibrations in the lungs.

The use of Intermittent Positive Pressure Breathing (IPPB) has declined as a therapeutic procedure over the past several years. While most hospitals across the country still perform IPPB therapy, its frequency of use is low.

Some IPPB equipment may also be used for adult mechanical ventilation. The use of these machines for this purpose is uncommon due to the variability of the delivered tidal volume. The discussion in this chapter will focus primarily on their usage for hyperinflation therapy.

The two primary manufacturers of IPPB equipment, Bird Products Corporation and Puritan Bennett Corporation, still manufacture some IPPB machines. This chapter will be devoted to those machines still manufactured or supported with parts. In this chapter you will learn about IPPB equipment, its principles of operation, and how to assemble and troubleshoot it.

Intrapulmonary Percussive Ventilation (IPV®), although not considered IPPB therapy, has some elements that are similar to IPPB therapy, warranting its inclusion in this chapter. IPV® combines a high-frequency, pneumatically driven, time-cycled flow interrupter with a dense aerosol administration device. The combination of percussive, pulsed gas delivery with aerosolized medication delivery facilitates endobronchial secretion mobilization. As of this writing, one company has devices approved for sale and distribution (Percussionaire Corporation's IPV®-1 and IPV®-2). Other companies have devices that are currently under clinical investigation for FDA approval.

In addition to volume enhancement, secretion mobilization is an important aspect of hyperinflation therapy. Various percussors are employed in the facilitation of secretion removal during chest physiotherapy and postural drainage. These devices, and their clinical application, are important for the practitioner to understand.

OBJECTIVES

After completing this chapter, the student will accomplish the following objectives:

PHYSICS OF HYPERINFLATION THERAPY EQUIPMENT

- Describe the two principles used by disposable incentive spirometers to measure inspired volumes.
- Describe how inspiratory flow and volume may be measured using a photoelectric sensor.
- Describe two ways gas pressure may be regulated with IPPB ventilators.
- Describe how needle valves may be used to regulate gas flow for IPPB ventilators.

INDICATIONS FOR INCENTIVE SPIROMETRY AND POSITIVE AIRWAY PRESSURE ADJUNCTS TO BRONCHIAL HYGIENE THERAPY

- Describe the indications for incentive spirometry.
- Describe the indications for Positive Expiratory Pressure (PEP) and flutter valve therapy.
- Discuss the use of inspiratory muscle resistance training.

INCENTIVE SPIROMETRY EQUIPMENT

- Describe the principles of operation, assembly and troubleshooting for the following incentive spirometers.
  - Hudson RCI
    - Voldyne
    - Triflo™ II
  - DHD Medical Coach® 2
  - Monaghan Spirocare

POSITIVE-EXPIRATORY-PRESSURE (PEP) AND FLUTTER VALVE THERAPY EQUIPMENT

- Describe how Positive-Expiratory-Pressure (PEP) and flutter valve therapy equipment works and how to use them.
- Describe the Scandipharm flutter valve oscillatory PEP therapy device, how it works, and how to clinically apply it.
- Describe the DHD Acapella oscillatory PEP therapy device, how it works, and how to clinically apply it.

INSPIRATORY MUSCLE TRAINING DEVICES

- Describe how inspiratory muscle training devices operate and how to instruct the patient on their use.

INDICATIONS FOR INTERMITTENT POSITIVE PRESSURE BREATHING (IPPB) THERAPY

- Describe the indications for IPPB therapy.

INTERMITTENT POSITIVE PRESSURE BREATHING (IPPB) EQUIPMENT

Bird IPPB Ventilators

- For the Bird Mark 7, 7A, and 8, identify the following components:
  - Ambient chamber
  - Pressure chamber
  - Center body
  - Venturi/venturi gate assembly
  - Ceramic switch/clutch plate assembly
  - Permanent magnets
- Describe the purpose and operation of the following controls on the Bird IPPB machines:
  - Sensitivity control
  - Flow rate control
  - Air mix control
  - Expiratory timer
  - Pressure control
  - Negative pressure control
  - Time/pressure cycle control
  - Apneustic time control
- Explain how adjustment of the controls affects F_IO_2, inspiratory time, expiratory time, and tidal volume.
- Trace the gas flow through the Bird circuit.
- Describe the steps in assembly and troubleshooting of the Bird machines and their circuits.

Bennett IPPB Ventilators

- Describe the operation of the Bennett valve.
- Differentiate between the AP-5 and PR-2 and the clinical application of both.
- Describe the purpose and operation of the following controls on the Bennett AP-5 IPPB machine:
  - Pressure
  - Nebulization

- Describe the purpose and operation of the following controls on the Bennett PR-2 ventilator:
  — Pressure
  — Air dilution
  — Rate
  — Expiration time
  — Nebulizer
  — Negative pressure
  — Sensitivity
  — Terminal flow
  — Peak flow
- Describe the function of the two pressure manometers on the Bennett PR-2 ventilator.
- Explain how adjustment of the controls affects F_IO_2, inspiratory time, expiratory time, and tidal volume.
- Trace the flow of gas through a Bennett circuit.
- Describe the steps in assembly and troubleshooting of the Bennett machines.

PERCUSSIONAIRE CORPORATION IPV® VENTILATORS

- Describe Intrapulmonary Percussive Ventilation (IPV®) and its clinical efficacy.

- Describe the Percussionator® and its function in IPV®.
- Describe the operation of the Phasitron® and the concept of fluid clutching.
- Differentiate between the Percussionaire IPV®-1 and IPV®-2 and their clinical applications and control features.
- Identify the components of the IPV® circuit and its correct assembly.
- Describe the steps in troubleshooting of the IPV® ventilators.

SECRETION MOBILIZATION DEVICES

- Describe the operation and clinical application of the following percussors:
  — Vibramatic
  — Flimm Fighter
  — MJ Percussor
  — Adjunctive equipment for manual chest percussion
- Define High-Frequency Chest Wall Oscillation (HFCWO) Therapy.
- Describe how to assemble and use the Vest® HFCWO airway clearance system.
- Describe the Emerson Coughassist™ MI-E device and its application.

KEY TERMS

Asynchronous ventilation
Atelectasis
Biofeedback
Exhalation valve
Flutter valve therapy
High Frequency Chest Wall Oscillation therapy (HFCWO)

Incentive Spirometry
Inspiratory time
Inspiratory-to-expiratory (I:E) ratio
IPPB ventilators
Needle valve
Percussors

Positive-Expiratory-Pressure (PEP) therapy
Sensitivity
Tidal volume
Ventilators

PHYSICS OF HYPERINFLATION THERAPY EQUIPMENT

MEASUREMENT OF INSPIRED VOLUMES

Incentive spirometry is a therapeutic modality that relies on a patient's voluntary effort to perform a hyperinflation maneuver. Incentive spirometry equipment measures the inspired volumes and provides **biofeedback** to the patient using the device. When the patient can observe the inspired volume, he or she can be encouraged to work to inhale more. As the patient's effort increases, the transpulmonary pressures become greater, causing an increased inspired volume. This therapy is considered to be effective in the prevention and reversal of **atelectasis** and the promotion of coughing in postoperative patients.

Several methods of volume measurement are used in the operation of incentive spirometers, including flow dependent methods, volume displacement, and photoelectric measurement. Accuracy varies, depending on the method employed.

Flow Dependent Methods

A flow of gas applied across the top of a tube will cause a sub-ambient pressure to be developed in the tube (Figure 4-1A). If a float device is added to the tube, the sub-ambient pressure will cause the float to rise (Figure 4-1B), overcoming gravity. The weight of the float and diameter of the tube determine how much flow is required to raise it. If the flow measuring device is accurate, a known flow rate can be translated into a volume. For example:

An incentive spirometer requires a flow of 275 mL/second to raise a float. A patient inhales, raising the float, and sustains the flow (float is held up) for 3 seconds. How much volume did the patient inhale?

Volume = Flow rate × Time
= 275 mL/sec. × 3 seconds
= 825 mL

Volume Displacement

A patient who inhales air from a bellows causes the bellows to collapse as the gas is removed from it (Figure 4-2). Since one side is fixed and cannot move, bellows displacement is proportional to the inspired volume. This method of measurement can be quite accurate and is also used in some pulmonary function spirometers.

Photoelectric Measurement

A photoelectric flow sensor consists of a turbine or other flow measurement device, a

Figure 4-2 *A functional diagram of a bellows-type incentive spirometer.*

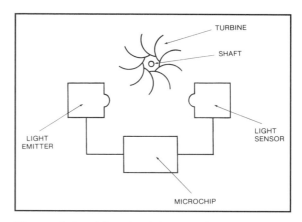

Figure 4-3 *A functional diagram of a photoelectric flow sensor.*

light emitting and sensing device, and an electronic circuit card or microchip. The turbine, when placed in the path of a light beam, will interrupt the beam as it turns (Figure 4-3). As the flow through the turbine increases, the light beam is interrupted at a faster rate.

Figure 4-1 *(A) Flow vertically through a tube causing reduced pressure. (B) Float rising in the tube in response to a pressure differential.*

The circuit card or microchip counts the rate at which the light beam is interrupted and translates it to a flow rate. By calibrating the sensing device, "X" number of interruptions can equal "Y" amount of flow. Volume can be measured by multiplying flow by the time the flow is sustained, as described above. This can all be accomplished electronically and virtually instantaneously.

GAS PRESSURE REGULATION

The reducing valves discussed in Chapter 1 are designed to reduce cylinder pressures to a working pressure of 50 psi. This pressure is too high to apply directly to a patient's lungs. **IPPB ventilators** reduce the pressure to between ambient pressure and 60 cmH$_2$O. Two different methods of reducing pressures are used by the manufacturers—a low pressure reducing valve (Puritan Bennett Corporation) and magnetic force opposing gas pressure (Bird Products Corporation).

Low Pressure Reducing Valve

Figure 4-4 shows a schematic of the Puritan Bennett reducing valve. Gas pressure entering the reducing valve displaces the diaphragm, opposing spring tension. When spring tension is overcome, the pivot closes the poppet valve. Gas escaping the pressure side reduces the pressure, causing spring tension to open the poppet valve again. This regulator functions in a way similar to those discussed in Chapter 1.

The spring tension may be varied by turning the knob on the face of the ventilator (pressure control). As spring tension is increased, the pressure from the regulator is also increased. Pressure is adjustable from zero to 45 cmH$_2$O.

Magnetic Attraction Opposing Gas Pressure

Figure 4-5 is a simplified schematic of the Bird IPPB ventilator's pressure chamber. Gas pressure within the chamber is conducted to a diaphragm through two holes in the center body. As gas pressure increases, the diaphragm moves to the left, causing a ceramic switch attached to it to close.

Magnetic attraction between a permanent magnet and a metal clutch plate opposes the movement of the diaphragm. Adjusting the pressure control causes the magnet to move closer to or farther from the metal clutch plate, varying the degree of magnetic attraction. If the magnet is moved closer to the clutch plate, it takes a greater pressure to move the diaphragm since magnetic attraction is greater.

GAS FLOW REGULATION

Needle valves are common devices used by manufacturers to regulate gas flow (Figure 4-6).

A needle valve designed to regulate gas flow operates much like a water faucet. Adjusting the valve by turning it moves the needle away from the valve seat (variable orifice), opening it and increasing gas flow. A larger opening allows more gas to pass through the valve seat in a given interval of time.

In addition to regulating flow, needle valves can be used to reduce pressure. Opening the

Figure 4-4 *The Puritan Bennett pressure control is a low pressure reducing valve. (A) Illustration showing the valve closed. (B) Illustration showing the valve open.*

Figure 4-5 *A full section of the Bird pressure chamber. Note the proximity of the magnet to the metal clutch plate.*

valve causes a pressure drop across the valve seat. The pressure proximal to the valve seat becomes greater than the pressure distal to it. This pressure difference can be used to reduce a higher pressure to a lower pressure.

INDICATIONS FOR INCENTIVE SPIROMETRY AND POSITIVE AIRWAY PRESSURE ADJUNCTS TO BRONCHIAL HYGIENE THERAPY

Incentive spirometry and positive airway pressure adjunctive therapy techniques have some commonalities in their application. Figures 4-7 and 4-8 are the AARC's Clinical Practice Guidelines for incentive spirometry and positive airway pressure adjuncts to bronchial hygiene therapy. Both techniques may be used to reverse or prevent atelectasis. Atelectasis is an airless state in the lung, either localized (segmental) or more wide spread (lobar). Both techniques facilitate lung expansion either through inspiratory effort (incentive spirometry) or positive pressure during exhalation (PEP or flutter valve therapy). In either case,

Figure 4-6 *A full section of a needle valve.*

the goal of therapy is hyperinflation or lung expansion. Both techniques rely on the patient's muscle effort to accomplish the clinical goal. Both techniques also require that the patient be alert, able to follow directions, and able to voluntarily accomplish the desired breathing pattern (inspiratory or expiratory).

The term sustained maximal inspiration (SMI) is often used in conjunction with incentive spirometry. SMI is simply the encouragement of a patient to inhale maximally and to briefly pause prior to exhalation. As stated in the clinical practice guideline, incentive spirometry and SMI are referred to synonomously.

AARC CLINICAL PRACTICE GUIDELINE
Incentive Spirometry

IS 1.0 PROCEDURE:
Incentive spirometry, also referred to as sustained maximal inspiration (SMI), is a component of bronchial hygiene therapy.

IS 2.0 DESCRIPTION/DEFINITION:
2.1 Incentive spirometry is designed to mimic natural sighing or yawning by encouraging the patient to take long, slow, deep breaths. This is accomplished by using a device that provides patients with visual or other positive feedback when they inhale at a predetermined flowrate or volume and sustain the inflation for a minimum of 3 seconds.

The objectives of this procedure are to increase transpulmonary pressure and inspiratory volumes, improve inspiratory muscle performance, and re-establish or simulate the normal pattern of pulmonary hyperinflation. When the procedure is repeated on a regular basis, airway patency may be maintained and lung atelectasis prevented and reversed.

2.2 Incentive spirometry should be contrasted with expiratory maneuvers (such as the use of blow bottles) that do not mimic the sigh and have been associated with the production of reduced lung volumes.

IS 3.0 SETTINGS:
3.1 Critical care
3.2 Acute care inpatient
3.3 Extended care and skilled nursing facility
3.4 Home care

IS 4.0 INDICATIONS:
4.1 Presence of conditions predisposing to the development of pulmonary atelectasis
4.1.1 upper-abdominal surgery
4.1.2 thoracic surgery
4.1.3 surgery in patients with chronic obstructive pulmonary disease (COPD)
4.2 Presence of pulmonary atelectasis
4.3 Presence of a restrictive lung defect associated with quadraplegia and/or dysfunctional diaphragm.

IS 5.0 CONTRAINDICATIONS:
5.1 Patient cannot be instructed or supervised to assure appropriate use of the device.
5.2 Patient cooperation is absent or patient is unable to understand or demonstrate proper use of the device.

5.3 IS is contraindicated in patients unable to deep breathe effectively (e.g., with vital capacity [VC] less than about 10 mL/kg or inspiratory capacity [IC] less than about one third of predicted).
5.4 The presence of an open tracheal stoma is not a contraindication but requires adaptation of the spirometer.

IS 6.0 HAZARDS AND COMPLICATIONS:
6.1 Ineffective unless closely supervised or performed as ordered
6.2 Inappropriate as sole treatment for major lung collapse or consolidation
6.3 Hyperventilation
6.4 Barotrauma (emphysematous lungs)
6.5 Discomfort secondary to inadequate pain control
6.6 Hypoxia secondary to interruption of prescribed oxygen therapy if face mask or shield is being used
6.7 Exacerbation of bronchospasm
6.8 Fatigue

IS 7.0 LIMITATIONS OF METHOD:
Evidence suggests that deep breathing alone without mechanical aides can be as beneficial as incentive spirometry in preventing or reversing pulmonary complications, and controversy exists concerning overuse of the procedure.

IS 8.0 ASSESSMENT OF NEED:
8.1 Surgical procedure involving upper abdomen or thorax
8.2 Conditions predisposing to development of atelectasis including immobility, poor pain control, and abdominal binders
8.3 Presence of neuromuscular disease involving respiratory musculature

IS 9.0 ASSESSMENT OF OUTCOME:
9.1 Absence of or improvement in signs of atelectasis
9.1.1 decreased respiratory rate
9.1.2 resolution of fever
9.1.3 normal pulse rate
9.1.4 absent crackles (rales) or presence of or improvement in previously absent or diminished breath sounds
9.1.5 normal chest x-ray
9.1.6 improved arterial oxygen tension (PaO_2) and decreased alveolar-arterial oxygen tension gradient, or $P(A\text{-}a)O_2$

Figure 4-7 *The American Association for Respiratory Care, Clinical Practice Guideline: Incentive Spirometry.*
(continues)

9.1.7 increased VC and peak expiratory flows

9.1.8 return of functional residual capacity (FRC) or VC to preoperative values, in absence of lung resection

9.2 Improved inspiratory muscle performance

9.2.1 attainment of preoperative flow and volume levels

9.2.2 increased forced vital capacity (FVC)

IS 10.0 RESOURCES:

10.1 Equipment

10.1.1 incentive spirometer

10.1.2 conclusive evidence to support the use of one type or brand of device over others is lacking

10.2 Personnel

10.2.1 Level I personnel should possess

10.2.1.1 mastery of techniques for proper operation and clinical application of device and understanding of the importance of effective postoperative pain relief and the absence of other impediments to patient cooperation (such as residual anesthetic or sensory impairment)

10.2.1.2 ability to instruct patient in proper technique and an under-standing of the importance of preoperative instruction and supervised practice

10.2.1.3 ability to respond appropriately to adverse effects

10.2.1.4 knowledge of and ability to implement Universal Precautions

10.2.2 Level II personnel, in addition to possessing knowledge and abilities described in 10.2.1.1–10.2.1.4, should have demonstrated ability to assess patient need for and response to therapy and recommend modifications and discontinuance as appropriate.

IS 11.0 MONITORING:

Direct supervision of every patient performance is not necessary once the patient has demonstrated mastery of technique; however, preoperative instruction, volume goals, and feedback are essential to optimal performance.

11.1 Observation of patient performance and utilization

11.1.1 frequency of sessions

11.1.2 number of breaths/session

11.1.3 inspiratory volume or flow goals achieved and 3- to 5-second breath-hold maintained

11.1.4 effort/motivation

11.2 Periodic observation of patient compliance with technique, with additional instruction as necessary

11.3 Device within reach of patient and patient encouraged to perform independently

11.4 New and increasing inspiratory volumes established each day

11.5 Vital signs

IS 12.0 FREQUENCY:

A number of authors suggest using the device 5–10 breaths per session, at a minimum, every hour while awake (i.e., 100 times a day). *Caregiver does not need to be present with each performance, and patient should be encouraged to perform independently.*

IS 13.0 INFECTION CONTROL:

13.1 Universal Precautions

13.2 Proper labeling and appropriate storage of devices between uses and appropriate cleaning of devices between patients

Reprinted with permission from *Respiratory Care* 1991; 36: 1402–1405. The complete AARC Clinical Practice Guidelines are available from the AARC Web site (*http://www.aarc.org*), from the AARC Executive Office, or from *Respiratory Care* journal.

Figure 4-7 *(continued)*

AARC CLINICAL PRACTICE GUIDELINE
Use of Positive Airway Pressure Adjuncts to Bronchial Hygiene Therapy

PAP 1.0 PROCEDURE:

Positive airway pressure (PAP) adjuncts are used to mobilize secretions and treat atelectasis and include continuous positive airway pressure (CPAP), positive expiratory pressure (PEP), and expiratory positive airway pressure (EPAP).

Cough or other airway clearance techniques are essential components of PAP therapy when the therapy is intended to mobilize secretions.

PAP 2.0 DEFINITION/DESCRIPTION:

During CPAP therapy, the patient breathes from a pressurized circuit against a threshold resistor (water-column, weighted, or spring loaded) that maintains consistent preset airway pressures from 5 to 20 cm H_2O during both inspiration and expiration. (By strict definition, CPAP is any level of above-atmospheric pressure.) CPAP requires a gas flow to the airway during inspiration that is sufficient to maintain the desired positive airway pressure.

During PEP therapy, the patient exhales against a fixed-orifice resistor, generating pressures during expiration that usually range from 10 to 20 cm H_2O. PEP does not require a pressurized external gas source.

During EPAP therapy the patient exhales against a threshold resistor, generating preset pressures of 10 to 20 cm H_2O.25-27 EPAP does not require a pressurized external gas source.

EPAP utilizing threshold resistors does not produce the same mechanical or physiologic effects that PEP does when a fixed orifice resistor is used. Further study is necessary to determine how these differences affect clinical outcome.

PAP 3.0 SETTINGS:

3.1 Critical care

3.2 Acute care inpatient

3.3 Extended-care and transitional-care facilities

3.4 Home care

3.5 Outpatient

PAP 4.0 INDICATIONS:

4.1 To reduce air trapping in asthma and COPD

4.2 To aid in mobilization of retained secretions (in cystic fibrosis and chronic bronchitis)

4.3 To prevent or reverse atelectasis

4.4 To optimize delivery of bronchodilators in patients receiving bronchial hygiene therapy

PAP 5.0 CONTRAINDICATIONS:

Although no absolute contraindications to the use of PEP, CPAP, or EPAP mask therapy have been reported, the following should be carefully evaluated before a decision is made to initiate PAP mask therapy.

5.1 Patients unable to tolerate the increased work of breathing (acute asthma, COPD)

5.2 Intracranial pressure (ICP) > 20 mm Hg

5.3 Hemodynamic instability

5.4 Recent facial, oral, or skull surgery or trauma

5.5 Acute sinusitis

5.6 Epistaxis

5.7 Esophageal surgery

5.8 Active hemoptysis

5.9 Nausea

5.10 Known or suspected tympanic membrane rupture or other middle ear pathology

5.11 Untreated pneumothorax

PAP 6.0 HAZARDS/COMPLICATIONS:

6.1 Increased work of breathing that may lead to hypoventilation and hypercarbia

6.2 Increased intracranial pressure

6.3 Cardiovascular compromise

6.3.1 myocardial ischemia

6.3.2 decreased venous return

6.4 Air swallowing, with increased likelihood of vomiting and aspiration

6.5 Claustrophobia

6.6 Skin break down and discomfort from mask

6.7 Pulmonary barotrauma

PAP 7.0 LIMITATIONS OF METHOD:

7.1 PAP therapies for bronchial hygiene require spontaneously breathing patients.

7.2 CPAP is an equipment-intensive procedure requiring an external positive pressure gas source or compressor and considerable training of personnel for proper setup and maintenance. These factors make CPAP more expensive and less portable than other PAP alternatives.

Figure 4-8 *The American Association for Respiratory Care, Clinical Practice Guideline: Use of Positive Airway Pressure Adjuncts to Bronchial Hygiene Therapy.* **(continues)**

PAP 8.0 ASSESSMENT OF NEED:
The following should be assessed together to establish a need for PAP therapy:

8.1 Sputum retention not responsive to spontaneous or directed coughing

8.2 History of pulmonary problems treated successfully with postural drainage therapy

8.3 Decreased breath sounds or adventitious sounds suggesting secretions in the airway

8.4 Change in vital signs-increase in breathing frequency, tachycardia

8.5 Abnormal chest radiograph consistent with atelectasis, mucus plugging, or infiltrates

8.6 Deterioration in arterial blood gas values or oxygen saturation

PAP 9.0 ASSESSMENT OF OUTCOME:

9.1 *Change in sputum production*—if PEP does not increase sputum production in a patient who produces > 30 mL/day of sputum without PEP, the continued use of PEP may not be indicated.

9.2 *Change in breath sounds*—with effective therapy, breath sounds may clear or the movement of secretions into the larger airways may cause an increase in adventitious breath sounds. The increase in adventitious breath sounds is often a marked improvement over no (or diminished) breath sounds. Note any effect that coughing may have had on the breath sounds.

9.3 *Patient subjective response to therapy*—the caregiver should ask the patient how he or she feels before, during, and after therapy. Feelings of pain, discomfort, shortness of breath, dizziness, and nausea should be considered in modifying and stopping therapy. Improved ease of clearing secretions and increased volume of secretions during and after treatments support continuation.

9.4 *Change in vital signs*—moderate changes in respiratory rate and/or pulse rate are expected. Bradycardia, tachycardia, increasingly irregular pulse, or a drop or dramatic increase in blood pressure are indications for stopping therapy.

9.5 *Change in chest radiograph*—resolution or improvement of atelectasis and localized infiltrates may be slow or dramatic.

9.6 *Change in arterial blood gas values or oxygen saturation*—normal oxygenation should return as atelectasis resolves.

PAP 10.0 RESOURCES:
10.1 Equipment:

10.1.1 *PEP*—Fixed orifice resistor capable of developing 10 to 20 cm H_2O pressure during passive expiration, with one-way valves allowing unobstructed inspiration.

10.1.2 *CPAP*—Threshold resistor capable of developing 5 to 20 cm H_2O pressure, with a source of gas flow sufficient to maintain the desired level of pressure during inspiration, at desired F_IO_2 (requiring flowrater or blender, reservoir bag on inspiratory line, or an adjustable demand valve)

10.1.3 *EPAP*—Threshold resistor capable of developing pressures of 10 to 20 cm H_2O, with a one-way valve that allows gas at ambient pressure to enter airway on inspiration and directs exhaled gas through the threshold resistor

10.1.4 Transparent mask or mouthpiece

10.1.5 Manometer for initial adjustments of resistor size and/or gas flow

10.1.6 Tissues and emesis basin or container for collecting or disposing of expectorated sputum

10.1.7 Gloves, goggles, gown, and mask

10.2 Personnel: A spectrum of education and skill levels is required for personnel who administer PEP, CPAP, or EPAP therapy. Different clinical situations warrant the degree of training necessary to provide optimal respiratory care:

10.2.1 Level-I personnel are responsible for ongoing assessment and care of unstable patients. Their demonstrated skills and knowledge should include

10.2.1.1 proper use and limitations of equipment;

10.2.1.2 ability to assess patient condition and response to therapy;

10.2.1.3 performance of physical examination (auscultation and vital signs);

10.2.1.4 understanding of effects of increased expiratory pressure on ventilation, perfusion, and sputum mobilization;

10.2.1.5 understanding of procedures, indications, and contraindications, and hazards for PEP, CPAP, and EPAP;

10.2.1.6 ability to demonstrate diaphragmatic breathing and relaxation, and to direct coughing;

10.2.1.7 ability to monitor effects of and subject response to changes in expiratory airway pressure;

10.2.1.8 understanding of and compliance with Universal Precautions and infection control standards related to cleaning equip-

Figure 4-8 *(continues)*

ment, maintaining equipment, and handling of secretions.

10.2.2 Level-II personnel should possess all Level-I skills and knowledge plus

10.2.2.1 ability to perform initial assessment of patient, initiate therapy and assess patient response and tailor therapy to patient needs.

10.2.2.2 ability to negotiate care plan and modifications with physician and health care team

10.2.2.3 ability to instruct patient, family, or caregiver in goals of therapy and

10.2.2.3.1 proper technique for administration,

10.2.2.3.2 proper use of equipment,

10.2.2.3.3 cleaning of equipment,

10.2.2.3.4 breathing patterns and cough techniques,

10.2.2.3.5 modification of technique in response to adverse reactions,

10.2.2.3.6 modification of duration or frequency in response to severity of symptoms.

10.2.3 Level III: Self-administration of PEP, EPAP, or CPAP—the patient who is to self-administer treatment should demonstrate

10.2.3.1 proper technique for administration,

10.2.3.2 proper use of equipment,

10.2.3.3 appropriate breathing patterns and cough techniques,

10.2.3.4 ability to modify technique in response to adverse reactions,

10.2.3.5 ability to modify duration or frequency in response to severity of symptoms.

PAP 11.0 MONITORING:

Items from the following list should be chosen as is appropriate for monitoring a specific patient's response to PAP.

11.1 Patient subjective response—pain, discomfort, dyspnea, response to therapy

11.2 Pulse rate and cardiac rhythm (if EKG is available)

11.3 Breathing pattern and rate, symmetrical lateral costal expansion, synchronous thoraco-abdominal movement

11.4 Sputum production (quantity, color, consistency, and odor)

11.5 Mental function

11.6 Skin color

11.7 Breath sounds

11.8 Blood pressure

11.9 Pulse oximetry (if hypoxemia with procedure has been previously demonstrated or is suspected); blood gas analysis (if indicated)

11.10 Intracranial pressure (ICP) in patients for whom ICP is of critical importance.

PAP 12.0 FREQUENCY:

12.1 *Critical Care*—from once per hour to once every 6 hours, for intermittent PAP as tolerated. PAP order should be re-evaluated at least every 24 hours based on assessment made during and following each treatment.

12.2 *Acute/Domiciliary Care*

12.2.1 Common strategies for PAP vary from twice to four times daily, with frequency determined by assessment of patient response to therapy.

12.2.2 PAP orders for acute care patients should be reevaluated at least every 72 hours based on patient response to therapy or with any change of patient status.

12.2.3 Domiciliary patients should be reevaluated periodically and with any change of status.

PAP 13.0 INFECTION CONTROL ISSUES:

13.1 Observe Universal Precautions as appropriate.

13.2 Follow guidelines for prevention of transmission of tuberculosis in health care settings.

13.3 Observe all infection control guidelines posted for specific patient.

13.4 Disinfect any reusable equipment (according to manufacturer's recommendations) between patients.

Reprinted with permission from *Respiratory Care* 1993; 38: 516–521. The complete AARC Clinical Practice Guidelines are available from the AARC Web site (*http://www.aarc.org*), from the AARC Executive Office, or from *Respiratory Care* journal.

Figure 4-8 *(continued)*

INCENTIVE SPIROMETRY EQUIPMENT

Several different types of incentive spirometers are employed in patient care. The majority are disposable, single-use devices. Others incorporate a permanent sensing/feedback device with disposable patient mouthpieces or flow sensors. All of the incentive spirometers in use today use one of the three principles of volume measurement discussed earlier in this chapter.

VOLDYNE

Hudson RCI makes the Voldyne incentive spirometer (Figure 4-9), which is a disposable device that operates by the application of sub-ambient pressure above a piston.

As the patient inhales, gas flows through a flow indication float, causing it to rise. The patient is encouraged to keep the yellow flow indicator centered in its chamber. The manufacturer maintains that keeping the float centered promotes a more uniform distribution of air throughout the lungs.

Movement of gas through the Voldyne causes pressure to be reduced above the volume indication piston. As pressure is reduced, the piston rises in its tube. The top of the piston indicates the level of inspired volume. The Voldyne's volume range is from 0 to 4000 milliliters.

A movable marker on the left side of the spirometer is adjusted to indicate to what volume the patient should inhale. The marker can be adjusted such that the patient is encouraged to work a little harder than normal, further expanding the lungs.

TRIFLO™ II

The Triflo™ II is a disposable incentive spirometer manufactured by Hudson RCI (Figure 4-10). Like the Voldyne, it is a flow-dependent device.

The patient's inspiratory flow is drawn across the top of three chambers, creating a sub-ambient pressure. If the patient's flow is greater than 800 milliliters per second but less than 1000 milliliters per second, the float in the first chamber will rise. As the flow increases to 1000 milliliters per second, the second float will rise. If the patient's flow exceeds 1200 milliliters per second, all three floats will be suspended. The respiratory care practitioner

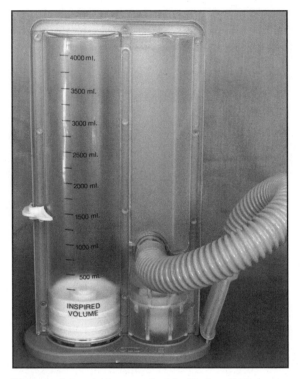

Figure 4-9 *A photograph of the Hudson RCI Voldyne incentive spirometer.*

Figure 4-10 *A photograph of the Hudson RCI Triflo incentive spirometer.*

should encourage the patient to sustain his inspiratory effort (flow), holding the float(s) up for at least 3 seconds. When the patient exhales, gravity pulls the floats back to the bottom of their chambers.

VOLUREX

DHD Medical manufactured and holds the trademark on the Volurex incentive spirometer (Figure 4-11), which is another disposable incentive spirometer that operates using volume displacement with a range of 0 to 4000 milliliters.

The Volurex incorporates a flexible bellows. As the patient inhales, volume is removed and the bellows rises.

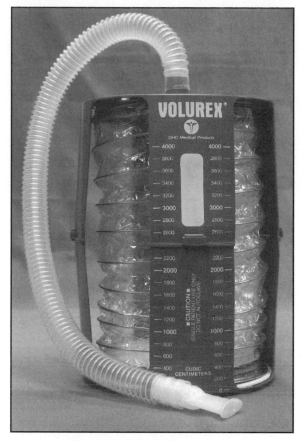

Figure 4-11 *The DHD Healthcare Corporation Volurex incentive spirometer.*

ASSEMBLY AND TROUBLESHOOTING

Assembly—Disposable Incentive Spirometers

1. Aseptically remove the Voldyne, flexible tubing, and mouthpiece from the package.

2. Attach the flexible tubing to the inlet of the spirometer.

3. Attach the mouthpiece to the free end of the flexible tubing.

4. Tip the spirometer to check for free movement of the flow indication float and the piston.

5. Instruct the patient on its use.

6. Adjust the volume pointer to the desired level.

Troubleshooting

Very little can go wrong with this relatively simple device. Check the tubing or mouthpiece for obstruction and ensure that the piston and flow indication float move freely. If the unit still fails to operate, replace it.

MONAGHAN SPIROCARE

Monaghan produces two models of the Spirocare spirometer (Figure 4-12). One model is small and is powered by batteries; the other is larger, operating from 110-volt electrical power.

Both Spirocares measure volume using the photoelectric principle discussed earlier in the chapter. The turbine is contained in a clear, disposable mouthpiece, positioned longitudinally along its axis. The patient's inspiratory flow causes the turbine to spin. The photoelectric transducer and receiver are located in the

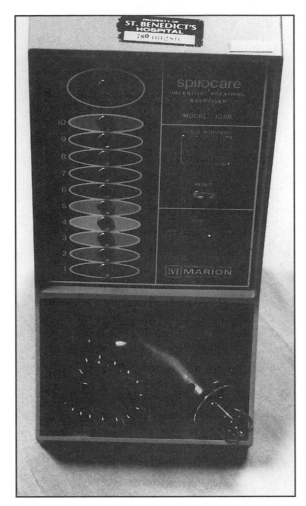

Figure 4-12 *The Monaghan Spirocare incentive spirometer.*

handle of the spirometer. The electronic circuitry that interprets the signals from the photoelectric cells is located in the spirometer housing.

Adjustment of the desired inspiratory volume (inside the side door for the larger unit and under the spirometer housing for the smaller unit) causes colored lights to illuminate on the right indicator panel. As the patient inhales, the row of lights on the left panel illuminates, indicating inspired volume. The patient is encouraged to match the goal indicated on the right-hand row of lights. When the patient reaches the goal, a breath hold light or clown light (early larger models for pediatric patients) illuminates for 3 seconds to encourage breath holding.

A counter keeps track of the number of times the patient achieves the desired goal (volume). In this way a patient may be encouraged to use the spirometer a specified number of times between therapy sessions.

POSITIVE-EXPIRATORY-PRESSURE AND FLUTTER VALVE THERAPY EQUIPMENT

Both Positive-Expiratory-Pressure (PEP) and flutter valve therapy apply positive expiratory pressure to mechanically splint the airways open, which facilitates the removal of secretions. Although they are both similar in the application of positive pressure during exhalation, they differ in that one provides continuous pressure while the other generates pressure pulses.

POSITIVE-EXPIRATORY-PRESSURE THERAPY EQUIPMENT

Positive-Expiratory-Pressure (PEP) therapy equipment consists of a mouthpiece, one-way valves, a T-assembly, a manometer, an adjustable resistance valve, and an optional nebulizer and reservoir (Figure 4-13). The PEP level is adjusted by varying the diameter of the resistance valve's orifice, increasing or decreasing expiratory resistance (10 to 15 cmH$_2$O). The patient is instructed to take a deeper than normal breath and to exhale actively against the resistance, observing the manometer to maintain the desired expiratory pressure. Following 10 to 20 breaths, the patient is then instructed to remove the PEP device and forcefully cough.

Figure 4-13 *A photograph of a PEP mask device. Note the attachment of an optional small-volume nebulizer for medication delivery.*

Oscillating PEP Therapy Devices

There are two distinct types of oscillating PEP therapy devices on the market: a weighted ball device and a counterweighted lever and magnet device. The **flutter valve** consists of a single, weighted ball valve, which rapidly opens and closes during exhalation, creating positive pressure and a rapidly oscillating pressure wave within the patient's airways (Figure 4-14).

Like PEP therapy, the patient takes a larger than normal tidal breath and then exhales against the flutter valve. This creates positive pressure in the airways in combination with an oscillating pressure wave caused by the valve's rapid opening and closing. Following 10 to 20 breaths, the patient is encouraged to vigorously cough.

DHD healthcare produces the Acapella oscillating PEP therapy device that employs a counterweighted lever and magnet that adjust the frequency and amplitude of the expiratory pressure wave (Figure 4-15). An adjustable knob on the base of the device is rotated, moving a magnet closer or further from the

Figure 4-15 *A photograph of the DHD Healthcare Corporation Acapella Oscillating PEP therapy device.*

counterweighted lever. This process adjusts the resistance to expiratory gas flow and adjusts the frequency and amplitude of the expiratory oscillations.

Like PEP therapy, the patient takes a larger than normal tidal breath and then exhales against the expiratory resistance. This creates positive pressure in the airways in combination with an oscillating pressure wave caused by the lever rapidly opening and closing a cone-shaped valve seat. Following 10 to 20 breaths, the patient is encouraged to vigorously cough.

INSPIRATORY MUSCLE TRAINING DEVICES

Inspiratory muscle training devices are designed to strengthen patient's inspiratory muscles by providing a variable resistance to gas flow during inspiration. These devices achieve the desired effect by adjusting a variable orifice (or replacing various inspiratory caps with different orifice sizes) to vary the inspiratory resistance to gas flow. As the orifice size decreases, the inspiratory resistance increases and more muscle effort is required to achieve a desired inspiratory volume. Most devices provide a port where inspiratory pressures may be monitored using a pressure manometer. To be effective, these devices should be used in conjunction with nose clips to encourage the patient to inhale through the inspiratory resistance device and not his or her nose. Figure 4-16 is an example of one of the inspiratory resistance devices currently being marketed.

Figure 4-14 *Photographs of a flutter valve. Note the weighted ball (top) with the expiratory cap removed.*

Figure 4-16   *A photograph of the DHD Healthcare Corporation inspiratory muscle trainer.*

INDICATIONS FOR INTERMITTENT POSITIVE PRESSURE BREATHING (IPPB) THERAPY

Figure 4-17 is the AARC Clinical Practice Guideline for IPPB therapy. The indications for IPPB therapy include the need to improve lung expansion (atelectasis or inability to clear secretions), short-term ventilatory support, and delivery of aerosol medications. The latter indication should not be the sole criteria for selection of IPPB therapy over another modality (SVN, MDI, DPI, etc.).

IPPB therapy does have some distinct hazards and complications. Therefore, it is imperative that the practitioner delivering therapy and using the ventilator understand how it operates and the physiological effects it has upon the patient. Careful monitoring and supervision is an important part of IPPB therapy.

INTERMITTENT POSITIVE PRESSURE BREATHING (IPPB) EQUIPMENT

Two common IPPB **ventilators** are made by two manufacturers: Puritan Bennett Corporation and the Bird Products Corporation. Currently only one model, the Mark 7A, is being produced by Bird Products Corporation, a division of Viasys Healthcare.

As indicated earlier in the chapter, the use of IPPB therapy has declined in the past several years. While it is still ordered and performed today, it is done so more selectively than it was in the past. It is still important to understand how the equipment functions and operates so that IPPB therapy can be administered safely and effectively.

AARC CLINICAL PRACTICE GUIDELINE
Intermittent Positive Pressure Breathing
2003 Revision & Update

IPPB 1.0 PROCEDURE:
Intermittent positive pressure breathing

IPPB 2.0 DESCRIPTION/DEFINITION:
The first American Association for Respiratory Care (AARC) clinical practice guideline (CPG) for Intermittent Positive Pressure Breathing (IPPB) was published in 1993. Since that time there have been additional studies, systematic overviews, and a meta-analysis that specifically addresses the efficacy of IPPB as compared to other hyperinflation and aerosol delivery techniques. Those studies have been added as references to this revised CPG. IPPB remains a technique used to provide short term or intermittent mechanical ventilation for the purpose of augmenting lung expansion, delivering aerosol medication, or assisting ventilation. A caveat, however, is that IPPB is not the therapy of first choice for delivering aerosol or as a method of lung hyperinflation in spontaneously breathing patients when other less expensive therapies can reliably meet the clinical objectives prescribed for the patient. It should be noted that noninvasive positive pressure ventilation (NPPV) may be considered as a form of IPPB to assist ventilation, although a review of this therapeutic modality was not included in this CPG.

   2.1 IPPB can include pressure- and time-limited, as well as pressure, time, and flow-cycled ventilation.

   2.2 IPPB may be delivered to artificial airways and nonintubated patients.

IPPB 3.0 SETTINGS:
IPPB can be administered in settings that include hospital, clinic, extended care facility, and home.

IPPB 4.0 INDICATIONS:
   4.1 The need to improve lung expansion

   4.1.1 The presence of clinically significant pulmonary atelectasis when other forms of therapy have been unsuccessful (incentive spirometry, chest physiotherapy, deep breathing exercises, positive airway pressure) or the patient cannot cooperate

   4.1.2 Inability to clear secretions adequately because of pathology that severely limits the ability to ventilate or cough effectively and failure to respond to other modes of treatment

   4.2 The need for short-term ventilatory support for patients who are hypoventilating as an alternative to tracheal intubation and continuous mechanical ventilation. Devices specifically designed to deliver noninvasive positive pressure ventilation (NPPV) should be considered.

   4.3 The need to deliver aerosol medication. (We are not addressing aerosol delivery for patients on long-term mechanical ventilation.)

   4.3.1 Some clinicians oppose the use of IPPB in the treatment of severe bronchospasm (acute asthma or status asthmaticus, and exacerbated COPD); however, a careful, closely supervised trial of IPPB as a medication delivery device when treatment using other techniques (metered-dose inhaler [MDI] or nebulizer) has been unsuccessful may be warranted.

   4.3.2 IPPB may be used to deliver aerosol medications to patients with fatigue as a result of ventilatory muscle weakness (e.g., failure to wean from mechanical ventilation, neuromuscular disease, kyphoscoliosis, spinal injury) or chronic conditions in which intermittent ventilatory support is indicated (e.g., ventilatory support for home care patients and the more recent use of nasal IPPV for respiratory insufficiency).

   4.3.3 In patients with severe hyperinflation, IPPB may decrease dyspnea and discomfort during nebulized therapy.

IPPB 5.0 CONTRAINDICATIONS:
There are several clinical situations in which IPPB should not be used. With the exception of untreated tension pneumothorax, most of these contraindications are relative:

   5.1 Tension pneumothorax (untreated)

   5.2 Intracranial pressure (ICP) > 15 mmHg

   5.3 Hemodynamic instability

   5.4 Recent facial, oral, or skull surgery

   5.5 Tracheoesophageal fistula

   5.6 Recent esophageal surgery

   5.7 Active hemoptysis

   5.8 Nausea

   5.9 Air swallowing

Figure 4-17 *The American Association for Respiratory Care, Clinical Practice Guideline: Intermittent positive Pressure Breathing–2003 Revision & Update.* **(continues)**

5.10 Active untreated tuberculosis
5.11 Radiographic evidence of bleb
5.12 Singulation (hiccups)

IPPB 6.0 HAZARDS/COMPLICATIONS:

6.1 Increased airway resistance and work of breathing
6.2 Barotrauma, pneumothorax
6.3 Nosocomial infection
6.4 Hypocarbia
6.5 Hemoptysis
6.6 Hyperoxia when oxygen is the gas source
6.7 Gastric distention
6.8 Impaction of secretions (associated with inadequately humidified gas mixture)
6.9 Psychological dependence
6.10 Impedance of venous return
6.11 Exacerbation of hypoxemia
6.12 Hypoventilation or hyperventilation
6.13 Increased mismatch of ventilation and perfusion
6.14 Air trapping, auto-PEEP, overdistended alveoli

IPPB 7.0 LIMITATIONS OF PROCEDURE OR DEVICE:

7.1 All of the mechanical effects of IPPB are short-lived, lasting £ an hour after treatment.
7.2 Based on the available literature, MDI or compressor-driven nebulizers should be considered the devices of choice for aerosol therapy to COPD and stable asthma patients.
7.3 Only a very small percentage of the aerosolized medication optimally deposits in the airway. Delivery of a therapeutic medication dose via IPPB may require as much as a tenfold increase in medication amount when compared to MDIs.
7.4 Efficacy of device for ventilation and aerosol delivery is technique-dependent (e.g., coordination, breathing pattern, selection of appropriate inspiratory flow, peak pressure, inspiratory hold).
7.5 Efficacy is dependent on the design of the device (e.g., flow, volume, and pressure capability as well as aerosol output and particle size).
7.6 IPPB is equipment- and labor-intensive as a method of delivery of aerosol.
7.7 Limited portability, lack of instruction, and/or lack of 50-psi gas source may affect patient compliance.

IPPB 8.0 ASSESSMENT OF NEED:

8.1 Presence of clinically significant atelectasis

8.2 Reduced pulmonary function as evidenced by reductions in timed volumes and vital capacity (e.g., FEV1 < 65% predicted, FVC < 70% predicted, MVV < 50% predicted, or VC < 10 mL/kg), precluding an effective cough
8.3 Neuromuscular disorders or kyphoscoliosis with associated decreases in lung volumes and capacities
8.4 Fatigue or muscle weakness with impending respiratory failure
8.5 Presence of acute severe bronchospasm or exacerbated COPD that fails to respond to other therapy
8.5.1 Based on proven therapeutic efficacy, variety of medications, and cost-effectiveness, the MDI with a spacing device or holding chamber should be the first method to consider for administration of aerosol.
8.5.2 Regardless of the type of delivery device used (MDI with spacer or small volume, large-volume, or ultrasonic nebulizer), it is important to recognize that the dose of the drug needs to be titrated to give the maximum benefit.
8.6 With demonstrated effectiveness, the patient's preference for a positive pressure device should be honored.
8.7 IPPB may be indicated in patients who are at risk for the development of atelectasis and are unable or unwilling to deep breathe without assistance.

IPPB 9.0 ASSESSMENT OF OUTCOME:

9.1 For lung expansion therapy, a minimum delivered tidal volume of at least ⅓ of the predicted IC (⅓ × 50 mL/kg) has been suggested. This corresponds to approximately 1200 mL in a 70 kg adult patient.
9.2 An increase in FEV1 or peak flow
9.3 Cough more effective with treatment
9.4 Secretion clearance enhanced as a consequence of deep breathing and coughing
9.5 Chest radiograph improved
9.6 Breath sounds improved
9.7 Favorable patient subjective response

IPPB 10.0 RESOURCES:

10.1 Equipment:
10.1.1 IPPB devices can be pneumatically driven or electrically powered. They are usually categorized as patient-triggered, pressure- or flow-cycled mechanical ventilators.
10.1.2 Most IPPB devices require a 45–55-psi gas pressure source (e.g., compressed gas cylinder, bulk gas system, external or internal air compressor).

Figure 4-17 *(continues)*

10.1.3 Single-use IPPB devices are now available for providing short-term or intermittent mechanical ventilation, augmenting hyperinflation and delivering aerosols.

10.1.3.1 Single-use IPPB devices are not equipped with a redundant pop-off valve and thus should not be used with an endotracheal tube, and used only cautiously with a mask.

10.1.3.2 Tidal volume may be determined by using the tidal volume chart included with single-use IPPB instructions.

10.1.3.3 For single-use IPPB equipment at home, the rental/purchase of a 50 psi gas source is usually necessary.

10.1.3.4 Limited research indicates that single-use IPPB may be a safe and effective method of delivering IPPB without the need for conventional IPPB capital equipment.

10.1.4 IPPB circuitry includes large bore and connective tubing, nebulizer, adapters, and patient connection (mouthpiece, lip seal, mask, 15-mm ETT connector), and if needed, nose clips.

10.1.5 Tissues, emesis basin, or sputum cup for collecting or disposing of expectorated sputum

10.1.6 Gloves, gown, goggles, and/or mask with face shield as indicated

10.1.7 Volume measuring device (handheld spirometer or other volume-collecting bag)

10.1.8 Oral and/or endotracheal suction equipment

10.2 Personnel: A continuum of education and skill levels is required for personnel who administer IPPB therapy. Different clinical situations warrant the degree of training necessary to provide optimal respiratory care.

10.2.1 Level I caregiver may be the provider of service after Level II personnel have established need for a specific device by patient assessment, and after the first administration has been completed. Level I personnel must demonstrate:

10.2.1.1 Ability to prepare, measure, and mix medication

10.2.1.2 Proper technique for administration of medication

10.2.1.3 Proper use of equipment, including adjustment of machine settings to meet patient demands

10.2.1.4 Effective cleaning of equipment

10.2.1.5 Proper disposal of wastes

10.2.1.6 Ability to encourage effective breathing patterns and coughing techniques

10.2.1.7 Ability to modify technique (after communication with physician) in response to recognized complications and adverse reactions or change in severity of symptoms as determined by observation, ausculation, and vitalsigns determination

10.2.1.8 Ability to implement Standard Precautions and use proper infection control

10.2.2 Level II Personnel must exhibit all Level I skills and demonstrate:

10.2.2.1 Ability to perform physical exam—auscultation, inspection, percussion, and vital signs

10.2.2.2 Ability to assess patient condition and patient response to therapy

10.2.2.3 Ability to perform peak expiratory flowrate, spirometry, and ventilatory mechanics measurement

10.2.2.4 Proper use and knowledge of limitations of IPPB equipment and aerosol device and ability to fit mask and/or identify best application device for particular patient

10.2.2.5 Ability to recognize and respond to therapeutic changes, adverse response, and complications of aerosol medications

10.2.2.6 Ability to modify dosage of medication and/or frequency of administration as prescribed in response to severity of symptoms

10.2.2.7 Ability to negotiate care plan and modifications with physician and health care team

10.2.2.8 Understanding of effects of increased pressure on ventilation, perfusion, and sputum mobilization

10.2.2.9 Ability to modify technique in response to adverse reactions

10.2.2.10 Ability to instruct patient/family/caregiver in goals of therapy, and:

10.2.2.10.1 Proper technique for administration

10.2.2.10.2 Proper use of equipment

10.2.2.10.3 Cleaning of equipment

10.2.2.10.4 Breathing patterns and coughing techniques

10.2.2.10.5 Recognition of communications and technique modification in response to adverse reactions

10.2.2.10.6 Frequency modification in response to severity of symptoms

10.2.2.11 Understanding and compliance with Standard Precautions and infection control issues related to cleaning and maintaining equipment and handling of secretions and hazardous waste

Figure 4-17 *(continues)*

10.2.3 Level III—Self-administration of IPPB. Patients who are to self-administer IPPB should demonstrate to the supervising clinician:

10.2.3.1 Proper technique for administration

10.2.3.2 Proper use of equipment

10.2.3.3 Proper cleaning of equipment

10.2.3.4 Ability to measure and mix medications

10.2.3.5 Optimal breathing patterns and coughing techniques

10.2.3.6 Technique modification in response to adverse reactions and duration or frequency modification in response to severity of symptoms

IPPB 11.0 MONITORING:

Items from the following list should be chosen as appropriate for the specific patient:

11.1 Performance of machine trigger sensitivity, peak pressure, flow setting, F_IO_2, inspiratory time, expiratory time, plateau pressure, PEEP

11.2 Respiratory rate

11.3 Delivered tidal volume

11.4 Pulse rate and rhythm from ECG if available

11.5 Patient subjective response to therapy: pain, discomfort, dyspnea

11.6 Sputum production: quantity, color, consistency

11.7 Mental function

11.8 Skin color

11.9 Breath sounds

11.10 Blood pressure

11.11 Arterial hemoglobin saturation by pulse oximetry (if hypoxemia is suspected)

11.12 Intracranial pressure (ICP) in patients for whom ICP is of critical importance

11.13 Chest radiograph

IPPB 12.0 FREQUENCY:

12.1 Critical care: Every 1 to 6 hours for IPPB as tolerated. IPPB order should be re-evaluated at least every 24 hours based on assessments during individual treatments.

12.2 Acute/home care patients:

12.2.1 Common strategies for IPPB vary from b.i.d. to q.i.d. Frequency should be determined by assessing patient response to therapy.

12.2.2 For acute care patients, order should be reevaluated based on patient response to therapy at least every 72 hours or with any change of patient status.

12.2.3 Home care patients should be re-evaluated/reinstructed periodically and with any change of status.

IPPB 13.0 INFECTION CONTROL:

13.1 Caregivers should implement Standard Precautions and appropriate guidelines for prevention of tuberculosis transmission.

13.2 Caregivers should observe all infection control guidelines posted for patient.

13.3 All reusable equipment should be disinfected between patients.

13.4 Nebulizers/IPPB circuits should be changed between patients, when visibly soiled, or according to institutional infection control policy.

13.5 IPPB machines/manifolds can be fitted with a scavenger or filter system to prevent aerosol from being released outside the immediate treatment areas.

13.6 Nebulizers should not be rinsed with tap water between treatments, but may be rinsed with sterile water or sterile saline and allowed to air dry.

Reprinted with permission from *Respiratory Care* 2003; 48: 540–546. The complete AARC Clinical Practice Guidelines are available from the AARC Web site (*http://www.aarc.org*), from the AARC Executive Office, or from *Respiratory Care* journal.

Figure 4-17 *(continued)*

BIRD IPPB VENTILATORS

The Bird Corporation developed an entire line of IPPB equipment based on the Mark 7. Figure 4-18 shows the most common Bird ventilators: the Mark 7, Mark 7A, and Mark 8.

Ventilator classification systems enable a practitioner to categorize different ventilators based upon common characteristics. These common characteristics include power source, what variable is controlled during inspiration, how the ventilator is triggered, and how the ventilator is cycled. The ventilator power source may be electric, pneumatic, or combined electric and pneumatic. The variable controlled during inspiration can be pressure, time, volume, or flow. How a ventilator triggers a breath, or begins inspiration, can include pressure, flow, volume, or time. How a ventilator is cycled, or ends inspiration, may include pressure, volume, flow, or time.

The Bird IPPB ventilators are classified as pneumatically powered pressure controllers.

Figure 4-18 *(A) Bird Mark 7; (B) Bird Mark 7A;* **(continues)**

Figure 4-18 *(continued)* *(C) Mark 8. (Reprinted with permission from Bird Products Corporation, Palm Springs, CA)*

The ventilators are pressure or time triggered and are pressure cycled.

Various modifications were made to the Mark 7 to accomplish new and varied clinical goals. By understanding the operation of the Mark 7, the other models can be readily learned and understood.

Basic Components of the Bird Ventilators

The basic components common to all of the Bird machines are the ambient chamber, pressure chamber, center body, venturi/venturi gate assembly, the ceramic switch/clutch plate assembly, and the permanent magnets. The ability to identify these components and to understand how they operate will enable you to apply these machines more effectively.

Ambient Chamber

As you face the front of the machine, the ambient chamber is the larger green transparent chamber on the left side of the machine. The ambient chamber is so named because it

remains at ambient pressure. Room air is drawn through the chamber and into the venturi/venturi gate assembly if the machine is operating in air mix mode. The ambient chamber also contains the pressure manometer, which indicates the pressure contained in the pressure chamber.

Pressure Chamber

The pressure chamber is located on the right side of the machine. Gas pressure from source gas (or source gas and room air) builds in this chamber and pressurizes the patient circuit, resulting in gas delivery to the patient.

Center Body

The center body is a narrow casting made from aluminum alloy that separates the ambient and pressure chambers. It contains the venturi/venturi gate assembly, ceramic switch/clutch plate assembly, timing cartridge, and other controls. The source gas supply attaches to the center body, where gas flow and its direction are controlled.

Venturi/Venturi Gate Assembly

The venturi/venturi gate assembly passes through the center body located at the top rear of the machine. When the machine is operating in air mix mode (Mark 7), source gas and room air mix in the venturi. The Mark 7A and Mark 8 operate using the venturi at all times.

The venturi gate is a spring-loaded gate that closes the distal end of the venturi with a spring tension equal to approximately 2 cmH$_2$O. This tension is necessary so that the patient's inspiratory effort will be sensed by the **sensitivity** system, and not be transmitted to the ambient chamber through the venturi. During ventilation when pressure in the pressure chamber reaches approximately 12 cmH$_2$O, the venturi gate closes. Once the gate closes, the only flow through the patient circuit is from the nebulizer.

Figure 4-19 *The Bird ceramic switch.*

Ceramic Switch/Clutch Plate Assembly

In the middle of the center body, passing through it, is the ceramic switch/clutch plate assembly (Figure 4-19). The assembly consists of the ceramic switch, diaphragm, two metal clutch plates, and the hand timing rod.

The ceramic switch is an on-off switch made of a ceramic material. The switch is contained in a cylindrical housing. The ceramic material offers the advantages of ease of sealing and operation with little friction.

When the switch is positioned to the right (Figure 4-20A), gas flows through it and the center body. When the switch is in the left position, no gas flow occurs (Figure 4-20B).

The diaphragm is located on the ambient side of the center body. It is attached to the ceramic switch assembly and moves back and forth with it. Pressure in the pressure chamber is communicated to the diaphragm through two holes in the center body. The diaphragm plays an important role in the sensitivity system, which will be discussed later in this chapter.

Attached to each end of the ceramic switch/clutch plate assembly are two metal clutch plates. One is located in each chamber (ambient and pressure). The clutch plates operate in conjunction with permanent magnets to regulate pressure and sensitivity.

The hand timing rod passes through the ambient chamber and protrudes through the center of the sensitivity control. Pushing the hand timing rod in moves the ceramic switch to the right and begins inspiration. Pulling the rod out moves the ceramic switch to the left and terminates inspiration. This rod provides a means for the operator to control the phase of ventilation (inspiration or expiration).

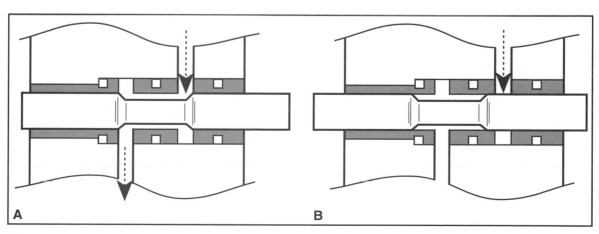

Figure 4-20 *A cross section of the Bird ceramic switch showing (A) the open (on) and (B) the closed (off) positions.*

Control Operation

A complete understanding of how the controls operate and interact with one another is essential in the safe operation of these IPPB machines. In this section, the controls will be individually discussed and their relation to other controls will be explained. The first four controls (sensitivity, flow rate, expiratory timer, and pressure control) are common to all of the Bird IPPB machines currently produced. The other controls in the discussion are unique to specific models.

Sensitivity Control

The sensitivity control is essentially a patient effort control. Adjustment of this control determines how much patient effort is required to initiate inspiration. The sensitivity ranges from 0 to 10 cmH$_2$O below ambient pressure.

The sensitivity control operates using the diaphragm, metal clutch plate (ambient side), and a permanent magnet. When the patient initiates a breath, the inspiratory effort (sub-ambient pressure) is communicated through the circuit and the pressure chamber to the diaphragm. The diaphragm responds to the change in pressure by flattening out, which moves the ceramic switch to the right, initiating inspiration (Figure 4-21).

Opposing the movement of the diaphragm is the magnetic attraction between the clutch plate and the permanent magnet. Adjustment of the sensitivity control moves the magnet closer or further from the clutch plate, varying the amount of magnetic attraction the patient must overcome. As the magnet gets closer to the clutch plate, it takes a higher or greater pressure (sub-ambient) to initiate inspiration.

When adjusting this control, the practitioner references the patient's inspiratory effort to the pressure manometer. The pressure manometer indicates the amount of negative pressure the patient must generate to initiate inspiration. Ideally, the control should be adjusted such that a pressure of 1 to 2 cmH$_2$O below ambient pressure will initiate inspiration.

Flow Rate Control

Gas entering the machine encounters the flow rate control first. It is located on the front of the center body (Figure 4-22) and is a needle valve. (The operation of needle valves was discussed in the Physics of Hyperinflation Therapy Equipment section earlier in this chapter.) Adjustment of the flow rate control regulates gas flow by opening and closing its valve seat. When the machine operates using the venturi, peak flows of up to 80 liters per minute are available.

Expiratory Timer

The expiratory timer is used to ventilate patients who are apneic. This control is not operated during IPPB therapy since it may cause **asynchronous ventilation**. An example of asynchronous ventilation is when a patient exhales while the machine delivers a breath.

The control operates using a timing cartridge, needle valve, and a timing arm.

During inspiration the cartridge is pressurized with source gas (Figure 4-23A). As the cartridge is pressurized, the diaphragm and spring opposite the inlet are compressed by the gas pressure. This increases the overall length of the cartridge slightly.

When the operator opens the needle valve (expiratory timer control), gas is allowed to

Figure 4-21 *A function diagram of the Bird sensitivity system.*

Figure 4-22 *The Bird center body with its controls labeled. (A) The gas inlet. (B) The flowrate control. (C) The air-mix switch. (D) Expiratory time for apnea.*

Figure 4-23 *A functional diagram of the Bird expiratory timer during (A) inspiration and (B) expiration.*

leak from the timing cartridge into the pressure chamber. The needle valve regulates how fast the cartridge empties, and therefore regulates the expiratory time and, indirectly, the respiratory rate.

As the timing cartridge empties, the spring pushes the diaphragm to the right, decreasing the cartridge's overall length (Figure 4-23B). Attached to the diaphragm is a rod that is connected to the timing arm. As the spring compresses the diaphragm, the timing arm contacts the clutch plate (ambient side) and pushes it to the right. The timing rod pushes the clutch plate and slides the ceramic switch to the open position, beginning inspiration, and the cycle is repeated.

Pressure Control

The pressure control is located on the right side of the machine. The control operates using the ceramic switch/clutch plate assembly and the permanent magnet in the pressure chamber.

Pressure building within the pressure chamber causes the diaphragm to distort and expand. As the diaphragm moves to the left, it also moves the ceramic switch. Once the switch moves far enough to the left, inspiration is terminated. Opposing the movement of the diaphragm is the magnetic attraction between the magnet and the clutch plate (pressure chamber).

Movement of the pressure control arm causes the magnet to be moved closer to or farther from the clutch plate. The magnet's

position varies the amount of magnetic attraction between it and the clutch plate (Figure 4-24). The closer the magnet is to the clutch plate, the greater the pressure needed to end inspiration, resulting in higher peak pressures.

Air Mix Control

The air mix control is unique to the Bird Mark 7. Essentially, it is an on-off switch that controls gas flow through the venturi/venturi gate assembly (see Figure 4-22).

In the out (on) position, source gas is conducted from the center body by plastic tubing to the venturi jet. If oxygen is the source gas, it is mixed with room air, diluting the oxygen. Oxygen percentage varies between 65% and 95% oxygen (depending on **tidal volumes** and peak pressures). Oxygen concentrations vary because, as pressure in the circuit increases, it causes less room air to be mixed with source gas (oxygen) through the venturi, increasing the oxygen concentration. Furthermore, when the spring-loaded venturi gate closes at approximately 12 H_2O, the only gas flow through the circuit is source gas through the nebulizer. When operated using the venturi, there is greater flow through the ventilator due to the additional air entrainment. The venturi causes a characteristic decelerating or tapered flow pattern (flow with respect to time). Flow throughout inspiration is not constant; it is greatest at the beginning of inspiration and decreases as inspiration proceeds.

When the control is pushed in, source gas alone powers the machine and the venturi/

Figure 4-24 *A function diagram of the Bird pressure control operation.*

venturi gate system is bypassed. Furthermore, when operated in this mode, flow rates are significantly reduced. Reduction in flow rate occurs due to the loss of the additional flow provided by air entrainment when the control is pulled out. Although flow rates are decreased when operating the ventilator on source gas, the flow is constant. This produces a characteristic flow versus time curve that is square in shape. Thus, the air-mix control affects the flow pattern during inspiration; with the venturi activated, a decelerating flow pattern is produced. With the venturi disengaged (100% source gas), a square wave pattern (constant flow) is produced.

Expiratory Flow Control (Negative Pressure Control)

The expiratory flow control is unique to the Bird Mark 8. Its function is to control the flow of gas through an accessory nipple during expiration. This flow of gas can be used to drive negative end expiratory pressure (NEEP) or positive end expiratory pressure (PEEP) devices. It also may be used to provide expiratory nebulization. These applications were primarily restricted to the "Q" and "J" circles used for infant ventilation. These circuits and negative pressure controls are no longer used in neonatal clinical practice. However, the controls remain on the ventilators as they were designed a few decades ago.

Activation of the control causes gas to be drawn from the expiratory flow cartridge, which is charged during inspiration. The control is a needle valve that adjusts the rate of flow.

Time/Pressure Trigger Control

This control was added to the Mark 7A and Mark 8 machines. It is a pneumatic switch that determines if the machine operates in a pressure-triggered mode (IPPB therapy) or a time-triggered mode (apneustic ventilation).

If the control is in the pressure-triggered mode, the machine will operate only when patient effort triggers it on. When the control is in the time-triggered mode, the timing cartridge determines the machine's triggering.

Apneustic Time Control

The purpose of this control is to provide an inspiratory hold or pause to improve gas distribution within the lungs. It is unique to the Mark 7A and Mark 8.

During inspiration, an apneustic flow cartridge is pressurized. If the control is activated, flow during expiration is directed from the cartridge to the nebulizer and auxiliary jets on the venturi. The additional flow from the nebulizer holds the exhalation valve shut while the venturi provides additional flow. The expiratory hold feature lasts between 0.3 and 3 seconds. Adjustment of the control moves a needle valve that regulates the flow rate from the apneustic cartridge.

How the Controls Affect Delivered F_IO_2

The Bird machines all employ the venturi/venturi gate assembly in their operation (provided the Mark 7 is operated with the air mix control pulled out). The way that back pressure distal to a venturi alters F_IO_2 was discussed in Chapter 1. As pressure distal to a venturi builds, air entrainment decreases, causing the F_IO_2 to increase.

When pressure in the pressure chamber reaches approximately 12 cmH$_2$O , the venturi gate closes and the only source of flow is from the nebulizer. Since the nebulizer is powered by source gas, this situation further increases the F_IO_2. These factors combine to cause a variation in the F_IO_2 delivered to the patient. This fluctuation in F_IO_2 is only true if the machine is powered by oxygen.

How the Controls Affect Inspiratory Time

Inspiratory time is affected by the pressure and flow rate controls. If these controls are improperly adjusted, it is possible to deliver inverse **(inspiratory-to-expiratory) (I:E) ratio** ventilation, which may have adverse effects on the patient. These effects may include cardiovascular compromise, increased intracranial pressure, and hypotension which is caused by a decrease in venous return. When the apneustic flow control is used on the Bird Mark 7A and Mark 8, it influences inspiratory time also.

If gas flows into a closed chamber at a constant rate, it will take longer to reach a high pressure than a low one. Therefore, if the pressure control is set to a higher pressure, a longer time period will pass before inspiration is terminated. The time from beginning to end of inspiration is termed the inspiratory time.

The flow rate control also affects inspiratory time. A closed chamber with a fixed size will fill faster at a higher flow rate than a low one. Increasing the setting of the flow rate control will shorten inspiratory time.

When the apneustic flow control is activated on the Mark 7A and Mark 8, an inspiratory pause occurs. The length of the inspiratory pause must be added to the inspiratory time to determine the total inspiratory time. One effect of this control is to lengthen inspiratory time, which may alter the I:E ratio.

How the Controls Affect Expiratory Time

Expiratory time is influenced when the expiratory timer is in operation. The expiratory timer control determines the length of expiratory time. Its operation was discussed earlier in the chapter.

How the Controls Affect Delivered Tidal Volume

Delivered tidal volume is the amount of gas delivered to the patient during a breath using the machine. One of the goals of IPPB therapy is hyperinflation, or the delivery of a breath larger than is possible spontaneously. Two controls on the machine can be adjusted to increase tidal volume.

The pressure control is the primary control influencing tidal volume. An increase in pressure causes more gas to be delivered before the machine pressure cycles into expiration (inspiration ceases). However, recall that an increase in pressure lengthens inspiratory time. To maintain the same inspiratory time at the higher pressure, the flow rate control must be increased.

Figure 4-25 *Gas flow through a Bird circuit during (A) inspiration and (B) expiration.*

The flow rate control may also influence delivered tidal volumes. If the flow rate is increased to the point where flow is turbulent, proximal pressure will build more rapidly. This may result in a lower volume delivery than is desired, since inspiration is terminated more quickly.

Gas Flow through the Bird Circuit

During inspiration, gas flows from the pressure compartment through the 22-mm large-bore tubing to the patient. This is sometimes referred to as "main flow" (Figure 4-25). It is this flow that is primarily responsible for the delivery of tidal volume to the patient. The gas flowing through the large-bore tubing also serves as the carrier gas for the medication nebulized in the nebulizer.

Source gas flows through small diameter tubing to the **exhalation valve** and to the nebulizer simultaneously with the main flow of gas.

The gas powering the exhalation valve either inflates a mushroom valve or pushes a diaphragm down, sealing the exhalation port. This prevents the gas from taking the path of least resistance away from the patient and out the exhalation port (Figure 4-26). The gas also flows to the nebulizer jet. The nebulizer works just like the jet nebulizers discussed in Chapter 3, using choked flow. The nebulizer is a small-volume nebulizer that is either a main stream (Bird permanent circuit) or sidestream (disposable circuit) nebulizer (Figure 4-27).

Figure 4-26 *A functional diagram of a typical exhalation valve during (A) inhalation and (B) exhalation.*

Figure 4-27 *An assembly drawing of the Bird circuit.*

ASSEMBLY AND TROUBLESHOOTING

Assembly—Bird IPPB Ventilator

Circuit Assembly:

1. Assemble the nebulizer drive line and exhalation valve drive line by attaching the adapter to the nebulizer nipple and the free end to the exhalation valve (see Figure 4-27).

2. Attach the short flexible tubing to the outlet of the manifold (nebulizer/exhalation valve assembly) and attach the mouthpiece to its free end. Figure 4-27 shows the circuit correctly assembled.

3. Connect the circuit to the machine by attaching the large-bore tubing to the machine outlet (disposable circuits may require an adapter) and the small diameter tubing to the accessory power line.

Ventilator Preparation:

1. Attach the machine to a 50-psi gas source with high pressure hose. If a cylinder is used, use a two-stage regulator.

2. Adjust the controls to the following settings for the patient's first breath:
   a. Pressure between 10 and 20 cmH$_2$O
   b. Flow at 15
   c. Sensitivity at 10
   d. Air mix control out (Mark 7)
   e. Expiratory time control off

3. Instruct the patient on the machine's use.

4. Make further adjustments based on exhaled tidal volumes and the patient's tolerance to therapy.

Troubleshooting

A complete explanation of all events that can cause a malfunction is beyond the scope of this text. The more common ones are listed below and may serve as a useful guide. When troubleshooting please follow the suggested troubleshooting algorithm (ALG 4-1).

Machine cycles prematurely:

1. Check the flow rate control to determine if it is set too high. Adjust the control to a lower setting.

2. The patient may be obstructing the mouthpiece with the tongue. Explain the proper use of equipment again.

3. Pressure may be set too low to achieve the desired volumes. Increase the pressure as required.

Machine cycles on and off rapidly:

1. Adjust the sensitivity control to a lower setting (more difficult to initiate inspiration).

2. Coach the patient, explaining how the machine works when it senses a breath.

Inspiratory time is too long:

1. Increase the flow rate.

2. Check for leaks:
   a. In the patient circuit.
   b. Around the patient's mouthpiece.
   c. In some cases, nose clips, a mouth seal or a mask may be required.

3. Decrease the pressure. However, recall that this will decrease delivered tidal volumes.

4. Coach the patient to wait longer between breaths in order to lengthen expiratory time.

The pressure manometer indicates high negative pressures prior to inspiration:

1. Increase the sensitivity, reducing the patient's inspiratory effort.

The pressure manometer hesitates or rises erratically during inspiration:

1. Flow is inadequate. Increase the flow rate using the flow rate control.

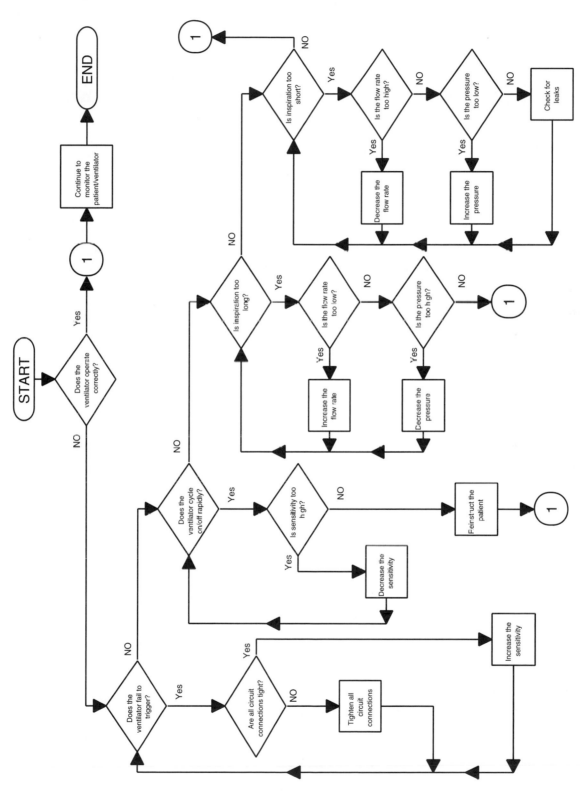

ALG 4-1 *A flowchart depicting troubleshooting of the Bird Mark 7 ventilator.*

BENNETT IPPB VENTILATORS

Puritan Bennett manufactured the AP-5 and the PR-2 models for sale and distribution.

The AP-5 shown in Figure 4-28 was designed for home use. It is an electrically powered ventilator with its own built-in compressor. The only other components required to operate the machine are a 120-volt power source and a patient circuit.

The Puritan Bennett PR-2 is a more complex machine designed for mechanical ventilation (Figure 4-29). It is a gas powered ventilator requiring a 50-psi source and is capable of ventilating an apneic patient.

The circuits are similar for both machines and will be discussed at the conclusion of this section.

The Bennett Valve

The Bennett valve functions as an on-off switch. The valve is flow sensitive and requires only 0.5 cmH$_2$O pressure to rotate it. Bennett literature describes the valve as "the valve that breathes with the patient."

The Bennett valve is composed of a drum, drum vane, counterweight, and front and back plates.

The drum is a cylinder that is closed at the front and rear. Windows located at the top and bottom of the drum permit gas to flow through it. The valve rotates on jeweled bearings at the front and rear. The bearings have serial numbers that match and each is machined individually for a near perfect fit. The precision bearings allow the valve to rotate with little

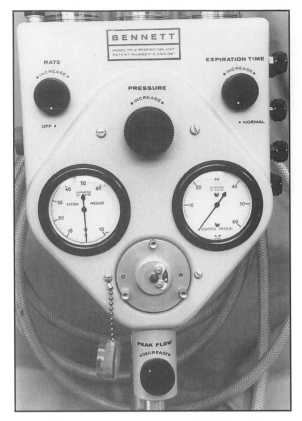

Figure 4-29 *The Puritan Bennett PR-2 ventilator.*

friction. Figure 4-30 shows the AP-5 and PR-2 Bennett valves; note that the PR-2 valve has two drum vanes.

As the patient begins inspiration, negative pressure is generated in the patient circuit and communicated to the Bennett valve. The reduced pressure rotates the valve (Figure 4-31).

Figure 4-28 *The Puritan Bennett AP-5 ventilator.*

Figure 4-30 *Two Bennett valves. The AP-5 valve on the left has only one drum vane while the PR-2 valve on the right has two drum vanes.*

Once the windows are aligned with the inlet and outlet of the valve, gas flows through it.

As pressure builds within the patient circuit, flow diminishes. When the flow is reduced to between 1 and 3 liters per minute, gravity pulls down on the counterweight closing the valve (Figure 4-32).

Bennett AP-5 Ventilator

As indicated earlier the Bennett AP-5 is primarily designed for home use; it is, however, used in some hospitals. The AP-5 ventilator is an electrically powered ventilator. It is a pressure controller that is pressure triggered and flow cycled. The controls and their operation were designed simply, so that the average patient would be able to use the machine effectively. There are three controls on the

Figure 4-32 *A functional diagram illustrating how the Bennett valve closes at the end of inspiration.*

Bennett AP-5: on-off switch, pressure control, and nebulizer control.

On-Off Switch

The on-off switch is located on the front of the machine below the pressure manometer. It is an electrical toggle switch that operates in a way similar to a light switch in your home.

Pressure Control

The pressure control on the AP-5 operates by using a spring-loaded disk that vents excess pressure to the atmosphere. Pressure output is limited to around 30 cmH$_2$O.

Gas pressure is supplied to the pressure control by an internal electric compressor.

Figure 4-31 *Functional diagrams of how the Bennett valve (AP-5) opens during inspiration.*

ASSEMBLY AND TROUBLESHOOTING

Assembly—Puritan Bennett Corporation AP-5

1. Connect the machine to a 120 volt power source.

2. Assemble the circuit. (Refer to the section discussing the Bennett circuits.)

3. Attach the 22-mm diameter large-bore tubing to the large outlet on the machine.

4. Attach the small-diameter tube without the flared (large-diameter) end to the exhalation valve nipple.

5. Attach the other small-diameter tube (with the flared end) to the nebulizer nipple.

6. Turn the machine on and aseptically occlude the mouthpiece. Adjust the pressure to the ordered level by manually cycling the Bennett valve and adjusting the pressure until the desired pressure is registered on the manometer.

7. Turn on the nebulizer flow until aerosol is visible coming out of the mouthpiece.

Troubleshooting

When troubleshooting, please follow the suggested troubleshooting algorithm (ALG 4-2).

1. If the nebulizer fails to operate:

 a. Check the circuit for correct assembly and any obstructions or kinks in the nebulizer drive line.

 b. Check to ensure that the nebulizer drive line is attached to the nebulizer nipple on the machine and the nipple on the circuit.

 c. Ensure that medication has been added to the nebulizer cup.

 d. Check for flow coming out of the nebulizer nipple. If flow is absent, take the machine to a qualified biomedical repair facility.

2. If the machine fails to cycle properly:

 a. Check the circuit for correct assembly and tighten all connections.

 b. Clean the Bennett valve. This must be performed carefully since the valve is quite delicate. Gently remove the front cover and lay it on a flat surface where it will not be accidentally dropped. Carefully remove the drum by grasping the handle protruding from the front of the drum (Figure 4-33). Gently clean the valve with an alcohol prep pad and allow the alcohol to evaporate. Replace the valve, carefully aligning it and replace the front cover.

 c. If a and b are satisfactory and the machine still fails to operate correctly, take it to a qualified biomedical repair facility.

Room air is drawn in through a 10-micron filter, compressed, then passed through a submicron filter. Flow is divided between the pressure control and the nebulizer.

Flow through the pressure control is augmented by a venturi. Ambient air enters the venturi through a 40-micron filter. The venturi boosts the flow out of the regulator providing total flow to the patient of between 75 and 90 liters per minute.

Nebulizer Control

The nebulizer on the AP-5 operates continuously (inspiration and expiration). Flow to the nebulizer is controlled by a needle valve. Opening the needle valve increases flow to the jet in the nebulizer, thus increasing the rate of nebulization.

Figure 4-33 *This photograph illustrates the correct way to handle the Bennett valve.*

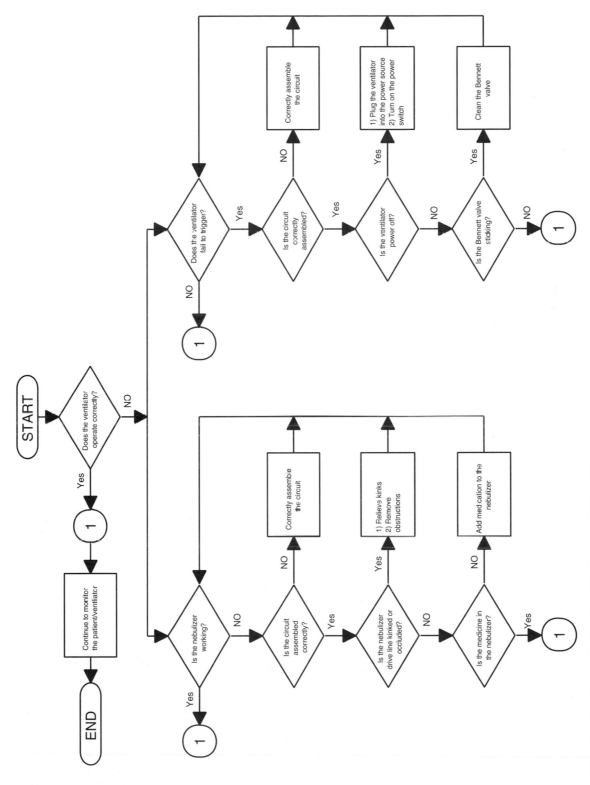

ALG 4-2 *A flowchart depicting troubleshooting of the Bennett AP-5 ventilator.*

The Bennett PR-2 Ventilator

The Bennett PR-2 has more controls than the AP-5 and is more complex in its operation. The PR-2 ventilator is one you will most likely encounter in the hospital environment. It is a pneumatically powered, pressure controller. The ventilator is pressure or time-triggered and is flow cycled.

Pressure Control

The purpose of the pressure control is to reduce the 50-psi line pressure to a safe level. It is located in the center of the ventilator (Figure 4-34). Pressure reduction is accomplished by a single-stage, low pressure reducing valve. The operation of this valve was discussed earlier in this chapter. The pressure output from the reducing valve is between 0 and 45 cmH$_2$O.

Air Dilution Control

The purpose of the air dilution control is identical to the air mix control on the Bird Mark 7. Adjustment of the control determines whether 100% source gas or source gas diluted with ambient air is delivered to the patient. Pushing in the air dilution control activates a venturi, delivering source gas mixed with ambient air to the patient. Pulling the control out delivers 100% source gas to the patient. Since the venturi is an integral part of the reducing valve (pressure control), it does not affect gas flow as the venturi in the Bird machines does (Figure 4-35).

When the control is pushed in, gas is channeled through a venturi that supplies pressure to the reducing valve. In the out position, the venturi channel is closed, and pure source gas enters the reducing valve through the poppet valve.

Rate Control

The rate control is not used for IPPB therapy. It is utilized only when ventilating an apneic patient.

The purpose of the rate control is to establish a respiratory rate for an apneic patient. Activation of the control will time-cycle the ventilator. The operation of this control is quite complex. A complete discussion of gas pathways and control is not required for most practitioners. Enough of the operation will be discussed to understand its function without becoming too complex. (Refer to "Operating Instructions, Bennett PR-2 Respiration Unit," Bennett Respiration Products, Santa Monica, CA, 1979, for more specific discussion.)

Figure 4-34 *The Bennett PR-2 ventilator. (A) Front panel controls; (B) side panel controls.*

Figure 4-35 *A functional diagram of the Bennett PR-2 pressure control and venturi system. Air dilution control (A) pulled out and (B) pushed in.*

Adjustment of the rate control opens or closes a needle valve. Gas flow from the needle valve is channeled to the left and right accumulators.

The accumulators are pneumatic timing switches that control the pathway of gas from many different lines. The PR-2 ventilator has three accumulators located on the top of the ventilator. Each accumulator has six ports (Figure 4-36). One port (number 6) supplies the gas pressure that drives the accumulator. Depending on the accumulator's position (up or down) gas is routed through ports 2, 3, and 5 (up position) or ports 2 and 4 (down position).

Gas flows from the left, and right accumu-

Figure 4-36 *This diagram of the PR-2 accumulators shows both the up and down positions.*

lators pass through the center accumulator that phases inspiration and expiration. Gas supply for the center accumulator originates from a port directly below the Bennett valve. The center accumulator is only pressurized during inspiration. During inspiration, the balloon at the top of the accumulator is inflated, pushing the shaft downward, opening the even numbered ports (2 and 4), and providing gas flow.

The number one accumulator (left most accumulator when facing the front of the ventilator), is phased to operate during expiration. The rate control is a needle valve, which directs gas flow to port 6 of the number one and number three accumulators. Port 6 of the number one accumulator is connected to an even port on the center accumulator. When the even ports of the center accumulator are blocked during expiration, gas can only flow to the left accumulator (port 6) and up the accumulator shaft and inflate the balloon at the top of the port, driving the piston down. Once the left accumulator piston reaches the bottom of its travel, gas from the low pressure reducing valve is directed out port 4 of the left accumulator to a port above the upper drum vane, triggering the ventilator into inspiration by rotating the Bennett valve open (Figure 4-37).

Adjustment of the rate control determines the speed at which the left most accumulator

Figure 4-37 *The Bennett PR-2 valve opening in response to gas flow above the upper drum vane.*

travels downward, and therefore the length of the expiratory time.

The number three accumulator (right most accumulator when facing the front of the ventilator) is phased to operate during inspiration. Port 6 of the right accumulator is connected to an odd port (port 1) on the center accumulator. During inspiration, the center accumulator piston moves down, blocking the odd ports. Since the gas pathway for the number 6 port of the right accumulator is blocked, gas flows up the piston, inflating the balloon and driving the piston downward. Once the piston reaches the bottom of its travel, gas flow from the low pressure reducing valve flows through port 4 of the right accumulator to a mushroom valve located at the outlet of the dilutor regulator assembly. Gas pressure inflates the mushroom valve, blocking gas flow from the dilutor regulator to the Bennett valve, cycling the ventilator into expiration. Functionally, the speed of the right accumulator's inflation determines the inspiratory time. Since the right accumulator only inflates on inspiration, it lags slightly behind the center phasing accumulator.

Expiration Time

The expiration time control, like the rate control, is not used for IPPB therapy. The expiration time control modifies the function of the rate control to lengthen the expiratory time.

Functionally the expiration time operates by closing a needle valve. Closing the expiration time needle valve reduces flow to the left accumulator, increasing expiratory time.

Nebulizer Controls

The PR-2 ventilator has the ability to nebulize medication during both inspiration and expiration independently. The intent of the expiration nebulizer control is to fill the flexible tubing, manifold, and mouthpiece with aerosol before inspiration begins. This is to ensure that the earliest part of inspiration (presumably the part that penetrates most deeply) contains aerosol.

The operation of these controls is regulated by an inflatable flapper valve, called a nebulizer pressure switch (Figure 4-38). During inspiration, the mushroom is inflated, directing gas to the needle valve. The needle valve controls the flow of gas to the nebulizer during inspiration.

During the expiration phase, gas no longer flows to inflate the mushroom valve in the nebulizer pressure switch. Hence, the valve is closed. Now gas flow may go to the expiration nebulizer needle valve only.

Negative Pressure Control

The negative pressure control is not used for IPPB therapy. Its use is primarily limited to the ventilation of neonates. The purpose of the control is to evacuate gas from the patient circuit. To operate, it requires an external attachment to the circuit.

The control operates by using the reduced lateral pressure from an internal venturi. The sub-ambient pressure (up to -6 cmH$_2$O) is applied to the patient circuit and also above the lower drum vane. The reduced pressure above the lower drum vane is to compensate for the application of reduced pressure below it (through the patient circuit) so the ventilator operates normally. Adjustment of the control varies the flow through the venturi and therefore the amount of reduced pressure generated. Application of negative pressure through special neonatal circuits using the PR-2 is no longer utilized in the modern newborn intensive care settings. The control however, remains as it was originally designed many years earlier.

Sensitivity

The sensitivity control on the PR-2 has the same function as the sensitivity control on the Bird ventilators. Both are patient effort controls.

The Bennett sensitivity control operates by using a needle valve. When the valve is opened, gas is directed to a port above the

Figure 4-38 *A functional diagram of the PR-2 nebulizer control during (A) inspiration and (B) expiration. Note how the flapper valve determines which needle valve is operating.*

upper drum vane. This gas flow assists in rotating the valve open during inspiration. The center accumulator ensures that the valve is only rotated in the inspiratory phase.

Terminal Flow Control

Terminal flow is used to help cycle the ventilator off when leaks are present. Leaks can occur in the circuit or around the patient's mouth. The terminal flow control will compensate for a leak of up to 15 liters per minute. If a leak is present, gas flow through the valve will not decrease sufficiently to close it. This control is very helpful when using the ventilator with a mask or mouth seal interface to provide therapy.

Activation of the terminal flow control directs gas to a venturi below the Bennett valve. The additional flow provides assistance in closing the Bennett valve.

The use of terminal flow adds mixed gas (source gas mixed with ambient air) distal to the Bennett valve. Addition of terminal flow with the air dilution control out (source gas setting) will dilute the delivered F_IO_2.

Peak Flow

Distal to the Bennett valve is a variable orifice that is attached to the peak flow control. The purpose of the control is to slow the flow of gas delivered from the ventilator. It only limits maximum flow from the ventilator and does not operate in the same way as the Bird's peak flow controls. By turning the peak flow control clockwise, the orifice is restricted limiting peak flow from the ventilator. During IPPB therapy the control is normally turned fully counterclockwise.

Pressure Manometers

The PR-2 ventilator has two pressure manometers, control pressure (right) and system pressure (left). The control pressure tells the operator what the internal machine pressure is. The left one reflects the pressure in the patient circuit.

The control pressure manometer is connected between the Bennett valve and the low pressure reducing valve (pressure control). This manometer reflects the pressure output from the reducing valve.

The system pressure control is connected to a port below the terminal flow control. This manometer only reflects pressure in the patient circuit.

How the Controls Affect Ventilation

Adjustment of the ventilator controls affects inspiratory time, expiratory time, and F_IO_2 in a way similar to that in which the Bird ventilator controls are interrelated.

F_IO_2. As discussed earlier, F_IO_2 will be diminished when using the source gas setting (air dilution control pulled out) and by using terminal flow.

As with the Bird ventilator, when the PR-2 is operating using the venturi system, F_IO_2 will vary. This is because increased pressure in the circuit will cause a decrease in ambient air entrainment through the venturi. Actual F_IO_2 will vary between 40% and 60%.

Inspiratory Time. The inspiratory time of the PR-2 is primarily related to the pressure set on the pressure control. As with the Bird, when pressure is set at a higher level, a longer time is required to deliver that pressure.

The peak flow control will decrease the flow of gas at a given pressure. The effect of this control is to lengthen inspiratory time. Normally this is not desired during IPPB therapy.

Expiratory Time. During IPPB therapy, expiratory time is largely a function of patient coaching. Patients must usually be told to deliberately slow their respiratory rate when using an IPPB ventilator. Hyperventilation is a common adverse effect of this therapy.

When using the ventilator to ventilate an apneic patient, the expiratory time control will increase expiratory time by decreasing flow through the rate control system.

Tidal Volume. Tidal volume delivered from the PR-2 is altered by using the pressure control. Care must be used to ensure that pressures do not become excessive or that inspiratory time does not become too long when trying to deliver specific tidal volumes.

Gas Flow Through the Bennett Circuit

The Bennett circuit is composed of three lines: (1) a 22-mm, large-diameter main flow line; (2) a small-diameter line to power the nebulizer; and (3) a small-diameter line to power the exhalation valve (Figure 4-39).

The large, 22-mm tubing is connected to the outlet of the ventilator (underside for the PR-2). Gas from the Bennett valve flows through this line to the patient. The majority of volume delivery occurs through this line and it also serves as a carrier gas for the aerosol from the nebulizer.

The exhalation valve is simultaneously powered during inspiration. Gas inflates a mushroom (permanent circuit) or depresses a diaphragm (disposable circuit) to close the exhalation port during inspiration. During the expiratory phase, pressure is released and the

Figure 4-39 *This diagram illustrates flow through the Bennett circuit during (A) inspiration and (B) exhalation.*

patient's exhaled air is conducted through the exhalation port. The exhalation valve line is the smaller of the two small-diameter lines in the circuit.

Flow to the nebulizer is delivered by the inspiration and expiration nebulizer controls. Output from the controls is conducted to the nebulizer by means of the small-diameter tubing. The nebulizer drive line is the larger of the two small-diameter lines in the Bennett circuit.

ASSEMBLY AND TROUBLESHOOTING

Assembly—Puritan Bennett Corporation PR-2 Ventilator

The following assembly procedure describes the use of the ventilator for IPPB therapy. For mechanical ventilation, a heated humidifier and monitoring equipment will need to be attached.

1. Assemble the circuit, as shown in Figure 4-40.

2. Connect the ventilator to a 50-psi gas source using high pressure hose.

3. Connect the circuit to the ventilator.

4. Adjust the following controls as indicated:
   a. Rate control fully counterclockwise (off).
   b. Expiration time fully counterclockwise (off).
   c. Peak flow fully counterclockwise (open).
   d. Terminal flow fully clockwise (off).
   e. Sensitivity fully counterclockwise (off).

f. Negative pressure fully clockwise (off).

g. Inspiration nebulizer counterclockwise about one-half turn (on).

h. Air dilution control pushed in (on).

5. Add the ordered amount and dilution of medication to the nebulizer.

6. Adjust the pressure control to the ordered level or between 10 and 20 cmH$_2$O.

7. Adjust the expiration nebulizer until aerosol is just visible coming out of the mouthpiece.

8. Instruct the patient on the ventilator's use.

9. Make further adjustment in the controls based upon the ordered tidal volume and patient's tolerance.

Troubleshooting

A complete explanation of all events that can cause a malfunction is beyond the scope of this text. The more common ones are listed below and may serve as a useful guide. Proficient application of IPPB therapy requires practice and experience. When troubleshooting, please follow the suggested troubleshooting algorithm (ALG 4-3).

Ventilator cycles prematurely:

1. The patient may be obstructing the mouthpiece with the tongue. Explain the use of ventilator again.

2. Pressure may be set too low to achieve the desired volumes. Increase the pressure as required.

Ventilator cycles on and off rapidly:

1. Coach the patient, explaining how the ventilator works when it senses a breath.

2. Check for obstructions in the main tubing or a kinked tube.

3. Sensitivity may be set too high. Decrease the sensitivity.

4. The rate control may be on. Turn the rate control off.

Inspiratory time is too long:

1. Check to ensure the peak flow control is fully clockwise.

2. Check for leaks:
   a. Check the patient circuit.
   b. Ensure the patient has a tight seal around the mouthpiece.
   c. In some cases nose clips, a mouth seal, or a mask may be required.

3. Decrease the pressure, recalling that delivered tidal volumes will decrease.

4. Coach the patient to wait longer between breaths in order to lengthen expiratory time.

Ventilator fails to cycle off:

1. Add terminal flow gradually to correct the problem.

2. Check for leaks in the patient circuit.

Figure 4-40 *An assembly drawing of a Bennett IPPB circuit.*

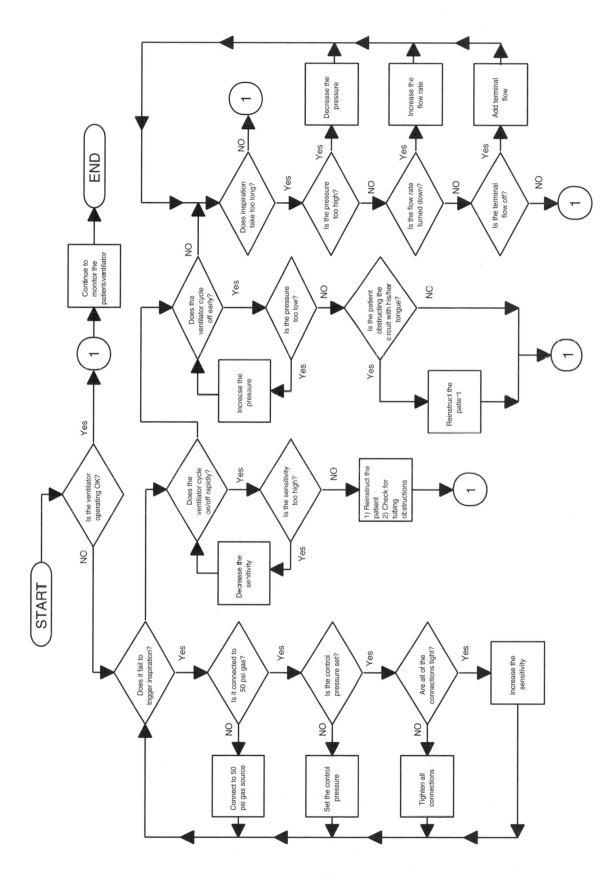

ALG 4-3 *A flowchart depicting troubleshooting of the Bennett PR-2 ventilator.*

PERCUSSIONAIRE CORPORATION IPV® VENTILATORS

Intrapulmonary Percussive Ventilation (IPV®) is a combination of high frequency phased pulse gas delivery (100–250 cycles per minute) and the administration of a dense aerosol. The high frequency pulsed delivery of a sub-tidal volume of gas causes a pressure wedge to be developed in the pulmonary system (Figure 4-41). This controlled wedge of pressure is caused by gas trapping due to the high ventilatory rate and precisely regulated I:E ratio of gas delivery. This increase in pressure helps to augment the volume of inspired gas and to stabilize or enlarge the caliber of the airways. The percussive effect of gas delivery helps to ventilate past obstructions and to deliver air to the distal portions of the lungs. Coughing following the percussive interval facilitates removal of retained secretions, further opening areas of the lung to ventilation.

The administration of a dense aerosol during IPV® allows the delivery of medications (vasoconstrictors, bronchodilators, and mucokinetic agents) to promote bronchial hygiene, reduce edema, and decrease bronchoconstriction.

The clinical effect of IPV® is to combine an intrapulmonary percussion (similar in effect to external chest clapping) with the delivery of a dense aerosol. Advantages of IPV® over conventional aerosol administration and chest clapping is that practitioner technique and fatigue are no longer factors in determining the effectiveness of therapy.

PERCUSSIONATOR®

The Percussionator® is the mechanical device that delivers the pulsed gas to the Phasitron® in the patient circuit. A pneumatic diagram of the IPV®-1C is shown in Figure 4-42. The Percussionator® is a pneumatically powered pressure controller that is time cycled. It is triggered by the patient when a thumb control is depressed.

Volume of pulsatile gas is controlled by adjusting the system pressure. Pressure is adjustable between 25 and 40 psi. As pressure is increased, volume delivery also is increased.

Frequency is controlled by the Impact control on the IPV®-1C and the frequency control (IPV-2). The frequency is adjustable between 100 and 250 pulses per minute. I:E ratios will vary from 1:1.5 (higher frequencies) to 1:3 (lower frequencies).

PHASITRON®

The Phasitron® provides a mechanical and pneumatic interface between the percussionator and the patient's airway. During delivery of pulsed gas flow as shown in Figure 4-43, gas pressure is applied to an orificed diaphragm. As the diaphragm distorts from the applied pressure, the sliding body of the venturi is advanced forward, closing the exhalation port. Simultaneously, gas is ejected through a nozzle into the throat of the venturi. The venturi entrains room air through the entrainment port at a ratio of 1:5 (source gas to ambient air). Aerosolized medication is admitted through the entrainment port and delivered to the patient's airway through the Phasitron®.

As the pressure wedge develops in the patient's airways, entrainment through the venturi is decreased due to increased pressure distal to the entrainment port. This reduction in total flow through the Phasitron® protects the patient from barotrauma, acting as a pneumatic buffer to the Percussionator®.

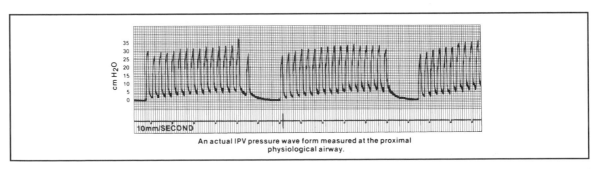

An actual IPV pressure wave form measured at the proximal physiological airway.

Figure 4-41   *Pressure versus time waveform of percussive ventilation while ventilating pulmonary structures (proximal airway pressure). (Courtesy Percussionaire Corporation, Sandpoint, ID)*

Figure 4-42 *A pneumatic diagram of the Percussionaire IPV®-1. (Courtesy Percussionaire Corporation, Sandpoint, ID)*

Figure 4-43 *A full section showing the Phasitron® during inspiration. (Courtesy Percussionaire Corporation, Sandpoint, ID)*

When the thumb button is released, the percussive gas delivery from the Percussionator® ceases. The coil spring in the Phasitron® slides the venturi body back against the diaphragm, opening the exhalation port as shown in Figure 4-44. The patient may then passively exhale. While the exhalation port is open, the patient is free to breathe aerosol passively from the nebulizer without any percussive effect.

PERCUSSIONAIRE IPV®-2

The Percussionaire IPV®-2 is the most complex of the IPV® ventilators produced by the company (Figure 4-45). It is an advanced postsurgical model intended for acute care use. It has the most control features giving the practitioner great flexibility in the clinical application of the device.

Figure 4-44 *A full section showing the Phasitron® during expiration. (Courtesy Percussionaire Corporation, Sandpoint, ID)*

Figure 4-45 *A photograph of the Percussionaire IPV®-2 ventilator. (Courtesy Percussionaire Corporation, Sandpoint, ID)*

Control Features

Master Switch

The master switch is an on/off valve that controls the operation of the IPV®-2 (Figure 4-46). In the on position, the IPV®-2 allows the practitioner to operate the ventilator delivering IPV® therapy, or IPV® therapy with continuous positive airway pressure (CPAP). This is termed oscillatory demand CPAP (OD-CPAP). In the off position, the ventilator delivers aerosolized medication with traditional demand CPAP.

Inspiratory Flow

Inspiratory flow may be regulated during percussive ventilation by using the Inspiratory flow control. The control regulates the flow of gas going out of the oscillator cartridge (See Figure 4-46). This control has the effect of reducing the percussive amplitude by modulating the output of the oscillator cartridge.

Inspiratory Time

The inspiratory time control gives the practitioner the ability to control the rate of inspiratory pressure rise during pulsed gas delivery. The control consists of a needle valve downstream from the oscillator (see Figure 4-46).

Frequency Control

The frequency control allows the practitioner to control the frequency of pulsed gas

Figure 4-46 *A pneumatic diagram of the IPV®-2 pneumatic circuit. (Courtesy Percussionaire Corporation, Sandpoint, ID)*

delivery to the Phasitron®. Frequencies from 100 to 250 cycles per minute are possible.

Source Pressure

The source pressure control is a pressure reducing valve that determines the impact velocity of the percussive pulses. Pressures are adjustable between 20 and 50 psi on the IPV®-2. It is recommended to begin therapy at pressures of 30 psi. The control is located on the side panel behind the hinged door on the front of the ventilator.

Nebulizer

The nebulizer control allows the practitioner to vary the output of the nebulizer in the patient circuit. A needle valve controls the flow of gas to the nebulizer.

Demand CPAP Control

The demand CPAP control is an adjustable regulator used to provide CPAP during oscillatory or demand ventilation. CPAP ranges are adjustable between 0 and 30 cmH₂O.

Manual Inspiration

The manual inspiration switch is located on the front panel to manually trigger the ventilator into the oscillatory mode. This is provided in the event the ventilator is used for cardiopulmonary resuscitation efforts.

PERCUSSIONAIRE IPV®-1C

The Percussionaire IPV®-1C (Figure 4-47) is an acute care IPV® ventilator with fewer control features than the IPV®-2. It is suitable for the management of patients with cardiopul-

Figure 4-47 *A photograph of the Percussionaire IPV®-1C ventilator. (Courtesy Percussionaire Corporation, Sandpoint, ID)* monary disease in which secretion mobilization is desirable.

Control Features

Source Pressure

The source pressure control is a pressure reducing valve that determines the impact velocity of the percussive pulses. Pressures are adjustable between 20 and 50 psi on the IPV®-2. It is recommended to begin therapy at pressures of 30 psi. The control is located on the side panel behind the hinged door on the front of the ventilator.

Impact Control

The impact control controls the frequency of the pulsed gas delivery to the Phasitron®. Frequencies are adjustable from 100 to 250 cycles per minute.

Manual Inspiration

The manual inspiration switch is provided on the front panel to manually trigger the ventilator into the oscillatory mode. This is provided in the event the ventilator is used for cardiopulmonary resuscitation efforts.

ASSEMBLY AND TROUBLESHOOTING

Patient Manifold (Phasitron® and Nebulizer)—Percussionaire Corporation IPV®

As you complete the following sequence, refer to Figure 4-48 to identify the components of the circuit you are assembling.

Phasitron®

1. Attach the orificed diaphragm onto the stem of the venturi cage socket.

2. Check the distal end of the Phasitron® (opposite the diaphragm) for a black "O" ring, which seals against the exhalation port. If the Phasitron® is missing the "O" ring, install one.

3. Slip the coil spring over the venturi body and insert the venturi body into the Phasitron® housing.

4. Complete the Phasitron® assembly by installing the threaded white end cap by rotating clockwise until it is seated.

5. Install a mouthpiece onto the proximal end of the Phasitron®.

Nebulizer

1. Remove the reservoir assembly from the nebulizer by rotating it counterclockwise.

2. Add the ordered medication to the nebulizer reservoir. The nebulizer can hold up to 20 ml of medication.

3. Reinstall the top of the nebulizer which contains the thumb switch to the nebulizer reservoir.

4. Mate the Phasitron® and the nebulizer together using the port on the side of the Phasitron® at its distal end (near the diaphragm).

5. Set the completed assembly aside, being careful not to spill medication from the Nebulizer.

Drive Line Assembly

The drive lines for the IPV® circuit are color coded, facilitating their assembly to thePercussionator® and Phasitron®.

Percussionator® Connections

1. Mate the red line to the red snap lock fitting on the Percussionator® labeled Gauge.

2. Mate the white line to the white snap lock fitting on the Percussionator® labeled Phasitron®.

3. Mate the green line to the green snap lock fitting on the Percussionator® labeled Remote.

4. Mate the yellow line to the yellow snap lock fitting on the Percussionator® labeled Nebulizer.

Phasitron® Connections

1. Mate the red line to the red snap lock fitting on the Phasitron®'s proximal airway port (at the proximal end).

Figure 4-48 *A photograph of the Percussionaire IPV® circuit. (Courtesy Percussionaire Corporation, Sandpoint, ID)*

2. Mate the white line to the white snap lock fitting on the Phasitron®'s white end cap.

3. Mate the Green line to the green snap lock fitting on the Phasitron®'s nebulizer cap opposite the thumb button.

4. Mate the Yellow line to the yellow snap lock fitting on the Phasitron®'s nebulizer at the base of the reservoir.

5. Finally connect red condenser tubing to the Phasitron®'s exhalation port to prevent aerosol from spraying yourself or the patient's clothing.

Operation of the IPV® Ventilator

1. If you are using an IPV®-1 or IPV®-2, connect the 50-psi gas inlet to a suitable 50-psi medical gas supply (typically oxygen).

2. If you are using the Spanker, connect the drive lines to their appropriate snap lock fittings on the regulator supplied in the kit. Ensure the regulator is attached to a medical gas cylinder with sufficient contents to deliver IPV® therapy.

3. When using the IPV®-1 or IPV®-2, adjust the operation pressure to 30 psi:
    a. Open the hinged door on the front of the ventilator.
    b. Depress the thumb button on the patient circuit, triggering pulsed gas delivery.
    c. Release the red locking ring on the Source Pressure adjustment control by pulling it out away from the body of the Percussionator®.
    d. Rotate the Source Pressure control clockwise to increase pressure or counterclockwise to decrease pressure. Monitor operational pressure adjustment by observing the pressure gauge on the top of the Percussionator® housing.

e. When the operational pressure is correctly set, lock the pressure adjustment by gently pushing the red locking ring, seating it against the Percussionator® housing.

4. IPV®-2 initial control settings:
   a. Rotate the Frequency control fully counterclockwise.
   b. Rotate the Insp. Time control fully clockwise.
   c. Rotate Insp. Flow control until the arrow is positioned at 12:00.
   d. Rotate the demand CPAP control clockwise to the "Off" position (inside the hinged door on the right of the Percussionator®).
   e. Rotate the Nebulizer control until the arrow points to the 12:00 position (inside the hinged door on the right of the Percussionator®).
   f. Rotate the Master Switch to the On position.
   g. Instruct the patient on IPV® therapy and carefully monitor the patient.

5. IPV®-1 initial control settings:
   a. Rotate the Impact control until the arrow is at the 12:00 o'clock position.
   b. Instruct the patient on IPV® therapy and carefully monitor the patient.

Troubleshooting

The IPV® unit fails to trigger delivering pulsed gas delivery. When troubleshooting, please follow the suggested troubleshooting algorithm (ALG 4-4).

1. Check to ensure that the IPV® unit is connected to a 50-psi medical gas power source.
2. Check for correct assembly of the drive circuit.
   a. Ensure that all color-coded lines match to the appropriately color coded snap locks on both the Phasitron® and the Percussionator®.
3. Check for correct operational pressure adjustment. Initial operational pressure should be set at 30 psi.

The nebulizer fails to generate any aerosol:

1. Check for correct assembly of the drive circuit.
   a. Ensure that all color-coded lines match to the appropriately color-coded snap locks on both the Phasitron® and the Percussionator®.
2. Check to ensure medication has been added to the nebulizer reservoir.
3. If using the IPV®-2, check to ensure that the Nebulizer control has been adjusted such that the nebulizer has sufficient output.

No pressure is indicated during percussive ventilation by the pressure manometer:

1. Check for correct assembly of the drive circuit.
   a. Ensure that all color-coded lines match to the appropriately color-coded snap locks on both the Phasitron® and the Percussionator®.

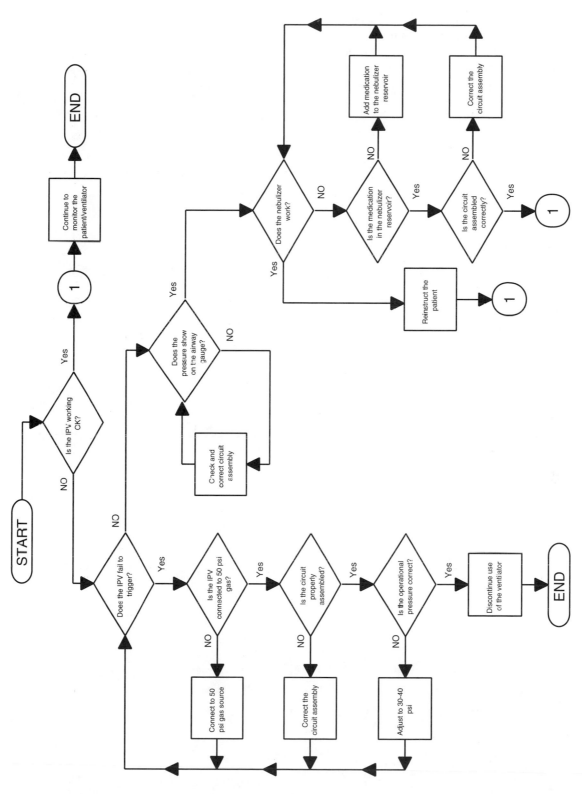

ALG 4-4 *A flowchart depicting troubleshooting of the Percussionaire IPV® ventilator.*

PERCUSSORS USED FOR CHEST PHYSIOTHERAPY

Chest physiotherapy involves clapping on a patient's chest using cupped hands. By trapping a small pocket of air under the hands, vibrations are induced in the lung parenchyma that loosen pulmonary secretions. Manual percussion, although effective, can be tiring. Mechanical **percussors** have been developed to facilitate administration of chest physiotherapy and to ensure that all patients receive effective therapy.

Percussors are either electrically powered or gas powered. Both types will be discussed in this text.

VIBRAMATIC

The General Physiotherapy company manufactures both the Vibramatic and Flimm Fighter percussors. Both machines are electrically powered. An electric motor turns a flexible shaft that causes the head or applicator to vibrate.

The Vibramatic incorporates a timer and a frequency control (Figure 4-49). The timer may be set for a specific time interval of therapy. Once the time has elapsed, the percussor turns off. The frequency control may be adjusted to increase or decrease the frequency at which the applicator vibrates, allowing for variations in patient tolerance.

FLIMM FIGHTER

The Flimm Fighter is primarily intended for home use (Figure 4-50). It is a small portable percussor that allows self-therapy by the patient. A velcro pad and strap allow the

Figure 4-50 *The Flimm Fighter percussor.*

Figure 4-49 *The Vibramatic percussor.*

patient to strap the applicator to his chest and then to assume the proper drainage position. Controls are limited to an "On/Off" switch.

MJ PERCUSSOR

The MJ Percussor is a gas powered percussor. The components of this percussor include a high pressure supply hose, control head, and applicator (Figure 4-51).

The high pressure hose is designed to use gas at 50 psi to power the unit. The gas may be oxygen or air. The use of air is recommended since one case of fire from an oxygen powered percussor has been reported.

The control head contains an electrically powered timing mechanism. The timing mechanism determines the frequency with which the gas powered piston is driven. The timer controls the operation of a solenoid valve that alternately applies gas pressure to the piston driving it. This electric control requires a 9-volt battery.

The applicator is a rubber suction cup. Disposable covers are available to promote aseptic usage of this device.

ASSEMBLY AND TROUBLESHOOTING

Assembly—Pneumatic and Electric Percussors

1. Connect the percussor to a 10-volt power source or 50-psi gas source.

2. Adjust the frequency control to the desired setting.

3. Set the timer for the ordered length of therapy.

4. Apply the percussor head (applicator) to the patient's chest. (Do not push on the applicator. The weight of the head is sufficient for good therapy.)

Troubleshooting

Troubleshooting these devices in the clinical setting is primarily limited to checking for proper power connection. Any other malfunction should be referred to a qualified biomedical repair center.

Figure 4-51 *The MJ Percussor.*

ADJUNCTIVE EQUIPMENT FOR MANUAL CHEST PERCUSSION

Chest percussion is frequently performed using a manual technique: cupping one's hand and clapping on the chest wall of the patient receiving therapy. The technique assists the patient in mobilizing secretions and expectorating them. It is a form of therapy that is highly technique dependent, requiring a lot of practice to become proficient.

Adjuncts have been developed to assist practitioners by providing a consistent cupped surface that strikes the patient's chest wall. These devices remove some of the technique-dependent aspects of the therapy. Most of these adjunctive devices are made from a soft silicone rubber that minimizes the potential trauma of using the device.

DHD HEALTHCARE PALM CUPS®

Figure 4-52 is a photograph of the four sizes of Palm Cups® manufactured and distributed by DHD Healthcare. The Palm Cups® are made of a soft vinyl rubber and are designed such that the raised portion of the Palm Cups® is placed between the first and second digits of one's hand. The Palm Cups® provide uniformity and consistency from one practitioner to another in their chest physiotherapy technique.

BALLARD® MANUAL PERCUSSOR FOR NEONATAL USE

Ballard® Medical, a division of Kimberly-Clark, manufactures and distributes a small, soft vinyl percussor mounted on a plastic wand designed for neonatal applications (Figure 4-53). Frequently, the chest wall size of a neonate is too small for using other adjunctive devices. The Manual Percussor is designed specifically for the small neonate's chest wall size. The flexibility of the plastic wand negates some of the impact when using the percussor and also alleviates some of the fatigue aspects of using such a small percussor head.

HIGH FREQUENCY CHEST WALL OSCILLATION (HFCWO) THERAPY

High Frequency Chest Wall Oscillation therapy (HFCWO) is the application of external chest wall compression using a self-inflating/deflating pneumatic vest. The patient applies the vest and performs self-therapy independent of any other caregiver. This therapy achieves the same effect as chest percussion as performed by a caregiver.

Figure 4-52 *A photograph of the four sizes of Palm Cups® manufactured and distributed by DHD Healthcare.*

Figure 4-53 *A photograph of the manual percussor for neonatal use manufactured and marketed by Ballard® Medical, a division of Kimberly-Clark.*

The Vest™ (Figure 4-54) consists of an air-pulse generator, two hoses, and a vest that the patient applies. The air-pulse generator creates inflation and deflation pulses that rapidly inflate and deflate the patient vest at frequencies between 5 and 25 times per second. Both the frequency and amplitude can be controlled by the patient for comfort and effectiveness. The pulsating inflation and deflation of the vest facilitates secretion mobilization and is indicated for mucous plugging, retained secretions, and chronic diseases such as cystic fibrosis.

The vest is contraindicated with unstable thoracic cage injuries. Disruption of unstable chest wall fractures could result in pneumothoracies or other complications.

The patient uses the device by first applying the vest using the Velcro® closures orienting the hose fittings where they are accessible on the front of the vest (Figure 4-55). Both hoses are then connected to the vest and the front of the air-pulse generator. The unit is connected to an appropriate electrical outlet and the foot switch depressed to turn the unit on. When pressure is released from the foot switch, oscillation stops. Patients can control the therapy to allow for coughing and expectoration.

Figure 4-54 *The Vest® High Frequency Chest Wall Oscillation (HFCWO) therapy device made by Advanced Respiratory, St. Paul, MN.*

THE EMERSON COUGHASSIST™ MI-E DEVICE

The Emerson Coughassist™ MI-E device is an electrically powered pneumatic insufflation/exsufflation device that applies positive and negative pressure to the patient's airway to assist the patient with coughing (Figure 4-56). The Coughassist™ may be applied by mask, or directly to an artificial airway. The device is capable of generating pressures of +60 cmH_2O

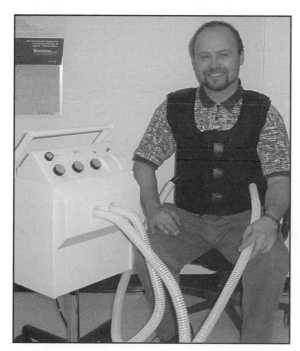

Figure 4-55 *The Vest® High Frequency Chest Wall Oscillation (HFCWO) therapy device correctly applied for therapy.*

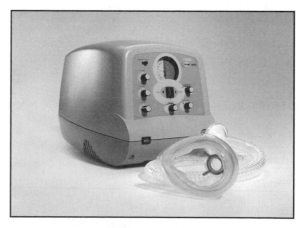

Figure 4-56 *The Emerson Coughassist™ MI-E device manufactured by J.H. Emerson Company, Cambridge, MA.*

pressure, both positive and negative, and flows of 10 liters/second during exhalation.

The Coughassist™ MI-E delivers a deep, positive pressure breath, followed by an expiratory flow to assist the patient in mobilizing secretions. The Coughassist™ MI-E device is indicated primarily for neuromuscular disorders and quadriplegia.

CLINICAL CORNER

Hyperinflation Equipment

1. You are asked to instruct a new adult postoperative patient on incentive spirometry. You learn in your review of her chart that she is blind. What incentive spirometer would you use and how you would instruct her?

2. Explain the advantages of flutter valve therapy as compared to chest physiotherapy for the ambulatory patient who is at home.

3. You are working with a 12-year-old cystic fibrosis patient, whom you are teaching to perform PEP therapy. During the session, he complains of being light-headed and adds that his fingers are numb. Explain what you should do and why.

4. You are asked to start an IPPB treatment on an elderly patient who wears a full set of dentures. The patient is not very cooperative and has a difficult time sealing his mouth around the mouthpiece. Describe what device or devices could help to improve the outcome of the IPPB treatment and how they would be used.

5. You are giving an IPPB treatment to a patient with chronic lung disease in the emergency room. You are using a Bird Mark 7, that is set on air mix with the ventilator powered by oxygen. Ten minutes into the treatment you notice that the patient's respiratory rate has decreased markedly since you started. What do you suspect is occurring, and what should you do about it?

6. A new physician in your area orders IPPB for a patient who is a new client of your home care company. Explain which IPPB unit would be the best for home use and what you would need to properly instruct and set up the new patient.

Self-Assessment Quiz

1. The most accurate method of measuring inspired volumes is:
   a. timing the duration of a flow of gas.
   b. volume displacement.
   c. photoelectric sensing.
   d. ultrasonic measurement.

2. Three methods of volume measurement used in incentive spirometers include:
   I. timing the duration of a flow of gas.
   II. volume displacement.
   III. photoelectric sensing.
   IV. ultrasonic measurement.
   V. measuring chest expansion.
   a. I, II, and III
   b. II, III, and IV
   c. I, III, and IV
   d. III, IV, and V

3. Gas pressure is regulated in the Bird ventilators by:
   a. a low-pressure reducing valve.
   b. needle valve.
   c. photoelectric sensing.
   d. magnetic attraction opposing gas pressure.

4. Gas pressure is regulated in the Bennett ventilators by:
   a. a low-pressure reducing valve.
   b. needle valves.
   c. magnetic attraction opposing gas pressure.
   d. two opposing flows of gas.
   e. using a venturi.

5. Needle valves are an effective way:
   a. to control gas temperature.
   b. to regulate gas pressure.
   c. to control gas flow.
   d. of lengthening inspiratory time.

6. Which of the following incentive spirometers operate by volume displacement?
   a. Voldyne
   b. Spirocare
   c. Volurex
   d. Triflow

7. Which of the following incentive spirometers operate using a photoelectric sensor?
   a. Voldyne
   b. Spirocare
   c. Volurex
   d. Triflow

8. A patient is using a flow-dependent incentive spirometer. The patient reaches a goal of 600 ml/second and holds that goal for 3 seconds. What inspired volume would you note in the patient's chart?
   a. 600 mL
   b. 1200 mL
   c. 1800 mL
   d. 2400 mL

9. An IPPB ventilator is failing to cycle off, and you suspect a leak. Possible places to check would include:
   I. the patient's ability to seal around the mouthpiece.
   II. all circuit connections.
   III. the exhalation valve.
   IV. the patient's nose.
   a. I
   b. I and II
   c. I, II, and III
   d. I, II, III, and IV

10. You are using a Bennett PR-2 ventilator to give an IPPB treatment. You want to increase the delivered tidal volume. You should:
    a. increase the pressure.
    b. increase the rate.
    c. increase the terminal flow.
    d. increase the peak flow.

11. When giving an IPPB treatment, the ventilator triggers on and cycles off rapidly. Which control should you adjust?
    a. pressure
    b. peak flow
    c. sensitivity
    d. rate

12. You are attempting to give an IPPB treatment with a Bird Mark 7 ventilator. The circuit has been assembled correctly, and the ventilator is connected to a 50-psi gas source. However, the ventilator will not trigger into inspiration in spite of your patient's cooperative efforts. What do you suspect is the problem?
    a. The flow rate has been turned off.
    b. The pressure is set too high.
    c. The sensitivity is set too low.
    d. The apnea control has been turned on.

13. The doctor wants an end inspiratory hold for his patient, who is receiving Albuterol via IPPB therapy. Which ventilator(s) can provide this?
    I. Bird Mark 7
    II. Bird Mark 7A
    III. Bird Mark 8
    IV. Bennett PR-2
    a. I and II
    b. I and III
    c. II and III
    d. II and IV

14. Which of the following controls will dilute the F_IO_2 delivered from a Bennett PR-2 operating in the source gas setting?
    a. rate control
    b. expiratory time control
    c. pressure control
    d. terminal flow control

15. When giving IPPB therapy using a Bird Mark 7, changes in the delivered F_IO_2 can be attributed to:
    I. the nebulizer.
    II. the venturi gate.
    III. the pressure.
    IV. the flow setting.
    a. I only
    b. I, II, and IV
    c. II and III
    d. I, II, and III

16. If an IPPB ventilator fails to cycle into exhalation (off), a common problem may be:
    a. too little pressure has been given.
    b. too much medication is in the nebulizer.
    c. that there is a leak.
    d. too much flow is going through the circuit.

17. A control on the Bennett PR-2 that is designed to compensate for leaks is the:
    a. rate control.
    b. peak flow control.
    c. pressure control.
    d. terminal flow control.

18. An IPPB ventilator designed primarily for home use is the:
    a. Bennett AP-5.
    b. Bennett PR-2.
    c. Bird Mark 7.
    d. Bird Mark 7A.

19. Ventilators that may be used to ventilate an apneic patient include the:
    I. Bennett AP-5.
    II. Bennett PR-2.
    III. Bird Mark 7.
    IV. Bird Mark 7A.
    V. Bird Mark 8.
    a. II only
    b. I and II
    c. I, II and III
    d. II, III, IV and V

20. When the patient attempts to trigger the IPPB ventilator on, a −8 cmH$_2$O is recorded on the pressure manometer. The respiratory care practitioner should:
    a. increase the flow.
    b. increase the pressure.
    c. increase the sensitivity.
    d. increase the terminal flow.

21. Intrapulmonary percussive ventilation:
    I. is a form of internal percussion.
    II. delivers an aerosol.
    III. is a form of IPPB.
    IV. xan only be used on apneic patients.
    a. I and II
    b. I and III
    c. I and IV
    d. II and IV

22. Which of the following delivers pulsed gas flow to the patient manifold on the Percussionaire IPV® ventilators?
    a. the Phasitron®
    b. the Nebulizer
    c. the Percussionator®
    d. the Spanker

23. Which of the following components of the Percussionaire IPV® units serves as a mechanical and pneumatic buffer to the high frequency generator?
    a. the Phasitron®
    b. the Nebulizer
    c. the Percussionator®
    d. the demand CPAP regulator

24. Which of the following components in the Percussionaire IPV® circuit has an orificed diaphragm and a sliding venturi?
    a. the Phasitron®
    b. the Nebulizer
    c. the Percussionator®
    d. the demand CPAP regulator

25. Which of the following controls governs the frequency of pulsed gas delivery when using the Percussionaire IPV®-1C?
    a. percussion
    b. inspiratory time
    c. impact
    d. inspiratory flow

26. Which of the Percussionaire IPV® units has CPAP capability?
    a. IPV®-1C
    b. IPV®-2
    c. demand CPAP regulator
    d. Mark 7

27. Which of the Percussionaire IPV® units can control the nebulizer output?
    a. IPV®-1C
    b. IPV®-2
    c. AP-5
    d. Mark 7

28. When troubleshooting the IPV®-1C, it fails to initiate percussive ventilation when the thumb button is depressed. Likely sources of the problem are:
    I. no line pressure.
    II. the electric power cord is unplugged.
    III. the circuit is assembled wrong.
    IV. the nebulizer drive is disconnected.
    a. I and II
    b. I and III
    c. II and III
    d. II and IV

29. Which mechanical percussor facilitates self-therapy?
    a. Vibramatic
    b. MJ Percussor
    c. Flimm Fighter
    d. manual percussion

30. Adjuncts for manual chest physiotherapy are primarily designed to:
    I. provide consistency of technique between practitioners.
    II. eliminate technique difficulties in maintaining correct hand positions.
    III. reduce fatigue.
    a. I
    b. I and II
    c. II and III
    d. I, II, and III

Selected Bibliography

American Association for Respiratory Care. (1993). AARC clinical practice guideline: Use of positive airway pressure adjuncts to bronchial hygiene therapy. *Respiratory Care, 38*, 516–521.

American Association for Respiratory Care. (2003). AARC clinical practice guideline: Intermittent positive pressure breathing—2003 revision & update. *Respiratory Care, 48*, 540–546.

American Association for Respiratory Care. (1991). AARC clinical practice guideline: Incentive spirometry, *Respiratory Care, 36*, 1402-1405.

Bennett Respiration Products. (1979). *Operating instructions, Bennett PR-2 respiration unit* (form 2131L). Santa Monica, CA.

Bird Corporation. *Instructions for operating the Mark 7 and Mark 8 respirators and Mark 10 and Mark 14 ventilators* (form 1718). Palm Springs, CA.

Bird Corporation. (1977). *Understanding the Bird Mark 7 and Mark 8 respirators with apneustic flow time (A) and the Bird ventilator* (form L929). Palm Springs, CA.

Bird, F. M. (1987). Intrapulmonary percussive ventilation. *Flying Physician, 30*(2), 4–9.

Cheeseborough-Ponds. (1982). *Valdyne product literature*. St. Louis, MO.

Fluck, R. R., Jr.. (1988). Intermittent positive-pressure breathing devices. In T. A. Barnes, et al. (Eds.), *Respiratory care practice*. Year Book Medical Publishers, Inc.

Indihar, F. F., et al. (1982). A prospective comparison of three procedures used in attempts to prevent postoperative pulmonary complications. *Respiratory Care, 27*(5), 564–568.

Mahlmeister, M. F., et al. (1991). Positive-expiratory-pressure mask therapy: Theoretical and practical considerations and a review of the literature. *Respiratory Care, 36*(11).

Mang, H., et al. (1989). Imposed work of breathing during sustained maximal inspiration: Comparison of six incentive spirometers. *Respiratory Care, 34*(12), 1122–1128.

McPherson, S. P. (1985). *Respiratory therapy equipment.* C. V. Mosby.

Miller, C. R., et al. (Jan./Feb. 1993). "IPV offers cost-effective method for self-administered therapy. *Advance,* 2–34.

Natale, J. E., et al. (1994). Comparison of intrapulmonary percussive ventilation and chest physiotherapy. A pilot study in patients with cystic fibrosis. *Chest, 105*(6), 1789–1793.

Percussionaire Corporation. (1993). *Intrapulmonary percussive ventilation, a twelve year learning curve 1980–1993.* Sandpoint, ID.

Percussionaire Corporation. (1985). *Manual of understanding, operations and clinical Restriction as they relate to the therapeutic protocol for Bird conceived intrapulmonary percussive ventilation (IPV) and the therapeutic device the Bird conceived IPV Percussionators® with the therapeutic breathing head assembly the Phasitron® and Percussive® Aerosol Generator manufactured by the Percussionaire Corporation.* Sandpoint, ID.

Reading, P. M., et al. (1984). Accuracy of incentive spirometer indicators (abstract). *Respiratory Care, 29*(10), 1025–1026.

Volsko, T. A, et al. (2003). Performance comparison of two oscillating positive expiratory pressure devices: Acapella versus flutter. *Respiratory Care, 48,* 124–130.

Wagener, J. S, et al. (2003). Cystic fibrosis: Current trends in respiratory care. *Respiratory Care, 48,* 234–247.

White, G. C. (2003). *Basic clinical lab competencies for respiratory care* (4th ed.). Clifton Park, NY: Thomson Delmar Learning.

CHAPTER 5

EMERGENCY RESUSCITATION EQUIPMENT

INTRODUCTION

This chapter will include discussions on artificial airways, manual resuscitators, vacuum regulation devices, and secretion removal devices. Almost all of this equipment may be employed in the emergency setting.

In addition to the emergency management equipment, airways and other devices are discussed in this chapter, including tracheostomy weaning devices. A thorough understanding of the function and application of this equipment is important in the practice of respiratory care.

OBJECTIVES

After completing this chapter, the student will accomplish the following objectives:

PHYSICS OF THE PRINCIPLES

- Explain how the surface area of an endotracheal tube or tracheostomy tube affects the force exerted against the tracheal mucosa.
- Describe how a cuff pressure manometer measures the pressure inside an endotracheal or tracheostomy tube's cuff.
- Describe the common valve configurations employed in manual resuscitators and how gas flows in the desired direction.
- Explain how Poiseuille's law affects artificial airways and suction catheters.
- Explain how vacuum is regulated in secretion evacuation devices.

POSITIONAL MANEUVERS TO OPEN THE AIRWAY

- Describe the manual maneuvers utilized to open the airway.
  - Head tilt and chin lift
  - Anterior mandibular displacement

ARTIFICIAL AIRWAYS

- Distinguish between the following artificial airways, their placement, and how they open the airway:
  - Oropharyngeal airway
  - Nasopharyngeal airway
  - Laryngeal mask airway
  - Combitube airway

MOUTH-TO-MASK VENTILATION DEVICES

- Describe the purpose and correct use of mouth-to-mask ventilation devices.
- Describe the advantages and disadvantages of mouth-to-mask ventilation devices.

MANUAL RESUSCITATORS

- Differentiate between the following self-inflating manual resuscitators and their valve configurations:
  - Laerdal
  - Hudson Lifesaver II
  - Puritan Bennett PMR 2

- Differentiate between the following disposable manual resuscitators:
  - Ambu® SPUR®
  - BagEasy
  - Pulmanex

INTUBATION EQUIPMENT

- Describe the types of laryngoscopes and blades used for intubation:
  - Fiber optic
  - Conventional
  - Miller
  - Macintosh
- Describe the two routes of intubation:
  - Oral route
  - Nasal route
- Describe the equipment used to assist in intubation:
  - Magill forceps
  - Stylet
  - Yankauer suction (tonsil tip)
  - Endtidal CO_2 detection equipment

ENDOTRACHEAL TUBES

- Identify and explain the importance of the following components of an oral endotracheal tube:
  - Murphy eye
  - Cuff
  - Pilot tube
  - Markings on the tube
  - Pilot balloon
  - 15-mm connector
  - Radiopaque line
- Describe the different types of endotracheal tubes:
  - Cuffed endotracheal tubes
  - Uncuffed endotracheal tubes
  - Specialized endotracheal tubes
    - Wire reinforced endotracheal tubes
    - Oral and nasal RAE tubes
    - Endobronchial endotracheal tubes

- Describe the application of the endotracheal tube exchanger

TRACHEOSTOMY TUBES

- Distinguish between the following tracheostomy tubes and their application:
  - Cuffed tracheostomy tube
  - Cuffed tracheostomy tube with a disposable inner cannula
  - Cuffed fenestrated tracheostomy tube
  - Hollinger or Jackson tracheostomy tube

CUFF PRESSURE MANOMETERS

- Differentiate between the following cuff pressure manometers and how each is used:
  - Manometer and a three-way stop cock
  - Posey Cufflator
  - DHD Cuff-Mate2
- Describe the use of the Respironics PressureEasy system.
- Describe the differences between the following tracheostomy weaning devices and their application:
  - Pitt speaking tube/Communi-Trach
  - Trach button
  - Kistner button
  - Passy-Muir valve
  - Olympic Trach-Talk

SECRETION EVACUATION DEVICES

- Differentiate between the following suction regulators and their operation:
  - Puritan Bennett
  - Ohmeda Surgical/Free-Flow
- Differentiate between the following suction catheters:
  - Whistle tip
  - Argyle Aeroflow
  - Coudé tip
  - Trach Care
- Describe the use of the Lukens trap during airway aspiration.

KEY TERMS

Anterior mandibular displacement
Carlens tube
Combitube airway
Communi-Trach (Pitt speaking tube)
Conventional laryngoscopes

Cuff
Disposable, self-inflating manual resuscitators
Endotracheal tubes
Fenestrated tracheostomy tube
Fiber-optic laryngoscopes

Flow-inflating manual resuscitators
Head tilt maneuver
Intubation
Kistner button
Lanz tube
Laryngeal mask airway

Lukens trap
Macintosh laryngoscope blade
Magill forceps
Miller laryngoscope blade
Minimal leak technique
Minimal occlusion volume
   (MOV)
Murphy eye
Nasopharyngeal airway
Olympic Trach-Talk™

Oral and nasal RAE®
   endotracheal tubes
Oropharyngeal airway
Passy-Muir tracheostomy
   valve
Pilot tube
Positive End Expiratory
   Pressure (PEEP)
Respironics PressureEasy
Robertshaw tube

Silver Jackson (or Hollinger)
   tracheostomy tube
Soft tissue obstruction
Stylet
Suction catheters
Trach button
Tracheostomy tube
Wire-wrapped reinforced
   endotracheal tube
Yankauer suction

PHYSICS OF THE PRINCIPLES

FORCES EXERTED BY ARTIFICIAL AIRWAY CUFFS

As you may recall from physics, pressure is equal to a unit of force divided by the area over which the force is applied.

$$PRESSURE = \frac{Force}{Area}$$

By rearranging the equation, force is a function of pressure multiplied by the area.

$$FORCE = PRESSURE \times AREA$$

As you can see in the second relationship, by increasing the surface area, a given force can be maintained at a lower pressure. This is the principle behind the design of the high-volume (increased surface area), low-pressure cuffs on **endotracheal tube** and **tracheostomy tubes**. By increasing the volume, and therefore the surface area, of the cuff, the pressure required to seal the tube against the tracheal wall is decreased. The force that is applied is distributed over a larger area, reducing pressure trauma to the sensitive mucosa of the trachea.

CUFF PRESSURE MANOMETERS

Cuff pressure manometers are devices designed to measure the pressure contained in the inflated cuffs of endotracheal tubes or

Figure 5-1 *A line drawing showing a cross section of a mechanical manometer. (Courtesy Thomson Delmar Learning,* Basic Clinical Lab Competencies for Respiratory Care *[3rd ed.], 1998)*

tracheostomy tubes. These manometers operate using simple diaphragms (mechanical manometer see Chapter 1), or a diaphragm in conjunction with a strain gauge.

The mechanical manometer records changes in pressure which are directly proportional to the expansion and contraction of the diaphragm contained inside of the manometer (Figure 5-1). The needle is connected to the diaphragm by gear set, such that the linear motion of the diaphragm is converted to a rotary motion (needle indicator). These manometers are calibrated so that atmospheric pressure measures zero on the instruments scale.

The strain gauge type manometer also uses a diaphragm, which changes shape with

Figure 5-2 *A schematic diagram of a strain gauge cuff manometer.*

pressure changes (Figure 5-2). As the diaphragm moves, the strain gauge elongates or contracts proportionally with the diaphragm. As the length of the strain gauge changes, electrical resistance increases or decreases. Therefore, a change in resistance is proportional to a change in pressure. Pressure is usually recorded digitally on a liquid crystal display (LCD).

RESUSCITATOR VALVE TYPES

Diaphragm or Leaf Type

The simplest type of resuscitator valve is the diaphragm valve. It is made of a flexible rubber or plastic that will distort when pressure is applied. This type of valve will change shape in response to small pressure changes,

which is advantageous in "sensing" a patient's spontaneous breathing efforts.

A diaphragm valve opens when pressure proximal to the valve seat distorts it (Figure 5-3A). The valve closes when pressure distal to the valve seat forces the valve against the seat closing it (Figure 5-3B).

Spring-and-Disk or Spring-and-Ball

This valve is composed of a rigid disk (diaphragm) or ball, spring, inlet, and outlet (Figure 5-4). When pressure proximal to the disk or ball compresses the spring, the valve opens (Figure 5-4A). When the pressure proximal to the disk decreases, spring tension overcomes gas pressure and the valve closes (Figure 5-4B).

A - INSPIRATION   B - EXHALATION

Figure 5-3 *The operation of a diaphragm-type resuscitator valve. (A) Inhalation. (B) Exhalation.*

INSPIRATION

EXHALATION

(A)

Figure 5-4 *A comparison of the (A) spring-and-disk and the (B) spring-and-ball resuscitator valves.* **(continues)**

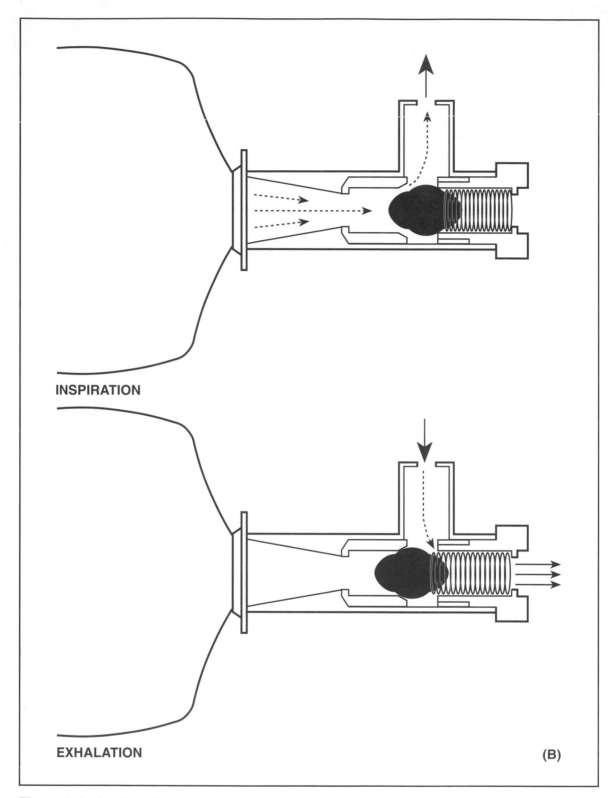

INSPIRATION

EXHALATION

(B)

Figure 5-4 *(continued)*

INSPIRATION   (A)

EXHALATION   (B)

Figure 5-5 *A duck bill–type resuscitation valve.*

Duck Bill Valve

The duck bill valve is made from a flexible silastic or plastic (Figure 5-5). It, like the diaphragm valve, is very responsive to changes in pressure and is therefore sensitive to patient efforts.

The valve opens when pressure proximal to the valve seat distorts it (Figure 5-5A). The valve closes when pressure distal to the valve seat forces the valve against the seat, closing it (Figure 5-5B).

THE IMPORTANCE OF POISEUILLE'S LAW

Poiseuille's law relates the diameter of a tube to the resistance imposed to gas flowing through it. This relationship is critical in both artificial airways and suction catheters.

A patient spontaneously breathing with a 6-mm internal diameter (ID) artificial airway will work harder than if using an 8.5-mm ID artificial airway. The imposed work of breathing from a narrow artificial airway can be significant. As the radius decreases by one-half, the resistance will increase 16 times. When a small artificial airway is placed, weaning from mechanical ventilation may be more difficult for that patient due to the increased work of breathing.

VACUUM REGULATION

The vacuum from the supply line in hospitals must be reduced to a safe physiological level for suctioning chest tubes and gastric tubes. Sub-ambient pressure of between 400 and 600 mmHg from the supply lines must be reduced to 20 to 120 mmHg for clinical use.

Single-stage reducing valves are incorporated into the vacuum regulators to accomplish this. The operation of reducing valves is discussed in Chapter 1.

UPPER AIRWAY OBSTRUCTION

Upper airway obstruction and cessation of ventilation can result in death within a few short minutes. Upper airway obstruction can be caused by soft tissue obstruction, laryngeal obstruction, central nervous system depression, drug overdose or anesthesia, cardiac arrest loss of consciousness, space-occupying lesions, edema, or foreign body aspiration. If left untreated, upper airway obstruction can quickly become a life-threatening emergency. The American Association for Respiratory Care has published a Clinical Practice Guideline: Management of Airway Emergencies, which has been partially reproduced in Figure 5-6.

AARC CLINICAL PRACTICE GUIDELINE
Management of Airway Emergencies

MAE 1.0 PROCEDURE:
Recognition of signs of an impending or actual airway emergency. Initial treatment and continued management of airway emergencies to minimize the likelihood of adverse outcomes, in adults, children, and infants.

MAE 2.0 DESCRIPTION/DEFINITION:
Management of airway emergencies (MAE) for the purpose of this guideline encompasses all care necessary to deal with sudden and often life-threatening events affecting natural and artificial airways and involves the identification, assessment, and treatment of patients in danger of losing or not being able to maintain an adequate airway, including the newborn. This includes (1) identification of the causes of airway emergencies; (2) management of airway emergencies prior to tracheal intubation; (3) use of adjunctive equipment and special techniques for establishing, maintaining, and monitoring effective ventilation; (4) translaryngeal tracheal intubation, including nasal and oral tracheal intubation; (5) transtracheal catheter ventilation, (6) percutaneous dilational cricothyrotomy, and; (7) surgical cricothyrotomy.

MAE 3.0 SETTING:
The guideline applies to a variety of settings including but not limited to hospitals and pre- or inter-hospital transport.

MAE 4.0 INDICATIONS:
4.1 Conditions requiring management of the airway, in general, are impending or actual (1) airway compromise, (2) respiratory failure, and (3) need to protect the air-

Figure 5-6 *The American Association for Respiratory Care, Clinical Practice Guideline: Management of Airway Emergencies.* **(continues)**

way. Specific conditions include but are not limited to

4.1.1 Airway emergency prior to endotracheal intubation

4.1.2 Obstruction of the artificial airway

4.1.3 Apnea

4.1.4 Acute traumatic coma

4.1.5 Penetrating neck trauma

4.1.6 Cardiopulmonary arrest and unstable dysrhythmias

4.1.7 Severe bronchospasm

4.1.8 Severe allergic reactions with cardiopulmonary compromise

4.1.9 Pulmonary edema

4.1.10 Sedative or narcotic drug effect

4.1.11 Foreign body airway obstruction

4.1.12 Choanal atresia in neonates

4.1.13 Aspiration

4.1.14 Risk of aspiration

4.1.15 Severe laryngospasm

4.1.16 Self-extubation

4.2 Conditions requiring emergency tracheal intubation include, but are not limited to

4.2.1 Persistent apnea

4.2.2 Traumatic upper airway obstruction (partial or complete)

4.2.3 Accidental extubation of the patient unable to maintain adequate spontaneous ventilation

4.2.4 Obstructive angioedema (edema involving the deeper layers of the skin, subcutaneous tissue, and mucosa)

4.2.5 Massive uncontrolled upper airway bleeding

4.2.6 Coma with potential for increased intracranial pressure

4.2.7 Infection-related upper airway obstruction (partial or complete)

4.2.7.1 Epiglottitis in children or adults

4.2.7.2 Acute uvular edema

4.2.7.3 Tonsillopharyngitis or retropharyngeal abscess

4.2.7.4 Suppurative parotitis

4.2.8 Laryngeal and upper airway edema

4.2.9 Neonatal- or pediatric-specific

4.2.9.1 Perinatal asphyxia

4.2.9.2 Severe adenotonsillar hypertrophy

4.2.9.3 Severe laryngomalacia

4.2.9.4 Bacterial tracheitis

4.2.9.5 Neonatal epignathus

4.2.9.6 Obstruction from abnormal laryngeal closure due to arytenoid masses

4.2.9.7 Mediastinal tumors

4.2.9.8 Congenital diaphragmatic hernia

4.2.9.9 Presence of thick and/or particulate meconium in amniotic fluid

4.2.10 Absence of airway protective reflexes

4.2.11 Cardiopulmonary arrest

4.2.12 Massive hemoptysis

4.3 The patient in whom airway control is not possible by other methods may require surgical placement of an airway (needle or surgical cricothyrotomy).

4.4 Conditions in which endotracheal intubation may not be possible and in which alternative techniques may be used include but are not limited to

4.4.1 restriction of endotracheal intubation by policy or statute;

4.4.2 difficult or failed intubation in the presence of risk factors associated with difficult tracheal intubations such as

4.4.2.1 Short neck, or bull neck

4.4.2.2 Protruding maxillary incisors

4.4.2.3 Receding mandible

4.4.2.4 Reduced mobility of the atlanto-occipital joint

4.4.2.5 Temporomandibular ankylosis

4.4.2.6 Congenital oropharyngeal wall stenosis

4.4.2.7 Anterior osteophytes of the cervical vertebrae, associated with diffuse idiopathic skeletal hyperostosis

4.4.2.8 Large substernal and/or cancerous goiters

4.4.2.9 Treacher-Collins syndrome

4.4.2.10 Morquio-Brailsford syndrome

4.4.2.11 Endolaryngeal tumors

4.4.3 when endotracheal intubation is not immediately possible

MAE 5.0 CONTRAINDICATIONS:

Aggressive airway management (intubation or establishment of a surgical airway) may be contraindicated when the patient's desire not to be resuscitated has been clearly expressed and documented in the patient's medical record or other valid legal document.

MAE 6.0 PRECAUTIONS/HAZARDS AND/OR COMPLICATIONS:

The following represent possible hazards or complications related to the major facets of management of airway emergencies:

6.1 Translaryngeal intubation or cricothyrotomy is usually the route of choice. It may be necessary occasionally to use a surgical airway. Controversy exists as to whether intubation is hazardous in the presence of an unstable injury to the cervical spine. In one series the incidence of serious cervical spine injury in a severely injured population

Figure 5-6 *(continues)*

of blunt trauma patients was relatively low, and commonly used methods of precautionary airway management rarely led to neurologic deterioration.

6.1.1 Failure to establish a patent airway

6.1.2 Failure to intubate the trachea

6.1.3 Failure to recognize intubation of esophagus

6.1.4 Upper airway trauma, laryngeal, and esophageal damage

6.1.5 Aspiration

6.1.6 Cervical spine trauma

6.1.7 Unrecognized bronchial intubation

6.1.8 Eye injury

6.1.9 Vocal cord paralysis

6.1.10 Problems with ETT tubes

6.1.10.1 Cuff perforation

6.1.10.2 Cuff herniation

6.1.10.3 Pilot-tube-valve incompetence

6.1.10.4 Tube kinking during biting

6.1.10.5 Inadvertent extubation

6.1.10.6 Tube occlusion

6.1.11 Bronchospasm

6.1.12 Laryngospasm

6.1.13 Dental accidents

6.1.14 Dysrhythmias

6.1.15 Hypotension and bradycardia due to vagal stimulation

6.1.16 Hypertension and tachycardia

6.1.17 Inappropriate tube size

6.1.18 Bleeding

6.1.19 Mouth ulceration

6.1.20 Nasal-intubation specific

6.1.20.1 Nasal damage including epistaxis

6.1.20.2 Tube kinking in pharynx

6.1.20.3 Sinusitis and otitis media

6.1.21 Tongue ulceration

6.1.22 Tracheal damage including tracheoesophageal fistula, tracheal innominate fistula, tracheal stenosis, and tracheomalacia

6.1.23 Pneumonia

6.1.24 Laryngeal damage with consequent laryngeal stenosis, laryngeal ulcer, granuloma, polyps, synechia

6.1.25 Surgical cricothyrotomy or tracheostomy specific

6.1.25.1 Stomal stenosis

6.1.25.2 Innominate erosion

6.1.26 Needle cricothyrotomy specific

6.1.26.1 Bleeding at insertion site with hematoma formation

6.1.26.2 Subcutaneous and mediastinal emphysema

6.1.26.3 Esophageal perforation

6.2 Emergency ventilation

6.2.1 Inadequate oxygen delivery

6.2.2 Hypo- or hyperventilation

6.2.3 Gastric insufflation and/or rupture

6.2.4 Barotrauma

6.2.5 Hypotension due to reduced venous return secondary to high mean intrathoracic pressure

6.2.6 Vomiting and aspiration

6.2.7 Prolonged interruption of ventilation for intubation

6.2.8 Failure to establish adequate functional residual capacity in the newborn

6.2.9 Movement of unstable cervical spine (more than by any commonly used method of endotracheal intubation).

6.2.10 Failure to exhale due to upper airway obstruction during percutaneous transtracheal ventilation.

MAE 7.0 LIMITATIONS OF PROCEDURE:

Despite adequate management of airway emergencies, desired outcome may not be achieved because of the patient's underlying condition and progression of the process leading to the need for emergency airway management.

MAE 8.0 ASSESSMENT OF NEED:

The need for management of airway emergencies is dictated by the patient's clinical condition. Careful observation, the implementation of basic airway management techniques, and laboratory and clinical data should help determine the need for more aggressive measures. Specific conditions requiring intervention include

8.1 Inability to adequately protect airway (e.g., coma, lack of gag reflex, inability to cough) with or without other signs of respiratory distress.

8.2 Partially obstructed airway. Signs of a partially obstructed upper airway include ineffective patient efforts to ventilate, paradoxical respiration, stridor, use of accessory muscles, patient's pointing to neck, choking motions, cyanosis, and distress. Signs of lower airway obstruction may include the above and wheezing.

8.3 Complete airway obstruction. Respiratory efforts with no breath sounds or suggestion of air movement are indicative of complete obstruction.

8.4 Apnea. No respiratory efforts are seen. May be associated with cardiac arrest.

8.5 Hypoxemia, hypercarbia, and/or acidemia seen on arterial blood gas analysis, oximetry or exhaled gas analysis.

Figure 5-6 *(continues)*

8.6 Respiratory distress. Elevated respiratory rate, high or low ventilatory volumes, and signs of sympathetic nervous system hyperactivity may be associated with respiratory distress.

MAE 9.0 ASSESSMENT OF PROCESS AND OUTCOME:

Timely intervention to maintain the patient's airway can improve outcome in terms of survival and level of function. Under rare circumstances, maintenance of an airway by nonsurgical means may not be possible. Despite optimal maintenance of the airway, patient outcomes are affected by patient-specific factors. Lack of availability of appropriate equipment and personnel may adversely affect patient outcome. Monitoring and recording are important to the improvement of the process of emergency airway management. Some aspects (e.g., frequency of complications of tracheal intubation or time to establishment of a definitive airway) are easy to quantitate and can lead to improvement in hospitalwide systems. Patient condition following the emergency should be evaluated from this perspective.

MAE 10.0 RESOURCES:

10.1 Personnel: All health professionals should be trained, evaluated at frequent intervals, and retrained as necessary in the skills of emergency clearance of foreign body airway obstruction and airway secretions. Health professionals who are primary members of resuscitation teams in acute care hospitals should be skilled in advanced management of airway emergencies, emergency cardiac care (ECC), and advanced cardiac life support (ACLS).

Emergency response system—a designated resuscitation team should be continuously available (24 hours/day, 7 days/week) to assist with the management of airway emergencies. Team members should be notified simultaneously. All hospital workers must know how to activate the hospital's emergency response system.

10.1.1 Level I

10.1.1.1 Training—all Level I personnel should be trained, evaluated by performance, and retrained as necessary in clearance of foreign-body airway obstruction, emergency airway-secretion evacuation techniques, and basic life support (BLS) at frequent intervals that do not exceed one year. Retraining should focus on identified deficiencies.

10.1.1.2 Responsibilities—Level I personnel are health professionals who assist the primary (Level II) members of the health-care team. They should be capable of assisting Level II personnel by (1) assessing patients for airway emergencies, respiratory, and/or cardiac arrest, (2) activating the resuscitation team, (3) administering BLS, (4) clearing the airway of foreign-body obstruction or material with the potential for obstruction, (5) providing mouth-to-mask ventilation, (6) assisting with tracheal intubation, (7) attaching pulse oximeter and capnograph, (8) moving adjunct airway equipment to the scene, (9) collecting arterial blood for analysis, (10) making a written record of resuscitation efforts.

10.1.1.3 Credentials—Level I health professionals should hold one or more of the following or equivalent credentials: RRT, CRTT, RN, MD, or DO; and have current BLS health-care provider-course completion card from the American Heart Association or a similar equivalent organization. Health professionals and hospital personnel not holding one of these Level I credentials should at a minimum be capable of assessing the patient for foreign-body airway obstruction, activating the resuscitation team, and administering BLS until the team arrives.

10.1.2 Level II

10.1.2.1 Training—Level II personnel should be trained, evaluated by performance, and retrained as necessary in advanced management of airway emergencies—ACLS and/or pediatric advanced life support (PALS) and/or neonatal resuscitation program (NRP)—as appropriate at intervals that should not exceed 1 year. To maintain operator competence, certain procedures (e.g., endotracheal intubation) need to be reinforced as often as every 3 months. Retraining should focus on identified deficiencies.

10.1.2.2 Responsibilities—Level II health professionals should be capable of serving as primary members of the resuscitation team. They may respond not only to airway emergency calls in their work areas but also to other areas of the hospital. They are skilled in the use of all adjunctive equipment and special techniques for ECC/ACLS, e.g., establishing, maintaining, and

Figure 5-6 (continues)

monitoring effective ventilation and circulation as described in more detail in the AARC Clinical Practice Guideline: Resuscitation in the Acute Care Hospital. They have the skills of Level I personnel and also the following capabilities: (1) advanced ECG monitoring and dysrhythmia recognition, (2) tracheal intubation and airway stabilization; (3) establishing ventilation via transtracheal catheter and cricothyrotomy; (4) emergency treatment of tension pneumothorax or hemothorax with large bore needle; (5) preparing patients for emergency transport; (6) use of continuous and transport mechanical ventilators, (7) evaluating oxygenation, ventilation and acid-base balance from blood gas reports.

10.1.2.3 Credentials—Level II health professionals should hold one or more of the following credentials: RRT, RN, MD, or DO; and current ACLS, PALS, and/or NRP course-completion card from the American Heart Association or a similar equivalent association.

10.2 Equipment should be rapidly available and functional. Durability, portability, reliability, and cost should be considered

10.2.1 Ventilation devices should comply with the recommendations made in the AARC Guideline: Resuscitation in the Acute Care Hospital.

10.2.2 Airway management devices should comply with the recommendations made in the AARC Guideline: Resuscitation in the Acute Care Hospital. Some other airway devices are available (e.g., laryngeal mask airway, esophageal obturator airway, combination esophageal-tracheal tubes) and may be acceptable and useful although they do not provide the airway control and protection afforded by an endotracheal tube.

10.2.2.1 The laryngeal mask airway (LMA) provides a low-pressure seal around the glottis. Although its size effectively prohibits its being inserted into either the trachea or the esophagus, it does not reliably protect the airway from aspirated gastric contents. It may cause less airway trauma than the endotracheal tube and less cardiovascular instability. Available in sizes 1–4, it works in children as well as adults. It may be easier to insert in patients with higher Mallampati classifications.

10.2.2.2 The esophageal obturator airway/esophageal gastric tube airway (EOA/EGTA) are considered together. Although researchers originally claimed it required less time for training than the endotracheal tube, this may not be the case. It is still widely used, primarily in prehospital care of adults. There have been several reports of the effectiveness of the EOA, but comparison is difficult due to variability in patients and in the medical supervision of the systems. Complications have been reported in many studies. While some believe it to be a useful second-line airway adjunct (for keeping gas out of the stomach and stomach contents out of the pharynx), others feel that the time used for training in EOA insertion would be better spent in training for endotracheal intubation or, failing that, placing more emphasis on basic airway maintenance and ventilation.

10.2.2.3 The pharyngeotracheal lumen airway (PTL) is a double-lumen tube that is inserted blindly into the pharynx. After the position of the tube has been assessed, the patient is ventilated through the appropriate lumen. A large pharyngeal balloon seals the airway and a smaller secondary balloon is then inflated. The published complication rate is low, but there has been relatively little evaluation of this device.

10.2.2.4 The esophageal tracheal Combitube (ETC) is the newest airway device to be developed. It is similar to the PTL in that it is a double-lumen tube that is inserted blindly into the oropharynx; the position of the tube is assessed; and the patient is ventilated through the appropriate lumen. It has both a low reported rate of complications and few published evaluations.

10.2.2.5 A 12–16 gauge intravenous catheter-over-the-needle device is used to initiate transtracheal catheter ventilation with the breathing mixture supplied at high pressure (30–50 psi). Because exhalation with this device must occur passively through the upper airway, CO_2 excretion is usually inadequate. This technique has potential for providing oxygen to the patient with a partially obstructed airway.

10.2.2.6 Percutaneous dilational cricothyrotomy is performed by making a small vertical incision and advancing a cricothyrotomy tube over a guidewire and dilator. If the catheter is improperly placed or becomes dislodged, ventilation and oxygenation will fail and barotrauma will occur (e.g., massive subcutaneous emphysema, pneumomediastinum, pneumothorax, bleeding).

Figure 5-6 *(continues)*

10.2.2.7 Surgical cricothyrotomy requires experience, skill, and specialized equipment and may be facilitated by a tracheal dilator or tracheal hook and a standard tracheostomy or endotracheal tube.

MAE 11.0 MONITORING:

11.1 Patient

11.1.1 Clinical signs-continuous observation of the patient and repeated clinical assessment by a trained observer provide optimal monitoring of the airway. Special consideration should be given to the following:

11.1.1.1 Level of consciousness

11.1.1.2 Presence and character of breath sounds

11.1.1.3 Ease of ventilation

11.1.1.4 Symmetry and amount of chest movement

11.1.1.5 Skin color and character (temperature and presence or absence of diaphoresis)

11.1.1.6 Presence of upper airway sounds (crowing, snoring, stridor)

11.1.1.7 Presence of excessive secretions, blood, vomitus, or foreign objects in the airway

11.1.1.8 Presence of epigastric sounds

11.1.1.9 Presence of retractions

11.1.1.10 Presence of nasal flaring

11.1.2 Physiologic variables—Repeated assessment of physiologic data by trained professionals supplements clinical assessment in managing patients with airway difficulties. Monitoring devices should be available, accessible, functional, and periodically evaluated for function. These data include but are not limited to:

11.1.2.1 Ventilatory frequency, tidal volume, and airway pressure

11.1.2.2 Presence of CO_2 in exhaled gas

11.1.2.3 Heart rate and rhythm

11.1.2.4 Pulse oximetry

11.1.2.5 Arterial blood gas values

11.1.2.6 Chest radiograph

11.2 Endotracheal tube position-Regardless of the method of ventilation used, the most important consideration is detection of esophageal intubation.

11.2.1 Tracheal intubation is suggested but may not be confirmed by

11.2.1.1 bilateral breath sounds over the chest, symmetrical chest movement, and absence of ventilation sounds over the epigastrium;

11.2.1.2 presence of condensate inside the tube, corresponding with exhalation

11.2.1.3 visualization of the tip of the tube passing through the vocal cords;

11.2.1.4 Esophageal detector devices may be useful in differentiating esopha-geal from tracheal intubation.

11.2.2 Tracheal intubation is confirmed by detection of CO_2 in the exhaled gas, although cases of transient CO_2 excretion from the stomach have been reported.

11.2.3 Tracheal intubation is confirmed by endoscopic visualization of the carina or tracheal rings through the tube.

11.2.4 The position of the endotracheal tube (i.e., depth of insertion) should be appropriate on chest radiograph.

11.3 Airway Management Process-a properly managed airway may improve patient outcome. Continuous evaluation of the process will identify components needing improvement. These include response time, equipment function, equipment availability, practitioner performance, complication rate, and patient survival and functional status.

MAE 12.0 FREQUENCY/AVAILABILITY/DURATION:

Because the need for management of airway emergencies occurs unpredictably, personnel need to be able to respond with the appropriate equipment within 3 minutes, 24 hours/day, 7 days/week. Additionally, a person capable of airway management in the infant should be present at every delivery. A Level-II practitioner should be present at every high-risk delivery.

MAE 13.0 INFECTION CONTROL:

13.1 Implement Universal Precautions including mouth-to-barrier devices and recommendations related to avoidance of the transmission of tuberculosis and other airborne diseases.

13.2 Observe all infection control guidelines posted for the patient.

13.3 Disinfect all equipment to be reused on other patients.

Reprinted with permission from *Respiratory Care* 1995; 40: 749–760. The complete AARC Clinical Practice Guidelines are available from the AARC Web site (*http://www.aarc.org*), from the AARC Executive Office, or from *Respiratory Care* journal.

Figure 5-6 *(continued)*

POSITIONAL MANEUVERS TO OPEN THE AIRWAY

Upper airway obstruction can be caused by soft tissue obstruction, laryngeal obstruction, or foreign body obstruction. **Soft tissue obstruction** is usually caused by the muscles of the tongue relaxing, resulting in the tongue falling posteriorly and obstructing the airway. Causes of loss of muscle tone can be due to loss of consciousness (trauma, cerebral vascular accidents (CVAs), or sedative or narcotic drugs) or central nervous system depression. The focus of positional maneuvers to open the upper airway is to reposition the airway such that the tongue is moved anteriorly away from the posterior pharynx, opening the upper airway.

HEAD TILT

Figure 5-7 illustrates two supine positions of the airway with the tongue having lost muscle tone. When the head is tilted backward, advancing the tongue anteriorly, the airway becomes opened. The **head tilt maneuver** is performed by tilting the head backward, thereby hyperextending the neck slightly. Sometimes this position is referred to as the "sniffing" position as if one were to sniff a rose. One hand is placed on the forehead and the head is tilted backward, advancing the mandible anteriorly opening the airway (Figure 5-8).

Caution must be used when performing this maneuver in that, if a cervical spine injury has been sustained, it may be worsened using this technique. The technique hyperextends the neck, which may displace an unstable fracture of the spine, which may in turn impinge upon the spinal cord.

ANTERIOR MANDIBULAR DISPLACEMENT

In the event a cervical spine injury is suspected, the **anterior mandibular displacement** maneuver can also open the airway without manipulation of the spine. Figure 5-9 illustrates this technique. The ramus of the mandible is grasped bilaterally, and the mandible is advanced anteriorly. As this maneuver is performed, the tongue is also displaced anteriorly, opening the airway.

Figure 5-7 *A comparison of the airway in two different head positions, the head is flexed neutral or slightly forward, and the head is hyperextended, opening the airway.*

Figure 5-8 *The head tilt maneuver to relieve upper airway obstruction.*

Figure 5-9 *Anterior mandibular displacement to relieve airway obstruction.*

Figure 5-10 *A variety of oropharyngeal airways. Berman airways, a Guedel airway, and a Cath-Guide Guedel airway are shown.*

ARTIFICIAL AIRWAYS

Artificial airways are specialized medical devices that are designed to maintain a patent, or open, airway. Depending on the device, it may only displace the tongue or it may be inserted directly into the trachea. Artificial airways work by bypassing areas of obstruction or preventing vomitus or foreign material from obstructing the airway. Airways may be placed to prevent or to relieve airway obstruction.

OROPHARYNGEAL AIRWAY

The **oropharyngeal airway** is designed to relieve obstructions in the unconscious patient caused by the tongue or other soft tissue. Its curved shape separates the tongue from the posterior wall of the pharynx when properly placed (Figure 5-10).

By inserting the airway with the tip pointing toward the hard palate, then advancing it and rotating the airway 180°, the tongue will be separated from the posterior pharynx. The patient does not breathe through the airway itself, but through the opening created between it and the soft tissues.

The correct sizing of the oropharyngeal airway is important. If the airway is too small, the tongue may not be adequately separated from the soft palate, resulting in continued airway obstruction. If the airway is too large, it may actually push the epiglottis against the larynx, closing the airway. When correctly sized, the posterior tip of the airway should be positioned at the base of the tongue (Figure 5-11).

Figure 5-11 *The correct placement of an oropharyngeal airway. Note how the distal tip of the airway rests at the base of the tongue.*

These airways are rarely tolerated by the conscious patient. The gag reflex may be strongly stimulated, which could result in vomiting and aspiration.

NASOPHARYNGEAL AIRWAY

Like the oropharyngeal airway, the **nasopharyngeal airway** will relieve obstructions in the conscious or semiconscious patient caused by the tongue. The nasopharyngeal airway is a narrow hollow tube (Figure 5-12)

Figure 5-12 *A nasopharyngeal airway.*

made from a soft pliable rubber or plastic. It, like the oropharyngeal airway, separates the tongue from the soft palate.

The nasopharyngeal airway is inserted through the nose and nasal passage until the tip rests between the tongue and the soft palate. Airflow can pass through the airway as well as through the space created between it and the soft tissues.

Nasopharyngeal airways have many diameters and lengths. To size the airway, insert the largest diameter that can be easily passed with minimal force or trauma. The length may be sized by placing the distal end of the airway at the tragus of the ear and the proximal end near the nose. The airway should span from the tragus of the ear to the tip of the nose.

As described with oropharyngeal airways, if the size is not correct, airway obstruction may continue to be a problem. If the airway is too small, the tongue may not be separated from the posterior oropharynx. If the airway is too large, the epiglottis may be pushed inferiorly against the larynx, closing the airway. When properly sized, the distal tip of the airway should rest at the base of the tongue (Figure 5-13).

LARYNGEAL MASK AIRWAY

The **laryngeal mask airway** is a small, triangular-shaped, inflatable mask secured to a tube, much like a cuff is secured to an endotracheal tube (Figure 5-14). The laryngeal mask is designed to be positioned such that when the mask is inflated, the tip rests against the upper esophageal sphincter and the sides face into the pyriform fossae and lie just under the base of the tongue (Figure 5-14). The laryngeal mask is designed to seal the esophagus, providing a more patent and easily maintained airway when compared with a conventional mask and oral airway combination.

Figure 5-13 *The correct placement of a nasopharyngeal airway. Note how the tip of the airway separates the tongue from the soft palate.*

Figure 5-14 *A photograph of the Laryngeal Mask Airway.*

Prior to insertion of the laryngeal mask airway, fully deflate the mask, using a syringe, and lubricate it well, using a water-soluble lubricant. Be certain to put on a pair of surgical gloves and wear appropriate personal protective equipment. Perform a manual head tilt maneuver and open the lower jaw widely, exposing the airway. With the aperture of the mask facing forward, guide it into the airway by holding it near where the mask joins the ventilation tube, just as one holds a pencil. Once the mask has advanced past the base of the tongue, use the ball of your finger to continue the mask's advance into position past the posterior portion of the pharynx, posterior to the tongue following the pharyngeal wall. Resistance will be felt when the mask rests against the isophageal sphincter. Inflate the mask and check for correct ventilation by observing chest rise and auscultation of the chest and by using exhaled carbon dioxide detection. Once ventilation is confirmed, secure the laryngeal mask in place using tape, and protect it with a bite block. When positioned correctly, the black line on the ventilation tube should always face the patient's upper lip; do not rotate the laryngeal mask from the optimal position.

COMBITUBE AIRWAY

The **Combitube airway** is a double lumen airway with the features of an esophageal gastric airway and an endotracheal tube (Figure 5-15).

The tube is designed to be inserted blindly (without visualization, using a laryngoscope).

Figure 5-15 *A photograph of the Combitube airway.*

Once inserted, two cuffs, one in the oropharynx and a second cuff at the distal end of the long tube, are inflated. The rescuer attempts ventilation through the shorter tube and observes the patient's chest for adequate expansion and condensate in the tube from exhaled air. If adequate ventilation is not observed, then the rescuer ventilates through the longer lumen of the airway. The patient is again observed for adequate ventilation (Figure 5-16).

If the long tube is in the esophagus, ventilation is accomplished by ventilating through the shorter tube. Air is directed into the trachea since the esophagus is occluded by the cuff at the distal end of the long tube. When used in this way, the PTL functions in a similar way to the esophageal obturator airway.

If the long tube has intubated the trachea, the airway performs in a similar way to an endotracheal tube. The cuff on the long tube seals the tracheal wall, facilitating positive pressure ventilation.

MOUTH-TO-MASK VENTILATION DEVICES

The Centers for Disease Control and the American Heart Association recommend the use of a barrier device when ventilating a patient prior to intubation, or the use of a manual resuscitator during cardiopulmonary resuscitation. These barrier devices are designed to protect the practitioner from microorganism transmission from contact

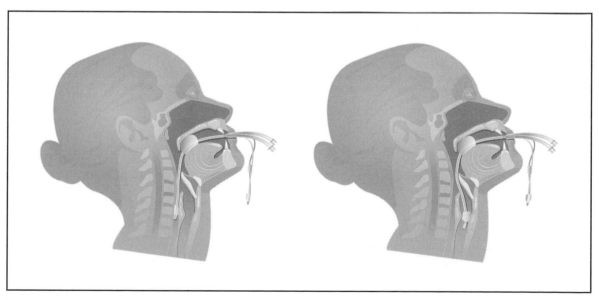

Figure 5-16 *A drawing showing the placement of the Combitube airway placed into the (A) esophagus and the (B) trachea.*

with the patient's saliva or body fluids during cardiopulmonary resuscitation efforts. These devices protect the practitioner by eliminating physical contact between the practitioner and the patient.

Mouth-to-mask devices incorporate a soft-seal mask for the patient and a one-way valve, or filter, to separate the patient from the practitioner (Figure 5-17). Additionally, some masks also incorporate an extension tube with a mouthpiece to further remove the practitioner physically from the patient. The masks are clear to allow for observation of vomiting. Some devices also have a port on the mask, or near the one-way valve, for supplemental oxygen administration during manual ventilation efforts. The use of a bacteria filter between the patient and the practitioner will further pro-

Figure 5-17 *A photograph of several mouth-to-mask devices for ventilation during cardiopulmonary resuscitation.*

Figure 5-18 *An illustration showing the correct use of the mouth-to-mask barrier devices. (A) Use of the thumbs to seal the mask. (B) Use of the thumbs and index fingers to seal the mask.*

tect the practitioner from microorganism transmission.

To use these devices, the practitioner should be at the patient's head, facing the patient's feet. Each hand should grasp the ramus of the patient's jaw, thrusting the jaw anteriorly. The mask should be placed over the patient's mouth and nose, using the thumbs or thumb and forefinger of each hand (Figure 5-18). It is important to keep a tight seal, in that leaks hamper the performance of these devices.

Supplemental oxygen may be connected to the oxygen enrichment port on the mask or delivery tubing. Use of supplemental oxygen can increase oxygen delivery to approximately 70%. If the mouth-to-mask device lacks an oxygen enrichment port, the practitioner may wear a nasal cannula to provide additional supplemental oxygen.

MANUAL RESUSCITATORS

Manual resuscitators or bags are used in the emergency setting to manually ventilate apneic patients. They may also be used during intrahospital patient transport when a patient is moved from an acute care area to another area of the hospital. An example of the type of transport is taking a patient to have a computerized tomography (CT) scan, magnetic resonance imaging (MRI) scan, or fluoroscopy procedure, or to transport the patient from the emergency room (ER) to the intensive care unit (ICU) or to the operating room (OR).

A manual resuscitator is classified based on inflation (flow-inflation or self-inflation) and whether it is disposable or permanent (reusable). The performance of these devices varies considerably and is well documented.

FLOW-INFLATING MANUAL RESUSCITATORS

As the name implies, **flow-inflating manual resuscitators** rely on gas flow to inflate them. Sometimes these devices are referred to as "anesthesia bags," due to their popularity in the operating theater. They are available as both permanent and disposable bags (Figure 5-19).

Oxygen flowing into the reservoir inflates it when the tail of the bag is pinched closed.

Figure 5-19 *A flow-inflating manual resuscitator. This may also be referred to as an anesthesia bag.*

When the bag is manually compressed (while pinching the tail), a breath is delivered to the patient. When the bag is released, the exhaled gas flows out through the tail of the bag.

Due to the design of the oxygen inlet at the elbow, it is possible to deliver 100% oxygen with these manual resuscitators. Furthermore, since the bag offers little resistance when compressed, it is easy to assess the patient's compliance when using the bag.

PERMANENT, SELF-INFLATING MANUAL RESUSCITATORS

Permanent, self-inflating manual resuscitators are designed to be cleaned and reused between patients. They are quite expensive and must be treated carefully to prevent unnecessary damage when used in the emergency setting. Several types are available for clinical use including the Laerdal, Hudson Lifesaver II, and Nellcor Puritan-Bennett resuscitators.

Laredal Resuscitator

The Laerdal resuscitator (Figure 5-20) is a permanent resuscitator made from silicone. It has a 2,600 milliliter reservoir that improves

Figure 5-20 *Three permanent manual resuscitators manufactured by Laerdal™ Medical, Inc. The three sizes include infant, child, and adult resuscitators. (Courtesy Laerdal™ Medical, Inc., Wappingers Falls, NY)*

the F_IO_2 delivery. This resuscitator uses the duck bill type of valve discussed earlier in this chapter. F_IO_2 delivery varies between .62 and 1.00 depending on oxygen flow, tidal volume and frequency.

Hudson RCI Lifesaver

The Hudson RCI Lifesaver is another permanent, self-inflating manual resuscitator. It is made with semi-transparent plastic and is capable of delivering up to 100% oxygen depending upon flow rate, tidal volume, and frequency. This resuscitator uses the duck bill type of valve described earlier. A vinyl oxygen reservoir helps to increase the delivered F_IO_2. All parts of the resuscitator except for the reservoir bag may be autoclaved to sterilize it.

Nellcor Puritan-Bennett PMR 2 Permanent Manual Resuscitator

Puritan-Bennett Corporation manufactures and markets a permanent manual resuscitator, the PMR 2 (Figure 5-21). The resuscitator uses a diaphragm and leaf valve combination. When used without the oxygen reservoir, an F_IO_2 level of .35 can be maintained. When used with the reservoir, an F_IO_2 of .94 can be achieved.

Positive End Expiratory Pressure (PEEP) Valves with Manual Resuscitators

Positive End Expiratory Pressure (PEEP) may be needed to improve the oxygenation of critically ill patients. When these patients are ventilated manually, PEEP must be provided to maintain the patient's Functional Residual Capacity (FRC). To facilitate this, there are several PEEP valves that may be attached to the manual resuscitator's exhalation port.

These valves operate using spring tension and a diaphragm to adjust the PEEP level or by using a metal disk and a magnet. In both designs, resistance is created during exhalation creating positive pressure in the lungs. At a set pressure (adjustable by the operator), the valve closes, retaining that amount of pressure in the lungs. Figure 5-22 shows a PEEP valve attached to a manual resuscitator. Rotation of the valve will cause an increase or decrease in PEEP levels. PEEP pressures should be verified and monitored during use by using a manometer attached to the exhalation port.

Figure 5-21 *A photograph of the PMR 2 manual resuscitator (Adult, Pediatric, Infant). (Courtesy Puritan-Bennett Corporation, Lenexa, KS)*

Figure 5-22 *A PEEP valve attached to the exhalation port of a manual resuscitator.*

DISPOSABLE, SELF-INFLATING MANUAL RESUSCITATORS

Disposable, self-inflating manual resuscitators have been available since 1985. Disposable resuscitators are effective, inexpensive, and reduce the threat of transmitting communicable diseases.

There are a variety of disposable, self-inflating resuscitators available today. Their performance varies from one type to the next. Since function and assembly of most disposable resuscitators are nearly the same, only two will be discussed in this text.

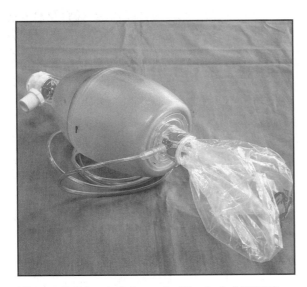

Figure 5-23 *A photograph of the Ambu® SPUR® disposable manual resuscitator.*

Ambu® SPUR® Disposable Resuscitator

Ambu Incorporated was one of the first companies to market a permanent manual resuscitator (Figure 5-23). In some areas the name Ambu is synonymous with a self-inflating manual resuscitator. The Ambu resuscitators are made from a semi-transparent vinyl material. The resuscitator is capable of delivering an F_1O_2 of between .4 and 1.00 depending on oxygen flow, rate, and tidal volume. The Ambu® SPUR® uses a diaphragm type of valve for its operation. (Diaphragm valves were discussed earlier in this chapter.)

BagEasy

The BagEasy resuscitator, manufactured by Respironics, Inc., is unique in that it is designed with a reservoir bag between the bag and the patient valve (Figure 5-24). This reservoir cannot be removed from the resuscitation bag. The bag delivers an F_1O_2 of between .52 and .93, depending upon oxygen flow rate.

Pulmanex

The Pulmanex disposable resuscitator is manufactured by Viasys Medical Systems (Figure 5-25). The bag is made from blue plastic and has a reservoir bag that attaches to the inlet of the bag. A duck bill valve is incorporated into the patient valve assembly. The F_1O_2 delivery varies between .38 and .86 depending upon oxygen liter flow and whether the reservoir is attached. Performance with the reservoir varies between .52 and .86.

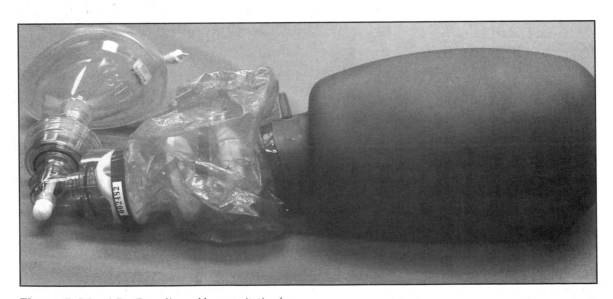

Figure 5-24 *A BagEasy disposable resuscitation bag.*

Figure 5-25 *A Pulmanex resuscitation bag.*

ASSEMBLY AND TROUBLESHOOTING

Assembly—Flow-Inflating Manual Resuscitators

1. Ensure that the resuscitation valve (duck bill, spring-and-ball, or diaphragm) is correctly assembled and functioning by blocking the patient airway connection and squeezing the resuscitation bag.

2. If the bag has a removable reservoir, install it.

4. Attach an appropriately sized mask to the patient connection (if the patient is not intubated or trached).

5. Connect an oxygen connecting tube between the bag and a flowmeter and set the oxygen flow to 10 to 15 liters per minute.

Troubleshooting

Troubleshooting this bag involves problems of improper assembly and loose connections. Careful inspection of the bag prior to use will eliminate many potential problems (ALG 5-1).

Assembly—Self-Inflating Manual Resuscitators

1. Connect a 3-liter anesthesia bag to the reservoir connection on the patient adapter. Be certain that the end of the 3-liter reservoir (tail) has been cut and is open to the atmosphere.

2. Connect an oxygen connecting tubing to the oxygen port on the patient adapter.

3. Attach the oxygen connecting tubing to a flowmeter and adjust the flow to 8 to 12 liters per minute.

4. Occlude the patient connection and observe for the bag to fill.

Troubleshooting

Troubleshooting this bag involves problems of improper assembly and loose connections. Careful inspection of the bag prior to use will eliminate many potential problems (ALG 5-1).

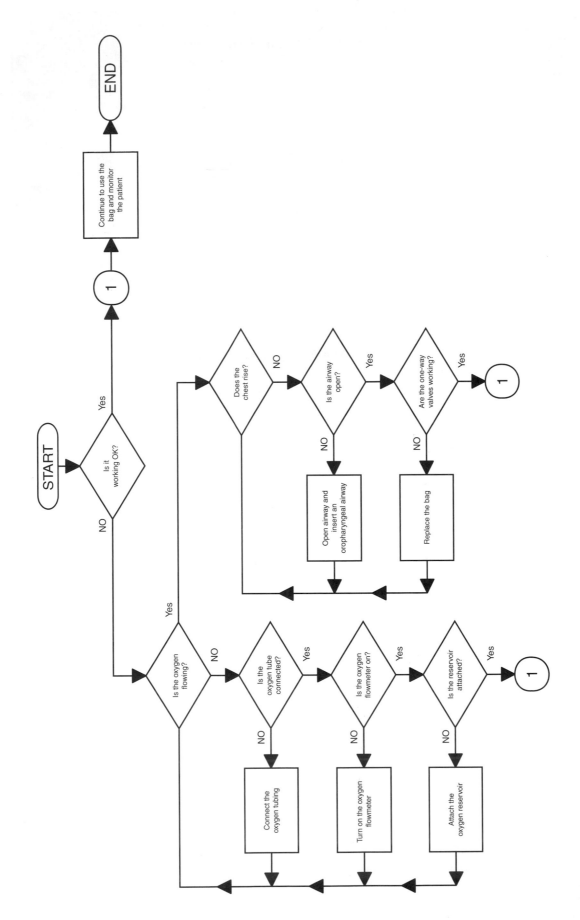

ALG 5-1 A flow chart depicting troubleshooting self-inflicting manual resuscitators.

INTUBATION EQUIPMENT

Intubation is the placement of an endotracheal tube into the trachea that secures an airway for protection and positive pressure ventilation. There are two routes of intubation: oral and nasal. Each route has its advantages and disadvantages, and the techniques for both will be discussed later in this chapter. The endotracheal tube passes through the posterior pharynx, the epigolottis, and the vocal cords with the tip resting 1.5 to 2.0 cm above the carina where the trachea bifurcates into the left and right mainstem bronchi.

Intubation is an invasive procedure with inherent risks and complications. To perform successful intubation with minimal complications, appropriate equipment must be on hand and ready for use.

LARYNGOSCOPES AND BLADES

Laryngoscopes

There are two types of laryngoscopes used to perform intubation: conventional and fiber-optic. **Conventional laryngoscopes** function much like a common flashlight (Figure 5-26). The handle contains two dry cell batteries and, when the blade is snapped into place and elevated into position, electrical current is conducted to the light at the end of the blade which illuminates. When the blade is at right angles to the handle, the light is on.

Fiber-optic laryngoscopes utilize fiber-optic bundles to transmit light to the distal end as well as fiber-optic bundles to conduct the image to the user's eyepiece for viewing. Like a bronchoscope, the tip of the fiber-optic laryngoscope can be manipulated up and down, and turned left or right to facilitate intubation of a tortuous or difficult airway. Frequently, the fiber-optic laryngoscope is first passed through the endotracheal tube, and then advanced into the airway. Caution must be used when using a fiber-optic scope. Should the patient bite on the scope, the bundles will be destroyed, and the scope is no longer of any use.

Laryngoscope Blades

There are two types of laryngoscope blades used with conventional laryngoscopes: the Miller and the Macintosh. The **Miller laryngoscope blade** is the straight blade. Several sizes of Miller blades are available from neonatal to adult sizes. Figure 5-27 illustrates three of the common Miller blade sizes. When using the Miller blade, the blade is inserted into the mouth diagonally, and the tongue is moved to the side while the blade is advanced down the airway. The epiglottis is lifted with the tip of the Miller blade, exposing the larynx and the vocal cords (Figure 5-28).

The **Macintosh laryngoscope blade** is curved (Figure 5-29). To use the Macintosh blade, introduce the blade into the mouth diagonally and move the tongue laterally as

Figure 5-26 *A photograph of a conventional laryngoscope with a Miller blade attached.*

Figure 5-27 *A photograph of different sizes of Miller blades.*

Figure 5-28 *A view of the airway as observed when using a Miller blade on a laryngoscope.*

Figure 5-29 *A photograph showing several different sizes of Macintosh laryngoscope blades.*

EQUIPMENT USED TO ASSIST IN INTUBATION

Magill Forceps

Magill forceps are long curved forceps that facilitate endotracheal tube placement by allowing the practitioner who is intubating to grasp the endotracheal tube to better guide its advancement into the airway (Figure 5-30). Magill forceps are frequently used when nasally intubating a patient, guiding the tip of the tube into the trachea. Magill forceps may also be used to remove foreign material from the airway, allowing the practitioner to grasp the object and remove it.

Stylet

The **stylet** (Figure 5-31) is a semi-rigid protected wire guide that is used to assist in the

Figure 5-30 *A photograph of Magill forceps.*

Figure 5-31 *A photograph of a stylet used during intubation to stiffen and shape the endotracheal tube.*

the blade is advanced. Keep advancing the blade along the base of the tongue until it stops and is resting in the vallecula (the space between the tongue and the epiglottis). By lifting the laryngoscope, the epiglottis is lifted, exposing the larynx and the vocal cords.

placement of an endotracheal tube during intubation. Occasionally, the airway is tortuous and difficult to intubate. The stylet facilitates shaping the endotracheal tube to more closely match the anatomy of the airway. It is inserted into the endotracheal tube and then bent into the desired shape. Care must be exercised so that the tip of the stylet does not project past the tip of the endotracheal tube. Once the stylet is correctly placed, some practitioners will make a right-angle bend where the stylet enters the endotracheal tube to prevent is further advancement down the tube.

Yankauer Suction (Tonsil Tip)

The **Yankauer suction** (tonsil tip) catheter is a rigid large-diameter plastic or metal catheter designed to quickly remove large amounts of liquid material from the airway (Figure 5-32). The Yankauer suction catheter should be connected to vacuum, ready and available when intubation is attempted. It is the best device to use to quickly clear an airway of secretions, blood, or vomitus.

Endtidal CO$_2$ Detection

Once the endotracheal tube is placed, breathsounds are auscultated bilaterally and an endtidal CO$_2$ detection device is placed on the airway to verify the presence of exhaled CO$_2$. Figure 5-33 is a photograph of a colormetric endtidal CO$_2$ detector that attaches to an artificial airway. Endtidal CO$_2$ detection equipment is discussed in further detail in Chapter 6.

Figure 5-32 *A photograph of the Yankauer suction catheter.*

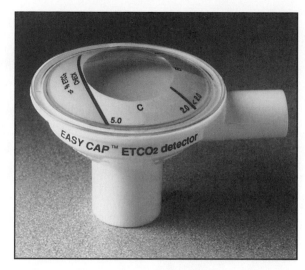

Figure 5-33 *A photograph of an Easy Cap® Endtidal CO$_2$ detection device that works on the colormetric (chemical) method of CO$_2$ detection.*

ENDOTRACHEAL TUBES

Endotracheal tubes are hollow pliable airways usually made from polyvinyl chloride (PVC) (Figure 5-34). The airway is inserted through the mouth or nose, through the larynx, and into the trachea. In proper position, the distal tip of the tube should be approximately 2 centimeters above the carina. Correct placement can be verified by examining the airway on a chest X-ray.

The endotracheal tube is hollow, allowing gas to flow through the airway. This type of airway may be used to bypass soft tissue obstructions. The component parts of an endotracheal tube include the cuff, pilot tube and pilot balloon, and Murphy eye.

Cuff

The **cuff** is a large inflatable balloon near the distal tip of the endotracheal tube. When inflated, it is designed to seal against the tracheal wall (Figure 5-35). Positive pressure ventilation may be accomplished once the cuff is inflated and a patent airway is established. Since pressure is exerted on the tracheal wall, modern cuffs are designed to be low-pressure, high-volume cuffs. Low-pressure, high-volume cuffs exert less pressure against the tracheal wall because the pressure is distributed over a greater area. The greater surface area also helps to seal the cuff. Pressure exerted by these cuffs is typically less than 25 cmH$_2$O.

Figure 5-34 *Two adult endotracheal tubes (8.0-mm ID). Note that one cuff is inflated and the other is not. Also note the markings visible on the tubes.*

Figure 5-35 *This illustration shows how an inflated cuff seals the trachea.*

If cuff pressures are too high, damage to the tracheal mucosa may result. High cuff pressures may occlude blood flow to the mucosa by compression of the capillaries in the tracheal mucosa. This can lead to ischemic damage to the mucosal wall. Once ischemic damage occurs, it can progress, resulting in tracheal stenosis, which causes a permanent narrowing of the tracheal lumen. These complications may be avoided by maintaining low cuff pressures and routinely monitoring the pressures within the cuff of the airway.

Another low-pressure cuff design is the foam cuff manufactured by Bivona. This cuff consists of a spongy foam covered with a thin silicone sheath (Figure 5-36). The cuff is exposed to ambient pressure (leaving the pilot tube uncapped), which allows the foam to expand to its normal size, thus sealing the tracheal wall. It is important not to inflate these cuffs with air like a conventional cuff. Addition of air will increase the pressure, defeating the purpose of the design. It is also important to size these tubes properly. If the tube is too small, insufficient pressure may be exerted against the tracheal wall to seal it.

The **Lanz tube** is another design that minimizes endotracheal cuff pressures. This design incorporates a regulating valve and a control balloon made of latex within the large pilot balloon. The regulation valve and balloon limit cuff pressures to between 16 and 18 mmHg. As additional volume is injected into the cuff, the control balloon assimilates it without transmitting additional pressure to the cuff of the tube.

Pilot Balloon and Pilot Tube

Attached to the cuff is the pilot tube. The **pilot tube** is a small-diameter tube that conducts air to the cuff for inflation. On the proximal end of the pilot tube is the pilot balloon. When the cuff is inflated, the pilot balloon contains air to indicate that the cuff is inflated.

The balloon therefore provides both a tactile and visual reference to whether the cuff is inflated. Close monitoring of cuff pressures is important to prevent adverse effects to the tracheal tissue.

Endotracheal Tube Markings

Endotracheal tubes have permanent markings to facilitate their usage. These markings include inside and outside diameters, length, and toxicity testing (see Figure 5-34).

The endotracheal tube's inside and outside diameters are indicated in millimeters. Endotracheal tubes are manufactured in sizes varying from 2.5- to 9-mm internal diameters. When sizing artificial airways, the internal diameter is the diameter that is referenced.

The length from the distal tip is indicated in centimeters. This provides a rough guide as to how far the tube has been inserted into the airway. A chest X-ray should be obtained to confirm the exact tube placement. Once the correct placement of the endotracheal tube has been confirmed by X-ray, it is common practice to document the length of the endotracheal tube, referenced to the patient's lips or incisors, in the patient's medical record. This documentation provides a reference in the event that the endotracheal tube advances down the airway or is displaced outward.

A radiopaque strip runs along the length of the tube from the proximal tip to the end of the tube. This strip makes the tube more visible on a chest X-ray.

Toxicity testing is indicated by the markings Z-79 or IT. One or both markings may be present. The Z-79 marking refers to the American National Standards Institute (ANSI) committee for anesthesia equipment. This committee requires specific cell culture testing to demonstrate a material's lack of human tissue toxicity. If the tube is marked IT (Implant Testing), a sample of the material was implanted into rabbit tissue to test for toxicity.

Figure 5-36 *A Bivona foam cuff on a tracheostomy tube.*

Murphy Eye

The **Murphy eye** provides an alternate pathway for gas to flow in the event the proximal tip becomes obstructed (Figure 5-37). If the tip becomes obstructed, air will continue to flow but resistance will increase, due to the decreased airway diameter.

Fifteen-Millimeter Connection

A 15-mm connection at the proximal end of endotracheal tubes and tracheostomy tubes provides a connection to manual resuscitators and other ventilation equipment. The connection is tapered so that all connections may be made by simply pressing the two parts together. The 15-mm size has been adopted as a standard for all resuscitation equipment so that all tubes will fit with all resuscitation equipment.

Radiopaque Line

A radiopaque line runs along the length of endotracheal and tracheostomy tubes. This thin line absorbs gamma rays emitted from an X-ray. The line facilitates the assessment of the artificial airway placement by appearing as a white (dense) line on a chest X-ray.

Mallinckrodt Hi-Lo® Evac Endotracheal Tube

The Mallinckrodt Hi-Lo® Evac endotracheal tube is a specialized endotracheal tube with an additional open lumen (suction lumen), which terminates proximal to the tube's cuff (Figure 5-38). The suction lumen has a separate suction line of its own and a fitting designed to interface with conventional suction lines. The purpose of the additional suction lumen is to evacuate secretions that pool above the endotracheal tube's cuff when inflated and therefore reduce the risk of their aspiration.

SPECIALIZED ENDOTRACHEAL TUBES

Wire Reinforced Endotracheal Tubes

Sometimes with a tortuous airway or in a case when intubation is only possible with a smaller-diameter endotracheal tube, kinking of the tube can become problematic. Endotracheal tubes can be reinforced with a heilical reinforcing wire imbedded into the PVC material such that the wire wrap helps to prevent

Figure 5-37 *The Murphy eye is at the distal end of an adult endotracheal tube.*

Figure 5-38 *Hi-Lo® Evac endotracheal tube. (Courtesy Mallinckrodt, Inc.)*

kinking. Figure 5-39 is a photograph of a **wire-wrapped reinforced endotracheal tube**. These tubes are also used in surgical cases when the patient's head is hyperexteneded or flexed, the patient is turned over following intubation

Figure 5-39 *A photograph of a reinforced wire-wrapped endotracheal tube.*

and anesthesia induction, or during head and neck procedures where the airway may become compromised.

Oral and Nasal RAE® Tubes

Oral and nasal RAE® endotracheal tubes have a preformed bend in their design (Figure 5-40). This bend is designed to remove the anesthesia/ventilator circuit from the patient's head. The preformed bend allows this positioning of the circuit without the risk of kinks or disconnects. Care must be used when inserting these tubes in that the bend may prevent the tube from intubating an individual with a long upper airway/trachea.

Endobronchial Endotracheal Tubes

Endobronchial endotracheal tubes are specialized tubes designed to intubate the left or right mainstem bronchus selectively. These are

Figure 5-40 *A photograph of an RAE® endotracheal tube.*

used in surgical cases where one lung is ventilated while the other is operated on or, on occasion, when differential lung ventilation is desired in the critical care setting. These tubes are large and fairly cumbersome to intubate with. Most often these tubes are inserted in the surgical setting where general anesthesia induction has been accomplished and the individual intubating the patient has optimal control and monitoring capability.

Carlens Tube

The **Carlens tube** is designed to intubate the left mainstem bronchus (Figure 5-41). The tube has two cuffs: one distal cuff and another cuff proximal. The distal cuff inflates against and seals the left mainstem bronchus, while the proximal cuff seals the trachea. The Carens tube has a carina hook that is designed to catch the carina upon insertion to facilitate its placement.

Robertshaw Tube

A **Robertshaw tube** is made for selective entry into either the right (Robertshaw right) or left (Robertshaw left) bronchus. Like the Carlens tube, it too is a double-cuffed endotracheal tube (Figure 5-42). The Robertshaw cuffs selectively seal the desired bronchus (right or left) and the trachea.

Endotracheal Tube Exchanger

Sometimes it is necessary to remove an endotracheal tube that is correctly placed, due to a cuff rupture, obstruction, or other complications. The endotracheal tube exchanger facilitates the removal of the endotracheal tube and replacement with a new one (Figure 5-43). The endotracheal tube exchanger is advanced through the existing endotracheal tube's lumen to just past the tube's tip. Centimeter markings on the endotracheal tube exchanger facilitate this process. The cuff on the existing tube is fully deflated, and then removed from the airway while the endotracheal tube exchanger remains in place. By first passing the endotracheal tube exchanger through the replacement endotracheal tube and then advancing the tube down the exchanger into the airway, it acts like a stylet, guiding the replacement endotracheal tube into correct position in the airway. Once the tube is placed, auscultate bilaterally for breath sounds, verify endtidal CO_2 and obtain a chest X-ray to confirm the new endotracheal tube's placement.

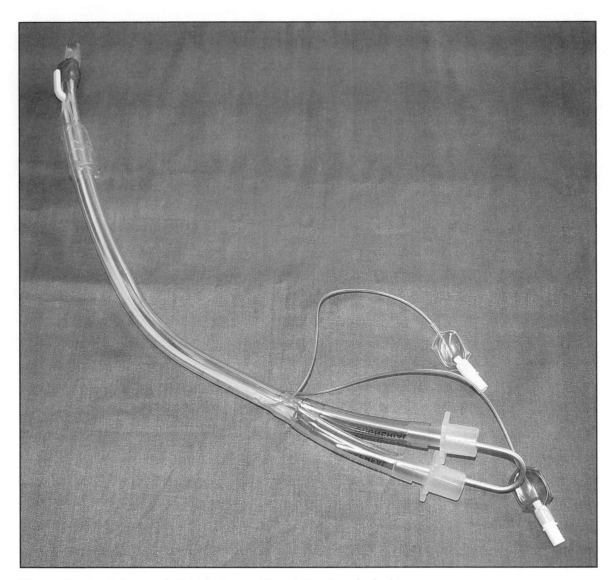

Figure 5-41   *A photograph of the Carlens endobronchial endotracheal tube.*

Figure 5-42   *A photograph of the Robertshaw endobroncheal endotracheal tube.*

Figure 5-43   *A photograph of an endotracheal tube exchanger designed to facilitate replacement of one endotracheal tube with another.*

TRACHEOSTOMY TUBES

A **tracheostomy tube** bypasses the entire upper airway. When a tracheostomy tube is placed, an incision is made between the second and third tracheal rings and the tube is inserted directly into the trachea. Tracheostomy tubes are made in differing configurations including cuffed, cuffed with a disposable inner cannula, uncuffed fenestrated tubes, Hollinger tubes, and Communi-Trach tubes.

Cuffed, Disposable Tracheostomy Tube

The cuffed, disposable tracheostomy tube is one of the most common types of tracheostomy tubes (Figure 5-44). The design of the cuffed tracheostomy tube is somewhat similar to an endotracheal tube, in that a cuff, pilot tube, and balloon are part of the design. This tracheostomy tube does not have a removable inner cannula; therefore, it is recommended to change the cannula periodically, when needed. Like the endotracheal tube, it is typically made from PVC, providing a flexible, nontoxic appliance.

Cuffed Tracheostomy Tube with a Disposable Inner Cannula

A variation on the cuffed tracheostomy tube is one with a disposable inner cannula (Figure 5-45). Frequent changes of the inner cannula will ensure that the airway remains patent. This design change eliminates the need to change the tube unless the patency of the cuff is compromised.

Fenestrated Tracheostomy Tube

The **fenestrated tracheostomy tube** has a removable inner cannula like the one just described. The outer cannula, however, has a fenestration, or hole, in it (Figure 5-46). With the inner cannula removed and the cuff deflated, the patient may breathe through the upper airway, via fenestration. This type of tracheostomy tube is frequently used for weaning purposes. In the event mechanical ventilation is required, the cuff can be inflated and the inner cannula replaced. In this configuration, the tube performs like a regular cuffed tracheostomy tube.

Figure 5-45 *An adult tracheostomy tube with a disposable inner cannula that may be replaced as required to maintain patency.*

Figure 5-44 *A disposable adult tracheostomy tube.*

Figure 5-46 *A fenestrated tracheostomy tube.*

Silver Jackson Tracheostomy Tube

The **silver Jackson (or Hollinger) tracheostomy tube** is frequently used as a permanent tracheostomy tube. It is made from sterling silver and is cuffless (Figure 5-47). A silver tube is more durable and easier to clean than a PVC tube.

Communi-Trach

The **Communi-Trach** or **Pitt speaking tube** is a tracheostomy tube that facilitates speech when the cuff is inflated. A second line and tube are attached to the tracheostomy tube, which directs oxygen flow above the cuff through small holes (Figure 5-48). This flow of gas allows the patient to use the vocal cords to communicate even when the cuff is inflated. The quality of the speech is different from normal communication, and the patient may initially have difficulty coordinating speech independent from diaphragmatic motion.

CUFF PRESSURE MEASUREMENT

As described earlier in this chapter, monitoring cuff pressure and maintenance of low cuff pressures are important to minimize some of the complications associated with endotracheal and tracheostomy tube cuffs. Two methods are frequently used to maintain the lowest cuff pressures while still allowing adequate positive pressure ventilation. These techniques are termed minimal occlusion volume and minimal leak techniques.

Minimal occlusion volume (MOV) is performed by slowly inflating or deflating the cuff during positive pressure ventilation. When cuff pressure is low, a leak can be heard at the patient's mouth. Once a leak is detected, enough air is added to the cuff to stop the leak. At this point, the cuff pressure is measured and recorded.

The **minimal leak technique** is performed by slowly removing air from the cuff until a very small leak is detected at the patient's mouth. At this point the cuff pressure is measured and recorded.

Cuff Pressure Manometers

Mechanical Manometer and Three-Way Stopcock

A mechanical manometer connected to a three-way stopcock and a syringe (Figure 5-49)

Figure 5-47 *A silver Jackson tracheostomy tube. This tube is permanent and is made from sterling silver.*

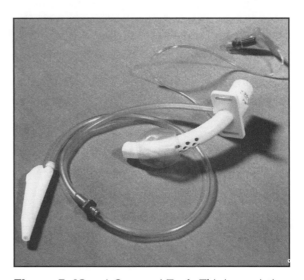

Figure 5-48 *A Communi-Trach. This is a variation of the Pitt speaking tube.*

Figure 5-49 *A photograph of a mechanical manometer, a syringe, and a three-way stopcock.*

is an effective way to measure and record cuff pressures. To effectively use this combination device, the practitioner must clearly understand which ports of the three-way stopcock are open as the valve is rotated (Figure 5-50).

When the valve is rotated toward the distal port, the manometer and the syringe are open to one another. When the valve is rotated pointing to the syringe, the manometer and the distal tip are open to one another. When the valve is rotated toward the manometer, the syringe and the distal port are open. When the valve is rotated pointing opposite the syringe, all three ports are open. It is critical to know these positions from memory, since rotation to the wrong port, if the system is connected to an endotracheal or tracheostomy cuff, may cause loss of pressure to the cuff.

To use this device, fill the syringe with 5–10 ml of air and attach it to the three-way stopcock. Rotate the valve so it points to the distal tip of the three-way stopcock. Slowly add air to the system until the manometer reads 18 cmH$_2$O. Attach the distal tip of the three-way stopcock to the pilot tube of the airway. Rotate the valve to a position opposite the syringe, opening all three ports. Perform the MOV or minimal leak technique and record the cuff pressure.

Posey Cufflator

The Posey Cufflator combines the syringe, stop cock assembly, and mechanical manometer into one easy-to-use device (Figure 5-51). A black rubber hand bulb replaces the syringe on this device. The silver port is connected to the pilot tube of the patient's airway. If there is insufficient air in the cuff, the bulb is gently squeezed, adding air to the cuff. Changes in pressure are recorded on the mechanical manometer. If too much air is in the cuff, depressing the red toggle valve on the side of the Cufflator allows air to be vented to the atmosphere, reducing pressure in the patient's cuff. MOV or minimal leak techniques may be performed with the Cufflator and the pressure may then be recorded.

DHD Cuff-Mate2

The DHD Cuff-Mate2 combines a syringe (piston) and a diaphragm strain gauge combi-

Figure 5-50 *A line drawing showing three of the four stopcock positions. (A) Off to the pilot tube. (B) Off to the syringe. (C) All three ports open.*

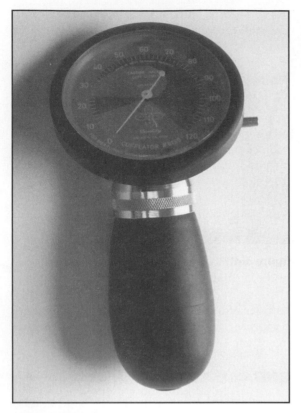

Figure 5-51   *A photograph of the Posey Cufflator.*

Figure 5-52   *The DHD Cuff-Mate2.*

Figure 5-53   *A photograph of the Respironics PressureEasy®.*

nation (Figure 5-52). To use the Cuff-Mate2, withdraw the piston by grasping the device in the palm of your hand and rotating the thumbwheel toward the digital display until the calibrated indicator reads between 0.0 and 5.0 cc. Connect the Cuff-Mate2 to the patient's pilot tube and depress the power switch (proximal to the digital display). Perform an MOV or minimal leak technique, by adding or subtracting air, using the thumbwheel to move the piston. When the desired condition is reached, record the pressure indicated on the digital display.

Respironics PressureEasy

The **Respironics PressureEasy** system (Figure 5-53) consists of a diaphragm spring assembly with a line that connects to the endotracheal tube via a T-piece assembly. The purpose of the PressureEasy is to maintain a low pressure in the endotracheal tube cuff during positive pressure ventilation. During inspiration when pressure increases in the patient circuit, a greater pressure is applied to the cuff (through the pilot line on the T assembly). During exhalation, that pressure is reduced. The system maintains cuff pressures at less than 27 cmH$_2$O, while minimizing volume loss during inspiration.

SPECIALIZED WEANING DEVICES

For many patients, it is desirable to remove the tracheostomy tube as their clinical course improves. Simply removing the tracheostomy tube and covering the stoma can be a difficult transition. Temporary devices have been developed to ease this transition. In the event that the weaning trial fails, these devices maintain the patency of the stoma and, if it is required, mechanical ventilation can be accomplished with some of these appliances.

Trach Button

The **trach button** (Figure 5-54) is one type of weaning device. It is made from Teflon and consists of an inner cannula, plug, IPPB adapter, and spacers. When the outer cannula is plugged, the stoma is closed and the patient is able to breathe through the upper airway (Figure 5-55).

With the IPPB adapter in place, mechanical ventilation may be accomplished. However, since this device is cuffless, some volume leakage will occur through the upper airway. The spacers allow the appliance to be adapted to different neck thicknesses.

Figure 5-54 *A tracheostomy button. Note the spacers, plug, and positive pressure adapter.*

Figure 5-55 *This drawing shows the placement of a trach button.*

Kistner Button

The **Kistner button** is similar to the trach button, only it is made from a more pliable plastic. This device does not have any provisions for mechanical ventilation or a removable plug (Figure 5-56). The Kistner button maintains the stoma as does the trach button. A removable cap with a one-way valve forces the patient to use his upper airway during exhalation. The cap assembly facilitates speech and also allows the patient to cough more effectively.

Olympic Trach-Talk™

The **Olympic Trach-Talk™** is an aerosol T with a spring-loaded, one-way valve (Figure 5-57). It is placed onto a tracheostomy tube (with the cuff deflated). A humidifier or aerosol

Figure 5-56 *A Kistner button.*

Figure 5-57 *A photograph of the Olympic Trach-Talk™.*

generator provides oxygen and humidification to the airway. During inspiration, the valve opens, allowing the patient to inhale through the Trach-Talk™ and tracheostomy tube. During the expiratory phase, the valve closes and the patient exhales through the upper airway. This appliance should only be used when the patient is awake and able to manage the secretions effectively.

Passy-Muir Valve

Passy-Muir, Inc., manufactures the **Passy-Muir tracheostomy valve** (Figure 5-58). This valve consists of a diaphragm valve which, during inspiration, allows the patient to inhale through the tracheostomy tube and, during exhalation, closes and forces air through the upper airway. When using this device it is important to deflate the cuff of the tracheostomy tube prior to placing the Passy-Muir valve onto the airway.

Figure 5-58 *A photograph of the Passy-Muir valve. (Courtesy Passy-Muir, Inc., Irvine, CA)*

SECRETION EVACUATION DEVICES

SUCTION REGULATORS

As discussed earlier in the chapter, suction regulators provide a means of reducing the high negative pressures from the supply line to safe physiological levels. Suction regulators operate using a single-stage regulator to control the pressure.

Puritan-Bennett Suction Regulator

The Puritan-Bennett suction regulator will control vacuum levels from 0 (off) to 200 mmHg (Figure 5-59). As discussed earlier, it controls vacuum using a single-stage reducing valve. Figure 5-60 shows a cross section of this regulator.

Note that the vacuum pressure opposes spring tension in much the same way that gas pressure in a cylinder opposes spring tension. Adjustment of the control increases or decreases spring tension, altering the vacuum level. Since the gauge is exposed to the same vacuum level at the outlet, the gauge measures the applied vacuum level.

In addition to the vacuum adjustment control, a safety lock on the side of the regulator prevents the accidental alteration of vacuum level when locked.

Ohmeda Surgical/Free-Flow

The Ohmeda Surgical/Free-Flow vacuum regulator is capable of regulating vacuum levels from 0 (off) to 200 mmHg (Figure 5-61). The regulator operates in a way similar to the Puritan-Bennett regulator, using a single-stage reducing valve.

A mode selector offers the choice of "full vacuum," "vacuum off," and "regulated vacuum." In addition, this regulator incorporates a squamper bar, which regulates the vacuum flow rate as vacuum levels fluctuate. This allows the regulator to provide high flows even if the central vacuum pressure diminishes.

Figure 5-59 *A Puritan Bennett suction regulator.*

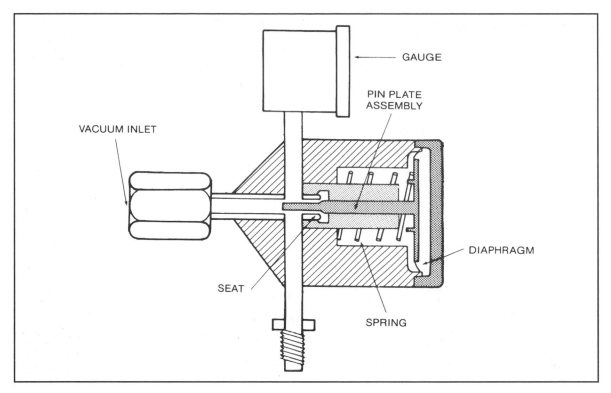

Figure 5-60   *A cross section showing the internal components of the Puritan Bennett suction regulator.*

Figure 5-61   *The Ohmeda Surgical/Free-Flow vacuum regulator. (Courtesy Ohmeda Critical Care, A Division of the BOC Group, Inc., Columbia, MD)*

ASSEMBLY AND TROUBLESHOOTING

Assembly—Suction Regulators

1. Attach the vacuum regulator to a vacuum source using a DISS or quick-connect fitting.

2. Occlude the outlet and adjust the regulator to the desired pressure.

3. If using the regulator for suctioning, attach a drainage trap to the inlet of the regulator to protect the piping system from contamination.

Troubleshooting

Troubleshooting primarily consists of checking for leaks (connection to the vacuum line or suction trap). Ensure that all connections are tight. If the regulator fails to operate properly, have it serviced by a qualified biomedical repair center.

SUCTION CATHETERS

Suctioning a patient is necessary if the patient's cough is not effectively removing pulmonary secretions. Suctioning may be required in the emergency setting when a patient is intubated, in acute care facilities, in long-term care facilities, or at home. Figure 5-62 is the AARC Clinical Practice Guideline: Endotracheal Suctioning of Mechanically Ventilated Adults and Children with Artificial Airways.

Suction catheters are long, narrow catheters specifically designed to remove secretions from the airway. The designs vary slightly, but the goal of efficient secretion removal with minimum trauma is common to all modern catheters. Suction catheters include the whistle tip, Argyle Aeroflow, Coudé tip, and the Trach Care.

When using a suction catheter to aspirate an endotracheal tube, or tracheostomy tube, it is important to properly size the suction catheter. Never use a suction catheter that is greater than half the inside diameter of the airway. Use of a larger catheter may result in excessive negative pressures applied to the lungs, causing atelectasis and hypoxemia (Poiseuille's law). Always use a catheter that is smaller than half the inner diameter of the airway.

AARC CLINICAL PRACTICE GUIDELINE
Endotracheal Suctioning of Mechanically Ventilated Adults and Children with Artificial Airways

ETS 1.0 PROCEDURE:

Endotracheal suctioning of mechanically ventilated adults and children with artificial airways

ETS 2.0 DESCRIPTION:

Endotracheal suctioning is a component of bronchial hygiene therapy and mechanical ventilation and involves the mechanical aspiration of pulmonary secretions from a patient with an artificial airway in place. The procedure includes patient preparation, the suctioning event(s), and follow-up care.

2.1 Patient Preparation:

2.1.1 In preparation for the suctioning event, the patient *should* receive hyperoxygenation by the delivery of 100% oxygen for > 30 seconds prior to the suctioning event. This may be accomplished by any of the following:

2.1.1.1 by adjusting the F_IO_2 setting on the mechanical ventilator.

2.1.1.2 by use of a temporary oxygen-enrichment program available on many microprocessor ventilators.

2.1.1.3 by manually ventilating the patient with an increased F_IO_2. (At least one study suggests that suctioning methods that use the ventilator for oxygenation and hyperinflation may be superior to use of the manual resuscitator.)

2.1.1.3.1 This technique has been shown to be ineffective for providing F_DO_2 of 1.0.

2.1.1.3.2 Practitioners should ensure that adequate PEEP levels are maintained while using this technique for patients requiring > 5 cm H_2O.

2.1.1.4 by the continuous or intermittent insufflation of oxygen through the suction catheter during the suction event—Devices designed for this purpose may be difficult to use and are expensive.

2.1.1.5 It has been shown that delivery of increased tidal volumes is difficult while using this technique.

2.1.2 In preparation for the suctioning event, the patient *may be* hyperventilated by delivery of an increased rate and/or tidal volume. Hyperventilation may be accomplished by temporarily increasing the mandatory rate on the mechanical ventilator prior to the suctioning event or by increasing the rate of ventilation with a manual resuscitator. (Note: Care should be taken to maintain an adequate expiratory time to allow for complete exhalation of the delivered tidal volume.)

2.1.3 In preparation for the suctioning event, the patient *may be* hyperinflated by the delivery of 'sigh' breaths prior to the suctioning event:

Figure 5-62 *The American Association for Respiratory Care, Clinical Practice Guideline: Endotracheal Suctioning of Mechanically Ventilated Adults and Children with Artificial Airways.* **(continues)**

2.1.3.1 by increasing the ventilator-set tidal volume to exceed the set tidal volume,

2.1.3.2 by manually triggering preset sigh breaths on mechanical ventilators that are equipped with a sigh feature, or

2.1.3.3 by manual ventilation with a resuscitation bag.

2.1.4 A closed-suction system may be used to facilitate continuous mechanical ventilation and oxygenation during the suctioning event.

2.1.5 A patient may be placed on a pulse oximeter to assess oxygenation during and following the procedure.

2.1.6 A patient may receive normal saline by instillation through the artificial airway to dilute and mobilize pulmonary secretions. The value of instilling other solutions appears to be based on anecdotal reports.

2.2 The Suctioning Event: The placement of a suction catheter through the artificial airway into the trachea and the application of negative pressure as the catheter is being withdrawn. Sterile technique should be employed. Each pass of the suction catheter into the artificial airway is considered a suctioning event. The duration of each suctioning event should be approximately 10–15 seconds. Suction pressure should be set as low as possible and yet effectively clear secretions. (Experimental data to support an appropriate maximum suction level are lacking. Some textbooks cite maximum safe limits of 100–150 torr but do not reference their recommendations.)

2.3 Follow-Up Care: Following the suctioning event,

2.3.1 the patient *should be* hyperoxygenated by delivery of 100% oxygen for > or = 1 minute by the same technique(s) used to preoxygenate the patient.

2.3.2 the patient *may be* hyperventilated by increasing the respiratory rate and/or tidal volume by the same technique(s) used prior to suctioning.

2.3.3 the patient *should be* monitored for adverse reactions.

ETS 3.0 SETTING:
Endotracheal suctioning may be performed by properly trained persons in a wide variety of settings that include (but are not limited to):

3.1 Hospital

3.2 Extended care facility

3.3 Home

3.4 Outpatient clinic

3.5 Physician's office

3.6 Transport vehicle

ETS 4.0 INDICATIONS:
4.1 The need to remove accumulated pulmonary secretions as evidenced by one of the following:

4.1.1 Coarse breath sounds by auscultation or 'noisy' breathing

4.1.2 Increased peak inspiratory pressures during volume-controlled mechanical ventilation or decreased tidal volume during pressure-controlled ventilation.

4.1.3 Patient's inability to generate an effective spontaneous cough.

4.1.4 Visible secretions in the airway

4.1.5 Changes in monitored flow and pressure graphics

4.1.6 Suspected aspiration of gastric or upper airway secretions

4.1.7 Clinically apparent increased work of breathing

4.1.8 Deterioration of arterial blood gas values

4.1.9 Radiologic changes consistent with retention of pulmonary secretions

4.2 The need to obtain a sputum specimen to rule out or identify pneumonia or other pulmonary infection or for sputum cytology

4.3 The need to maintain the patency and integrity of the artificial airway

4.4 The need to stimulate a patient cough in patients unable to cough effectively secondary to changes in mental status or the influence of medication

4.5 Presence of pulmonary atelectasis or consolidation, presumed to be associated with secretion retention

ETS 5.0 CONTRAINDICATIONS:
Endotracheal suctioning is a necessary procedure for patients with artificial airways. Most contraindications are relative to the patient's risk of developing adverse reactions or worsening clinical condition as result of the procedure. When indicated, there is no absolute contraindication to endotracheal suctioning because the decision to abstain from suctioning in order to avoid a possible adverse reaction may, in fact, be lethal.

ETS 6.0 HAZARDS/COMPLICATIONS:
6.1 Hypoxia/hypoxemia

6.2 Tissue trauma to the tracheal and/or bronchial mucosa

Figure 5-62 *(continues)*

6.3 Cardiac arrest

6.4 Respiratory arrest

6.5 Cardiac dysrhytmias

6.6 Pulmonary atelectasis

6.7 Bronchoconstriction/bronchospasm

6.8 Infection (patient and/or caregiver)

6.9 Pulmonary hemorrhage/bleeding

6.10 Elevated intracranial pressure

6.11 Interruption of mechanical ventilation

6.12 Hypertension

6.13 Hypotension

ETS 7.0 LIMITATIONS OF METHOD:

Endotracheal suctioning is not a benign procedure, and operators should remain sensitive to possible hazards and complications and take all necessary precautions to ensure patient safety. Secretions in peripheral airways are not directly removed by endotracheal suctioning.

ETS 8.0 ASSESSMENT OF NEED:

Qualified personnel should assess the need for endotracheal suctioning as a routine part of a patient/ventilator system check.

ETS 9.0 ASSESSMENT OF OUTCOME:

9.1 Improvement in breath sounds

9.2 Decreased peak inspiratory pressure (PIP) with narrowing of PIP - Pplateau; decreased airway resistance or increased dynamic compliance; increased tidal volume delivery during pressure-limited ventilation

9.3 Improvement in arterial blood gas values (ABGs) or saturation as reflected by pulse oximetry (SpO_2)

9.4 Removal of pulmonary secretions

ETS 10.0 RESOURCES:

10.1 Necessary Equipment:

10.1.1 Vacuum source

10.1.2 Calibrated, adjustable regulator

10.1.3 Collection bottle and connecting tubing

10.1.4 Sterile disposable gloves

10.1.5 Sterile suction catheter of appropriate caliber. Diameter of the suction catheter should not exceed more than one half of the internal diameter of the artificial airway. For selective main stem suctioning, a curved-tip catheter may be helpful. The information related to the effectiveness of head turning for selective suctioning is inconclusive.

10.1.6 Sterile water and cup

10.1.7 Sterile normal saline, if instillation is desirable

10.1.8 Goggles, mask, and other appropriate equipment for Universal Precautions

10.1.9 Oxygen source with a calibrated metering device

10.1.10 Manual resuscitation bag equipped with an oxygen enrichment device

10.1.11 Stethoscope

10.2 Optional Equipment:

10.2.1 EKG monitor

10.2.2 Pulse oximeter

10.2.3 Sterile sputum trap for culture specimen

10.2.4 Closed suction system

10.2.5 Oxygen insufflation device

10.2.5.1 Double-lumen suction catheter for continuous oxygen insufflation

10.2.5.2 Control valve device to alternate suction and oxygen insufflation to the suction catheter

10.3 Personnel: Personnel responsible for performing endotracheal suctioning should demonstrate the following—

10.3.1 Knowledge of proper use and assembly of all equipment used

10.3.2 Ability to recognize abnormal breath sounds by auscultation

10.3.3 Knowledge and understanding of the patient's history, disease process, and goals of treatment

10.3.4 Knowledge and understanding of basic physiology and pathophysiology

10.3.5 Knowledge and understanding of ventilation, mechanical ventilators, and their alarm systems

10.3.6 Knowledge and understanding of all artificial airways and adjuncts used

10.3.7 Ability to monitor vital signs, assess the patient's condition, and appropriately respond to complications or adverse reactions to the procedure

10.3.8 Ability to modify techniques and equipment in response to complications or adverse reactions

10.3.9 Knowledge of basic EKG interpretation

10.3.10 Ability to assess the need for and provide cardiopulmonary resuscitation

10.3.11 Ability to evaluate and document the effectiveness and patient response to the procedure

10.3.12 Knowledge and understanding of the CDC guidelines for Universal Precautions

Figure 5-62 *(continues)*

10.3.13 Knowledge of signs and symptoms of decreased cardiac output, oxygenation, and perfusion

10.3.14 Ability to teach lay-persons the procedure for home and extended care

10.3.15 Lay-persons responsible for endotracheal suctioning outside the hospital should demonstrate:

10.3.15.1 Knowledge, skill, and understanding of the assembly, use, maintenance, and cleaning of all equipment used

10.3.15.2 Ability to assess the need for and patient response to the procedure

10.3.15.3 Ability to perform the proper suctioning technique

10.3.15.4 Ability to assess the need for and provide cardiopulmonary resuscitation

ETS 11.0 MONITORING:

The following should be monitored prior to, during, and after the procedure:

11.1 Breath sounds

11.2 Oxygen saturation

11.2.1 Skin color

11.2.2 Pulse oximeter, if available

11.3 Respiratory rate and pattern

11.4 Hemodynamic parameters

11.4.1 Pulse rate

11.4.2 Blood pressure, if indicated and available

11.4.3 EKG, if indicated and available

11.5 Sputum characteristics

11.5.1 Color

11.5.2 Volume

11.5.3 Consistency

11.5.4 Odor

11.6 Cough effort

11.7 Intracranial pressure, if indicated and available

11.8 Ventilator parameters

11.8.1 Peak inspiratory pressure and plateau pressure

11.8.2 Tidal volume

11.8.3 Pressure, flow, and volume graphics, if available

11.8.4 F_IO_2

11.9 Arterial blood gases, if indicated and available

ETS 12.0 FREQUENCY:

Endotracheal suctioning should be performed whenever clinically indicated, with special consideration for the potential complications associated with the procedure. Endotracheal suctioning may be required at some minimum frequency in order to maintain the patency of the artificial airway used.

ETS 13.0 INFECTION CONTROL:

13.1 CDC Guidelines for Universal Precautions should be adhered to.

13.2 All equipment and supplies should be appropriately disposed of or disinfected.

Reprinted with permission from *Respiratory Care* 1993; 38: 500–504. The complete AARC Clinical Practice Guidelines are available from the AARC Web site (*http://www.aarc.org*), from the AARC Executive Office, or from *Respiratory Care* journal.

Figure 5-62 *(continued)*

Whistle Tip

The whistle tip catheter has the tip cut at an angle and one or more side ports above the tip (Figure 5-63). An advantage of this design is that vacuum will be applied through the side ports even if the tip becomes occluded. Also, if the tip becomes lodged against the mucosal wall, the side ports will relieve vacuum levels and minimize tissue trauma.

Figure 5-63 *A whistle tip suction catheter. Note the eyes a short distance proximal to the tip of the catheter.*

Argyle Aeroflow

The Argyle Aeroflow catheter incorporates a ring at the tip with multiple side ports above it (Figure 5-64). The ring keeps the catheter separated from the mucosal wall when it is parallel to the airway. If the distal tip becomes occluded, the side ports relieve the vacuum applied at the tip. This type of catheter demonstrates less tissue trauma than other types.

Coudé Tip

The Coudé tip catheter incorporates a special bend at the distal end of the catheter. It is also known as a directional tip catheter (Figure 5-65).

The bend in the catheter allows the practitioner to selectively enter the right or left main stem bronchus by rotating and redirecting the catheter. Although it is not assured that the desired airway will be entered, chances are improved with this design.

Figure 5-64   *The Argyle Aeroflow catheter. Note the doughnut shaped ring at the tip of the catheter and the multiple eyes for pressure relief.*

Closed Suction Systems

Closed suction systems consist of a control valve, suction catheter, sealed plastic sheath and a modified aerosol T (Figure 5-66).

The closed system design allows the catheter to be used multiple times, reducing costs. One would assume that, with reuse of the catheter, infection would be a concern. However, this type of catheter has shown no increased risk of infection when compared to other types of catheters.

The sealed plastic sheath allows the practitioner to use the catheter without having to glove up to maintain aseptic technique. How-

Figure 5-65   *A Coudé tip suction catheter. Note the angled catheter tip.*

Figure 5-66   *An example of a closed suction system manufactured by Ballard Medical, Inc.*

ever, as when performing all patient care, universal precautions should be taken, which assumes gloving using examination gloves for this procedure.

Additionally, the specialized aerosol T permits suctioning without having to disconnect the patient from oxygen to mechanical ventilation. This is advantageous because decrease of oxygen saturation can be minimized. Patients tend to desaturate less when suctioned without disconnection from mechanical ventilation or PEEP.

The control valve regulates the application of suction (on or off) and, additionally, incorporates a locking mechanism that is activated by lifting and turning the control valve.

Lukens Trap

The **Lukens trap** is a specimen trap that can be placed in the vacuum circuit when suctioning a patient to obtain a sample for culture and analysis (Figure 5-67). Place the Lukens trap between the suction tubing and the suction catheter by connecting the surgical tubing on the trap to the suction catheter and the suction tubing to the tapered fitting on the lid of the trap. Collected material will flow into the

Figure 5-67 *An illustration of a Lukens trap attached to a suction catheter for collection of endobronchial secretions.*

Lukens trap and will not be aspirated through the suction tubing. Once a sufficient sample has been collected, remove the suction tubing and catheter from the trap and bend the surgical tubing over, attaching it to the suction tubing port. Once accomplished, the unit is now sealed and ready to be placed in a biohazard bag for transport to your facility's laboratory.

CLINICAL CORNER

Emergency Resuscitation Equipment

1. You are a respiratory care practitioner in a small rural hospital. You are paged overhead to the emergency room. Upon your arrival, you learn that a patient who is en route via ambulance is in full cardiopulmonary arrest. Explain what equipment you would prepare and how you would organize it for the patient's arrival. Then answer questions (2) through (5) by referring to this patient.

2. The patient described in situation (1) has arrived. He is an elderly male who is being bag mask–ventilated by emergency medical technicians. The patient still has upper and lower dentures in place, and it is obvious that the mask is not sealing well. What should you do when you assume responsibility for the patient's ventilation?

3. You are successfully ventilating the patient, but the emergency room physician asks you to increase the respiratory rate to a rate twice as fast as what you are currently providing. Why does the physician want this increase?

4. You are asked to intubate the patient. Your facility uses Bivona endotracheal tubes. Describe how you would prepare a tube for insertion and how you would correctly secure it after placement.

5. After placing the endotracheal tube, you notice that it has become more difficult to bag the patient. The chest rise is not as great as before, and the patient appears to be doing less well. Explain how you would evaluate the situation and what you could do.

6. You are measuring the cuff pressure on a patient who is on mechanical ventilation and has a disposable tracheostomy tube. Using a mechanical manometer, you find the cuff pressure to be only 5 cmH$_2$O. You add air to the cuff, and then you note that the pressure gradually falls. What can you do to evaluate and correct the problem?

Self-Assessment Quiz

1. Which type(s) of manual resuscitation valves open in response to a patient's spontaneous effort(s)?
   I. diaphragm
   II. duck bill
   III. spring-and-disk
   IV. spring-and-ball
   a. I only
   b. II only
   c. I and II
   d. II and III

2. An increase in work of breathing caused by placement of an artificial airway that is too small is an application of:
   a. Charles' law.
   b. Poiseuille's law.
   c. Boyle's law.
   d. Bernoulli's principle.

3. Vacuum regulation is accomplished by:
   a. single-stage regulators.
   b. bleeding off excessive vacuum.
   c. needle valves.
   d. Bernoulli's principle.

4. Simple, cuffless airways designed for use with a manual resuscitator or to facilitate suctioning include a(an):
   I. nasopharyngeal airway.
   II. oropharyngeal airway.
   III. endotracheal tube.
   a. I
   b. I and II
   c. II and III
   d. I and III

5. Airway(s) that relieve laryngeal obstruction include a(an):
   I. nasopharyngeal airway.
   II. oropharyngeal airway.
   III. endotracheal tube.
   IV. combitube airway.
   a. I only
   b. III only
   c. IV only
   d. III and IV

6. Which of the following airways are inserted into the trachea?
   I. nasopharyngeal airway
   II. oropharyngeal airway
   III. endotracheal tube
   IV. tracheostomy tube
   a. I and II
   b. I and III
   c. II and III
   d. III and IV

7. The marking Z-79 on an endotracheal tube refers to:
   a. the fact that it was implanted into rabbit tissue to test for toxicity.
   b. the type of material it is made from.
   c. the serial number of the tube.
   d. the ANSI anesthesia subcommittee culture test.

8. Examples of low-pressure endotracheal tube cuffs include:
   I. low-pressure, high-volume.
   II. Bivona foam cuff.
   III. Lanz tubes.
   a. I only
   b. II and III
   c. I and III
   d. I, II, and III

9. Tracheal damage caused by endotracheal tube cuffs may be minimized by:
   I. correctly sizing the tube.
   II. maintaining cuff pressures less than 25 cmH2O.
   III. adding only 3 ml more air after the cuff has sealed.
   a. I only
   b. II only
   c. I and II
   d. I, II, and III

10. A type of tracheostomy tube that allows communication when the cuff is inflated is the:
    a. cuffed tracheostomy tube.
    b. cuffed tracheostomy tube with a disposable inner cannula.
    c. Hollinger tube.
    d. Communi-Trach.

11. A type of tracheostomy tube used for a permanent tracheostomy is the:
    a. cuffed tracheostomy tube.
    b. cuffed tracheostomy tube with a disposable inner cannula.
    c. Hollinger tube.
    d. Communi-Trach.

12. A device designed to preserve the patency of the stoma and allow weaning from a tracheostomy is the:
    a. cuffed tracheostomy tube.
    b. cuffed tracheostomy tube with a disposable inner cannula.
    c. Communi-Trach.
    d. trach button.

13. Advantages of disposable self-inflating resuscitation bags over permanent resuscitators include:
    I. cost savings.
    II. infection control.
    III. durability.
    IV. ease of cleaning.
    a. I only
    b. I and IV
    c. I and II
    d. I, II, III, and IV

14. Which of the following suction catheters allows the suctioning of a patient without disconnection from oxygen or ventilation?
    a. whistle tip
    b. Coudé tip
    c. Argyle Aeroflow
    d. Trach Care

15. The primary purpose of mouth-to-mask resuscitation devices is:
    a. to improve effectiveness of CPR efforts.
    b. infection control.
    c. to increase oxygen delivery.
    d. to open the airway.

16. Besides the use of the one-way valve or filter incorporated into the design of mouth-to-mask devices, it is recommended that the practitioner also use:
    a. an oropharyngeal airway.
    b. a bacteria filter.
    c. a nasopharyngeal airway.
    d. a PTL airway.

17. In order for the mouth-to-mask devices to be effective, it is important that the practitioner:
    I. maintain a tight seal at the mask.
    II. use good positional techniques to open the airway.
    III. use both hands.
    IV. utilize the supplemental oxygen fitting and supplemental oxygen if available.
    a. I
    b. I and II
    c. I, II, and III
    d. I, II, III, and IV

18. Use of supplemental oxygen through the oxygen enrichment port can increase oxygen delivery when using mouth-to-mask devices to:
    a. 40%.
    b. 50%.
    c. 60%.
    d. 70%.

19. An endotracheal tube cuff with a large surface area:
    I. applies more pressure to the tracheal wall.
    II. applies less pressure to the tracheal wall.
    III. causes increased pressure trauma.
    IV. causes decreased pressure trauma.
    a. I
    b. I and IV
    c. II
    d. II and IV

20. You are checking a cuff pressure on a patient's endotracheal tube. You deflate the cuff until a small audible leak is detected at the mouth. This technique is termed:
    a. maximal pressure technique.
    b. minimum seal technique.
    c. minimal leak technique.
    d. minimal occlusion volume.

21. When using a mechanical manometer and a three-way stopcock, the patient's cuff suddenly deflates. A probable cause is:
    a. The valve was turned the wrong way.
    b. There is a leak at the pilot line.
    c. There was too much pressure in the manometer.
    d. The patient coughed.

22. Which of the following combines a mechanical manometer with an inflation bulb?
    a. mechanical manometer and a three-way stopcock
    b. a Posey Cufflator
    c. a DHD Cuff Mate2
    d. the Puritan-Bennett PMR 2

23. Prior to removal of a Combitube airway, which of the following should be performed?
    I. Intubate the patient.
    II. Ensure that the gastric tube is functioning.
    III. Have suction supplies handy.
    IV. Ensure the endotracheal tube cuff is inflated.
    a. I
    b. I and II
    c. I, II, and III
    d. I, II, III, and IV

24. When using the Combitube airway, you ventilate through the short tube and you don't see any chest rise. Which of the following should you perform?
    I. Ensure that both cuffs are inflated.
    II. Attempt to ventilate through the long tube.
    III. Remove the airway and intubate.
    IV. Continue to ventilate through the short tube.
    a. I
    b. I and II
    c. III
    d. II

25. When using the Respironics PressureEasy, advantages include:
    I. decreased volume loss during inspiration.
    II. lower applied cuff pressure during exhalation.
    III. cuff pressures of less than 27 cmH$_2$O.
    a. I
    b. II
    c. I and II
    d. I, II, and III

26. When using the Passy-Muir valve, the practitioner must:
    a. inflate the cuff before use.
    b. deflate the cuff before use.
    c. connect supplemental oxygen to the valve.
    d. verify that the cuff pressure is less than 25 cmH$_2$O.

27. When using the Olympic Trach-Talk, you neglect to deflate the patient's cuff. Which of the following will occur?
    a. The patient can inhale but not exhale.
    b. The patient cannot inhale.
    c. The patient will breathe normally.
    d. Coughing will be easier.

28. If an oral airway is too large or too small, which of the following may occur?
    I. The epiglottis may occlude the larynx.
    II. The airway obstruction may not be relieved.
    III. The esophagus may be intubated.
    IV. The cuff may not fit.
    a. I
    b. I and II
    c. I, II, and III
    d. I, II, III, and IV

29. When sizing a suction catheter for use in an endotracheal tube, the diameter of the catheter should not exceed what portion of the inner diameter of the endotracheal tube?
    a. ⅓
    b. ½
    c. ¾
    d. ⅘

30. From auscultating the patient's chest you know more secretions are on the left side than the right side. What suction catheter will improve your chances of aspirating the left side?
    a. Argyle Aeroflow
    b. whistle tip
    c. Coudé tip
    d. Trach Care

Selected Bibliography

American Association for Respiratory Care. (1995). Clinical practice guideline: Management of airway emergencies. *Respiratory Care, 40*, 749–760.

American Association for Respiratory Care. (1993). Clinical practice guideline: Endotracheal suctioning of mechanically ventilated adults and children with artificial airways. *Respiratory Care, 38*, 500–504.

American Association for Respiratory Care. (1992). Clinical practice guideline: Nasotracheal suctioning. *Respiratory Care. 37*, 898–901.

Barnes, T. A. (1982). Oxygen delivery performance of four adult resuscitation bags. *Respiratory Care, 27*(2), 139–146.

Barnes, T. A., et al. (1983). Oxygen delivery performance of old and new designs of the laerdal, vitalograph, and AMBU adult manual resuscitators. *Respiratory Care, 28*(9), 1121–1128.

Barnes, T. A., et al. (1989). Evaluation of five adult disposable operator-powered resuscitators. *Respiratory Care, 34*(4), 254–261.

Demers, R. R.. (1982). Complications of endotracheal suctioning procedures. *Respiratory Care, 27*(4), 453–457.

DHD Diemolding Healthcare Division. *Cuff-Mate2 owner's manual.* Canastota, NY.

Finucane, B. T., et al. (1988). *Principles of airway management.* F. A. Davis Company.

Fitzmaurice, M. W. (1980). Oxygen delivery performance of three adult resuscitation bags. *Respiratory Care, 25*(9), 928–936.

Gensia Pharmaceuticals, Inc. (1996). *The Intavent Laryngeal Mask instruction manual.* San Diego, CA.

Hess, D. (1987). The effects of two-hand versus one-hand ventilation of volumes delivered during bag-valve ventilation at various resistances and compliances. *Respiratory Care, 32*(11), 1025–1028.

Hess, D., et al. (1989). Evaluation of mouth-to-mask ventilation devices. *Respiratory Care, 34*(3), 191–195.

Hess, D., et al. (1993). Resistance to flow through the valves of mouth-to-mask ventilation devices. *Respiratory Care, 38*(2), 183–188.

Johannigman, J. A., et al. (1991). Oxygen enrichment of expired gas for mouth-to-mask resuscitation. *Respiratory Care, 36*(2), 99–103.

Jung, R., et al. (1976). Comparison of tracheobronchial suction catheters in humans. *Chest, 69*(2), 179–181.

Kester, L., et al. (1986). Fire in a pneumatic percussor (letter). *Respiratory Care, 31*(4), 343–345.

LeBouef, L. L. (1980). Assessment of eight adult manual resuscitators. *Respiratory Care, 25*(11), 1136–1142.

Michael, T. A., et al. (1980). The esophageal obturator airway: A new device in emergency cardiopulmonary resuscitation. *British Medical Journal, 281,* 1531–1534.

Naigow, D., et al. (1977). The effect of different endotracheal suction procedures on arterial blood gases in a controlled experimental model. *Heart and Lung, 6*(5), 808–815.

Neff, T., et al. (1983). A new monitoring tool—the ratio of the tracheostomy tube cuff diameter to the tracheal air column diameter (C/T ratio). *Respiratory Care, 28*(10), 1287–1290.

Off, D., et al. (1983). Efficacy of the minimal leak technique, of cuff inflation in maintaining proper intracuff pressure for patients with cuffed artificial airways. *Respiratory Care, 28*(9), 1115–1120.

Puritan Bennett Corporation. *PMR 2 owner's manual.* Lenexa, KS.

Ritz, R., et al. (1986). Contamination of a multiple-use suction catheter in a closed-circuit system compared to contamination of a disposable, single-use catheter. *Respiratory Care, 31*(11), 1086–1091.

Smith, J. P., et al. (1983). The esophageal obturator: A review. *Journal of the American Medical Association, 250,* 1081–1084.

White, G. C. (1993). *Basic clinical lab competencies for respiratory care: An integrated approach* (2nd ed.). Clifton Park, NY: Thomson Delmar Learning.

CHAPTER 6

PHYSIOLOGICAL MEASUREMENT AND MONITORING DEVICES

INTRODUCTION

Physiological measurement and monitoring devices are very important in the medical field. Many of these monitors are employed at the bedside and provide instantaneous information about the patient's condition. These devices allow the measurement of physiological parameters to diagnose disease entities, alert practitioners to dangerous physiological changes, and analyze inspired, expired, and dissolved gases.

The use of microprocessors has increased in recent years, providing this data nearly instantaneously. Therefore, more rapid and sophisticated monitoring systems have proliferated in the management of critically ill patients. This chapter will focus on measurement principles and how they apply to equipment used today.

OBJECTIVES

After completing this chapter, the student will accomplish the following objectives.

PULMONARY MEASUREMENT DEVICES

- Describe the methods used to measure inspired or expired gas volume and flows including:
  — Volume displacement
  — Body plethysmography
  — Flow measurement

OXYGEN ANALYZERS

- Describe the three physical principles of oxygen analysis and give an example of a specific oxygen analyzer using that principle:
  — Physical
  — Electrical
  — Electrochemical

BLOOD GAS ELECTRODES

- Explain the principle of operation for the following blood gas electrode systems:
  — pH
  — PCO_2 (Severinghaus electrode)
  — PO_2 (Clark electrode)
- Describe how the blood gas electrode

systems have been incorporated into a sensor block assembly, reducing routine maintenance requirements.
- Describe the operation of a transcutaneous O_2 and CO_2 electrode.
- Describe the four hemoglobin variants including those that can combine reversibly with oxygen.
- Describe how a pulse oximeter measures oxygen saturation.
- Describe what signal extraction technology (SET) is and how it improves pulse oximetry accuracy.
- Describe how a CO-oximeter differs from a pulse oximeter.
- Describe the operation of an infrared end tidal CO_2 monitor.
- Describe the colormetric principle of carbon dioxide measurement.
- Describe how nitrogen oxides are measured and monitored.
- Describe the principles of operation and how to set up bedside indirect calorimetry equipment.
- Describe the operation and setup of apnea monitors.
- Describe the operation and setup of home sleep monitors.

KEY TERMS

Apnea monitors	Indirect calorimetry	Shift
Body plethysmograph	Inductive plethysmography	Stead-Wells water seal
Calibration	Kymograph	spirometer
Capnography	Levey-Jennings chart	Thermal anemometer
Capnometry	Peak flowmeter	Tonometry
Clark electrode	pH glass	Trend
Dry rolling seal spirometer	Pitot tube flow sensor	Venturi pneumotachometer
Fleisch pneumotachometer	Pneumotachometers	Vortex sensor
Home sleep monitors	Quality control	Water seal spirometers
Impedance plethysmography	Severinghaus electrode	Wheatstone bridge

PULMONARY MEASUREMENT DEVICES

Pulmonary measurement devices measure lung volumes and flow rates. Several different principles are used in this measurement. These include volume displacement, body plethysmography, and flow measurement. Each will be discussed and examples of these devices will be given.

VOLUME DISPLACEMENT DEVICES

Volume displacement devices rely on the patient's exhaled volume or gas to expand a bellows and move a bell or a piston. The amount of movement (displacement) is proportional to the volume exhaled.

Water Seal Spirometers

Water seal spirometers have been the industry standard for many years. The patient's exhaled gas enters a counterweighted bell, displacing it upward. Figure 6-1 illustrates a Collins water seal spirometer. The counterweighted bell moves in proportion to the volume of gas entering the chamber below it. Linear movement of the counterweighted bell may be converted to a volume by multiplying the distance the bell moved by the bell factor (20.73 mL/mm or 41.27 mL/mm). Lined paper is available that is scaled correctly such that the volumes may be read directly from the paper.

The CO_2 absorber takes up the exhaled carbon dioxide, preventing it from being rebreathed during repeated maneuvers. Soda lime is a typical absorbing agent. An indicator turns a violet color when the soda lime needs to be changed.

A **kymograph** (moving pen recorder) turns at a specific speed (32 mm/min, 160 mm/min, and 1,920 mm/min) that allows the measurement of flows as well as of volumes. If a patient exhales 3.0 liters in 32 mm while the kymograph is moving at 1,920 mm/min, the expired flow rate is 3 liters per second (there are 60 32-mm intervals in 1,920 mm; therefore, 32 mm = 1 second).

Another type of water seal spirometer is the **Stead-Wells water seal spirometer** (Figure 6-2). It differs from the Collins spirometer in that it uses a lightweight plastic bell that is not

Figure 6-1 *A cross section of a Collins water seal spirometer.*

Figure 6-2 *A Stead-Wells spirometer.*

counterweighted. Since the mass of the plastic bell is less than the counterweighted metal bell, it is less susceptible to inertial effects. The Stead-Wells spirometer is more sensitive to subtle flow changes, when compared to the counterweighted spirometer, because of its lower mass and increased frequency response.

Dry Rolling Seal Spirometers

The best way to describe a **dry rolling seal spirometer** is to say that it operates like a frictionless piston (Figure 6-3). A volume of gas entering the spirometer causes the piston to be displaced. The piston moves on very low friction bearings, so that motion is not impeded.

Figure 6-3 *A functional diagram of a dry rolling seal spirometer.*

Lightweight plastic seals seal the walls of the cylinder with the piston, folding or unfolding as the piston moves. Oriented horizontally, mass is not a factor with the dry rolling seal spirometer. Therefore, counterweights are not required.

The recording pen can be directly attached to the piston rod, but more commonly a potentiometer is used instead. As the potentiometer rotates, electrical resistance changes. Therefore, a change in resistance is proportional to a change in volume. The output from the potentiometer may be directly connected to an X-Y recorder for Flow-Volume loop recording or digitized by an analog to digital (A/D) conversion card in a microcomputer.

Bellows Spirometers

A bellows also may be used as a volume displacement device. Gas entering the bellows (Figure 6-4) causes it to expand. The bellows expansion is proportional to the change in volume. A pen attached to the bellows records its linear movement. The Vitalograph spirometer, which is an example of a wedge-type bellows spirometer, has the addition of a moving chart table. This allows the measurement of flows as well as volumes. These devices are usually employed as bedside screening tools.

BODY PLETHYSMOGRAPHS

A **body plethysmograph** is a device that relies on Boyle's law to measure thoracic volume changes (Figure 6-5). A body plethysmograph completely encloses the patient in an airtight sealed chamber. As the patient's lungs expand and contract, the volume (V) that they occupy in the box increases and decreases ($P_1 \times V_1 = P_2 \times V_2$). The pressure (P) in the box will also change, providing that the tem-

Figure 6-5 *A schematic diagram of a body plethysmograph.*

perature remains constant. By measuring the pressure change in the box, one can calculate the volume change of the thorax. This is accomplished by means of two pressure transducers. One transducer measures the pressure within the box and the other measures mouth pressures when a shutter is closed.

A pneumotachometer at the patient's mouth measures exhaled or inhaled gas flow. This pressure versus flow measurement ultimately yields the airway resistance (change in pressure divided by flow).

When the shutter is closed, the patient's airway is occluded. Pressure measurements in the box and at the patient's mouth are made

Figure 6-4 *A functional diagram of a bellows spirometer.*

directly, as he or she attempts to breathe. The box volume (pressure) versus mouth pressure measurement provides data that yield the functional residual capacity. The following relationships may be used to calculate the Functional Residual Capacity (FRC).

$$P \times V = P \times V$$

$$P \times V = (P + \Delta P) \times (V + \Delta V)$$

$$V = (P + \Delta P) \times \frac{\Delta V}{\Delta P}$$

$$V = P \times \frac{\Delta V}{}$$

The final form of the equation assumes that the change in pressure (ΔP) produced by the patient's inspiratory efforts is small when compared to the atmospheric pressure. The change in volume divided by the change in pressure ($\Delta V / \Delta P$) is the slope observed on an oscilloscope or X-Y tracing. This method reflects the total gas volume within the thorax.

PNEUMOTACHOMETERS

Pneumotachometers are devices that measure gas flow. If volume is obtained, it is obtained indirectly by the following relationship.

VOLUME = FLOW × TIME

Time is measured by the computer (sample rate), and is further subdivided into inspiratory and expiratory times. Pneumotachometers operate using different principles. These devices may be employed in freestanding pulmonary function equipment or portable spirometers, or incorporated into mechanical ventilators. It is important to understand the principles of operation of the various types of pneumotachometers and any limitations each design might have.

Thermal Anemometer

A **thermal anemometer** uses a heated element, elements, or a grid positioned in the gas flow (Figure 6-6). The heated element is maintained at a constant temperature by a sensitive thermostat. As gas flows past the element, it is cooled by convection. When the temperature of the element drops, additional current is called for by the thermostat circuit to maintain the constant temperature. Therefore, current flow is proportional to gas flow.

SensorMedics Corporation employs another type of thermal anemometer that uses two elements heated to different temperatures

Figure 6-6 *A schematic diagram of a thermal anemometer. (Courtesy Thomson Delmar Learning, Inc., Madama,* Pulmonary Function Testing and Cardiopulmonary Stress Testing, *1993)*

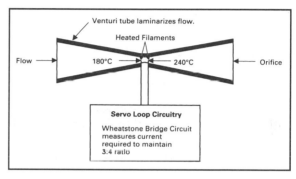

Figure 6-7 *A schematic diagram of the SensorMedics mass flow sensor. (Courtesy SensorMedics Corporation, Yorba Linda, CA)*

(Figure 6-7). By using two elements in series at different temperatures, gas composition and humidity cannot affect the accuracy of the measurements. Only the rate of gas flow influences the current flow through the device.

Fleisch Pneumotachometer

The **Fleisch pneumotachometer** relies on a pressure differential to measure flow (Figure 6-8). The heated capillary tubes cause a resistance to gas flowing through the pneumotachometer. The resistance grid is heated to prevent moisture from condensing on the grid, altering the resistance to gas flow. Gas flowing through the device will create a pressure difference before and after the resistance grid (the pressure differential is proportional to flow). A differential pressure transducer is employed to measure the pressure difference. (For a discussion of differential pressure transducers, refer to Chapter 7.) Microprocessors convert the differential pressure to a flow. If sample time is known, volume then is a function of time.

Fleisch pneumotachometers are frequently employed in laboratory type pulmonary func-

Figure 6-8 *A schematic diagram of a Fleisch pneumo-tachometer.*

tion equipment. The output from the differential pressure transducer is easily interfaced with microprocessors to provide accurate data reduction.

Venturi Pneumotachometers

A **venturi pneumotachometer** incorporates a venturi tube and a differential pressure transducer (Figure 6-9). By placing pressure taps distal to the throat of a venturi and at the venturi throat, it is possible to measure flow. As gas flows through the venturi, the gas velocity is a maximum where the cross sectional area is a minimum (refer to Chapter 1 to review a discussion of venturi tubes). At the point of maximum flow, pressure within the tube is at a minimum. Therefore, the difference in pressure between the proximal pressure port and the port at the venturi throat is proportional to the flow of gas through the tube.

The differential pressure transducer converts the pressure difference to an electrical signal. The voltage difference then becomes directly proportional to flow. The data can be displayed as an analog output (meter or digital display), or it can be converted to digital information by a computer's analog to digital conversion card (A/D card).

Pitot Tube Flow Sensors

A **pitot tube flow sensor** is another pneumotachometer that measures flow based upon a differential pressure. One set of ports is directly exposed to the on-coming gas (Figure 6-10). These pressure ports are frequently termed the ram pressure ports, since the pressure the ports see is the on-coming gas flow or ram air pressure. The other set of ports is on the side of the pneumotachometer and measures static pressure (ambient pressure). Since gas flow adjacent to the surface is stationary, those ports reflect the ambient or static pressure. The pressure difference between the ram air pressure and the static pressure is proportional to flow.

Vortex Sensor

A **vortex sensor** is a device that uses the vortex shedding principle to measure flow. The transmission of ultrasonic waves is impeded by turbulent gas flow. In a vortex sensor, struts are strategically placed in a smooth-walled tube to induce vortices distal to the struts (Figure 6-11). An ultrasonic transducer and receiver are placed into the vortex stream to measure their intensity. An increase

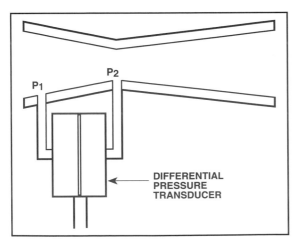

Figure 6-9 *A schematic diagram of a venturi pneumotachometer.*

Figure 6-10 *A photograph of a pitot tube pneumo-tachometer.*

Figure 6-11 *A schematic diagram of a vortex sensor pneumotachometer employing the vortex shedding principle. (Courtesy Bear Medical Systems, Inc., Riverside, CA)*

Figure 6-12 *A schematic diagram of a Wright respirometer.*

in turbulence causes the strength of the ultrasonic energy to diminish. Therefore, the decrease in strength is proportional to the gas flow through the tube.

VANE-TYPE RESPIROMETERS

Wright Respirometer

The Wright respirometer is a portable respirometer that uses rotating vanes and a gear mechanism to measure exhaled volumes (Figures 6-12 and 6-13). The rotating vane turns a gear mechanism, causing a dial to move and to indicate a change in volume. The gear mechanism resembles a watch. Directional vanes divert the gas flow in only one direction. This is advantageous, because the use of one-way valves is not required for tidal volume and minute volume measurements. These devices are most accurate between 10

and 20 liters per minute. Coaching is important to ensure that the patient will not blow hard into the respirometer, potentially damaging the unit. Flow rates in excess of 300 L/min can damage the delicate rotating vane.

A disadvantage of these respirometers is that inertia acting on the rotating vane may cause some inaccuracy in the measurement. Once an object is in motion, it tends to remain in motion unless acted upon (Newton's first law). This law applies to the rotating vane. Once it is in motion (caused by the gas flow), it tends to remain in motion, even if the flow stops. Therefore, at a high flow rate, actual volumes may be lower than those measured. Inertia also causes a slight lag, since at low flows (early inspiration) there is insufficient energy to rotate the vane.

Figure 6-13 *Wright and Haloscale respirometers.*

ASSEMBLY AND TROUBLESHOOTING

Assembly—Portable Respirometers

1. It is recommended that a disposable bacteria filter be attached between the patient's mouthpiece and the respirometer. This will help to prevent contamination of the respirometer as the patient exhales into it.

2. Connect the mouthpiece/bacteria filter assembly to the respirometer inlet. Instruct the patient on how to perform the desired respiratory maneuver (tidal volume or vital capacity).

3. Place nose clips on the patient's nose to ensure that all exhaled gas is directed through the respirometer.

4. Have the patient hold the respirometer and place the mouthpiece into his or her mouth.

5. When measurement is desired, turn the on/off switch on to record the exhaled volume.

Troubleshooting

1. Check all connections for leaks by hand tightening them.

2. If the spirometer fails to operate, verify that the on/off switch is in the on position.

3. If the spirometer still fails to function properly, send it to an authorized biomedical repair facility.

PEAK FLOWMETERS

A **peak flowmeter** is a type of pneumotachometer that is used at the bedside to measure peak expiratory flow rates. Peak expiatory flows are useful in determining the effectiveness of a bronchodilator and the reversibility of airway obstruction.

A peak flowmeter is schematically represented in Figure 6-14. Exhaled flow displaces the diaphragm (spring loaded), opening a slot for the exhaled gas to escape. As the slot is progressively opened, more flow is required to move the diaphragm. Therefore, linear movement of the diaphragm is proportional to flow. The slot is calibrated and linear movement is read directly as a flow rate.

Other disposable devices are available that utilize a calibrated Thorpe tube to measure exhaled flows. As the patient exhales forcefully, a ball rises in the tube, which displaces an indicator marker. As the diameter of the Thorpe tube increases, greater flow is required to suspend the ball within the tube. These devices operate in a way similar to the Thorpe tube flowmeter described in Chapter 1.

Wright Peak Flowmeter

The Wright peak flowmeter is a permanent reusable peak flowmeter (Figure 6-15). It is commonly used at the bedside to assess the effectiveness of bronchodilator therapy. This device operates using a spring and a diaphragm. Linear motion of the diaphragm is proportional to the peak expiratory flow.

Mini-Wright Peak Flowmeter

The Mini-Wright peak flowmeter is a less expensive version of the Wright peak flowmeter. It is made from molded plastic components while the larger Wright peak flowmeter has cast metal parts. The Mini-Wright peak flowmeter operates using a principle similar to the larger peak flowmeter (Figure 6-16). The exhaled gas pushes against a spring-loaded diaphragm. Linear motion of the diaphragm is proportional to peak expiratory flow. The

WRIGHT PEAK FLOW

Figure 6-14 *A schematic drawing of the Wright peak flowmeter.*

Figure 6-15 *The Wright peak flowmeter. (Courtesy Thomson Delmar Learning, Inc., Madama,* Pulmonary Function Testing and Cardiopulmonary Stress Testing, *1993)*

Figure 6-17 *A photograph of the Assess disposable peak flowmeter.*

Figure 6-16 *A schematic diagram of the Mini-Wright peak flowmeter.*

Mini-Wright peak flowmeter, being made of molded plastic, is much lighter weight and easier for patients to use and handle.

Assess Peak Flowmeter

The Assess peak flowmeter is a disposable single-patient use peak flowmeter manufactured by Healthscan Products, Inc. This peak flowmeter operates using a spring-loaded diaphragm, which is oriented vertically (Figure 6-17). Linear motion of the diaphragm is proportional to peak expiratory flow. A single-patient use peak flowmeter eliminates the need for processing and cleaning the device between patients. Each patient requiring peak expiratory flow assessment may be given a peak flowmeter for individual use.

ASSEMBLY AND TROUBLESHOOTING

Assembly—Peak Flowmeters

1. Attach a large diameter mouthpiece to the peak flowmeter inlet.

2. If required, move the flow indicator to the base of the calibrated track.

3. Instruct the patient on how to perform the desired expiratory maneuver.

4. Use nose clips to ensure that all exhaled gas flow is directed through the peak flowmeter.

5. Have the patient exhale forcefully (Forced Vital Capacity) into the peak flowmeter and record the results.

6. Reset the indicator, and if the patient has the pulmonary reserve, take the best of three attempts.

Troubleshooting

Very little can go wrong when using these devices. Problems can arise when the patient is not instructed thoroughly prior to performing the measurement. If the device fails to operate, replace it.

OXYGEN ANALYZERS

Oxygen analyzers are used clinically to verify and adjust the F_IO_2. These analyzers employ three main principles of operation: (1) physical, (2) electrical, and (3) electrochemical. The electrochemical analyzers may be further subdivided into galvanic and polarographic types.

PHYSICAL OXYGEN ANALYZER

The physical oxygen analyzer uses the Pauling principle or the principle of paramagnetism to measure oxygen concentration. Gases are either paramagnetic (attracted to a magnetic field, aligning with flux lines) or diamagnetic (not aligned with magnetic flux lines). Oxygen is a paramagnetic gas. Therefore, if a magnetic field is present, oxygen will be attracted to it and its molecules will align themselves with the north–south magnetic flux lines.

The physical oxygen analyzer consists of two fixed permanent magnets with a hollow dumbbell filled with nitrogen between them (Figure 6-18). The dumbbell is suspended by a very fine quartz fiber. Attached to the quartz fiber is a mirror. Rotation of the dumbbell/fiber causes the mirror to rotate with the fiber. A light shines its beam onto the mirror, which is then reflected onto a scale on the front of the analyzer. Rotation of the mirror results in a deflection of the reading to a different part of the scale. The scale shows both partial pressure and fractional concentration, so it can be used at altitude when properly calibrated.

When oxygen is drawn into the sensing cell, it is attracted to the magnetic field and the molecules align with the magnetic field, aligning with the poles. As the magnetic field is altered, the dumbbell rotates with changes in the field intensity. The degree of rotation is proportional to the oxygen concentration (partial pressure).

Disadvantages of this analyzer include: (1) it cannot continuously measure a flowing gas sample; (2) the gas sample must be anhydrous; and (3) it is very delicate and expensive to purchase and repair. Silica gel containing a cobalt chloride indicator is used as a desiccant to remove water vapor from the sample gas. The cobalt chloride indicator shows when the silica gel has been saturated with water vapor by changing color. If the silica gel is blue, the silica gel is still able to absorb water vapor. If it changes to a pink color, it must be replaced. An example of this type of oxygen analyzer is the Beckman D-2.

ELECTRICAL OXYGEN ANALYZER

Another type of oxygen analyzer is one that uses the principle of thermoconductivity to measure oxygen percentage. The principle of thermoconductivity states that a molecule of greater mass has a better ability to conduct

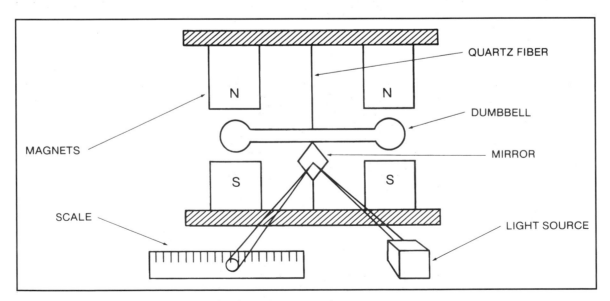

Figure 6-18 *A functional diagram of a physical oxygen analyzer.*

Figure 6-19 *A schematic diagram of an electrical oxygen analyzer.*

heat. Oxygen has a greater mass, and therefore better thermoconductivity, than nitrogen, which is the primary gas in ambient air. Therefore, if more oxygen is present, there is a greater overall heat transfer.

An electrical oxygen analyzer uses four temperature sensitive resistors (thermistors) arranged into a circuit known as a Wheatstone bridge (Figure 6-19). The **Wheatstone bridge** is a special electrical circuit used to detect small changes of resistance. A small change in the resistance of one limb of the circuit will cause a change in current, which may be easily measured.

The electrical oxygen analyzer in Figure 6-19 exposes one limb to ambient air, and the other to the sample gas (containing oxygen). The side exposed to the greater oxygen concentration cools, resulting in an unbalanced bridge state. Therefore, a current change is measured that is proportional to the oxygen concentration (percentage). A disadvantage of this analyzer is that it may only analyze static gas samples (moving samples would result in further cooling). Also, due to the heat and electrical components, these are not suitable for a flammable anesthetic agent environment. An example of this type of analyzer is the OEM.

ELECTROMECHANICAL OXYGEN ANALYZER

Electrochemical oxygen analyzers rely on a chemical reaction to produce a flow of electrons (current). The electrochemical analyzers may be further subdivided into galvanic and polarographic types.

Galvanic Oxygen Analyzers

The galvanic oxygen analyzer (Figure 6-20) relies on the chemical reaction that takes place when oxygen combines with water and electrons from the negative electrode (cathode) to form hydroxyl ions (OH^-). This is a reduction reaction. The hydroxyl ions migrate to the positive lead electrode (anode). At the lead anode, oxidation of the lead occurs to form PbO_2, free electrons, and water.

$$O_2 + 2H_2O + 4e^- \leftrightarrows 40H^- + 2Pb \leftrightarrows 2H_2O + 2PbO_2 + 4e^-$$

The free electrons flow through a sensitive meter (current meter), which measures the electrical current that is proportional to the partial pressure of oxygen. Although partial pressure is being measured, the analyzer's scale is calibrated in oxygen percentage. The

Figure 6-20 *A schematic diagram of a galvanic oxygen analyzer.*

Polarographic Oxygen Analyzers

A polarographic analyzer is similar to a galvanic analyzer. The differences lie in the composition of the electrodes and the fact that a battery is used to polarize the system. The battery speeds the reduction reaction; therefore, the response time is faster.

The polarographic oxygen analyzer is shown in Figure 6-22. Oxygen passes through the semipermeable membrane while other gases do not. Electrons from the cathode combine with water and oxygen to form hydroxyl ions (OH^-) and free electrons.

Figure 6-22 *A functional diagram of a polarographic oxygen analyzer.*

semipermeable membrane ensures that only oxygen can pass through and other gases cannot. An example is the Hudson galvanic oxygen analyzer (Figure 6-21). An advantage of this type of analyzer is that moving gas samples may be analyzed. A disadvantage is that the chemicals in the fuel cell are continuously used, and the cell must be periodically replaced.

Figure 6-21 *The Hudson galvanic oxygen analyzer.*

$$O_2 + 2H_2O + 4e^- \leftrightharpoons 40H^- + 2Ag \leftrightharpoons$$
$$2H_2O + 2AgO_2 + 4e^-$$

The hydroxyl ions migrate to the positive anode, where the silver is reduced to AgO, water, and free electrons. The free electrons result in a current flow measured by the current meter. The electrical current changes in proportion to the partial pressure of oxygen. This analyzer measures the partial pressure and displays its reading as an oxygen percentage. An example of this type of analyzer is the Teledyne Ted 60 (Figure 6-23). The advantages and disadvantages are similar to the galvanic analyzers, with the difference being response time (discussed earlier).

Teledyne Ted 60 Oxygen Analyzer

The Teledyne Ted 60 is an example of a polarographic oxygen analyzer (Figure 6-23). As described earlier, this analyzer uses a battery to polarize the electrodes, speeding the reduction reaction. This type of oxygen analyzer is used clinically to measure inspired oxygen concentrations for patient's receiving supplemental oxygen.

Figure 6-23 *The Teledyne Ted 60 polarographic oxygen analyzer.*

ASSEMBLY AND TROUBLESHOOTING

Assembly—Oxygen Analyzers

1. Open the battery compartment and install a 9-volt battery if the analyzer is not equipped with one. Most analyzers use a standard 9-volt transistor radio battery.

2. If you are installing a new polarographic sensor, turn the analyzer on/off switch to the off position. Install the new sensor cell. Place the on-off switch in the on position, and verify the analyzer's operation.

3. Calibrate the analyzer at room air (21%) and 100% oxygen. The final calibration point should be close to the value you are attempting to verify. For example, if you are attempting to verify 30% oxygen, the last calibration point should be 21%. If you are attempting to verify 80% oxygen, the last calibration point should be 100%.

4. Place the analyzer probe in the desired position to analyze the patient's inspired oxygen concentration and record the results.

Troubleshooting

When troubleshooting, please follow the suggested troubleshooting algorithm (ALG 6-1).

1. If the reading appears to be significantly different from what you expected, recalibrate the analyzer and measure the oxygen concentration once again.

2. If the analyzer fails to respond to calibration attempts, check the battery and replace it as required.

3. If the battery is good, the fuel cell may be bad. If the fuel cell is disposable, replace it.

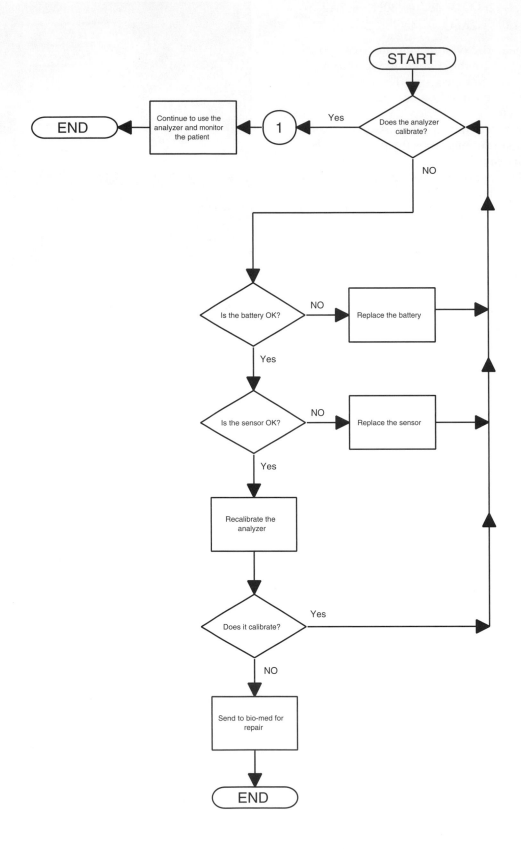

ALG 6-1 *A flowchart for troubleshooting oxygen analyzers.*

BLOOD GAS ELECTRODES

Blood gas analysis has become an essential component in the management of critically ill patients. Over the years blood gas analysis (measurement of oxygen and carbon dioxide tension and pH) has become rapid and reliable.

Blood gas information is indicated to assess a patient's ventilatory ($PaCO_2$), acid-base (pH), and oxygenation (PaO_2 and HbO_2) status. The American Association for Respiratory Care has published a Clinical Practice Guideline: Blood Gas Analysis and Hemoximetry: 2001 Revision & Update, which has been reproduced in this text (Figure 6-24). The measurement of blood gases relies on three separate electrode systems, the pH, the PCO_2, and the PO_2.

AARC CLINICAL PRACTICE GUIDELINE
Blood Gas Analysis and Hemoximetry
2001 Revision & Update

BGA 1.0 PROCEDURE:
Blood gas and pH analysis and hemoximetry (i.e., CO-oximetry)

BGA 2.0 DESCRIPTION:
Analysis of arterial and/or mixed venous blood provides information concerning the oxygenation, ventilatory, and acid-base status of the subject from whom the specimen was obtained. Analysis of samples from other sources (i.e., capillary, peripheral venous, umbilical venous samples, and pH measured from other body fluids) may provide limited information The variables most generally measured are the partial pressures for carbon dioxide and oxygen (PCO_2 and PO_2), and hydrogen ion concentration (pH). Additional clinically useful variables are the concentration of total hemoglobin (tHb), oxyhemoglobin saturation (O_2Hb), and saturations of the dyshemoglobins (carboxyhemoglobin, or COHb, and methemoglobin, or metHb), and other calculated or derived values such as plasma bicarbonate and base excess/deficit.

BGA 3.0 SETTING:
Analysis should be performed by trained individuals in a variety of settings including, but not limited to:
  3.1 hospital laboratories,
  3.2 hospital emergency areas,
  3.3 patient-care areas,
  3.4 clinic laboratories,
  3.5 laboratories in physicians' offices.

BGA 4.0 INDICATIONS:
Indications for blood gas and pH analysis and hemoximetry include:

4.1 the need to evaluate the adequacy of a patient's ventilatory ($PaCO_2$), acid-base (pH and $PaCO_2$), and/or oxygenation (PaO_2 and O_2Hb) status, the oxygen-carrying capacity (PaO_2, O_2Hb, tHb, and dyshemoglobin saturations) and intrapulmonary shunt (Q_{sp}/Q_t);
4.2 the need to quantitate the response to therapeutic intervention (e.g., supplemental oxygen administration, mechanical ventilation) and/or diagnostic evaluation (e.g., exercise desaturation);
4.3 the need to monitor severity and progression of documented disease processes.

BGA 5.0 CONTRAINDICATIONS:
Contraindications to performing pH-blood gas analysis and hemoximetry include:
5.1 an improperly functioning analyzer;
5.2 an analyzer that has not had functional status validated by analysis of commercially prepared quality control products or tonometered whole blood or has not been validated through participation in a proficiency testing program(s);
5.3 a specimen that has not been properly anticoagulated;
5.4 a specimen containing visible air bubbles;
5.5 a specimen stored in a plastic syringe at room temperature for longer than 30 minutes, stored at room temperature for longer than 5 minutes for a shunt study, or stored at room temperature in the presence of an elevated leukocyte or platelet count (PaO_2 in samples drawn from subjects with very high leukocyte counts can decrease rapidly. Immediate chilling and analysis is necessary).
5.6 an incomplete requisition that precludes adequate interpretation and documentation

---

Figure 6-24 *The American Association for Respiratory Care, Clinical Practice Guideline: Blood Gas Analysis and Hemoximetry, 2001 Revision & Update.* **(continues)**

of results and for which attempts to obtain additional information have been unsuccessful. Requisitions should contain

5.6.1 patient's name or other unique identifier, such as medical record number; birth date or age, date and time of sampling;

5.6.2 location of patient;

5.6.3 name of requesting physician or authorized individual;

5.6.4 clinical indication and tests to be performed;

5.6.5 sample source (arterial line, central venous catheter, peripheral artery);

5.6.6 respiratory rate and for the patient on supplemental oxygen, fractional concentration of inspired oxygen (F_IO_2) or oxygen flow;

5.6.7 ventilator settings for mechanically ventilated patients (tidal volume, respiratory rate, F_IO_2, mode);

5.6.8 signature of person who obtained sample.

It may also be useful to note body temperature, activity level, and working diagnosis. Test requisition should be electronically generated or handwritten and must be signed by the person ordering the test. Oral requests must be supported by written authorization within 30 days.

5.7 an inadequately labeled specimen lacking the patient's full name or other unique identifier (e.g., medical record number), date, and time of sampling.

BGA 6.0 HAZARDS/COMPLICATIONS:

Possible hazards or complications include:

6.1 infection of specimen handler from blood carrying the human immunodeficiency virus, or HIV, hepatitis B, other blood-borne pathogens;

6.2 inappropriate patient medical treatment based on improperly analyzed blood specimen, or from analysis of an unacceptable specimen, or from incorrect reporting of results.

BGA 7.0 LIMITATIONS OF PROCEDURE/ VALIDATION OF RESULTS:

7.1 Limitations of technique or methodology can limit value of the procedure. Erroneous results can arise from

7.1.1 sample clotting due to improper anticoagulation or improper mixing;

7.1.2 sample contamination by

7.1.2.1 air,

7.1.2.2 improper anticoagulant and/or improper anticoagulant concentration,

7.1.2.3 saline or other fluids (specimen obtained via an indwelling catheter),

7.1.2.4 inadvertent sampling of systemic venous blood;

7.1.3 deterioration or distortion of variables to be measured resulting from

7.1.3.1 delay in sample analysis (Section 5.5);

7.1.3.2 inappropriate collection and handling (Accurate total hemoglobin concentration measurement depends on homogeneous mixture of specimen, appropriate anticoagulant concentration and specimen-size ratio, and absence of contamination of specimen by analyzer solutions or calibration gases. The concentration measured may also be dependent on the method incorporated by the specific analyzer.);

7.1.3.3 incomplete clearance of analyzer calibration gases and previous waste or flushing solution(s);

7.1.4 Hyperlipidemia causes problems with analyzer membranes and may affect CO-oximetry.

7.1.5 Appropriate sample size is determined by the type of anticoagulant and the sample requirements of the analyzer(s). Attempts should be made to keep sample sizes as small as is technically feasible to limit blood loss, particularly in neonates.

7.1.6 Some calculated values may be in error (e.g., calculated SaO_2 may not reflect O_2Hb in the presence of COHb and/or metHb and with changes in 2,3 DPG concentration).

7.1.7 Arterialized capillary samples may be adequate to assess acid-base disorders but may not adequately reflect patient oxygenation.

7.1.8 The laboratory must have a defined procedure for temperature correction of the measured results. Errors in the measurement of the patient's temperature may cause erroneous temperature-corrected results. If temperature-adjusted results are reported, the report should be clearly labeled as such, and the measured results at 37°C must also be reported.

7.2 Results of analysis can be considered valid if

7.2.1 analytic procedure conforms to recommended, established guidelines and follows manufacturer's recommendations;

7.2.2 results of pH-blood gas analysis fall within the calibration range of the analyzer(s) and quality control product ranges. If a result outside of the usual calibration

Figure 6-24 *(continues)*

range is obtained (e.g., PaO_2 measured as 250 torr, but analyzer calibrated to 140 torr), the analyzer should be recalibrated to accommodate this unusual value (using "calibration override" function and high- or 100%-oxygen standard gas).

7.2.3 laboratory procedures and personnel are in compliance with quality control and recognized proficiency testing programs.

7.3 If questionable results are obtained and are consistent with specimen contamination:

7.3.1 the labeling of the blood sample container should be rechecked for patient's full name, medical record number (patient identifier), date and time of acquisition, and measured F_IO_2 (or supplemental oxygen liter flow);

7.3.2 the residual specimen should be reanalyzed (preferably on a separate analyzer);

7.3.3 an additional sample should be obtained if the discrepancy cannot be resolved;

7.3.4 results of analysis of discarded samples should be logged with reason for discarding.

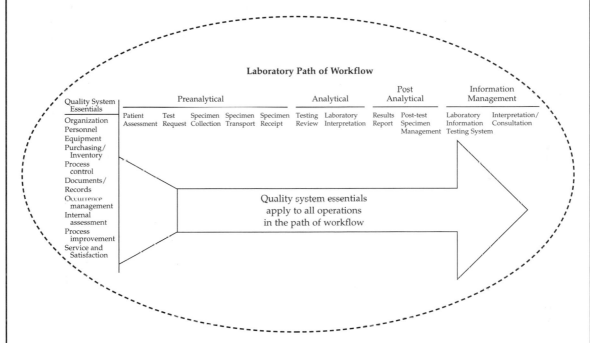

Figure 1.   Structure for a Quality System Model for a Laboratory Service. Adopted from NCCLS document GP26-A—Quality System Model for Health Care; Approved Guideline.

BGA 8.0 ASSESSMENT OF NEED:

The presence of a valid indication (BGA 4.0) in the subject to be tested supports the need for sampling and analysis.

BGA 9.0 ASSESSMENT OF QUALITY OF TEST AND VALIDITY OF RESULTS:

The consensus of the committee is that all diagnostic procedures should follow the quality model described in the NCCLS GP26-A Quality System Model for Health Care. (Figure 1) The document describes a laboratory path of workflow model that incorporates all the steps of the procedure. This process begins with patient assessment and the generation of a clinical indication for testing through the application of the test results to patient care. The quality system essentials defined for all healthcare services provide the framework for managing the path of workflow. A continuation of this model for respiratory care services is further described in NCCLS HS4-A A Quality System Model for Respiratory Care. In both quality models the patient is the central focus.

9.1 General considerations include:

9.1.1 As part of any quality assurance program, indicators must be developed to monitor areas addressed in the path of workflow.

9.1.2 Each laboratory should standardize procedures and demonstrate intertechnologist reliability. Test results can be considered

Figure 6-24 *(continues)*

valid only if they are derived according to and conform to established laboratory quality control, quality assurance, and monitoring protocols.

9.1.3 Documentation of results, therapeutic intervention (or lack of) and/or clinical decisions based on testing should be placed in the patient's medical record.

9.1.4 The mode of ventilation, the oxygen concentration, and the oxygen delivery device and the results of the pretest assessment should be documented.

9.1.5 Report of test results should contain a statement by the technician performing the test regarding test quality (including patient understanding of directions and effort expended) and, if appropriate, which recommendations were not met.

9.1.6 Test results should be interpreted by a physician, taking into consideration the clinical question to be answered.

9.1.7 Personnel who do not meet annual competency requirements or whose competency is deemed unacceptable as documented in an occurrence report should not be allowed to participate, until they have received remedial instruction and have been re-evaluated.

9.1.8 There must be evidence of active review of quality control, proficiency testing, and physician alert, or 'panic' values, on a level commensurate with the number of tests performed

9.2 Blood gas-pH analysis and hemoximetry are beneficial only if no preanalytical error has occurred.

9.3 Considerations related to equipment quality control and control materials:

9.3.1 For internal-equipment quality control using commercial controls:

9.3.1.2 Establish the mean and standard deviation (SD) for each constituent (i.e., pH, PCO_2, PO_2) in each level for a new lot number of commercial quality control material prior to expiration of the old lot number. The laboratory director or designee should determine the acceptable range for quality control results based on statistically relevant or medical-needs criteria.

9.3.1.3 The frequency of each control run and number of levels is dependent on regulatory requirements and manufacturer's recommendations beyond a minimum of 1 level every 8 hours and 2 levels each day that the instrument is in operation.

9.3.1.4 Quality control results outside predefined acceptability limits should trigger equipment troubleshooting. Quality control must be verified to be "in control" prior to analysis of specimens. Appropriate documentation of actions taken and results of verification are required.

9.3.1.5 Duplicate specimen analysis (i.e., twice on one instrument or once on two instruments) may also be performed on a regular basis as an additional method of quality control. Duplicate analysis of the same analytes on different models of equipment is generally required by accrediting agencies.

9.3.1.6 Tonometry is the reference procedure to establish accuracy for blood PO_2 and PCO_2. If issues of true accuracy arise, tonometry should be available.

9.3.1.7 Electronic quality control monitors only the equipment performance. The use of nonelectronic controls at periodic intervals should also be employed to evaluate the testing process.

9.3.1.8 Recordkeeping. Summarize all quality control data for a specified lot number. Maintain and generate reports according to regulatory and institutional policy.

9.3.2 External quality control or proficiency testing considerations:

9.3.2.1 Proficiency testing is required by the Clinical Laboratory Amendments of 1988 (CLIA '88) for each regulated analyte. Specimens of unknown values from an external source are to be analyzed a minimum of 3 times a year.

9.3.2.2 Proficiency-testing materials should be obtained from an approved source to meet regulatory requirements.

9.3.2.3 The proficiency-testing survey report should be carefully reviewed by the medical director and laboratory supervisor. If the results are suboptimal, the medical director and supervisor should promptly review their equipment, procedures, and materials to ascertain the cause of the poor performance.

9.3.3 With new equipment installation:

9.3.3.1 CLIA '88 requires the evaluation of equipment accuracy and imprecision prior to analysis of patient samples.

9.3.3.2 Tonometry is the reference method for establishing accuracy for PaO_2 and $PaCO_2$, but unless the entire tonometry process is of the highest quality, it, too, can have errors.

Figure 6-24 *(continues)*

9.3.3.3 When an existing instrument is replaced, duplicate analysis must be performed to compare the new instrument to the existing instrument.

9.3.4 Calibration verification

9.3.4.1 Calibration verification is performed prior to initial use and at 6-month intervals. Calibration verification is completed by analyzing a minimum of 3 levels of control material to verify the measuring range of the analyzer. A fourth level should be considered if samples with high O_2 levels are analyzed on the instrument.

9.3.4.2 Frequency of calibration verification may vary according to regulatory agencies under which the laboratory is accredited or licensed [i.e., College of American Pathologists (CAP), CLIA '88 or Joint Commission on Accreditation of Healthcare Organizations (JCAHO)].

9.4 Testing (analytical phase) is carried out according to an established proven protocol, conforming to manufacturer recommendations. The following aspects of analysis should be monitored and corrective action taken as indicated:

9.4.1 detection of presence of air bubbles or clots in specimen, with evacuation prior to mixing and sealing of syringe;

9.4.2 assurance that an uninterrupted (i.e., solid or continuous) sample is aspirated (or injected) into analyzer and that all of the electrodes are covered by the sample (confirmed by direct viewing of sample chamber if possible;

9.4.3 assurance that 8-hour quality control and calibration procedures have been completed and that instrumentation is functioning properly prior to patient sample analysis;

9.4.4 assurance that specimen was properly labeled, stored, and analyzed within an acceptable period of time (see Section 5.5).

9.5 Post-testing (post-analytical phase) The results should validate or contradict the patient's clinical condition (i.e., the basis for ordering the test).

9.5.1 Documentation of results, therapeutic intervention (or lack of), and/or clinical decisions based upon the pH-blood gas measurements should be available in the patient's medical record and/or be otherwise readily accessible (e.g., at the testing area) for at least 2 years.

9.5.2 Reference intervals and 'critical values' must be determined for each analyte prior to sample analysis. If the reference interval is determined by transference, the interval should be validated. Defining and determining reference intervals is described in NCCLS document C24-A2.

BGA 10.0 RESOURCES:

Federal regulations stipulate that requirements relative to personnel (levels of education and training), documentation procedures, and equipment be fulfilled. Blood gas instrumentation is classified as being either moderately or highly complex. Persons performing blood gas analysis should be conversant with applicable federal regulations (CLIA '88) and appropriately qualified.

10.1 Recommended equipment:

10.1.1 Automated or semiautomated pH-blood gas analyzer with related calibration gases, electrodes, membranes, electrolytes, reagents, and accessories.

10.1.2 Fixed, multiple wavelength spectrophotometer (hemoximeter or CO-oximeter) or other device for determining total hemoglobin and its components.

10.1.3 Protective eye wear as necessary and outer wear, protective gloves, impenetrable needle container, face mask and/or faceshield.

10.1.4 Quality control and proficiency testing materials.

10.2 Personnel:

The following recommendations are for tests of moderate complexity, as designated by CLIA '88. Persons at either of the levels described should perform pH-blood gas analysis under the direction and responsibility of a laboratory director and technical consultant (may be the same individual) who possess at least a baccalaureate degree and who have specific training in blood gas analysis and interpretation.

10.2.1 Level I: Personnel should be specifically trained in pH-blood gas analysis, oxygen delivery devices, and related equipment, record keeping, and hazards and sources of specimen and handler contamination(s) associated with sampling and analysis. Such persons should be, at minimum, high school graduates (or equivalent) with strong backgrounds in mathematics, and preferably with one or more years of college courses in the physical and

Figure 6-24 (continues)

biological sciences. Such persons must have documented training and demonstrated proficiency in pH-blood gas analysis, preventive maintenance, troubleshooting, instrument calibration, and awareness of the factors that influence test results, and the skills required to verify the validity of test results through the evaluation of quality-control sample values, prior to analyzing patient specimens and reporting results. Performance of pH-blood gas analysis must be supervised by a Level-II technologist.

10.2.2 Level II: Level-II personnel supervise Level-I personnel and are health care professionals specifically trained (with proven, documented proficiency) in all aspects of blood gas analysis and hemoximetry:

10.2.2.1 quality control, quality assurance, and proficiency testing;

10.2.2.2 operation and limitations, including instrument troubleshooting and appropriate corrective measures.

10.2.2.3 Level-II personnel should be cognizant of various means for specimen collection and the causes and impact of preanalytical and instrument error(s).

10.2.2.4 Level-II personnel should be trained in patient assessment, acid-base and oxygenation disorders, and diagnostic and therapeutic alternatives. A baccalaureate, or higher, degree in the sciences or substantial experience in pulmonary function technology is preferred. Although, 2 years of college in biological sciences and mathematics, plus 2 years of training and experience, or equivalent may be substituted for personnel supervising arterial pH-blood gas analysis. A recognized credential (MT, MLT, CRT, RRT, CPFT, RPFT) is strongly recommended.

BGA 11.0 MONITORING:

Monitoring of personnel, sample handling, and analyzer performance to assure proper handling, analysis, and reporting should be ongoing during the process.

BGA 12.0 FREQUENCY:

Frequency of execution of procedures depends upon the sample load of the laboratory and the requirements of agencies that specify quality control maneuvers.

BGA 13.0 INFECTION CONTROL:

13.1 The staff, supervisors, and physician-directors associated with the pulmonary laboratory should be conversant with "Guideline for Isolation Precautions in Hospitals" made by the Centers for Disease Control and the Hospital Infection Control Practices Advisory Committee (HICPAC) and develop and implement policies and procedures for the laboratory that comply with its recommendations for Standard Precautions and Transmission-Based Precautions.

13.2 The laboratory's manager and its medical director should maintain communication and cooperation with the institution's infection control service and the personnel health service to help assure consistency and thoroughness in complying with the institution's policies related to immunizations, post-exposure prophylaxis, and job- and community-related illnesses and exposures.

13.3 Primary considerations include

13.3.1 adequate handwashing,

13.3.2 provision of prescribed ventilation with adequate air exchanges,

13.3.3 careful handling and thorough cleaning and processing of equipment,

13.3.4 the exercise of particular care in scheduling and interfacing with the patient in whom a diagnosis has not been established.

BGA 14.0 AGE-SPECIFIC ISSUES:

This document applies to samples from neonatal, pediatric, adult, and geriatric populations.

Reprinted with permission from *Respiratory Care* 2001; 46: 498–505. The complete AARC Clinical Practice Guidelines are available from the AARC Web site (*http://www.aarc.org*), from the AARC Executive Office, or from *Respiratory Care* journal.

Figure 6-24 *(continued)*

THE pH SYSTEM

In this text the term "system" is used rather than "electrode" because, to an electrochemist, an electrode is the point at which electrical current enters or leaves the electrochemical cell. The pH system is in reality made up of two electrodes (half-cells) acting together to measure potential differences (voltage) that we term pH. Two electrodes or electrochemical cells make up the pH system: the reference cell and the measuring cell.

Reference Cell (Electrode)

The reference cell's purpose is to provide a constant potential or voltage. Several processes must occur so that the reference potential is constant: (1) the electrochemical reaction must be reversible; (2) the electrochemical reaction must be reproducible (it must be the same each time); and (3) the system must be stable. If all three requirements are met, a consistent voltage will be produced by a cell to serve as a reference. Common reference cells or systems include the calomel and the silver/silver chloride cells.

The calomel reference cell is composed of a metal and metallic paste electrode in contact with a salt solution. Figure 6-25 is an illustra-

tion of a calomel reference cell. The base of the electrode is a mercurous chloride paste (calomel) with a porous plug at the bottom. The calomel paste is blended into mercury metal. Finally, a wire conducts electrical current from the cell. The electrode itself is in a salt solution of saturated potassium chloride (KCl). The reaction that drives the cell is as follows:

$$KCl \rightleftharpoons K^+ + Cl^-$$

$$Hg \rightleftharpoons Hg^+ + e^-$$

$$2Hg^+ + 2Cl^- \rightleftharpoons Hg2Cl_2$$

As can be seen, the dissociation of mercury results in the formation of free electrons, and therefore a potential difference (voltage), which drives the cell. The electrons are conducted by the wire to a galvanometer (sensitive voltmeter), which measures the potential when compared with something else (serving as a reference). The calomel reference cell is the most common "reference electrode" used in clinical blood gas instruments.

The silver/silver chloride cell is depicted in Figure 6-26. It is simpler in design than the calomel reference cell. A silver wire has its end coated with silver chloride. The entire conductor is immersed in a solution of soluble chlo-

Figure 6-25 *A schematic diagram of a calomel reference electrode.*

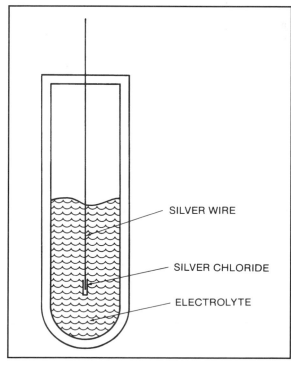

Figure 6-26 *A schematic of a silver/silver chloride reference electrode.*

ride. The reaction that drives the cell is as follows:

$$Ag \leftrightharpoons Ag^+ + e^-$$

$$Ag + Cl^- \leftrightharpoons AgCl$$

The dissociation of silver produces electrons. As with the calomel reference cell, the silver/silver chloride cell produces free electrons creating a potential difference (voltage) that may be compared with something else.

pH Glass

One key component in the pH system is pH glass. The **pH glass** is said to be permeable to hydrogen ions (H^+). The exact method of ion or electrical transfer is not well understood. However, a potential difference (voltage) may be produced by placing two solutions of differing pH on opposite sides of the glass. This potential difference may be used to determine the pH of an unknown solution.

pH System (or Cell)

One reference electrode and one sample electrode are placed on opposite sides of pH glass to measure the pH of a solution. This complete cell (two reference half-cells combined) is known as a pH cell or system (Figure 6-27).

The reference half-cell is immersed in its KCl bath and provides a constant reference voltage. The measuring half-cell has a known buffer solution on one side of the pH glass and an unknown pH solution (blood) on the other. The KCl bridge serves to complete the electrical contact between the reference half-cell and the measuring half-cell. The potential difference (voltage) between the buffer solution (known pH) and the unknown pH of the blood is proportional to the pH of the blood. The display is usually calibrated in pH units rather than voltage.

THE PCO$_2$ MEASURING SYSTEM

If the reader understands the pH measuring system, the CO$_2$ system will be easy to understand. This is because the PCO$_2$ system is a pH system modified to measure PCO$_2$. The modern PCO$_2$ system was developed by John Severinghaus in 1958. Sometimes the PCO$_2$ is referred to as a **Severinghaus electrode.** You may recall from your study of human physiology that the following reaction occurs in the blood.

$$CO_2 + H_2O \leftrightharpoons H_2CO_3 \leftrightharpoons H + HCO_3^-$$

Carbon dioxide combines with water and

Figure 6-27 *A schematic diagram of the pH system in a blood gas analyzer.*

BLOOD

WATER BATH

MEMBRANE

ELECTRODES

pH GLASS

ELECTROLYTE

NYLON MESH

Figure 6-28 *A schematic diagram of a PCO$_2$ system in a blood gas analyzer.*

forms carbonic acid, which dissociates to free hydrogen ions and bicarbonate ions. The PCO$_2$ cell is a system that takes advantage of this reaction to measure pH (which, as you will see, is proportional to PCO$_2$).

The PCO$_2$ cell consists of two measuring half-cells (silver/silver chloride), as shown in Figure 6-28. The tip of the electrode has two special coverings. The inner one is a nylon mesh that allows only a thin film of sodium bicarbonate buffer to exist between the pH glass and the membrane. If the layer of buffer is thin, small changes in pH will produce a rapid change in hydrogen ions. The membrane is permeable only to carbon dioxide.

Carbon dioxide diffuses across the membrane from the blood and reacts with the sodium bicarbonate buffer and water to produce hydrogen ions. The hydrogen ions cause a measurable potential (voltage) to be produced between the buffer solution and the pH electrode. The voltage change (potential) is proportional to the partial pressure of dissolved carbon dioxide in the blood.

THE PO$_2$ MEASURING SYSTEM

The modern PO$_2$ system was developed by Leland Clark in 1958 (Figure 6-29). Frequently, the PO$_2$ electrode system is referred to as a **Clark electrode.**

The PO$_2$ cell is composed of a platinum

cathode and silver/silver anode. The tip of the electrode is covered with a membrane that is permeable only to oxygen. Oxygen diffuses from the blood across the membrane and reacts with the potassium hydroxide buffer to drive the following reaction.

$$2O_2 + 2H_2O + 4e^- \leftrightarrows 4OH^-$$

As you can see, four electrons will be consumed to form 4 hydroxide ions. The platinum cathode provides the electrons to drive the reaction and the hydroxide ions migrate to the silver/silver chloride reference cell (anode). The current flow from the anode to the cathode is measurable, and is proportional to the oxygen tension in the blood.

BLOOD

WATER BATH

ELECTROLYTE

SILVER ANODE

PLATINUM CATHODE

MEMBRANE

Figure 6-29 *A schematic diagram of a PO$_2$ system in a blood gas analyzer.*

BLOOD GAS SENSOR BLOCKS

The conventional blood gas electrodes have been reduced in size and can be combined together to from sensor blocks (Figure 6-30). The sensor block for each electrode is about one-third the size of a conventional electrode. Furthermore, membranes, electrolyte solutions, and other consumable components have been eliminated. The service life of these sealed systems is much greater than that of the conventional electrode.

CALIBRATION AND QUALITY CONTROL OF BLOOD GAS SYSTEMS

Life-and-death decisions in the management of critically ill patients are made from information provided by blood gas systems. To ensure clinical accuracy, calibration, and quality control of the pH, PO_2 and PCO_2 systems are essential. **Calibration** is the process of comparing a measuring device (blood gas system) with a known physical standard. Periodic calibration of the blood gas instrument is one important part of ensuring clinical accuracy. **Quality control** is the application of statistical analysis with standardized control samples. Random testing is used to identify random errors that may affect clinical accuracy. A comprehensive calibration and quality control program will ensure that a blood gas instrument is accurate and that gross errors will not jeopardize patient safety.

Calibration

Blood gas instrument calibration involves the use of precision gases with concentrations known to within ±.05% and known buffer solutions. Gas mixtures (O_2, CO_2, and N_2) are used to calibrate the PO_2 and PCO_2 systems, and buffer solutions are used to calibrate the pH system. To use the precision gases, the barometric pressure at the instrument must be known. Most laboratories have a mercury barometer to measure the barometric pressure. In some locations in the United States, barometric pressures can vary significantly with the passage of frontal weather systems. It is therefore important to check the barometric pressure frequently when weather changes are observed.

To determine the expected calibration readings for the PO_2 and PCO_2 systems, Dalton's law of partial pressures must be applied.

Example: Given the following gas mixture and barometric pressure, determine the calibration points for PO_2 and PCO_2.

Calibration Gas Mixture: 5% oxygen, 20% carbon dioxide, balance nitrogen

Barometric Pressure: 745 mmHg

Step 1: Since the blood gas instrument is at body temperature (37°C) and physiological solutions are being measured, water vapor pressure must be accounted for. The calibration gases are humidified with water creating a fourth gas (PH_2O), or water vapor. Subtract the water vapor pressure from the barometric pressure.

$$\begin{array}{r} 745 \text{ mmHg} \\ - \ 47 \text{ mmHg} \\ \hline 698 \text{ mmHg} \end{array}$$

Step 2: Apply Dalton's law using the corrected barometric pressure.

$$O_2 .05 \times 698 \text{ mmHg} = 34.9 \text{ mmHg}$$
$$CO_2 .20 \times 698 \text{ mmHg} = 139.6 \text{ mmHg}$$
$$N_2 .75 \times 698 \text{ mmHg} = 523.5 \text{ mmHg}$$

Since nitrogen is not measured, the value may be ignored. The values for PO_2 and PCO_2 are 34.9 mmHg and 139.6 mmHg, respectively.

Modern blood gas instruments will introduce a known buffer solution and the gases simultaneously to calibrate the instrument. Knowing the pH of the buffer and the calibration points for PO_2 and PCO_2, the instrument can be accurately calibrated to these known physical standards.

Figure 6-30 *A photograph of a sensor block for the pH and pH reference system.*

Both a high calibration and a low calibration are used to calibrate blood gas instruments. The difference between the two points is the gas concentrations and the buffer solutions used. Two common calibration points are listed below for one instrument manufacturer.

High Calibration		Low Calibration	
pH	6.840	pH	7.384
PCO_2	5%	PCO_2	12%
PO_2	0%	PO^2	10%

By calibrating at the high and low points of the physiological normals expected, the accuracy of the instrument between the two points is assured.

Quality Control

A quality control program involves random sampling of known solutions and statistical analysis to identify analytical variations that may impact the accuracy of a clinical instrument. The purpose of a quality control program is to differentiate between random analytical errors or variation and systematic, technical errors or variation. Quality controls are run following calibration and randomly with patient specimens according to the instrument manufacturer's approved quality control schedule.

Reference materials are manufactured by the blood gas instrument manufacturers and other companies for the purpose of quality control. The majority of these materials are aqueous solutions of a known pH with known partial pressures of dissolved gases (O_2 and CO_2). These materials are produced under very strict standards to ensure their accuracy and reproducibility in the clinical setting. Most companies manufacture aqueous solutions with different pH values and gas concentrations. Most manufacture three levels (different mixtures), ensuring that the instrument is tested over a wide physiological range of values. Some laboratories also employ tonometry of whole blood samples in their quality control programs.

Tonometry is the rapid equilibration of known gas samples with whole blood samples. An instrument known as a tonometer rapidly mixes a known gas mixture with whole blood until the gases are dissolved in the plasma. If the barometric pressure is known, and the gas mixture is also known, expected results may be calculated in a way similar to that described in the calibration section.

Statistical Analysis of the Results

As described earlier, statistical analysis plays an important role in a quality control program. When establishing a quality control program one must: (1) establish the allowable limits for variation, due to random analytical error; (2) evaluate all laboratory control data using those established limits; and (3) take corrective action in the event the limits are exceeded.

The limits for variation are established using the Gaussian distribution. The standard deviation is a measure of the distribution of values around the mean. The acceptable limits are established using plus and minus two standard deviations from the mean (±2 SD). Variations due only to random analytical error will follow a Gaussian distribution; other kinds of errors will not. The ±2 SD confidence limits are the cutoff between random analytical errors versus mistakes in technique or systematic errors. If a control's value is less than ±2 SD from the established mean, then there is at least a 5% chance that a random error was the cause. If a control's value is greater than ±2 SD from the mean, there is less than a 5% chance of random analytical error being the cause. Therefore, there is a greater chance of technical or systematic error causing the deviation, and the result is out of control. The following example will illustrate how to calculate the mean and standard deviation given a set of data. The set of data represents 10 replicate assays of the same quality control sample. Normally at least 30 data points, collected over a period of time, are needed to establish the mean and standard deviation for a given lot number of quality control materials.

Number	Result (PCO_2)
1	20.4
2	21.6
3	19.8
4	20.8
5	20.2
6	20.4
7	21.0
8	20.8
9	20.5
10	20.6

$$\text{Mean} = \frac{\Sigma x}{n} = \frac{206.1}{10} = 20.61$$

The mean is the arithmetic average of the results. To find the mean, add all of the results and divide the sum (x) by the number of results (n). The standard deviation is found using the following formula.

$$SD = \frac{\sqrt{\Sigma(X_1 - X)^2}}{n - 1}$$

To calculate the standard deviation (SD), one must first find the mean and then find the difference between each result and the mean. The sum of the differences is then squared and divided by the number of results (n) minus one. The square root of this number then becomes the standard deviation. To compute the standard deviation, it is convenient to work in columns as illustrated in the following example.

Number	Result	Mean	Difference	(Difference)²
1	20.4	20.61	−.21	.0441
2	21.6	20.61	.99	.9801
3	19.8	20.61	−.81	.6561
4	20.8	20.61	.19	.0361
5	20.2	20.61	−.41	.1681
6	20.4	20.61	−.21	.0441
7	21.0	20.61	.39	.1521
8	20.8	20.61	.19	.0361
9	20.5	20.61	−.11	.0121
10	20.6	20.61	−.01	.0001

The next step is to add all of the differences that were squared.

$$\Sigma \text{(differences)}^2 = 2.129$$

To complete the calculation of the standard deviation, divide the sum of the differences squared by the number of results minus one and take the square root of this result.

$$SD = \sqrt{\frac{2.129}{9}} = 0.486$$

If ±2 standard deviations is chosen as the acceptable limit, 95.5% of all values will be contained within these limits.

The standard deviation is used in conjunction with the mean to create a **Levey-Jennings chart** for graphing the quality control results. The sample data set analyzed earlier is shown plotted on a Levey-Jennings chart (Figure 6-31). All results are plotted, indicating their relationship to the mean and whether they fall within the limit of ±2 standard deviations. The Levey-Jennings chart is advantageous for quickly assessing whether a control value falls within the acceptable limits of variation but is used mainly for detecting shifts and trends. Levey-Jennings charts are available for the pH, PO_2, and PCO_2 results at each control level.

Not all quality control results will fall within the limit of limit of ±2 standard deviations. Of those that do not, 5% may be due to

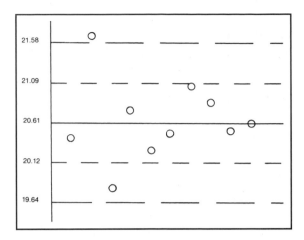

Figure 6-31 *The data points plotted on a Levey-Jennings chart showing the distribution about the mean.*

random analytical error. The greatest probability is that they represent either technical or systematic error. These results are out of control. Not only will a single quality control result vary, but as a group, a set of results may display a predictable pattern (known as a trend or a shift) when compared to the mean.

A **trend** is six or more results that show an increasing or decreasing pattern (Figure 6-32). A trend may start on one side of the mean and cross over to the other side. Trends may be caused by worn electronic components, protein contamination on the electrodes, or deterioration of reagents.

A **shift** is defined as six or more results falling on the same side of the mean (Figure 6-33). A shift is also an out-of-control result even though the results fall within the limit of ±2 standard deviations. Shifts may be caused by use of a new standard (new lot number of control materials), electronic component deterioration, use of new reagents, or an incorrect calibration.

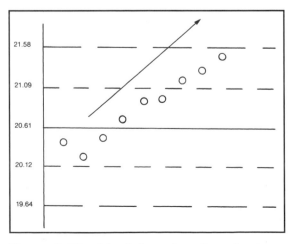

Figure 6-32 *A trend observed on a Levey-Jennings chart.*

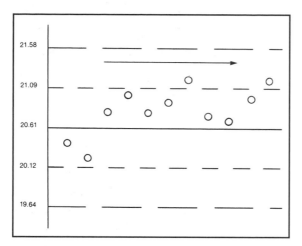

Figure 6-33 *A shift observed on a Levey-Jennings chart.*

Once an out-of-control condition has been recognized, corrective action must be taken. Corrective action may include changing membranes, removing protein contamination, changing reagents, changing electrodes, and recalibration. Once the corrective action has been completed, repeat quality control results should be run to ensure accuracy and reproducibility.

TRANSCUTANEOUS ELECTRODES

The clinical measurement of dissolved gases in the arterial blood depends on the ability to draw an arterial blood sample for analysis. The operation of these systems were described in the previous section. In some cases, repeated sampling may be detrimental to the patient. Furthermore, real time monitoring, trending, and immediate information regarding the patient's status are not available. Fortunately, a means to quantify dissolved oxygen and carbon dioxide transcutaneously (across the skin) is available. The transcutaneous carbon dioxide and oxygen electrodes are modifications of their blood gas counterparts. These systems provide immediate information as to the partial pressures of O_2 and CO_2 dissolved in the blood. They are used clinically at the bedside for monitoring and trending the patient's status, especially in the newborn intensive care setting. The American Association for Respiratory Care has published a Clinical Practice Guideline: Transcutaneous Blood Gas Monitoring for Neonatal & Pediatric Patients (Figure 6-34).

AARC CLINICAL PRACTICE GUIDELINE
Transcutaneous Blood Gas Monitoring for Neonatal & Pediatric Patients

TCM 1.0 PROCEDURE:
Transcutaneous monitoring of oxygen (PtcO$_2$) and carbon dioxide (PtcCO$_2$) in neonates, infants, and small children—this guideline does not address the application of transcutaneous monitoring in adults and older children.

TCM 2.0 DESCRIPTION/DEFINITION:
Transcutaneous monitoring measures skin-surface PO$_2$ and PCO$_2$ to provide estimates of arterial partial pressure of oxygen and carbon dioxide (PaO$_2$ and PaCO$_2$). The devices induce hyperperfusion by local heating of the skin and measure the partial pressure of oxygen and carbon dioxide electrochemically.

TCM 3.0 SETTING:
Transcutaneous monitoring may be performed by trained personnel in a variety of settings including (but not limited to) hospitals, extended care facilities, and patient transport.

TCM 4.0 INDICATIONS:
4.1 The need to monitor the adequacy of arterial oxygenation and/or ventilation
4.2 The need to quantitate the response to diagnostic and therapeutic interventions as evidenced by PtcO$_2$ and/or PtcCO$_2$ values

TCM 5.0 CONTRAINDICATIONS:
In patients with poor skin integrity and/or adhesive allergy, transcutaneous monitoring may be relatively contraindicated.

TCM 6.0 HAZARDS/COMPLICATIONS:
PtcO$_2$ and/or PtcCO$_2$ monitoring is considered a safe procedure, but because of device limitations, false-negative and false-positive results may lead to inappropriate treatment of the patient. In addition, tissue injury may occur at the measuring site (e.g., erythema, blisters, burns, skin tears).

Figure 6-34 *The American Association for Respiratory Care, Clinical Practice Guideline: Transcutaneous Blood Gas Monitoring for Neonatal & Pediatric Patients.* **(continues)**

TCM 7.0 DEVICE LIMITATIONS/ VALIDATION OF RESULTS:

$PtcO_2$ is an indirect measurement of PaO_2 and, like PaO_2, does not reflect oxygen delivery or oxygen content. Complete assessment of oxygen delivery requires knowledge of hemoglobin, saturation, and cardiac output. In a similar way, $PtcCO_2$ is an indirect measurement of $PaCO_2$, but knowledge of delivery and content is not necessary to use $PtcCO_2$ as an indicator of adequacy of ventilation.

7.1 Factors, agents, or situations that may affect readings, limit precision, or limit the performance or application of a transcutaneous monitor include

7.1.1 Technical:

7.1.1.1 The procedure may be labor intensive, although newer designs make application quicker and simpler.

7.1.1.2 Prolonged stabilization time is required following electrode placement.

7.1.1.3 Manufacturers state that electrodes must be heated to produce valid results; however, clinical studies suggest that valid results may be obtained with $PtcCO_2$ electrodes operated at lower than recommended temperatures or with no heat.

7.1.1.4 The theoretical basis for mandatory heating of the $PtcO_2$ electrode is established.

7.1.1.5 Improper calibration is possible and may be difficult to detect.

7.1.2 Clinical: The following factors may increase the discrepancy between arterial and transcutaneous values—

7.1.2.1 The presence of hyperoxemia (PaO_2 > 100 torr),

7.1.2.2 The presence of a hypoperfused state (shock, acidosis),

7.1.2.3 Improper electrode placement or application,

7.1.2.4 Vasoactive drugs,

7.1.2.5 The nature of the patient's skin and subcutaneous tissue (skinfold thickness, edema).

7.2 Validation: Arterial blood gas values should be compared to transcutaneous readings taken at the time of arterial sampling in order to validate the transcutaneous values. This validation should be performed initially and periodically as dictated by the patient's clinical state.

7.2.1 During validation studies in patients with functional shunts, electrode site and arterial sampling site should be on the same side of the shunt.

7.2.2 When disparity exists between transcutaneous and arterial values and the clinical presentation of the patient, possible causes should be explored before results are reported. Discrepancies may be reduced by monitoring at alternate sites, recalibration, or appropriate substitution of instruments. If such steps do not remedy the disparity, transcutaneous results should not be reported; instead a statement describing the corrective action should be included in the patient's chart and some other mode of monitoring should be established (e.g., pulse oximetry and/or arterial blood analysis). The absolute limits that constitute unacceptable disparity vary with patient condition and specific device. Clinical judgment must be exercised.

7.3 To help assure consistency of care based on transcutaneous blood gas readings, the operator should verify that

7.3.1 High- and low-limit alarms are set appropriately;

7.3.2 Appropriate electrode temperature is set;

7.3.3 Electrode placement is appropriate and systematic electrode-site change occurs;

7.3.4 Specific manufacturer's recommendations for maintenance, operation, and safety are complied with.

TCM 8.0 ASSESSMENT OF NEED:

8.1 When direct measurement of arterial blood is not available or accessible in a timely fashion, $PtcO_2$ and/or $PtcCO_2$ measurements may temporarily suffice if the limitations of the data are appreciated.

8.2. Transcutaneous blood gas monitoring is appropriate for continuous and prolonged monitoring (e.g., during mechanical ventilation, CPAP, and supplemental oxygen administration).

8.3 $PtcO_2$ values can be used for diagnostic purposes as in the assessment of functional shunts (e.g., persistent pulmonary hypertension of the newborn, PPHN, or persistent fetal circulation) or to determine the response to oxygen challenge in the assessment of congenital heart disease.

TCM 9.0 ASSESSMENT OF OUTCOME:

9.1 Results should reflect the patient's clinical condition (i.e., validate the basis for ordering the monitoring).

9.2 Documentation of results, therapeutic intervention (or lack of), and/or clinical decisions based on the transcutaneous measurements should be noted in the medical record.

Figure 6-34 *(continues)*

TCM 10.0 RESOURCES:

10.1 Equipment: Transcutaneous monitor, electrodes, calibration gases, and associated expendable supplies-the monitor should have been validated by the manufacturer, using appropriate quality control procedures and clinical reliability studies.

10.2 Personnel: Licensed or credentialed respiratory care practitioners or other credentialed persons with equivalent training and demonstrated ability to exercise the necessary clinical judgment, assess the patient, and perform the essential tasks of calibration and application

TCM 11.0 MONITORING:

The monitoring schedule of patient and equipment during transcutaneous monitoring should be integrated into patient assessment and vital signs determinations. Results should be documented in the patient's medical record and should detail the conditions under which the readings were obtained:

11.1 The date and time of measurement, transcutaneous reading, patient's position, respiratory rate, and activity level;

11.2 Inspired oxygen concentration or supplemental oxygen flow, specifying the type of oxygen delivery device;

11.3 Mode of ventilatory support, ventilator, or CPAP settings;

11.4 Electrode placement site, electrode temperature, and time of placement;

11.5 Results of simultaneously obtained PaO_2, $PaCO_2$, and pH when available;

11.6 Clinical appearance of patient, subjective assessment of perfusion, pallor, and skin temperature.

TCM 12.0 FREQUENCY:

Transcutaneous blood gas monitoring should be continuous for development of trending data. So-called spot checks are not appropriate.

TCM 13.0 INFECTION CONTROL:

No special precautions are necessary, but Universal Precautions (as described by the Centers for Disease Control) are recommended.

13.1 The device probe should be cleaned between patient applications according to manufacturer recommendations.

13.2 The external portion of the monitor should be cleaned according to manufacturer's recommendations whenever the device remains in a patient's room for prolonged periods, when soiled, or when it has come in contact with potentially transmissible organisms.

Reprinted with permission from *Respiratory Care* 1994; 39: 1176–1179. The complete AARC Clinical Practice Guidelines are available from the AARC Web site (*http://www.aarc.org*), from the AARC Executive Office, or from *Respiratory Care* journal.

Figure 6-34 *(continued)*

TRANSCUTANEOUS PCO₂ ELECTRODE

The transcutaneous PCO_2 electrode is essentially the same as a Severinghaus electrode but modified slightly. The electrode incorporates pH glass formed into a flat surface that is perpendicular to the skin surface, separating the measuring and reference electrodes (Figure 6-35). A heater and a thermocouple maintain the electrode at 44°C to increase the circulation to the skin, "arterializing" the blood. The thermocouple near the skin adjusts the heater to maintain a constant skin temperature. The electrode must be moved frequently to prevent skin burns. Like the Severinghaus blood gas electrode, a semipermeable membrane separates the electrode from the area of measurement (gases diffusing across the skin). An airtight seal around the electrode base prevents ambient air from entering the electrode, causing erroneous readings.

The reaction of carbon dioxide with water to ultimately form hydrogen ions and bicarbonate ions is the same. The H^+ concentration is proportional to the CO_2 concentration.

Figure 6-35 *A schematic diagram of a transcutaneous CO_2 electrode. (Courtesy Novametrix Medical Systems, Wallingford, CT)*

Therefore a change in pH is proportional to the amount of carbon dioxide present.

Calibration

Calibration of transcutaneous PCO_2 monitors is performed in a way similar to that of blood gas electrode systems. Two gases of known CO_2 concentration (typically 5% and 10%) are used to calibrate the instrument. Knowing the barometric pressure, calibration values may be calculated. The known gas samples are introduced and the instrument is calibrated.

TRANSCUTANEOUS PO_2 MEASUREMENT

The transcutaneous PO_2 electrode also bears a strong resemblance to its blood gas counterpart (Figure 6-36). The electrode is a Clark electrode, modified with the addition of thermocouples and a heating element.

The heating element raises the skin temperature to 44°C, and the thermocouple maintains it there. The thermocouple near the skin adjusts the heater to maintain a constant skin temperature. The electrode must be moved frequently to prevent skin burns. Gases diffuse across the skin surface (circulation is improved with heating), and oxygen diffuses across the membrane. An airtight seal around the electrode base prevents ambient air from falsifying the reading. The oxygen tension is then measured in the same way it is measured in a blood gas analyzer.

The oxygen combines with water to form hydroxide ions, consuming electrons. The electron flow (current) is proportional to the oxygen tension.

Calibration

Like the transcutaneous PCO_2 electrode, the transcutaneous PO_2 electrode must also be calibrated at two points. A zero solution, which contains no oxygen (usually sodium sulfite), is used. A drop is placed on the electrode and the instrument is calibrated at the zero point. The instrument is then calibrated using room air (21% oxygen).

NOVAMETRIX MEDICAL SYSTEMS MODEL 840 $PtcO_2/PtcCO_2$ MONITOR

Novametrix Medical Systems, Inc. manufactures a transcutaneous $PtcO_2/PtcCO_2$ monitor (Figure 6-37), model 840 VFD (Vacuum Fluorescent Display). This instrument combines both the oxygen and carbon dioxide electrode into one electrode, which is attached to the patient's skin. The single electrode monitors both transcutaneous oxygen and carbon dioxide noninvasively. The combined electrode is similar to the individual transcutaneous electrodes discussed earlier, but both have been combined into one electrode with a common heating element.

Controls

The Novametrix 840 VFD monitor uses a vacuum fluorescent display and four soft keys to control the many functions of the monitor. By depressing the appropriate soft key, alarm limits, calibration, temperature selection and other features may be adjusted or entered. The lower portion of the display is reserved for soft key labeling and for adjusting limits when working through the various menus.

Figure 6-36 *A schematic diagram of a transcutaneous PO_2 electrode. (Courtesy Novametrix Medical Systems, Wallingford, CT)*

Figure 6-37 *The Novametrix Model 840 $PtcO_2/PtcCO_2$ Monitor. (Courtesy Novametrix Medical Systems, Wallingford, CT)*

Temperature Selection

To operate the monitor, the sensor temperature must be adjusted to the desired temperature. For monitoring $PtcO_2/PtcCO_2$ the recommended temperature setting for both adults and neonates is 44°C. To adjust the temperature, depress the Temp soft key in the main menu. The set temperature is displayed in the upper left portion of the display. The temperature may be adjusted up or down, by depressing the appropriate soft key (Up or Down Arrow). Once the desired set temperature is displayed, press the Main Menu key to exit the temperature menu.

Calibration

The 840 VFD monitor is calibrated by using the Model 898 Portable Gas Calibrator. To calibrate the monitor, connect the model 898 Portable Gas Calibrator to the AUTOCAL connector on the front panel of the monitor.

Once the sensor has reached the desired operating temperature, lift the black sensor port cover away from the calibrator to expose the calibration chamber. Place the sensor into the calibration chamber and release the cover. Make certain that the sensor fits tightly into the calibration chamber.

From the Main Menu, depress the Cal soft key. Depress the Start soft key from the calibration submenu. Verify the correct calibration values by referring to the precision gas calibration chart. During low calibration (approximately 2 minutes), an asterisk will flash on the display panel. Once calibration is complete, the monitor will display the calibration value, beep, and automatically begin the high point calibration. A similar sequence will follow for the high point calibration. Once the sensor has calibrated, "Cal Done—Press Run" will be shown on the display. By depressing the RUN soft key, the monitor will return to the Main Menu. With each calibration, the site timer alarm will be reset to zero and will begin timing unless it is disabled.

Limits

The high and low alarm limits can be adjusted on the 840 VFD by depressing the LIM soft key from the main menu. Limits may not be adjusted any closer than 5 mmHg from one another. Once the LIM soft key is depressed, "O_2 Low Limit" will be displayed. The value may be adjusted by depressing the Up/Down Arrow soft key until the desired

value is reached. Depressing the Next soft key advances the limit adjustment to the "High Limit" parameter.

Once the oxygen limits are set, depress the Next soft key to advance to the CO_2 Low and High limits. Adjust the CO_2 limits by using the Up/Down Arrow soft keys and the Next soft key to advance to the next limit.

Once all limits are adjusted, depress the Main Menu Key to capture the settings and return to the main menu. The new settings will be displayed to the left of the current $PtcO_2$ and $PtcCO_2$ displays. If the current value exceeds the set limits for more than 30 seconds, an audio and visual alert will sound.

Sensor Site Timer

The 840 VFD monitor has a built-in timer to alert the practitioner of the need to change the site of the transcutaneous electrode. Since the electrode is heated to enhance arterialization of the skin, prolonged exposure to one site may result in burns. The risk of a burn is dependent upon the temperature of the sensor and the length of time the sensor has been applied. Since the recommended temperature for monitoring $PtcO_2$ and $PtcCO_2$ is 44°C, it is recommended that the site be changed every 2 to 4 hours.

To set the site timer, while in the main menu press Next. Depress the Timer soft key. The current Set time may be increased, or decreased, in 0.5 hour increments by depressing the Up/Down Arrow soft keys until the desired time is reached. Depress the Prev soft key to capture the value and return to the main menu.

Two Minute Silence

The Two Minute Silence button will disable the audio alarm for two minutes after depressing this key. Once two minutes have passed, the alarm will be automatically reactivated.

Audio Off

This key disables the audible alarm. When this key is depressed, only the visual alerts will indicate if displayed values are outside of the set limits.

Audio Volume

The audio volume of the monitor may be adjusted by depressing the Next soft key from the Main Menu. Once in the Next submenu, depress the Vol soft key. The volume may be adjusted up or down by using the Up/Down

Arrow soft keys. When the desired level is set, depress the Prev soft key to capture the value and return to the main menu.

Display Brightness

The brightness of the Vacuum Fluorescent Display can be adjusted from the Next sub-menu. Depress the Next soft key from the Main menu, then depress the Disp soft key. The brightness may be adjusted up or down by depressing the Up/Down Arrow soft keys. When the desired level is reached, depress the Prev soft key to capture the value and return to the main menu.

ASSEMBLY AND TROUBLESHOOTING

Assembly—Transcutaneous Monitors

1. Connect the monitor to an appropriate electrical power outlet. In the NICU/ICU environment, select an outlet that has backup power capability in the event of a housewide power failure.

2. Connect the O_2/CO_2 sensor to the monitor by pushing the cable connector into the appropriate connector on the monitor. Make sure the power is turned off.

3. Prepare the sensor for use:
   a. Remove the old membrane and, using an appropriate solution (supplied by the manufacturer), clean the electrode.
   b. Apply a new membrane to the electrode following the manufacturer's instructions.

4. Turn the monitor on and calibrate the unit following the manufacturer's recommended procedures.

5. Apply the sensor to the patient.
   a. The selected site should be well perfused, flat, and absent of any bony or fat deposits. Typical locations include the following:
      (1) Upper chest
      (2) Abdomen
      (3) Inner thigh
      (4) Inner aspect of the arm (adults and pediatrics)
   b. Attach an adhesive ring to the membrane and calibrated sensor by pressing the self-adhesive ring onto the membrane assembly.
   c. Place a drop of transcutaneous contact gel onto the center of the sensor face. Distilled water may be substituted for the transcutaneous gel.
   d. Thoroughly clean the desired site with an alcohol prep pad. Allow the site to dry before applying the sensor.
   e. Pull the protective facing off of the adhesive ring, exposing the second self-adhesive side.
   f. Firmly press the sensor assembly onto the desired location on the patient's skin. Press around all of the edges of the adhesive disk to form a complete seal.
   g. To help stabilize the sensor, the sensor cable may be taped approximately one sensor assembly diameter away from the sensor head. Alternatively, a small roll of gauze may be used to stabilize the cable by placing it under the cable.

6. Set the temperature setting to the desired range (42–45 degrees Celsius) if there are provisions for temperature selection and adjustment.

7. Adjust the alarm limits and audio level, and adjust the sensor timer as required.

Troubleshooting

1. The sensor readings fluctuate or are significantly different from blood gas results.
   a. The sensor needs to be re-membraned.
   b. The site may need to be changed.
   c. Edema may be present at the sensor site.
   d. Medications may be affecting perfusion (vasopressors).
   e. An air leak is present around the self-adhesive ring.

2. It is important in neonates to avoid burns from transcutaneous monitoring, therefore, changing the sensor site regularly is important.

OXYGEN SATURATION MEASUREMENT

HEMOGLOBIN

Hemoglobin is contained in the red blood cell and is capable of reversibly binding with oxygen. When hemoglobin binds with oxygen, it is termed oxyhemoglobin (HbO2). When the hemoglobin molecule binds with oxygen forming oxyhemoglobin, it changes color to a bright red or scarlet.

When the hemoglobin molecule is not bound with oxygen, it is termed deoxyhemoglobin. Deoxyhemoglobin is also referred to as reduced hemoglobin (RHb). The term reduced hemoglobin does not imply that electrons have been added to the hemoglobin molecule, but rather that the molecule has not bound with or has released oxygen. Both oxyhemoglobin and deoxyhemoglobin exist in the Fe^{++} state. Deoxyhemoglobin has a darker bluish color when compared to the color of oxyhemoglobin. Since both oxyhemoglobin and deoxyhemoglobin can reversibly bind with oxygen, they are called functional hemoglobin.

Besides oxyhemoglobin and deoxyhemoglobin, there are two other common hemoglobin variants. These variants are carboxyhemoglobin and methemoglobin. These variants cannot combine reversibly with oxygen, and are therefore termed dysfunctional hemoglobin.

Carboxyhemoglobin (COHb) is hemoglobin that is bound to carbon monoxide. Hemoglobin has a strong affinity for carbon monoxide (CO). Its affinity for CO is 200–250 times greater than for oxygen. Once CO binds to and saturates a hemoglobin molecule, oxygen cannot be carried on that molecule.

Methemoglobin (MetHb) is oxidized hemoglobin that has oxidized to the Fe^{+++} state. Like COHb, MetHb is not able to bind with oxygen. Oxidation of hemoglobin causes it to change color from red to brown.

Since the majority of oxygen carried in the blood is bound to hemoglobin, measurement of hemoglobin saturation provides useful clinical information. The saturation of hemoglobin is most often expressed as a percentage. Oxygen saturation can be determined two ways, fractional (HbO$_2$ in proportion to total Hb) or functional (HbO$_2$ in proportion to functional Hb).

$$Fractional\ SaO_2 = \frac{HbO_2}{RHb + MetHb + COHb + HbO_2}$$

$$Functional\ SaO_2 = \frac{HbO_2}{RHb + HbO_2} \times 100$$

CO-OXIMETRY

A CO-oximeter is an instrument that is able to measure all hemoglobin variants and therefore determines oxygen saturation as a fraction of the total hemoglobin. A CO-oximeter measures hemoglobin saturation using spectrophotometry.

Each hemoglobin variant has a different absorption spectrum for red and infrared light (Figure 6-38). By using multiple wavelengths, the concentration of each hemoglobin variant may be determined.

At 548 nm, Hb, HbO$_2$, and HbCO all absorb the same degree of light. Since all three variants absorb the same degree of light at this wavelength, it is termed an isosebestic point. Any wavelength where two or more variants have the same absorbance is termed an isosebestic point. At 568 nm, HbO$_2$ and RHb have the same absorbance while HbCO has a greater absorbance. At 581 nm, HbCO and RHb have the same absorbance while HbO$_2$ has a greater absorbance. By comparing the isosebestic points where two variants have the same absorbance with the third variant, its concentration can be determined.

Point A – All three absorbances are equal
Point B – HbCO has the single greatest absorbance
Point C – HbO$_2$ has the single greatest absorbance

Figure 6-38 *The absorption spectrophotometry for hemoglobin. (Courtesy Thomson Delmar Learning, Inc., Madama,* Pulmonary Function Testing and Cardiopulmonary Stress Testing, *2nd ed. 1998)*

The 548-nm wavelength is used to determine changes in total hemoglobin. Since CO-oximetry measures the fractional saturation, the SaO_2 reported is the HbO_2 in proportion to the total hemoglobin.

A CO-oximeter requires a blood sample to measure the HbO_2 and all of the Hb variants. The red blood cells are hemolyzed (cell membranes are broken) by using chemicals or by bombarding them with ultrasonic waves. This releases the hemoglobin and provides a uniform distribution of hemoglobin in the sample for spectrophotometric analysis.

PULSE OXIMETRY

Pulse oximetry is a non-invasive method of measuring hemoglobin saturation. Being non-invasive, it does not require a blood sample to obtain a result. Furthermore, pulse oximetry may be performed continuously, providing real-time information regarding oxygen saturation, thus enhancing its usefulness at the bedside. The American Association for Respiratory Care has published a Clinical Practice Guideline: Pulse Oximetry listing the indications, contraindications and resources required to perform the procedure (Figure 6-39).

AARC CLINICAL PRACTICE GUIDELINE
Pulse Oximetry

PO 1.0 PROCEDURE:
Pulse Oximetry (SpO_2)

PO 2.0 DESCRIPTION/DEFINITION:
Pulse oximetry provides estimates of arterial oxyhemoglobin saturation (SaO_2) by utilizing selected wavelengths of light to noninvasively determine the saturation of oxyhemoglobin (SpO_2).

PO 3.0 SETTING:
Pulse oximetry may be performed by trained personnel in a variety of settings including (but not limited to) hospitals, clinics, and the home.

PO 4.0 INDICATIONS:
4.1 The need to monitor the adequacy of arterial oxyhemoglobin saturation
4.2 The need to quantitate the response of arterial oxyhemoglobin saturation to therapeutic intervention or to a diagnostic procedure (e.g., bronchoscopy)
4.3 The need to comply with mandated regulations or recommendations by authoritative groups

PO 5.0 CONTRAINDICATIONS:
The presence of an ongoing need for measurement of pH, $PaCO_2$, total hemoglobin, and abnormal hemoglobins may be a relative contraindication to pulse oximetry.

PO 6.0 HAZARDS/COMPLICATIONS:
Pulse oximetry is considered a safe procedure, but because of device limitations, false-negative results for hypoxemia and/or false-positive results for normoxemia or hyperoxemia may lead to inappropriate treatment of the patient. In addition, tissue injury may occur at the measuring site as a result of probe misuse (e.g., pressure sores from prolonged application or electrical shock and burns from the substitution of incompatible probes between instruments).

PO 7.0 DEVICE LIMITATIONS/VALIDATION OF RESULTS:
7.1 Factors, agents, or situations that may affect readings, limit precision, or limit the performance or application of a pulse oximeter include
7.1.1 motion artifact
7.1.2 abnormal hemoglobins (primarily carboxyhemoglobin [COHb] and methemoglobin [metHb])
7.1.3 intravascular dyes
7.1.4 exposure of measuring probe to ambient light during measurement
7.1.5 low perfusion states
7.1.6 skin pigmentation
7.1.7 nail polish or nail coverings with finger probe
7.1.8 inability to detect saturations below 83% with the same degree of accuracy and precision seen at higher saturations
7.1.9 inability to quantitate the degree of hyperoxemia present
7.1.10 Hyperbilirubinemia has been shown *not* to affect the accuracy of SpO_2 readings.

Figure 6-39 *The American Association for Respiratory Care, Clinical Practice Guideline: Pulse Oximetry.*
(continues)

7.2 To validate pulse oximeter readings, incorporate or assess agreement between SpO_2 and arterial oxyhemoglobin saturation (SaO_2) obtained by direct measurement—these measurements should be initially performed simultaneously and then periodically re-evaluated in relation to the patient's clinical state.

7.3 To help assure consistency of care (between institutions and within the same institution) based on SpO_2 readings, assess

7.3.1 selection of proper probe and appropriate placement (the probe is attached to its intended site);

7.3.2 for continuous, prolonged monitoring, the Hi/Low alarms are appropriately set;

7.3.3 specific manufacturer's recommendations are complied with, the device is applied and adjusted correctly to monitor response time and electrocardio-graphic coupling;

7.3.4 strength of plethysmograph waveform or pulse amplitude strength; assure that device is detecting an adequate pulse.

7.4 SpO_2 results should be documented in the patient's medical record and should detail the conditions under which the readings were obtained:

7.4.1 date, time of measurement, and pulse oximeter reading; patient's position, activity level, and location; during monitoring, assure that patient's activity is according to physician's order;

7.4.2 inspired oxygen concentration or supplemental oxygen flow, specifying the type of oxygen delivery device;

7.4.3 probe placement site and probe type;

7.4.4 model of device (if more than one device is available for use);

7.4.5 results of simultaneously obtained arterial pH, PaO_2, and $PaCO_2$, and directly measured saturations of COHb, MetHb, and O_2Hb_4 (if direct measurement was not simultaneously performed, an additional, one time statement must be made explaining that the SpO_2 reading has not been validated by comparison to directly measured values);

7.4.6 stability of readings (length of observation time and range of fluctuation, for continuous or prolonged studies, review of recording may be necessary);

7.4.7 clinical appearance of patient—subjective assessment of perfusion at measuring site (e.g., cyanosis, skin temperature);

7.4.8 agreement between patient's heart rate as determined by pulse oximeter and by palpation and oscilloscope.

7.5 When disparity exists between SpO_2, SaO_2 readings, and the clinical presentation of the patient, possible causes should be explored before results are reported. Discrepancies may be reduced by monitoring at alternate sites or appropriate substitution of instruments or probes. *If such steps do not remedy the disparity, results of pulse oximetry should not be reported*; instead, a statement describing the corrective action should be included in the patient's medical record, and direct measurement of arterial blood gas values should be requested. The absolute limits that constitute unacceptable disparity vary with patient condition and specific device. Clinical judgment must be exercised.

PO 8.0 ASSESSMENT OF NEED:

8.1 When direct measurement of SaO_2 is not available or accessible in a timely fashion, a SpO_2 measurement may temporarily suffice if the limitations of the data are appreciated.

8.2 SpO_2 is appropriate for continuous and prolonged monitoring (e.g., during sleep, exercise, bronchoscopy).

8.3 SpO_2 may be adequate when assessment of acid-base status and/or PaO_2 is not required.

PO 9.0 ASSESSMENT OF OUTCOME:

The following should be utilized to evaluate the benefit of pulse oximetry:

9.1 SpO_2 results should reflect the patient's clinical condition (i.e., validate the basis for ordering the test).

9.2 Documentation of results, therapeutic intervention (or lack of), and/or clinical decisions based on the SpO_2 measurement should be noted in the medical record.

PO 10.0 RESOURCES:

10.1 Equipment: pulse oximeter and related accessories (probe of appropriate size)—the oximeter should have been validated by the manufacturer by a comparison of its values (and consequently its calibration curve) with directly measured oxyhemoglobin saturation.

10.2 Personnel: Pulse oximetry is a relatively easy procedure to perform. However, if the procedure is not properly performed or if it is performed by persons who are not cognizant of device limitations or applica-

Figure 6-39 *(continues)*

tions, spurious results can lead to inappropriate intervention.

10.2.1 Level I—personnel trained in the technical operation of pulse oximeters, oxygen delivery devices and related equipment, measurement of vital signs, and record keeping—may perform and record results of pulse oximetry but should be supervised by Level II personnel.

10.2.2 Level II—health care professionals trained in patient assessment, disorders of acid-base, oxygenation and ventilation, and diagnostic and therapeutic alternatives—evaluate patients and recommend and/or make changes in therapy based on assessment.

PO 11.0 MONITORING:

The clinician is referred to *Section 7.0 Validation of Results*. The monitoring schedule of patient and equipment during continuous oximetry should be tied to bedside assessment and vital signs determinations.

PO 12.0 FREQUENCY:

After agreement has been initially established between SaO_2 and SpO_2, the frequency of SpO_2 monitoring (i.e., continuous vs 'spot check') depends on the clinical status of the patient, the indications for performing the procedure and recommended guidelines. For example, continuous SpO_2 monitoring may be indicated throughout a bronchoscopy for detecting episodes of desaturation, whereas a spot check may suffice for evaluating the efficacy of continued oxygen therapy in a stable postoperative patient. However, it must be emphasized that direct measurement of SaO_2 is necessary whenever the SpO_2 does not confirm or verify suspicions concerning the patient's clinical state.

PO 13.0 INFECTION CONTROL:

No special precautions are necessary, but Universal Precautions (as described by the Centers for Disease Control) are recommended.

13.1 If the device probe is intended for multiple patient use, the probe should be cleaned between patient applications according to manufacturer recommendations.

13.2 The external portion of the monitor should be cleaned according to manufacturer's recommendations whenever the device remains in a patient's room for prolonged periods, when soiled, or when it has come in contact with potentially transmissible organisms.

Reprinted with permission from *Respiratory Care* 1992; 37: 918–922. The complete AARC Clinical Practice Guidelines are available from the AARC Web site (*http://www.aarc.org*), from the AARC Executive Office, or from *Respiratory Care* journal.

Figure 6-39 *(continued)*

Like CO-oximetry, pulse oximetry uses spectrophotometry to measure hemoglobin saturation. The pulse oximeter uses two wavelengths of light, one red and one infrared. At 660 nm (red), deoxyhemoglobin (RHb) has an absorbance ten times greater than HbO_2 (Figure 6-40). At 940 nm (infrared), HbO_2 has an absorbance two to three times greater than RHb. Using only two wavelengths of light, only the functional hemoglobin variants may be determined (HbO_2 and RHb).

Pulse oximeters use two light emitting diodes (LEDs) to transmit light through a capillary bed to a silicone photodiode detector. One diode emits light at 660 nm while the other emits light at 940 nm. The ratio of the two absorbencies forms the basis by which oxygen saturation is determined.

$$R = \frac{A_{660}nm}{A_{940}nm}$$

A calibration curve is determined by calculating various R values for different oxygen saturations from 0.00 to 100%. The calculated R values are compared to actual values and a calibration curve is then constructed.

Since the light passes through all tissue (venous, lymphatic, fat, skin, etc.), the pulse oximeter must be able to distinguish between light absorbed by hemoglobin and light absorbed by other tissues. In a capillary bed, the capillaries are subjected to two distinct states, venous (V) during diastole and arterialized (A) during systole. The light absorbance between these two states varies.

During the venous state (V), the capillaries are the smallest in diameter and are not pulsating. During this state, light absorbance is constant, having a fixed value.

During the arterialized state (A), the vessels expand with blood, changing the absorbance of the tissue. The pulsating action of the capillary bed modulates light absorption (Figure 6-41).

The basis of oxygen saturation accounting for venous and arterialized states now becomes as follows:

$$R = \frac{A_{660}/V_{660}}{A_{940}/V_{940}}$$

This new ratio allows the oximeter to eliminate changes in absorbance by other tissues other than the arterialized blood.

Pulse oximetry is heavily dependent upon microprocessor technology. The microprocessor in the oximeter cycles the LEDs on and off at a rate of between 400 and 500 Hz. First the 660-nm LED is activated, then the 940-nm LED is activated, and then both are turned off. This rapid cycling allows the instrument to measure the RHb and HbO$_2$ and compensate for changes in ambient light (when both LEDs are off). The microprocessor also permits the instrument to make rapid measurements so that real-time monitoring is possible.

Comparison of Pulse Oximetry with CO-Oximetry

Pulse oximetry measures functional saturation while CO-oximetry measures fractional saturation (%HbO2 compared to all hemoglobin variants). When comparing the results of

pulse oximetry with the values obtained by CO-oximetry, one must convert the fractional saturation (CO-oximetry value) to functional saturation in order to compare the results from the two different instruments.

$$\%SaO_2\,func = \left[\frac{\%SaO_2\,frac}{100-(\%COHb+\%MetHb)}\right] \times 100$$

The percent COHb and Met Hb may be obtained from the CO-oximetry data and then applied in the above equation to convert the fractional saturation to the functional saturation. Once the factional saturation has been converted to functional saturation, the two instruments can be accurately compared with one another.

Signal Extraction Technology (SET)

Masimo Corporation has developed adaptive filtration technology that helps to eliminate motion and low peripheral perfusion artifacts from pulse oximetry signals. By actively calculating various optical density ratios for arterial and venous saturations through the normal physiologic range and using the resulting reference signals in combination with active filtration, undesired signals (artifact) can be actively cancelled from the physiologic (patient) signal. This technology enables more accurate measurement of oxygen saturation during patient motion and low perfusion resulting in fewer false alarms for low oxygen saturation. This technology has been incorporated into many manufacturers' pulse

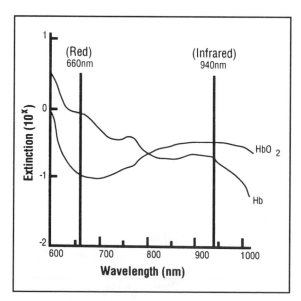

Figure 6-40 *Two-wavelength absorption spectrophotometry for hemoglobin. (Courtesy Ohmeda Critical Care, a Division of the BOC Group, Inc., Columbia, MD)*

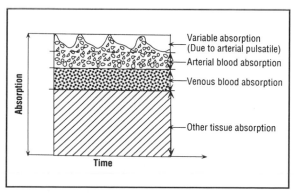

Figure 6-41 *A composite showing signal modulation with diastole and systole. (Courtesy Ohmeda Critical Care, a Division of the BOC Group, Inc., Columbia, MD)*

oximeters, including Ohmeda and Respironics, for example.

Pulse Oximetry Sensors

There are several different types of sensors employed in pulse oximetry. All sensors have some things in common. They all have two LEDs and one silicone photodiode. All sensors must transmit light through a capillary bed and receive that light on the opposite side of the capillary bed. Different sensors have been designed for adult, pediatric, and neonatal patients (Figure 6-42).

When using a probe that is a wraparound type (usually self-adhesive), it is important to ensure that the LEDs and the silicone photodiode are opposite one another. Misalignment of the photodiode and LEDs can result in poor operation and signal strength or may result in not obtaining a signal at all.

Similarly, when using a finger probe, it is important not to force the finger or digit too far into the probe. This also may result in a misalignment of the LEDs and the photodiode (Figure 6-43).

Figure 6-43   *A finger probe for a pulse oximeter misaligned by inserting the finger too far. (Courtesy Ohmeda Critical Care, a Division of the BOC Group, Inc., Columbia, MD)*

Figure 6-42   *Different types of pulse oximeter sensors. (Courtesy Ohmeda Critical Care, a Division of the BOC Group, Inc., Columbia, MD)*

When selecting a sensor site, convenience or access is only one consideration. The site should also be assessed for adequate circulation. Check the desired site for good skin color. Perfusion may be assessed by performing a capillary refill test. Depress the area firmly between your thumb and index finger for a few seconds. Once released, observe for rapid color return. If color does not rapidly return, this may be indicative of poor circulation, and therefore the site may not be the best for monitoring.

Limitations of Pulse Oximetry

Sensor Position

As stated earlier, it is important to position the LEDs opposite the photodiode. If there is a significant misalignment, the result may be poor signal quality or the inability to measure saturation. If a sensor does not fit the patient or site well, select a different sensor to optimize LED/photodiode position.

Oxyhemoglobin Dissociation Curve

The oxyhemoglobin dissociation curve is not linear (Figure 6-44). There can be a significant change in PaO_2 between a saturation of 85% and 95%. As the patient's PaO_2 falls on the portion of the curve where it plateaus, changes in SpO_2 may not be a good indicator of the patient's pending hypoxemia. Only

when the PaO_2 falls far enough to cause significant changes in saturation will the SpO_2 be reflective of the hypoxemia. Therefore, measurements from pulse oximetry may not provide adequate warning of hypoxemia when the saturation and PaO_2 fall on the upper portion of the oxyhemoglobin dissociation curve.

Hemodynamics

The operation of the pulse oximeter depends upon adequate circulation to the site being monitored. Conditions such as shock, inadequate cardiac output, peripheral vasoconstriction, and other conditions that affect peripheral perfusion and circulation may affect the accuracy of pulse oximeters. Many of these conditions will be encountered when caring for critically ill patients. Therefore, it is important to understand the patient's hemodynamics and how that may be influencing the accuracy of the pulse oximeter. When in doubt, obtain results from CO-oximetry, which is less dependent upon peripheral hemodynamics.

Motion Artifact

With patient motion, the motion may amplify the difference the instrument perceives between the venous and arterialized states. This amplification may result in inaccuracies in both SpO_2 and heart rate measurements. Often motion artifact is more common in pediatric and neonatal patients. The use of sensors that have self-adhesive characteristics can help to reduce motion artifact.

Exogenous Dyes and Nail Polish

Since pulse oximetry relies on spectrophotometry to measure SpO_2 changes, the use of intravenous dyes can create an artifact. Dyes such as methylene blue, indigo, carmine, and indocyanine green have similar absorption spectra as deoxyhemoglobin. Therefore, when these dyes are used diagnostically, the performance of the pulse oximeter will be affected. If you are in doubt, obtain arterial blood gases to accurately assess the patient's status.

Nail polish can also act as an additional filter to the light transmission through the capillary bed. If the pulse oximeter shows a poor signal strength or if the values obtained do not match the patient's clinical appearance, select another site or remove the nail polish. Often an ear or a toe may be used if the patient refuses to have the nail polish removed.

Figure 6-44 *The Oxyhemoglobin dissociation curve.* *(Courtesy Thomson Delmar Learning, Inc., Des Jardins,* Cardiopulmonary Anatomy and Physiology, 3rd ed., *1998)*

Ohmeda 3800 Pulse Oximeter

The Ohmeda 3800 pulse oximeter is one example of many pulse oximeters in clinical use (Figure 6-45). It uses the principle of spectrophotometry (described earlier in this section) to measure SpO_2 and also incorporates TruTrak®+ technology to minimize motion and perfusion artifact. TruTrak®+ technology is a signal processing algorithm similar to the SET technology described earlier in this chapter. The oximeter may be used to monitor adult, pediatric, and neonatal patients when employed with the correct sensor.

Controls

The Ohmeda 3800 pulse oximeter uses several hard keys (keys located below and left and right of the LCD display) and a large LCD display to operate the many functions of the pulse oximeter. By selecting the appropriate key and using the Menu, all features of the oximeter may be accessed and utilized. By

Figure 6-45 *The Datex-Ohmeda 3800 pulse oximeter. (Courtesy Datex-Ohmeda, Inc., part of GE Medical Systems, Madison, WI)*

using a large screen and hard key format, the number of controls has been reduced.

The display screen is split into two sections (Figure 6-46). The majority of the screen displays the plethysmographic waveform of the SpO_2, while the upper secton of the screen is reserved for message displays. In this display mode, saturation and pulse rate are displayed numerically to the left of the plethysmograph tracing. Alarm setting ranges are displayed to the right of the plethysmographic display.

Control Operation

Power/Standby Button

The power/standby button is located near the lower right of the front panel. The button toggles between on (operational mode) and off (standby mode). When in the off position, the internal battery recharges itself as long as the unit is connected to an AC power source.

Display Contrast

A slide switch located on the lower right of the unit can be used to adjust the display contrast of the LED plethysmographic display. This can aid in viewing the display from unusual angles.

Alarm/Pulse Volume Controls

The alarm/pulse volume controls are located to the left of the numeric SpO_2 and heart rate displays. Pressing the volume switch + or – sides increases or decreases the audio tone volume. The alarm volume cannot be set to OFF.

Figure 6-46 *The screen display of the Datex-Ohmeda 3800 pulse oximeter. (Courtesy Ohmeda Critical Care, a Division of the BOC Group, Inc., Columbia, MD)*

Alarm Silence

The alarm silence button is a button located at the upper left of the control panel. Depressing the button once will silence the audible alarm for two minutes. During the alarm silence period, the flashing red or yellow alarm light becomes a steady nonflashing display.

To continuously silence the audible alarm, the all mute button function can be activated by depressing the alarm silence button three times within a three-second interval. Once the system is activated, the all mute symbol flashes on the right of the screen and any alarm condition is indicated by the alarm button flashing and a message display above the plethysmographic waveform display. No audible alarms will result when the all mute feature is being used.

Alarm Settings

Alarm settings for the SpO_2 and pulse rate may be adjusted using switches on the right of the control panel. As the switches are pressed, upper and lower alarm limits change and are displayed to 100% or OFF on the alarm limits section of the LED display to the right of the plethysmographic display. The SpO_2 limits may be set between 50% to 100% or OFF (high limit) and 50 % (low limit). The heart rate limits may be set from 30 BPM to 235 BPM or OFF (high limit) and off to 30 BPM to 235 BPM or OFF (low limit).

Nellcor N-180 Pulse Oximeter

The Nellcor N-180 pulse oximeter is another freestanding pulse oximeter that uses spectrophotometry to determine oxygen saturation (SpO_2). The Nellcor N-180 is a micro-processor controlled monitor that allows real-time monitoring of oxygen saturation and heart rate (Figure 6-47). The monitor uses two LED displays for heart rate and SpO_2 and an LED bar graph for signal strength. The monitor also has built-in alarms for high and low SpO_2 and heart rate.

Controls

On/Off Switch

The main power switch is located on the back panel of the monitor. Toggling the switch to the on position delivers power to the monitor. Prior to turning on the power, connect a sensor probe to the sensor connector on the front panel of the monitor.

On/Stdby Switch

The On/Stdby switch turns the monitor on or places the monitor in standby mode. When turned on, the monitor has full capability. In the standby mode, all displays are inactive and power consumption is minimized (extends battery life when not in use). When the switch is toggled to the on position, the monitor automatically performs a self-diagnostic test. When the test is completed, the monitor displays measurements and the pulse amplitude bar graph indicator rises and falls with each heartbeat.

Control Knob

On the right front panel is a large round control knob. Its function is that it changes the instrument functions and allows you to adjust alarms setting desired values.

Figure 6-47 *The Nellcor N-180 pulse oximeter. (Courtesy Nellcor, Incorporated, Pleasanton, CA)*

High and Low Sat Buttons

By depressing the appropriate button (High or Low Sat), the alarm setting is displayed in the oxygen saturation LED display. The alarm settings may be changed by depressing the appropriate button (High or Low Sat) and simultaneously rotating the control knob clockwise or counterclockwise to adjust the display to the desired setting. Once the button is released, the new alarm parameter will have been set.

High and Low Rate Buttons

By depressing the appropriate button (High or Low Rate), the alarm setting is displayed in the pulse rate LED display. The alarm settings may be changed by depressing the appropriate button (High or Low Rate) and simultaneously rotating the control knob clockwise or counterclockwise to adjust the display to the desired setting. Once the button is released, the new alarm parameter will have been set.

Alarm Volume

To adjust the audio alarm volume, press the High Sat and Low Sat buttons simultaneously and hold them down. Rotate the control knob clockwise to increase the volume and counterclockwise to decrease the volume. Once the volume has been adjusted, release the High and Low Sat buttons.

Alarm Silence and Alarm Off

The audio alarm may be temporarily silenced by depressing the Audio Alarm Off button. When depressed, the audio alarm will remain off for 60 seconds before it is reactivated. The duration of the alarm silence may be adjusted by holding the Audio Alarm Off button down and rotating the control knob until the desired time interval is displayed in the Oxygen Saturation Display. The time interval may be adjusted between 30 and 120 seconds.

The audio alarm may be disabled by holding down the Audio Alarm Off button and rotating the control knob clockwise until "OFF" appears in the Oxygen Saturation Display.

Novametrix Oxypleth Pulse Oximeter Model 520A

Novametrix Medical Systems manufactures a pulse oximeter, the Oxypleth Model 520A, that utilizes the principle of spectrophotometry to measure oxygen saturation and heart rate. It is a microprocessor controlled monitor with many features including alarms and the ability to monitor saturation and heart rate continuously (Figure 6-48).

Controls

The Novametrix Oxypleth uses a large liquid crystal display (LCD) and several soft keys to control the many features of the oximeter. The display screen is divided into a main menu (Alert, Trend, and Menu) and several submenus. By depressing the soft key directly under the desired selection, the appropriate submenu will appear.

System Menu

By depressing the "Menu" soft key from the main menu, the "System Menu" will be displayed on the main LCD display screen. From the "System Menu," you may adjust audio volumes, display screen brightness, and SpO_2 averaging times by depressing the appropriate soft keys.

To adjust the Alert Volume, press the "Menu" soft key from the main menu display. Select the "Audio" soft key from the "System Menu" screen display. Press the "Alert" soft key from the "Audio Features" menu. Adjust the volume by pressing the Up/Down Arrow to reach the desired setting. Press "Run" to return to the main menu.

To adjust the "Beep" volume, press the "Menu" soft key from the main menu display. Select the "Audio" soft key from the "System Menu" screen display. Press the "Set Pulse Volume" soft key from the "Audio Features" menu. Adjust the volume by pressing the Up/Down Arrow soft keys until the desired setting is reached. Press the "Run" soft key to return to the main menu.

To adjust the screen brightness, press the "Menu" soft key from the main menu display. Select the "Lite" soft key from the "System Menu" screen display. The "Lite" soft key will switch the background between bright and dim settings. To return to the main menu, press the "RUN" soft key.

Alert Menu

The alert menu allows the operator to adjust the limits for SpO_2 and pulse rate. Each of these alerts can be adjusted by the user to match the patient's condition and needs.

To set the SpO_2 High or Low limit, press the "Alert" soft key from the main menu. Use

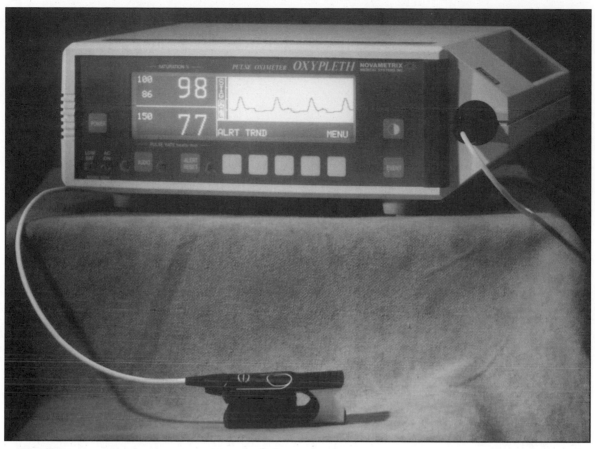

Figure 6-48 *The Novametrix Oxypleth Model 520A pulse oximeter. (Courtesy Novametrix Medical Systems, Inc., Wallingford, CT)*

the Sel soft key to move the cursor to the desired limit (SpO$_2$ High or Low limit). Use the Up/Down Arrow soft key to adjust the limit to the desired value. Note that limits may not be set closer than five digits of one another. To adjust the High or Low Pulse rate limit, follow the same procedure as described, only use the Sel soft key to select the desired pulse rate limit. When the limits have been adjusted, press the "Run" soft key to return to the main menu.

ASSEMBLY AND TROUBLESHOOTING

Assembly— "Table Top" Bedside Pulse Oximeters

1. Connect the power cord to a 110 volt, 60 Hz electrical outlet. In the critical care environment, select an electrical outlet with backup power capability in the event of a housewide power failure.

2. Connect the oximeter probe to the monitor by plugging it into the appropriate connection.

3. Turn on the power switch. Verify that the unit passes all self-diagnostic tests upon application of power.

4. Wipe the probe clean with an alcohol prep pad prior to applying it to the patient.

5. Apply the probe to the patient.

6. Observe for an adequate signal indicated by a good waveform and adequate signal strength. Compare the heart rate to an ECG monitor or count the radial pulse.

7. Set the alarms to the desired values.

Troubleshooting

ALG 6-2 will serve as a useful guide when troubleshooting the various alarm conditions for pulse oximeters.

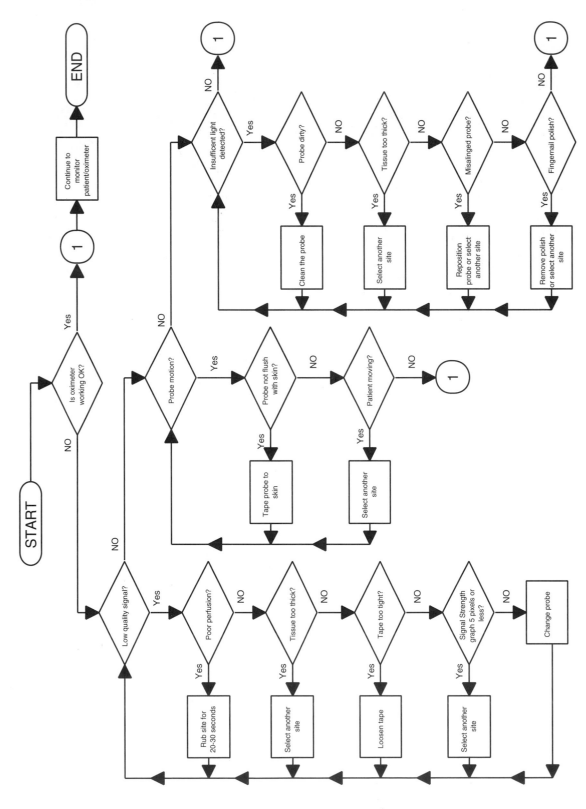

ALG 6-2 *A flowchart to assist in troubleshooting the Ohmeda Model 3800 pulse oximeter.*

Alert Reset and Audio Keys

The "Alert Reset" key located below the numeric displays is used to reset alert conditions that may have corrected themselves. If the probe becomes disconnected from the patient, pressing the "Alert Reset" key will silence the alarms until the probe can be reconnected and the monitor is able to detect appropriate signals from the sensor.

The "Audio" key is used to silence the audio portion of a limit or alarm. To silence the audio portion for two minutes, press and release the "Audio" key. To disable the audio alarms, press and hold the "Audio" key until the audio off indicator illuminates.

BCI International 3301 Oximeter

BCI International manufacturers a handheld battery operated portable oximeter (Figure 6-49). Weighing less than one pound, including batteries, it can be easily carried or inserted into a lab jacket pocket, making it ideal for "spot checks" or patient transport

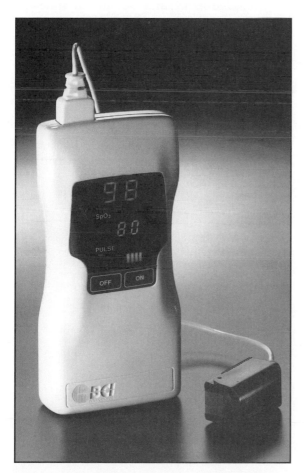

Figure 6-49 *The BCI Model 3301 handheld pulse oximeter. (Courtesy BCI International, Waukesha, WI)*

settings. The oximeter uses the principle of spectrophotometry to measure oxygen saturation and pulse rate. The oximeter may be used with a permanent finger probe or disposable self-adhesive probes for adult, pediatric, and infant patients.

Controls and Displays

On/Off Keys

The On/Off keys are the only user-activated keys on the oximeter. Depressing the appropriate key turns the oximeter on or off.

Displays

The SpO_2 and pulse are displayed on an LED display. Both are real-time displays.

A pulse strength bar graph indicator is located below the digital displays. The bar graph indicates the signal strength of the site selected for monitoring. To the left of the signal strength bar graph is a Low Battery Indicator. The Low Battery Indicator will illuminate when approximately two hours of battery life are left.

Nonin Model 8500M Pulse Oximeter

Nonin Medical manufacturers a handheld, battery operated, portable oximeter (Figure 6-50). Weighing only 10 ounces, including batteries, it can be easily carried or inserted into a lab jacket pocket, making it ideal for "spot checks" or patient transport settings. The oximeter uses the principle of spectrophotometry to measure oxygen saturation and pulse rate. The oximeter may be used with a permanent finger probe or disposable self-adhesive probes for adult, pediatric, and infant patients.

Controls and Displays

On/Off Keys

The On/Off keys on the oximeter are marked 1 and 0. Depressing the appropriate key turns the oximeter on or off.

Display Intensity

By depressing the display intensity button, the intensity of the digital LED displays may be adjusted. The brightness of the display may

Figure 6-50 *The Nonin 8500M handheld pulse oximeter. (Courtesy Nonin Medical, Inc., Plymouth, MN)*

be altered by using this feature. The display intensity will cycle through the entire intensity range as long as the button is depressed. Once the desired brightness is obtained, release the button.

Perfusion LED Indicator

The perfusion LED indicator will blink with each heartbeat. The indicator has three colors: green, yellow, and red. Each color signifies to the operator the condition of the signal strength at the selected monitoring site.

If the indicator is green, the signal strength is good and the SpO_2 and pulse rate are accurate. If the indicator is yellow, the signal is of marginal quality and the operator should consider selecting an alternate site. The data obtained may be acceptable, however, even if the indicator is blinking yellow. If the indicator is red, there is insufficient signal strength for a reliable reading.

SpO₂ and Heart Rate Displays

The SpO_2 and pulse are displayed on LED displays. Both are real-time displays.

Battery Low Display

If the numerical displays blink off and on, this is an indicator that the battery power is low and the batteries should be changed.

Nonin 9500 Onyx Pulse Oximeter

Nonin Medical, Inc. manufacturers and distributes a small, portable finger probe oximeter (Figure 6-51). The finger probe contains the red/infrared LEDs, display, microprocessor, and two AAA batteries that power the unit.

When placed on a finger or toe, the unit turns on when the two parts of the probe move apart. The oximeter searches for a sufficient pulsatile signal, and then displays the heart rate and SpO_2. A green indicator light will flash red (insufficient signal), yellow (marginal signal), or green (good signal) indicating the adequacy of the pulsatile signal for oximetry measurement. Being so compact, the unit is ideal for ambulatory, transport, and portable use.

Figure 6-51 *A photograph of the 9500 Nonin Onyx pulse oximeter (Courtesy Nonin Medica, Plymouth MN).*

ASSEMBLY AND TROUBLESHOOTING

Assembly— Handheld Pulse Portable Oximeters

1. Open the battery compartment and install the appropriate size alkaline batteries, following the polarity indicated in the battery compartment. Once the batteries are installed, replace the battery compartment cover.

2. Select an appropriate sensor probe and connect it to the sensor probe connector on the oximeter (if required).

3. Connect the probe to the patient at the selected monitoring site and turn on the oximeter.

4. Observe the display for appropriate signal strength, the SpO_2, and the pulse rate.

Troubleshooting

ALG 6-3 will provide a useful guide when troubleshooting handheld oximeters.

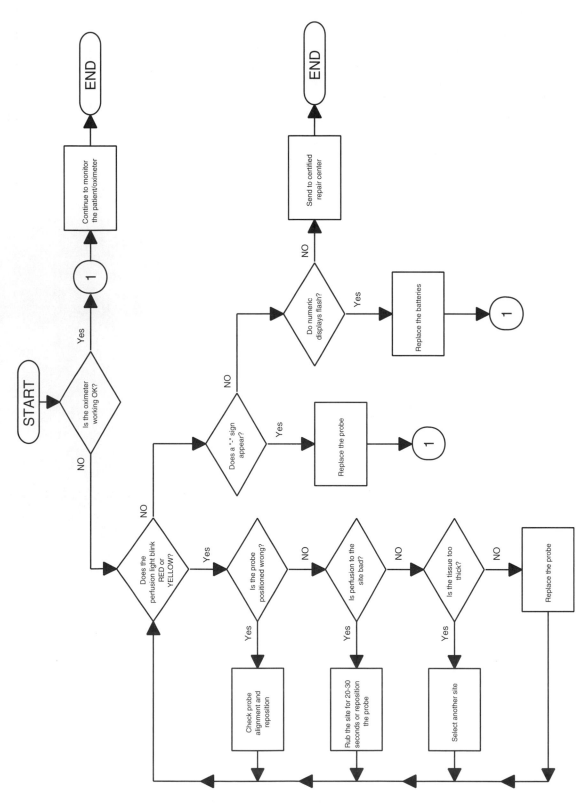

ALG 6-3 *A flowchart to troubleshoot the Nonin Model 8500M pulse oximeter.*

END TIDAL CO₂ MONITORING

End tidal carbon dioxide monitoring allows continuous and instantaneous measurement of the exhaled carbon dioxide. Furthermore, contemporary equipment allows a concentration versus time curve to be plotted graphically on liquid crystal diode (LCD) displays. The morphology (shape of the waveform) has been shown to be more significant clinically in patient management than the actual end tidal carbon dioxide value.

CAPNOGRAPHY

Terms Used during End Tidal CO₂ Monitoring

Capnography is the graphic display of CO_2 concentration versus time (Figure 6-52). As described earlier, the shape of the waveform is more important clinically than the actual concentration displayed numerically. The capnograph (waveform) can be displayed at both fast and slow speeds. The fast speed is useful for trending data, while the slow speed is useful in the evaluation of the waveform's morphology or shape.

Capnometry is the measurement of end tidal CO_2 concentration. This data is a numeric display that changes with time and the venti-

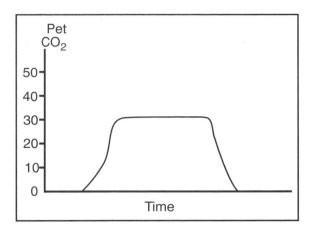

Figure 6-52 *A capnograph showing the relationship of exhaled carbon dioxide tension and time.*

latory cycle. A capnometer is the instrument that provides this numeric information.

Most often, capnometry and capnography are combined in the same instrument. This has the advantage of providing both types of data simultaneously. When combined, the validity of the numeric display can be verified by comparing it to the graphic display. The American Association for Respiratory Care has published a Clinical Practice Guideline: Capnometry/Capnography During Mechanical Ventilation (Figure 6-53), listing the indications, contraindications, hazards, and resources required for the procedure.

AARC CLINICAL PRACTICE GUIDELINE
Capnography/Capnometry during Mechanical Ventilation
2003 Revision & Update

CO₂ MV 1.0 PROCEDURE:
Capnography comprises the continuous analysis and recording of carbon dioxide concentrations [CO_2] in respiratory gases. Although the terms capnography and capnometry are sometimes considered synonymous, capnometry suggests measurement (i.e., analysis alone) without a continuous written record or waveform. Capnographic waveforms may be time-based or volume-based.

CO₂ MV 2.0 DESCRIPTION/DEFINITION:
For the purposes of this Guideline, capnography refers to the evaluation of the [CO_2] in the respiratory gases of mechanically ventilated

patients. A capnographic device incorporates one of two types of analyzers: mainstream or sidestream. Mainstream analyzers insert a sampling window into the ventilator circuit for measurement of CO_2; whereas a sidestream analyzer aspirates gas from the ventilator circuit, and the analysis occurs away from the ventilator circuit. Analyzers utilize infrared, mass or Raman spectra, or a photoacoustic spectra technology. Flow measuring devices are utilized in volume-based capnographs.

CO₂ MV 3.0 SETTING:
This procedure may be performed by trained health care personnel in any setting in which

---

Figure 6-53 *The American Association for Respiratory Care Clinical Practice Guideline: Capnometry/Capnography during Mechanical Ventilation 2003 Revision & Update.* **(continues)**

mechanically ventilated patients are found—for example, the hospital, the extended care facility, or during transport.

CO$_2$ MV 4.0 INDICATIONS:

On the basis of available evidence, capnography should not be mandated for all patients receiving mechanical ventilatory support, but it may be indicated for:

4.1 Evaluation of the exhaled [CO$_2$], especially end-tidal CO$_2$, which is the maximum partial pressure of CO$_2$ exhaled during a tidal breath (just prior to the beginning of inspiration) and is designated PetCO$_2$

4.2 Monitoring severity of pulmonary disease and evaluating response to therapy, especially therapy intended to improve the ratio of dead space to tidal volume (YD/YT) and the matching of ventilation to perfusion (Y/Q) and, possibly, to increase coronary blood flow

4.3 Use as an adjunct to determine that tracheal rather than esophageal intubation has taken place (low or absent cardiac output may negate its use for this indication) Colorimetric CO$_2$ detectors are adequate devices for this purpose.

4.4 Continued monitoring of the integrity of the ventilatory circuit, including the artificial airway

4.5 Evaluation of the efficiency of mechanical ventilatory support by determination of the difference between the arterial partial pressure for CO$_2$ (PaCO$_2$) and the PetCO$_2$

4.6 Monitoring adequacy of pulmonary, systemic, and coronary blood flow

4.6.1 Estimation of effective (nonshunted) pulmonary capillary blood flow by a partial rebreathing method

4.6.2 Use as an adjunctive tool to screen for pulmonary embolism (Evidence for the utility of dead space determinations as a screening tool for pulmonary embolism is at present not conclusive.)

4.6.3 Monitoring the matching of ventilation to perfusion during independent lung ventilation for unilateral pulmonary contusion

4.7 Monitoring inspired CO$_2$ when CO$_2$ gas is being therapeutically administered

4.8 Graphic evaluation of the ventilator-patient interface; evaluation of the shape of the capnogram may be useful in detecting rebreathing of CO$_2$, obstructive pulmonary disease, waning neuromuscular blockade ('curare cleft'), cardiogenic oscillations, esophageal intubation, cardiac arrest, and contamination of the monitor or sampling line with secretions or mucus.

4.9 Measurement of the volume of CO$_2$ elimination to assess metabolic rate and/or alveolar ventilation

CO$_2$ MV 5.0 CONTRAINDICATIONS:

There are no absolute contraindications to capnography in mechanically ventilated patients provided that the data obtained are evaluated with consideration given to the patient's clinical condition.

CO$_2$ MV 6.0 HAZARDS/COMPLICATIONS:

Capnography with a clinically approved device is a safe, noninvasive test, associated with few hazards. With mainstream analyzers, the use of too large a sampling window may introduce an excessive amount of dead space into the ventilator circuit. Care must be taken to minimize the amount of additional weight placed on the artificial airway by the addition of the sampling window or, in the case of a sidestream analyzer, the sampling line.

CO$_2$ MV 7.0 LIMITATIONS OF PROCEDURE OR DEVICE:

Capnography, when performed using a device calibrated and operated as recommended by the manufacturer, has few limitations. It is important to note that although the capnograph provides valuable information about the efficiency of ventilation (as well as pulmonary, systemic, and coronary perfusion), it is not a replacement or substitute for assessing the PaCO$_2$. The difference between PetCO$_2$ and PaCO$_2$ increases as dead-space volume increases. In fact, the difference between the PaCO$_2$ and PetCO$_2$ has been shown to vary within the same patient over time. Alterations in breathing pattern and tidal volume may introduce error into measurements designed to be made during stable, steady-state conditions. Interpretation of results must take into account the stability of physiologic parameters such as minute ventilation, tidal volume, cardiac output, ventilation/perfusion ratios and CO$_2$ body stores. Certain situations may affect the reliability of the capnogram. The extent to which the reliability is affected varies somewhat among types of devices (infrared, photoacoustic, mass spectrometry, and Raman spectrometry). Limitations include:

7.1 The composition of the respiratory gas mixture may affect the capnogram (depending on the measurement technology incorporated).

Figure 6-53 *(continues)*

7.1.1 The infrared spectrum of CO_2 has some similarities to the spectra for both oxygen and nitrous oxide. High concentrations of either or both oxygen or nitrous oxide may affect the capnogram, and, therefore, a correction factor should be incorporated into the calibration of any capnograph used in such a setting.

7.1.2 The reporting algorithm of some devices primarily mass spectrometers) assumes that the only gases present in the sample are those that the device is capable of measuring. When a gas that the mass spectrometer cannot detect (such as helium) is present, the reported values of CO_2 are incorrectly elevated in proportion to the concentration of helium present.

7.2 The breathing frequency may affect the capnograph. High breathing frequencies may exceed the response capabilities of the capnograph. In addition, breathing frequency above 10 breaths/min has been shown to affect devices differently.

7.3 The presence of Freon (used as a propellant in metered dose inhalers) in the respiratory gas has been shown to artificially increase the CO_2 reading of mass spectrometers (i.e., to show an apparent increase in $[CO_2]$). A similar effect has not yet been demonstrated with Raman or infrared spectrometers.

7.4 Contamination of the monitor or sampling system by secretions or condensate, a sample tube of excessive length, a sampling rate that is too high, or obstruction of the sampling chamber can lead to unreliable results.

7.5 Use of filters between the patient airway and the sampling line of the capnograph may lead to lowered $PetCO_2$ readings.

7.6 Low cardiac output may cause a false-negative result when attempting to verify endotracheal tube (ETT) position in the trachea. False-positive results have been reported with ETT position in the pharynx and when antacids and/or carbonated beverages are present in the stomach.

7.7 Decreased tidal volume delivery is possible during volume modes, some dual control modes, and time-cycled pressure limited ventilation with low continuous flowrates if the sampling flowrate of a sidestream analyzer is too high, especially in neonates and pediatrics.

7.8 Inaccurate measurement of expired CO_2 may be caused by leaks of gas from the patient/ventilator system preventing collection of expired gases, including

7.8.1 Leaks in the ventilator circuit

7.8.2 Leaks around tracheal tube cuffs or uncuffed tubes

CO_2 MV 8.0 ASSESSMENT OF NEED:

Capnography is considered a standard of care during anesthesia. The American Society of Anesthesiologists has suggested that capnography be available for patients with acute ventilatory failure on mechanical ventilatory support. The American College of Emergency Physicians recommends capnography as an adjunctive method to ensure proper ETT position. The international guidelines for emergency cardiovascular care recommend use of capnography to verify ETT placement in all age groups. Assessment of the need to use capnography with a specific patient should be guided by the clinical situation. The patient's primary cause of respiratory failure and the acuteness of his or her condition should be considered.

CO_2 MV 9.0 ASSESSMENT OF OUTCOME:

Results should reflect the patient's condition and should validate the basis for ordering the monitoring. Documentation of results (along with all ventilatory and hemodynamic variables available), therapeutic interventions, and/or clinical decisions made based on the capnogram should be included in the patient's chart.

CO_2 MV 10.0 RESOURCES:

10.1 Equipment: The capnograph and accessories (e.g., airway adapter, sampling tube, depending on capnograph). The capnograph should be calibrated as recommended by the manufacturer.

10.2 Personnel: Licensed or credentialed respiratory care practitioners or individuals with similar credentials (e.g., MD, RN) who have the necessary training and demonstrated skills to correctly calibrate and evaluate the capnograph, assess the patient and the patient-ventilator system, and the ability to exercise appropriate clinical judgment.

CO_2 MV 11.0 MONITORING:

During capnography the following should be considered and monitored:

11.1 Ventilatory variables: tidal volume, respiratory rate, positive end-expiratory pressure, inspiratory-to-expiratory time ratio

Figure 6-53 *(continues)*

(I:E), peak airway pressure, and concentrations of respiratory gas mixture

11.2 Hemodynamic variables: systemic and pulmonary blood pressures, cardiac output, shunt, and ventilation-perfusion imbalances

CO₂ MV 12.0 FREQUENCY:

Capnography (or, at least, capnometry) should be available during endotracheal intubation. Capnography is not indicated for very mechanically ventilated patient; however, hen it is used, the measurement period should be long enough to allow determination of the $PaCO_2$-$PetCO_2$ difference, note changes in $PaCO_2$-$PeCO_2$ difference as a result of therapy, and allow interpretation of observed trends.

CO₂ MV 13.0 INFECTION CONTROL:

No specific precautions are necessary although Standard Precautions (as described by the Centers for Disease Control & Prevention) and precautions designed to limit the spread of tuberculosis should always be implemented during patient care.

13.1 The sensor (the portion of the device contacting the patient's airway) should be subjected to high-level disinfection between patients, according to the manufacturer's recommendations.

13.2 The monitor (the portion not contacting the patient or the patient's airway) should be cleaned as needed according to the manufacturer's recommendations.

Reprinted with permission from *Respiratory Care* 2003; 48: 534–539. The complete AARC Clinical Practice Guidelines are available from the AARC Web site (*http://www.aarc.org*), from the AARC Executive Office, or from *Respiratory Care* journal.

Figure 6-53 *(continued)*

Principle of Operation

End tidal CO_2 monitors rely on nondispersive infrared technology to detect the concentration of CO_2 in a gas sample. When infrared light at a specific wavelength is passed through a sample containing carbon dioxide, the gas absorbs some of the infrared light. If a detector is placed opposite the light source, infrared light transmission is proportional to CO2 concentration in the sample.

At a wavelength of 4.26 μm (infrared light), CO_2 absorption of light is at maximum. Two other gases (CO and N_2O) have absorption spectra very close to CO_2. These two gases may be differentiated from CO_2 by using a very narrow band-pass filter, which only passes the 4.26-μm wavelength, allowing the instrument only to detect changes in transmission that are proportional to the CO_2 concentration.

WAVEFORM MORPHOLOGY

The normal capnograph has a distinct shape (Figure 6-54). The capnograph can be divided into four distinct phases. Phase I contains no exhaled CO_2. The first part of the capnograph shows an absence of CO_2 because it originates from the conducting zone of the lungs, which is primarily dead-space gas, and therefore does not participate in ventilation (gas exchange). Phase II has a steep slope as

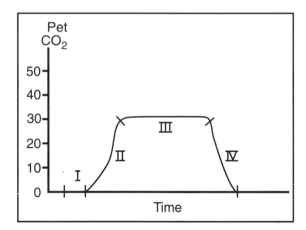

Figure 6-54 *The four phases of a capnograph. (I) Anatomical dead space. (II) Mixed dead space and alveolar gas. (III) Alveolar gas. (IV) Inspiration.*

the exhaled CO_2 concentration increases. This gas is mixed dead-space gas and alveolar gas. Since some of the gas in this phase has participated in ventilation, the CO_2 concentration rises. Phase III represents alveolar gas. The concentration of CO_2 plateaus as the alveoli empty their contents during this part of the expiratory phase. The maximum concentration at the end of the alveolar plateau (phase III), is the end tidal CO_2 concentration. The CO_2 concentration rapidly falls to zero once inspiration begins. Phase IV represents the inspiratory portion of the capnograph.

Abnormal Capnograph Morphology

As described earlier, the morphology of the capnograph can be important in interpreting changes in the patient's status. Changes in ventilation and distribution can be detected by observing the capnograph morphology.

Hypoventilation

Hypoventilation may be caused by a decrease in respiratory rate, tidal volume, or both. Increases in metabolic rate or a rapid rise in body temperature will also cause a patient to produce higher than normal CO_2 concentrations. The morphology of hypoventilation is illustrated in Figure 6-55. Notice how the concentration (height) of the capnograph has increased.

Hyperventilation

Hyperventilation may be caused by an increase in respiratory rate, tidal volume, or both. Decreases in metabolic rate or a decrease in body temperature will also cause the CO_2 concentration to fall. The morphology of hyperventilation is illustrated in Figure 6-56. Notice the decrease in the height (concentration) of the capnograph.

Rebreathing

If a patient is rebreathing part of his or her exhaled gas, CO_2 concentrations in the exhaled gas will rise. This may be performed intentionally (addition of dead space) or not intentionally. Inadvertent causes of rebreathing can include insufficient expiratory time (inverse I:E ratios), faulty exhalation valves of ventilator circuits, or inadequate inspiratory flow. Note how the baseline of Phase I increases from zero with rebreathing (Figure 6-57).

Obstruction

Obstruction is characterized on a capnograph by a decrease in the slope of phase II (Figure 6-58). Obstruction may be caused by pulmonary pathophysiology (emphysema, asthma, bronchitis, etc.), a foreign body in the airway, partial obstruction of ventilator tubing, kinking of the endotracheal tube, or bronchospasm.

Esophageal Intubation

Esophageal intubation is characterized by a sudden decrease in CO_2 concentrations (Figure 6-59). Since the stomach has little or no

Figure 6-55 *Hypoventilation. Note how the carbon dioxide tension is greater than normal. (Courtesy Novametrix Medical Systems, Inc., Wallingford, CT)*

Figure 6-56 *Hyperventilation. Note how the carbon dioxide tension is less than normal. (Courtesy Novametrix Medical Systems, Inc., Wallingford, CT)*

Figure 6-57 *Rebreathing. Note how the baseline of the capnograph has become elevated. (Courtesy Novametrix Medical Systems, Inc., Wallingford, CT)*

Figure 6-58 *Obstruction. Note how the slope of phase II has become decreased. Obstruction can be at the level of the circuit or airway or can be related to bronchospasm. (Courtesy Novametrix Medical Systems, Inc., Wallingford, CT)*

Figure 6-59 *A capnograph illustrating esophageal intubation. (Courtesy Novametrix Medical Systems, Inc., Wallingford, CT)*

CO_2, the capnograph quickly plateaus to zero in a few breaths. When the endotracheal tube is repositioned properly, a normal capnograph will result.

SENSOR POSITION

The sensor for a capnometer may be positioned in one of three ways (Figure 6-60), mainstream, sidestream, and proximal diverting. Each sensor position has advantages and disadvantages.

The mainstream sensor is positioned directly at the patient's airway in line with the inspired and expired gases. The sensor must be very lightweight to prevent torsion or traction on the endotracheal tube or tracheostomy tube. This sensor position results in the most instantaneous and well-defined capnographs.

The sidestream sensor position is where the sensor/monitor is removed from the patient and exhaled gas is diverted to the sensor through small-diameter tubing. This sensor position has an advantage in that a heavy sensor is not applying force or torque on the airway. However, the small-diameter line may become occluded with mucous or secretions, disrupting flow. Also an adequate flow rate must be maintained to the sensor to prevent artifact from showing on the capnograph.

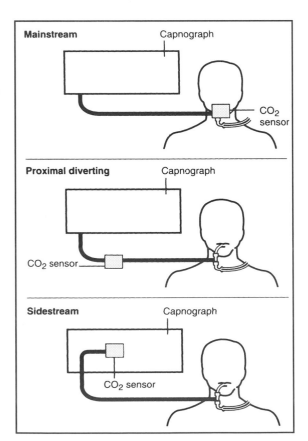

Figure 6-60 *The three positions for the capnograph sensor. (1) Mainstream. (2) Proximal diverting. (3) Sidestream. (Copyrights Nellcor, Incorporated, Pleasanton, CA)*

The proximal diverting position places the sensor adjacent to the airway, where some of the exhaled gas is diverted to the sensor. This combines some of the best features of the mainstream and sidestream positions while attempting to minimize the disadvantages.

END TIDAL CO₂ MONITORING EQUIPMENT

Novametrix Capnogard 1265

Novametrix Medical Systems manufactures an end tidal CO_2 monitor that operates using nondispersive infrared technology (Figure 6-61). The monitor provides capnometry, capnography, and alarms for $EtCO_2$ and respiratory rate.

Principle of Operation

The Capnogard Model 1265 uses a lightweight solid-state sensor (Capnostat) that can be used in the mainstream or sidestream sampling position. The Capnostat (Figure 6-62) uses a pulsed infrared light source that cycles at a frequency of 86 Hz. The pulsed infrared light passes through the airway adapter to a beam splitter. The beam splitter splits the infrared light beam into two beams. Each infrared light beam passes through an optical filter. One filter only passes light at 4.2 μm and the other only passes light at 3.7 μm. A detector then converts the transmitted light into an electrical signal.

The two signals from each sensor are compared electronically. During the time that the infrared light source is off, the signals are forced to be zero. During the time the infrared light source is on, the ratio between the 3.7- and 4.2-μm sensors are compared. The 4.2-μm wavelength is absorbed in proportion to any CO_2 present in the sample. The 3.7-μm wavelength is unaffected by any respiratory gases (including CO and N_2O). The ratio of the two signals is therefore proportional to the CO_2 concentration in the gas sample.

Controls

The Novametrix Medical Systems Capnogard Model 1265 uses a cold cathode display (CCD) to present numeric data (capnometry and respiratory rate) and graphic data (capnography). The monitor is controlled by soft keys and is menu driven.

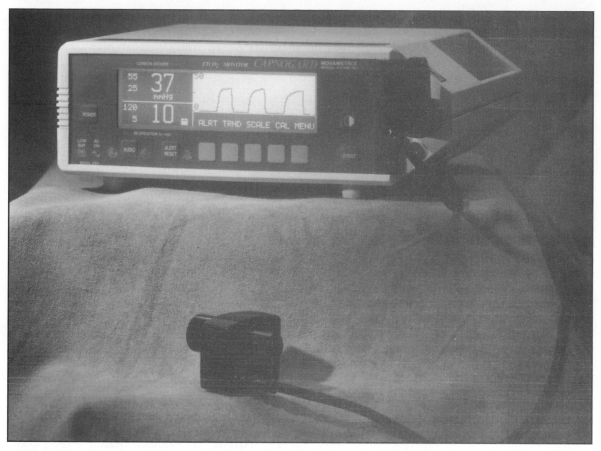

Figure 6-61 *The Novametrix Capnogard 1265. (Courtesy Novametrix Medical Systems, Inc., Wallingford, CT)*

Figure 6-62 *A schematic drawing of the Novametrix Capnostat sensor. (Courtesy Novametrix Medical Systems, Inc., Wallingford, CT)*

Main Menu

The main menu consists of the following selections: Alert, Trend, Scale, Calibration, and Menu. By depressing the appropriate soft key, the desired submenu can be accessed.

Alert Settings

The alert settings are adjusted by depressing the Alert soft key from the main menu. Once accessed, "Set Alert Limits" appears on the display. By using the "Select" soft key, the cursor can be moved to the desired limit (High, Low, Respiration Rate) and then that limit may be adjusted using the Up/Down Arrow soft keys. Once the desired value is obtained, press the "Run" soft key to capture that value and return to the main menu.

The alert volume may be adjusted by depressing the "Menu" soft key from the main menu display. Once pressed, "CO_2 Options" appears in the display. Press the "Next" soft key and the next submenu "System Options" will appear. Select the "Audio" soft key and adjust the volume using the Up/Down Arrow soft key to the desired level. Press the "Run" soft key to capture the value and return to the main menu.

Display Brightness

The brightness of the CCD display may be user adjusted between bright and dim. From the main menu select the "Menu" soft key. Once pressed, "CO_2 Options" appears in the display. Press the "Next" soft key and the next submenu, "System Options," will appear. Press the "Lite" soft key. Pressing the key will toggle the display from bright to the dim settings. Once the desired brightness has been selected, press the "Run" soft key to return to the main menu.

Scale

The vertical scale of the capnogram can be adjusted from 0 to 50 mmHg or 0 to 75 mmHg. To set the scale, press the "Scale" soft key from the main menu. Once the desired scale has been set, press the "Run" soft key to return to the main menu.

Calibration

To calibrate the Capnogard, place the Capnostat sensor into the Zero cell. Press the "Cal" soft key from the main menu. Once pressed, a "Time Remaining" counter is displayed. After the counter has timed out, place the Capnostat on the Reference cell (furthest from the monitor face). The prompt "Checking Calibration" should be displayed. "Calibration Verified" will appear on the display when calibration is complete.

Nellcor Ultra Cap™ N-6000

Nellcor, Inc. manufacturers the Ultra Cap™ N-6000 pulse oximeter and capnograph monitor (Figure 6-63). This monitor combines pulse oximetry with end tidal CO_2 monitoring into one monitor. The monitor can display the plethysmographic waveform of end tidal CO_2 or SpO_2 and numeric data for pulse rate, respiratory rate, and end tidal CO_2. All information is displayed on a large vacuum fluorescent display. Alarm systems are incorporated for both the pulse oximetry and end tidal carbon dioxide monitors.

Principle of Operation

The pulse oximeter uses the principle of spectrophotometry to measure the hemoglobin saturation. The N-6000 monitor may be interfaced with any compatible Nellcor oximeter probe.

The capnograph uses nondispersive infrared technology to measure the end tidal CO2 concentration. The sensor consists of a light source, airway adapter, filter, chopper wheel, and a photodiode detector (Figure

Figure 6-63 *The Nellcor Ultra Cap™ N-6000 monitor. (Photo courtesy Nellcor Incorporated, Pleasanton, CA)*

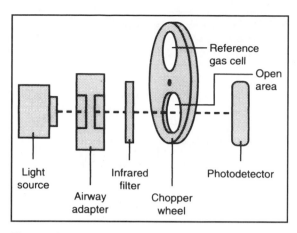

Figure 6-64 *A schematic drawing of the Nellcor Ultra Cap N-6000 CO_2 sensor. (Copyrights Nellcor Incorporated, Pleasanton, CA)*

6-64). The infrared light passes from the light source, through the airway adapter and filter, to the chopper wheel, and then to the photodetector. The optical filter ensures transmission of the specific wavelength for carbon dioxide, while filtering other infrared wavelengths.

The chopper wheel is motor driven and rotates. The photodiode alternately senses no light transmission (solid areas between the reference and open areas), light transmitted through the sample gas (airway), and light transmitted through the reference-plus-sample. The concentration of $EtCO_2$ becomes a ratio between reference-plus-sample and sample measurements (reference + sample / sample).

Controls

The Nellcor Ultra Cap™ N-6000 uses a large vacuum fluorescent display and several function keys or soft keys to control the many features of the monitor. The main monitoring display screen is shown in Figure 6-65. From this display screen, the operator may select from several submenus using the Menu key or the soft keys along the lower part of the monitoring screen. Figure 6-65 illustrates the four primary menus or screens and their respective submenus using a branching directory tree.

System Screen

The system screen allows the operator to perform the following: select what parameters will be monitored, set the monitor to compensate for nitrous oxide or high F_IO_2 levels, dis-

able the graphics display to conserve power when running on batteries, or adjust system variables.

To select what parameter you wish to monitor, press the Menu key and from the menu screen, press the System key. The operator may turn off the SpO_2 display, $EtCO_2$ display or monitor both parameters simultaneously from the system screen by pressing the Monitored Parameters key until the desired option is selected. Once the desired option has been selected, press the Menu key to return to the monitoring screen.

To compensate for the presence of nitrous oxide or high F_IO_2 levels, press the Menu key and press the System key from the display. Select the COMP. key and press the key until the desired parameter is displayed. Press the Menu key to return to the monitoring screen. It is recommended that compensation be used for F_IO_2 levels greater than 0.60.

Alarm Screen

By depressing the Menu key and then the Alarms key, the alarm screen can be selected. From the alarm screen you may set limits, configure the alarms (silence, volume, time periods), or disable alarms.

To set the alarm limits, press the Menu key and then the Alarms key. Once the alarms screen is displayed, press the Set Limits soft key. You may scroll through the various alarm parameters by pressing the Select soft key. Continue pressing the Select soft key until the desired alarm limit is highlighted. Press the increase or decrease soft key to adjust the alarm to the desired level. Press the Menu key to return to the monitoring screen.

To configure the alarms, press the Menu key and then the Alarms key. Select Configure by pressing the appropriate soft key. From the configure alarms screen, the length of alarm silence, alarm volume, and apnea periods may be adjusted. Press the Menu key to return to the monitoring screen.

The Disable key from the Alarms screen allows the operator to disable the audible portion of an alarm for any of the monitored parameters. To disable an alarm, press the Disable soft key from the Alarms screen display. Use the Select soft key to move through the screen until the desired parameter is highlighted. Press the Change soft key to change the alarm status. Press the Menu key to return to the monitoring screen.

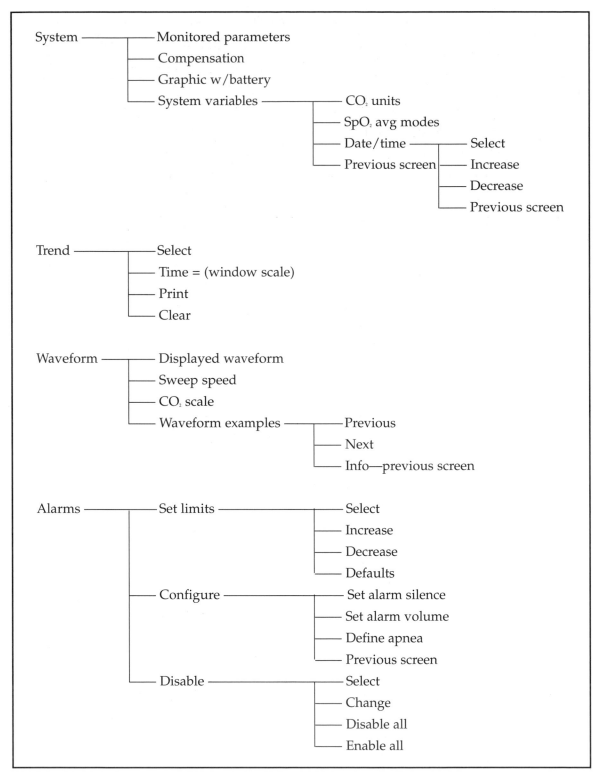

Figure 6-65 *The Nellcor Ultra Cap™ N-6000 main monitoring menu tree. (Copyright Nellcor Incorporated, Pleasanton, CA)*

Waveform Screen

The waveform screen allows the operator to adjust what waveform is displayed, the sweep speed, and CO_2 scales. To enter the waveform screen, press the Menu key and then the Waveform soft key.

To select the waveform display, press the Displayed Waveform soft key and continue depressing the soft key until the desired waveform is highlighted. Press the Menu key to capture your selection and return to the monitoring screen.

Sweep speed is adjustable from 6.25 to 50 mm/sec. To adjust the sweep speed, press the Sweep SPD soft key from the waveform screen until the desired speed is selected. Press the Menu key to capture the parameter and return to the monitoring screen.

The CO_2 scale may be adjusted from 0.00 to 50 mmHg to a maximum of 0.00 to 99.00 mmHg.

To adjust the scale of the screen, press the CO_2 Scale soft key from the Waveform screen display. Continue to press the soft key until the desired scale is highlighted. Press the Menu soft key to return to the monitoring screen.

Trend

The Trend function may be used to record trends for SpO_2, $EtCO_2$, pulse rate, and respiratory rate. The trends may be displayed individually or in any combination. Use the Select key to display the desired trend(s). Press the Menu key to return to the monitoring screen.

To select the time scale for monitoring the trend, press the Time soft key from the Trend screen. Continue pressing the soft key until the desired time interval is highlighted (2, 4, 8, 12, and 24 hours). To return to the monitoring screen, press the Menu key.

ASSEMBLY AND TROUBLESHOOTING

Assembly— End Tidal Capnographs

1. Connect the monitor to a 115 volt, 60 Hz electrical outlet. Ensure that the monitor is off. In the critical care environment, select an electrical outlet with backup power capability in the event of a housewide electrical failure.

2. Select an airway adapter to use with the sensor.

3. Interface the sensor with the airway adapter (mainstream or sidestream).

5. Calibrate the monitor as described earlier.

6. Place the capnostat in the mainstream position or, if using in the sidestream position, the airway adapter at the patient's airway, and route the monitoring tubing to the sensor located away from the patient.

7. Turn the monitor's main power on.

8. Adjust the alert limits, scale, and screen brightness to the desired levels as described earlier.

Troubleshooting

ALG 6-4 will assist you in troubleshooting end tidal capnograph monitors.

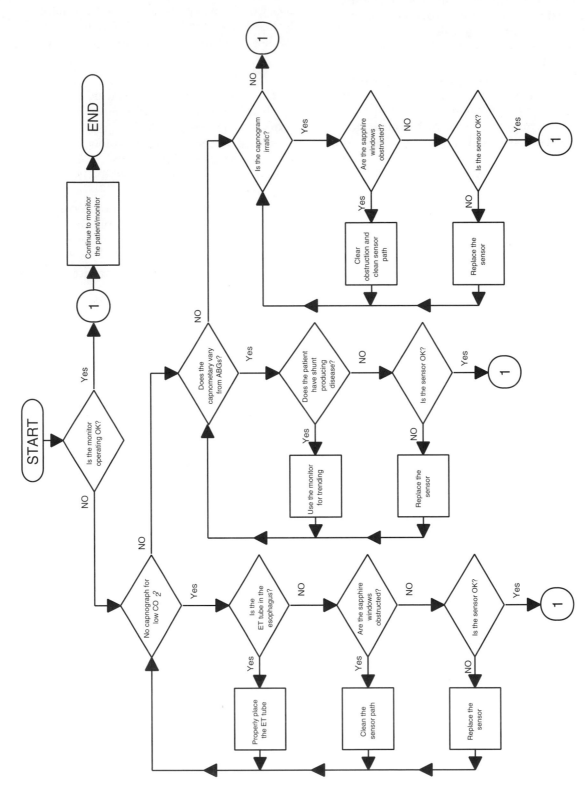

ALG 6-4 A flowchart for troubleshooting the Nellcor Ultra Cap™ N-6000 CO₂ monitor.

Colormetric End Tidal CO$_2$ Determination

Besides nondispersive infrared spectroscopy to detect CO$_2$, a chemical method may be used to detect end tidal CO$_2$. When a chemical with a color indicator is exposed to CO$_2$, and the color changes are due to the chemical used for detection, the reaction is reversible, allowing breath-to-breath determination. Nellcor markets a colormetric detector called "Easy Cap™."

Easy Cap™ (Figure 6-66) is a disposable single-patient use, nonelectronic monitor that measures EtCO$_2$ using a chemical reaction and color change (colormetric). It is designed to be used following intubation to detect esophageal intubation (no exhaled CO$_2$). To use the Easy Cap™, place it on the airway following intubation and observe for a color change from purple to yellow in the center of the monitor. If the color changes from inspiration (purple) to yellow (expiration), the endotracheal tube is in the trachea and CO$_2$ has been detected. If the color in the center remains purple, esophageal intubation has occurred.

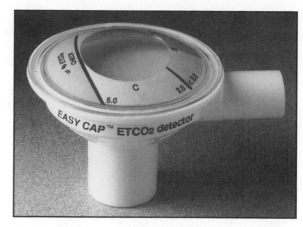

Figure 6-66 *The Nellcor Easy Cap™ colormetric CO$_2$ monitor. (Photo courtesy Nellcor Incorporated, Pleasanton, CA)*

NITRIC OXIDE MEASUREMENT AND MONITORING

Inhaled nitric oxide is administered to treat persistent pulmonary hypertension in newborns and, experimentally, in adults with ARDS. Administration of inhaled nitric oxide can cause adverse effects, methemoglobinemia, and toxicity. Therefore, the monitoring of inhaled concentrations is important in maintaining both safety and therapeutic levels of this gas. Nitric oxide is measured using either electrochemical analyzers or chemiluminescence analyzers.

ELECTROCHEMICAL ANALYZERS FOR NITRIC OXIDE

Electrochemical analyzers operate in a way similar to oxygen fuel cell analyzers. The nitric oxide reacts with a reactive electrolyte, releasing free electrons. The current generated between electrodes then becomes proportional to the concentration of nitric oxide.

These analyzers are small, portable, and easy to calibrate. The response time, however, is fairly slow (30–40 seconds) and may be used in both sidestream and mainstream applications. The accuracy of these sensors can be affected by humidity and pressure.

CHEMILUMINESCENCE NITRIC OXIDE ANALYZERS

Chemiluminescence nitric oxide analyzers operate by measuring photon emissions. Nitric oxide reacts with ozone (O$_3$) to form nitrogen dioxide (NO$_2$) with a free electron in an excited state. When the electron decays, a photon is released. The analyzer measures luminescent intensity and converts it to an electrical signal that is proportional to the nitric oxide concentration. Chemiluminescence analyzers are very accurate (parts per billion). They also have a faster response time when compared with electrochemical analyzers.

INDIRECT CALORIMETRY

Indirect calorimetry assessment is frequently performed at the bedside to obtain data that is used to assess a patient's nutritional status and to modify either the enteral or parenteral feeding of the patient. Indirect calorimeters measure inhaled and exhaled oxygen and carbon dioxide, minute volume, and tidal volume. This data is then used to calculate the respiratory quotient (VCO$_2$/VO$_2$)

and the resting energy expenditure (REE) using the Weir equation.

$$REE =$$
$$[VO_2(3.941) + VCO_2(1.11)]1440 \text{ min/day}$$

By correctly determining the patient's energy (nutritional) requirements, costs of parenteral nutrition may be reduced (if the patient is being overfed) and CO_2 production in ventilator patients may be reduced by altering the caloric substrate. The American Association for Respiratory Care has published a Clinical Practice Guideline: Metabolic Measurement using Indirect Calorimetry during Mechanical Ventilation (Figure 6-67), listing the indications, contraindications, and equipment required for the procedure.

Indirect calorimeters may be further classified into closed-circuit or open-circuit systems. The closed-circuit system is one in which the patient breathes from a closed reservoir containing a known quantity of oxygen with or without mixing chambers, depending upon the system. The oxygen consumption is determined by measuring the volume consumed by the patient during the interval of the study or by how much oxygen must be added to the system during the study to maintain the original oxygen concentration.

Open-circuit calorimeters may utilize gas dilution measurement, mixing chambers, or breath-by-breath measurement of exhaled gases, depending upon the system. Gas dilution measurement introduces a bias flow of gas (typically room air) to move the patient's exhaled gas to the sampling chamber and analyzers. The oxygen and carbon dioxide concentration of the bias flow of gas is compensated for prior to measurement of the patient's gas sample.

AARC CLINICAL PRACTICE GUIDELINE
Metabolic Measurement using Indirect Calorimetry during Mechanical Ventilation

MMMV 1.0 PROCEDURE:

Metabolic measurements using indirect calorimetry for determination of oxygen consumption (VO_2), carbon dioxide production (VCO_2), respiratory quotient (RQ), and resting energy expenditure (REE) as an aid to patient nutritional assessment and management; assessment of weaning success and outcome; and assessment of the relationship between O_2 delivery (DO_2) and VO_2—this guideline addresses metabolic measurement during mechanical ventilation.

MMMV 2.0 DESCRIPTION/DEFINITION:

Metabolic measurements use an indirect calorimeter to measure VO_2 and VCO_2 via expired gas analysis. The measurements of VO_2 and VCO_2 are used to calculate RQ (VCO_2/VO_2) and REE using the Weir equation:

REE = [VO_2(3.941) + VCO_2(1.11)] 1440 min/day.

The measurement of REE in mechanically ventilated patients has been shown to be more accurate than published formulas used to predict REE, to reduce the incidence of overfeeding and underfeeding, and to decrease costs associated with total parenteral nutrition (TPN). Measurement of REE and RQ has been shown to be helpful in designing nutritional regimens to reduce VCO_2 in patients with chronic obstructive pulmonary disease (COPD) and in patients requiring mechanical ventilation. Despite this evidence, studies demonstrating improved outcome, improved weaning success, or shorter ICU/hospital stay are lacking.

The objectives of metabolic measurements by indirect calorimetry are

2.1 To accurately determine the REE of mechanically ventilated patients to guide appropriate nutritional support;

2.2 To accurately determine RQ to allow nutritional regimens to be tailored to patient needs;

2.3 To accurately determine REE and RQ to monitor the adequacy and appropriateness of current nutritional support;

2.4 To allow determination of substrate utilization when urinary nitrogen values are concomitantly measured;

Figure 6-67 *The American Association for Respiratory Care Clinical Practice Guideline: Metabolic Measurement Using Indirect Calorimetry during Mechanical Ventilation.* **(continues)**

2.5 To determine the O_2 cost of breathing as a guide to the selection of ventilator mode, settings, and weaning strategies;

2.6 To monitor the VO_2 as a guide to targeting adequate DO_2.

MMMV 3.0 SETTING:

3.1 Mechanically ventilated patients

3.1.1 In the hospital

3.1.2 In the extended care facility

MMMV 4.0 INDICATIONS:

Metabolic measurements may be indicated

4.1 In patients with known nutritional deficits or derangements. Multiple nutritional risk and stress factors that may considerably skew prediction by Harris-Benedict equation include

4.1.1 neurologic trauma,

4.1.2 paralysis,

4.1.3 COPD,

4.1.4 acute pancreatitis,

4.1.5 cancer with residual tumor burden,

4.1.6 multiple trauma,

4.1.7 amputations,

4.1.8 patients in whom height and weight cannot be accurately obtained,

4.1.9 patients who fail to respond adequately to estimated nutritional needs,

4.1.10 new patients on home TPN,

4.1.11 patients who are unable to eat and who require mechanical ventilation for > 5 days,

4.1.12 transplant patients,

4.1.13 morbidly obese patients,

4.1.14 severely hypermetabolic or hypometabolic patients.

4.2 When the desire or perceived need is present to measure the O_2 cost of breathing in mechanically ventilated patients.

4.3 When the need exists to assess the VO_2 in order to evaluate the hemodynamic support of mechanically ventilated patients.

MMMV 5.0 CONTRAINDICATIONS:

When a specific indication is present, there are no contraindications to performing a metabolic measurement using indirect calorimetry unless short-term disconnection of ventilatory support for connection of measurement lines results in hypoxemia, bradycardia, or other adverse effects.

MMMV 6.0 HAZARDS/COMPLICATIONS:

Performing metabolic measurements using an indirect calorimeter is a safe, noninvasive procedure with few hazards or complications. Under certain circumstances and with particular equipment the following hazards/complications may be seen.

6.1 Closed circuit calorimeters may cause a reduction in alveolar ventilation due to increased compressible volume of the breathing circuit.

6.2 Closed circuit calorimeters may decrease the trigger sensitivity of the ventilator and result in increased patient work of breathing.

6.3 Short-term disconnection of the patient from the ventilator for connection of the indirect calorimetry apparatus may result in hypoxemia, bradycardia, and patient discomfort.

6.4 Inappropriate calibration or system setup may result in erroneous results causing incorrect patient management.

MMMV 7.0 LIMITATIONS OF PROCEDURE:

Limitations of the procedure include

7.1 Accurate assessment of REE and RQ may not be possible because of patient condition or certain bedside procedures or activities.

7.2 Inaccurate measurement of REE and RQ may be caused by leaks of gas from the patient/ventilator system preventing collection of expired gases including:

7.2.1 leaks in the ventilator circuit,

7.2.2 leaks around tracheal tube cuffs or uncuffed tubes,

7.2.3 leaks through chest tubes or bronchopleural fistula.

7.3 Inaccurate measurement of REE and RQ occurs during peritoneal and hemodialysis due to removal across the membrane of CO_2 that is not measured by the indirect calorimeter.

7.4 Inaccurate measurement of REE and RQ during open circuit measurement may be caused by

7.4.1 instability of delivered oxygen concentration (FDO_2) within a breath or breath-to-breath due to changes in source gas pressure and ventilator blender/mixing characteristics;

7.4.2 $FDO_2 > 0.60$;

7.4.3 inability to separate inspired and expired gases due to bias flow from flow-triggering systems, IMV systems, or specific ventilator characteristics;

Figure 6-67 *(continues)*

7.4.4 the presence of anesthetic gases or gases other than O_2, CO_2, and nitrogen in the ventilation system;

7.4.5 the presence of water vapor resulting in sensor malfunction;

7.4.6 inappropriate calibration;

7.4.7 connection of the indirect calorimeter to certain ventilators, with adverse effect on triggering mechanism, increased expiratory resistance, pressure measurement, or maintenance of the ventilator.

7.4.8 total circuit flow exceeding internal gas flow of indirect calorimeter that incorporates the dilutional principle.

7.5 Inaccurate measurement of REE and RQ during closed circuit measurement may be caused by

7.5.1 short duration of the measurement period (a function of CO_2 absorber life and VCO_2) that may not allow REE state to be achieved;

7.5.2 changes in functional residual capacity (FRC) resulting in changes in spirometer volume unassociated with VO_2;

7.5.3 leaks drawing gas into the system during spontaneous breathing measurements that adds volume to the system and cause erroneously low VO_2 readings;

7.5.4 increased compressible volume in the circuit that prevents adequate tidal volume delivery resulting in alveolar hypoventilation and changes in VCO_2/VO_2;

7.5.5 increased compressible volume and resistance that results in difficulty triggering the ventilator and increased work of breathing.

MMMV 8.0 ASSESSMENT OF NEED:

Metabolic measurements should be performed only on the order of a physician after review of indications (MMMV 4.0) and objectives.

MMMV 9.0 ASSESSMENT OF TEST QUALITY AND OUTCOME:

9.1 Test quality can be evaluated by determining whether

9.1.1 RQ is consistent with the patient's nutritional intake;

9.1.2 RQ rests in the normal physiologic range (0.67 to 1.3);

9.1.3 measured VO_2 is within ±10% of the mean value, and measured VCO_2 within ±6% of the mean value;

9.1.4 REE has been defined as the value obtained with the patient lying in bed, awake and aware of his or her surroundings. (This state should have been observed for 10–15 minutes associated with results in 9.1.3.)

9.2 Outcome may be assessed by the interpretation and confirmation/manipulation of patient nutritional support regimen by a physician or nutritionist based on the measurement results.

9.3 Outcome may be assessed by the successful manipulation of the mechanical ventilator settings and/or hemodynamic management based on the measurement of the VO_2.

MMMV 10.0 RESOURCES:

10.1 Indirect calorimeter, open- or closed-circuit design.

10.1.1 The calibration gas mixture should be relevant to the concentration of gas to be measured clinically.

10.1.2 The indirect calorimeter should be calibrated on the day of measurement and more often if errors in measurement are suspected.

10.1.3 When the measurement results are suspect and/or when repeated calibration attempts are marked by instability, the indirect calorimeter may be tested via an independent test method (burning ethanol or other substance with a known RQ or adding known flows of CO_2 and nitrogen to simulate VO_2 and VCO_2).(52-55) As a simple test, ventilation of a leak-free system should yield VO_2 and VCO_2 values of near 0. Routinely scheduled measurement of normal control subjects (volunteers) may be useful.

10.2 A method of stabilizing FDO_2 during open-circuit measurements should be available and may include

10.2.1 an air-oxygen blender connected between the gas source and the ventilator inlets for high pressure gas;

10.2.2 an inspiratory mixing chamber between the ventilator main flow circuit and the humidifier.

10.3 An isolation valve, double-piloted exhalation valve, or other device to separate inspiratory and expiratory flow should be incorporated when using continuous flow in the ventilator circuit.

10.4 Personnel: Due to the level of technical and patient assessment skills required, metabolic measurements using indirect calorimeters should be performed by individuals trained in and with the demonstrated and documented ability to

Figure 6-67 *(continues)*

10.4.1 calibrate, operate, and maintain an indirect calorimeter;

10.4.2 operate a mechanical ventilator, including knowledge of the air-oxygen blending system, the spontaneous breathing mechanisms, and the alarm and monitoring functions; .

10.4.3 recognize metabolic measurement values within the normal physiologic range and evaluate the results in light of the patient's current nutritional and clinical status;

10.4.4 assess patient hemodynamic and ventilatory status and make recommendations on appropriate corrective/therapeutic maneuvers to improve or reverse the patient's clinical course.

A relevant credential (e.g., RRT, CRTT, RN, or RPFT) is desirable.

MMMV 11.0 MONITORING:

11.1 The following should be evaluated during the performance of a metabolic measurement to ascertain the validity of the results:

11.1.1 clinical observation of the resting state (MMMV 9.1.4);

11.1.2 patient comfort and movement during testing;

11.1.3 values in concert with the clinical situation;

11.1.4 equipment function;

11.1.5 results within the specifications listed in 9.1.3.

11.2 Measurement data should include a statement of test quality and list the current nutritional support, ventilator settings, and vital signs.

MMMV 12.0 FREQUENCY:

12.1 Metabolic measurements should be repeated according to the clinical status of the patient and indications for performing the test. The literature suggests that more frequent measurement may be necessary in patients with a rapidly changing clinical course as recognized by

12.1.1 hemodynamic instability,

12.1.2 spiking fevers.

12.2 Patients in the immediate postoperative period and those being weaned from mechanical ventilation may also need more frequent measurement.

MMMV 13.0 INFECTION CONTROL:

Metabolic measurements using indirect calorimetry are relatively safe procedures, but a remote possibility of cross-contamination exists either via patient-patient or patient-caregiver interface. The following guidelines should be followed when a metabolic measurement is performed.

13.1 Universal Precautions should be exercised whenever equipment (isolation valves) is contaminated with blood or other body fluids.

13.2 Appropriate use of barriers and hand washing is recommended.

13.3 Tubing used to direct expiratory gas from the ventilator to the indirect calorimeter should be disposed of or cleaned between patients.

13.4 Connections used in the inspiratory limb of the circuit proximal to the humidifier should be wiped clean between patients; equipment distal to the humidifier should be disposed of or subjected to high-level disinfection between patients.

13.5 Bacteria filters may be used to protect equipment in both the inspired and expired lines, but caution should be used that moisture does not increase filter resistance resulting in poor gas sampling flow or increased resistance to exhalation.

Reprinted with permission from *Respiratory Care* 1994; 9: 1170–1175. The complete AARC Clinical Practice Guidelines are available from the AARC Web site (*http://www.aarc.org*), from the AARC Executive Office, or from *Respiratory Care* journal.

Figure 6-67 *(continued)*

Figure 6-68 *A schematic of a mixing chamber that is designed to homogenize a gas sample prior to analysis.*

Mixing chambers are baffled chambers that are designed to homogenize the exhaled gas sample (Figure 6-68). The exhaled gas sample must follow a convoluted pathway through the baffles, which ensure that the exhaled gas is homogenous prior to being analyzed. A vacuum pump extracts the sample gas from the mixing chamber and moves it to the analyzer section of the instrument.

Breath-by-breath analysis is performed using rapid response gas analyzers. The patient's exhaled gas is directed through the rapid response gas analyzer and a pneumotachometer where the oxygen, carbon dioxide, and volumes are measured (Figure 6-69).

Figure 6-69 *A photograph of a pneumotachometer with a sampling port for breath-by-breath analysis of oxygen and carbon dioxide.*

PATIENT INTERFACES

Indirect calorimetry may be performed on patients being mechanically ventilated or on patients breathing spontaneously. When performing indirect calorimetry on ventilated patients, the exhaled gas must be isolated from the inspired gas. Most contemporary ventilators have incorporated the exhalation valve internally within the confines of the ventilator and have removed it from the patient circuit. The gas must be sampled far enough from the patient wye to prevent inspired gas from entering the sample or mixing chamber. Ideally, the gas should be sampled where the exhalation tubing interfaces with the ventilator's exhalation port (Figure 6-70).

Fluctuation in F_IO_2 and bias flow during flow triggering are other potential complications of performing indirect calorimetry on ventilated patients. Fluctuation in F_IO_2 levels should ideally vary no more than +0.1%, especially at concentrations greater than 0.85. The denominator of the Haldane equation $(1 - F_IO_2)$ becomes very small at high oxygen concentrations, and approaches zero, which can result in division by zero or infinity.

Bias flow during flow triggering must also be accounted for and compensated for prior to data collection using indirect calorimetry. Most software systems allow for compensation for elevated oxygen concentrations and flows during bias flow gas delivery through the ventilator circuit.

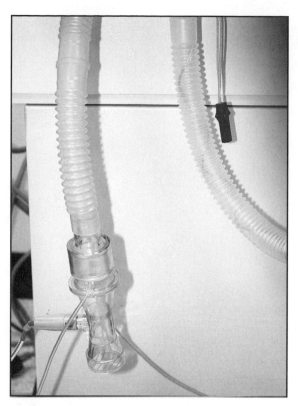

Figure 6-70 *A photograph illustrating how to connect an indirect calorimeter to the exhalation port of a mechanical ventilator.*

Figure 6-71 *A photograph of a canopy being used for metabolic measurement on a spontaneously breathing patient.*

MOUTHPIECE AND CANOPY COLLECTION

A mouthpiece and nose clips can be used to collect exhaled gas from a spontaneously breathing patient during indirect calorimetry. However, the presence of the mouthpiece (SCUBA-type mouthpiece) can adversely affect the breathing pattern of the patient, which can in turn affect the data. It may take some time for the patient to "settle down" and reach a true resting state when using a mouthpiece and nose clips.

A canopy is shown in Figure 6-71. The canopy eliminates some of the breathing pattern anomalies associated with the use of a mouthpiece and nose clips. A bias flow through the canopy ensures that the exhaled gas is collected and the oxygen concentration and flow rate can be compensated for by the calorimeter's software. Most spontaneously breathing patients rapidly adjust to the canopy collection system when compared with mouthpiece and nose clips.

APNEA MONITORS

Apnea monitors operate either using inductive plethysmography or impedance plethysmography. **Inductive plethysmography** apnea monitors consist of two elastic bands that are positioned around the abdomen and around the chest. As the chest expands and contracts, coiled wires within the bands expand and contract. These wire bands are connected to an oscillator that provides about a 20-millivolt signal at about 300 kilohertz. As the cross-sectional area of the bands changes with thoracic or abdominal motion, the frequency of the oscillations changes due to inductance. A microprocessor converts the frequency change to an analog voltage, which is then displayed graphically or digitally as a respiratory rate.

Impedance plethysmography units rely on the placement of two ECG leads on the anterior chest wall along the midaxillary line. As the chest wall expands and contracts, the impedance between the two electrodes changes. Therefore, a voltage difference can be measured between the two electrodes. The monitor then uses the analog voltage signal to measure respiratory rate. Impedance monitoring can be affected by body position changes and other movement. Most units are small and typically have high and low respiratory rate alarms that can be operator set (Figure 6-72).

Figure 6-72 *A photograph of an impedance plethysmograph apnea monitor.*

ASSEMBLY AND TROUBLESHOOTING

Assembly—Apnea Monitors

1. Prepare the electrodes:
   a. Attach the leads to the electrodes by placing each electrode on a flat surface and snapping the lead wire into place.
   b. The black lead wire will be connected to the electrode on the left side of the chest and the white lead wire will be connected to the electrode on the right side of the chest.
   c. Place the electrodes on the belt with the lead wires facing toward the bottom of the belt. Position the electrodes such that, when the belt is applied to the chest, the electrodes will be placed along the midaxillary line.

2. Secure the belt snugly around the patient's chest. You should only be able to place one finger between the belt and the patient's chest.

3. Connect the lead wires to the appropriate connections on the monitor.

4. Turn the monitor on and adjust the apnea period to the desired setting.

Troubleshooting

ALG 6-5 will assist you in troubleshooting apnea monitors.

1. If the monitor alarms, the following steps should be taken:
   a. Respond as quickly as possible (within 10 seconds).
   b. Check the patient first. If the patient's color is not good or if they are not breathing, stimulate them. If they do not respond, initiate CPR.
   c. If the patient is breathing and the patient's color appears good, check the electrodes, lead wires, and cable to determine the cause of the false alarm.
   d. If the alarm is steady, it is typically a lead or battery problem.
   e. If the alarm is intermittent, it is likely to be an event (apnea or hypopnea).

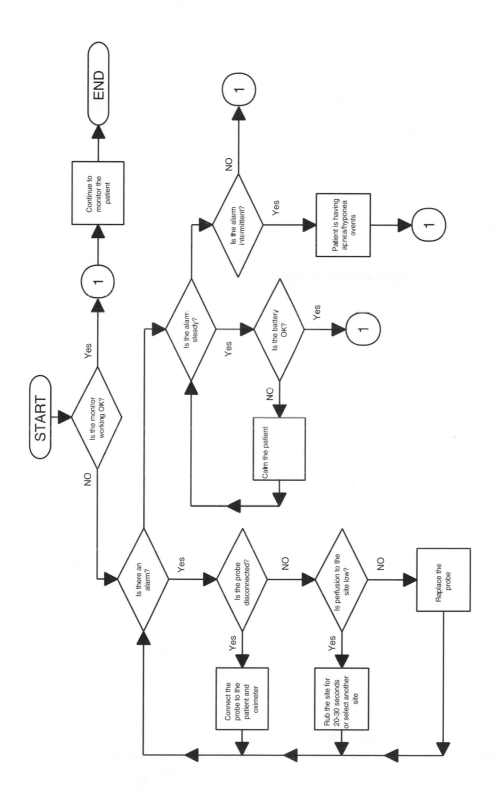

ALG 6-5 *A flowchart for troubleshooting the BCI Model 3301 handheld pulse oximeter.*

HOME SLEEP MONITORS

Home sleep monitors have become more prevalent in the diagnosis of obstructive sleep apnea. Typically, the patient is instructed on how to set up and apply the monitor in an outpatient setting. The patient then goes home with the monitor and applies it upon retiring for bed. Most home monitors are four-channel units consisting of ECG, snoring microphone, oximeter, and an airflow thermister (Figure 6-73).

The ECG electrodes are placed on the anterior chest along the midaxillary line. Once the ECG electrodes have been placed, the appropriate left and right leads are attached to the electrodes.

The snoring microphone is taped adjacent to the larynx. In the event the patient snores, the microphone picks up the vibrations and records it. In the event of obstructive apnea, frequently a loud snort is heard upon the airway becoming patent following the obstructive event.

The oximeter probe is placed on the patient's finger. Like a standard oximeter, the probe consists of a red and infrared LED that determines the oxygen saturation.

The airflow thermister is similar to a small nasal cannula. The probes are taped just under the nares. As the patient exhales, the thermister detects the warm, exhaled gas and the analog temperature signal (cold to warm) is converted to a voltage and used to measure airflow or lack of airflow in the event of an obstructive event.

Figure 6-74 is an example of a four-channel printout from a home monitor. The upper channel is the heart rate, the next lower channel is the impedance channel (abdominal motion), the next channel down is the airflow channel, and the lowest channel is the oxygen saturation. Note how oxygen saturation periodically falls. The drop in saturation is preceded by a cessation of airflow accompanied by respiratory efforts (obstructive apnea event).

Figure 6-73 *A schematic drawing showing the components of a four-channel home sleep apnea monitor.*

Figure 6-74 *An example of a tracing from a home sleep study printed from a four-channel monitor.*

ASSEMBLY AND TROUBLESHOOTING

Assembly—Home Sleep Monitors

1. Patient preparation:
   a. ECG electrodes
      (1) Place the ECG electrodes between the collar bone and the fourth rib space along the midaxillary line.
      (2) Connect the leads to the electrodes (white on the right, black on the left).
   b. Wrap the belt around the patient's abdomen snuggly (one finger width between the cable and the abdomen), with the sensor block positioned mid-line anteriorly.
   c. Attach the snore microphone adjacent to the larynx using the self-adhesive disk. Back up the adhesive disk with a small strip of tape. Make sure the microphone lead is attached to the appropriate port on the sensor block.
   d. Connect the oximeter finger probe to the patient's finger. Wrap the adhesive strip around the finger securing it. Make certain that the LED transmitter and receiver are opposite one another.
   e. Attach the airflow sensor to the patient's upper lip securing it under the nose with the self-adhesive strip on the back of the sensor. Make sure that the sensor probes are positioned near the patient's nares similar to a nasal cannula. Connect the airflow sensor's lead to the sensor block.

2. Connect the main cable from the sensor block to the bedside recording unit.
   a. If the patient needs to get up during the night, instruct the patient to disconnect the cable from the bedside recorder and not to remove leads or electrodes from the abdomen or face.

3. Turn the recorder on. The patient can now "settle down" for the night.

CLINICAL CORNER

Pulmonary Measurement Equipment

1. You are using a standard range peak flowmeter to assess an asthmatic patient in your emergency room. The peak flowmeter is calibrated from 60 to 800 L/min. The patient is unable to achieve even 60 L/min. What should you report for peak flow, and what other device could you use?

Oxygen Analyzing Equipment

1. You are checking the F_IO_2 on a Nellcor Puritan Bennett 7200ae ventilator using a polarographic oxygen analyzer. The oxygen percent control is set at 60%, and your oxygen analyzer reads 67%. Describe the steps you should take to verify the oxygen concentration.

2. You are using a polarographic oxygen analyzer to measure the F_IO_2 on a heated nebulizer. While attempting to use the analyzer, it fails to calibrate. You suspect the battery is low, so you change it, but the analyzer still fails to calibrate. Describe the steps you should take to troubleshoot the analyzer.

Blood Gas–Analyzing Equipment

1. You are performing quality control on your blood gas instrument. The control results for the oxygen electrode fail to come in within plus-or-minus two standard deviations. Upon review of the Levey-Jennings chart, you note a trend. What could you do to bring the electrode back into plus-or-minus two standard deviations?

Transcutaneous Monitoring Equipment

1. You are tending a $PtcCO_2$ monitor with a patient's blood gases. The monitor values are drifting away from the blood gas results. What could you do bring the monitor more closely in line with the current blood gas results?

Pulse Oximetry Equipment

1. The pulse oximeter you just connected to a patient's finger is indicating that the signal strength is poor. What can you do to improve the ability of the oximeter to give you the desired results, and what other means can you use to verify the signal strength?

End Tidal CO_2 Equipment

1. You are resuscitating a patient in the emergency room, and the emergency room physician asks you to intubate. How can you verify placement of the endotracheal tubes before the chest X-ray returns? Discuss at least three ways.

Apnea Monitoring Equipment

1. You are responding to an apnea alarm. The patient's color is poor, and you don't see any chest rise or movement. What steps should you take?

Home Sleep Monitoring Equipment

1. The airflow tracing from a four-channel home monitor shows no airflow for an extended period of time (several minutes). The heart rate and SpO_2 channels appear normal. What could cause this?

Self-Assessment Quiz

1. Which of the following pulmonary function measuring devices are volume displacement devices?
   I. Collins spirometer
   II. Vortex shedding pneumotachometer
   III. Stead-Wells spirometer
   IV. Fleisch pneumotachometer
   a. I and II
   b. I and III
   c. II and III
   d. III and IV

2. A body plethysmograph measures thoracic volume by:
   I. changes in pressure.
   II. flow measurements.
   III. temperature changes.
   IV. rotating vanes.
   a. I only
   b. II only
   c. III only
   d. II and III

3. A type of pneumotachometer that depends upon a resistive element that causes a pressure drop is:
   a. the Fleisch pneumotachometer.
   b. the vortex shedding pneumotachometer.
   c. the venturi pneumotachometer.
   d. the Wright respirometer.

4. A pneumotachometer that is susceptible to damage from high flow rates is:
   a. the vortex shedding pneumotachometer.
   b. the venturi pneumotachometer.
   c. the Wright respirometer.
   d. the Wright peak flowmeter.

5. Which gas law is used in the body plethysmograph to measure lung volumes?
   a. Charles' law
   b. Gay-Lussac's law
   c. Henry's law
   d. Boyle's law

6. A type of pneumotachometer that is dependent upon a temperature change to measure flow is:
   a. a vortex sensor.
   b. a thermal anemometer.
   c. a vane respirometer.
   d. a Fleisch pneumotachometer.

7. A venturi pneumotachometer works by measuring:
   a. a difference in ultrasonic energy.
   b. a difference in voltage.
   c. a difference in current.
   d. a difference in pressure.

8. A physical oxygen analyzer measures oxygen using:
   a. the chemical reaction of oxygen-forming hydroxyl ions.
   b. the paramagnetic property of oxygen.
   c. the chemical reaction of oxygen-forming hydrogen ions.
   d. the principle of thermoconductivity.

9. An electrical oxygen analyzer measures oxygen using:
   a. the chemical reaction of oxygen-forming hydroxyl ions.
   b. the paramagnetic property of oxygen.
   c. the chemical reaction of oxygen-forming hydrogen ions.
   d. the principle of thermoconductivity.

10. A galvanic oxygen analyzer measures oxygen using:
    a. the chemical reaction of oxygen-forming hydroxyl ions.
    b. the paramagnetic property of oxygen.
    c. infrared absorption.
    d. the principle of thermoconductivity.

11. A polarographic oxygen analyzer is similar to a galvanic analyzer with the exception of:
    a. the addition of a battery.
    b. the deletion of an anode.
    c. a separate reference and sample chamber.
    d. the addition of a quartz fiber.

12. The most common reference half-cell for the pH system is:
    a. the silver/silver chloride cell.
    b. the calomel cell.
    c. the polarographic cell.
    d. a platinum cathode.

13. The PCO_2 blood gas electrode directly measures:
    a. PCO_2.
    b. hydrogen ion concentration.
    c. carbon dioxide percentage.
    d. hydroxyl ions.

14. The PO_2 blood gas electrode measures oxygen by:
    a. changes in electrical current.
    b. changes in mass.
    c. using a photospectrometer.
    d. using an infrared analyzer.

15. A blood gas PO_2 electrode measures oxygen:
    a. percentage.
    b. mass.
    c. tension.
    d. weight.

16. A transcutaneous carbon dioxide electrode is a modified:
    a. Clark electrode.
    b. galvanic electrode.
    c. Severinghaus electrode.
    d. polarographic electrode.

17. A transcutaneous carbon dioxide electrode directly measures:
    a. PCO_2.
    b. hydrogen ion concentration.
    c. carbon dioxide percentage.
    d. hydroxyl ions.

18. Both an end tidal carbon dioxide monitor and a pulse oximeter work using:
    a. changes in electrical current.
    b. changes in mass.
    c. a photospectrometer.
    d. an infrared analyzer.

19. The occurrence of six or more blood gas quality control results that show an increasing pattern is termed a:
    a. shift.
    b. trend.
    c. standard deviation.
    d. drift.

20. The presence of six or more blood gas quality control results on the same side of the mean is termed a:
    a. shift
    b. trend
    c. standard deviation
    d. drift

21. Which of the following hemoglobin variants are unable to combine reversibly with oxygen?
    I. oxyhemoblobin
    II. reduced hemoglobin
    III. methemoglobin
    IV. carboxyhemoglobin
    a. I and II
    b. I and III
    c. I and IV
    d. III and IV

22. Which of the following hemoglobin variants exists in the Fe^{+++} state?
    a. oxyhemoblobin
    b. reduced hemoglobin
    c. methemoglobin
    d. carboxyhemoglobin

23. The term functional hemoglobin refers to which of the following variants?
    I. oxyhemoblobin
    II. reduced hemoglobin
    III. methemoglobin
    IV. carboxyhemoglobin
    a. I and II
    b. II and III
    c. I and IV
    d. III and IV

24. Which of the following factors may influence the accuracy of a pulse oximeter?
    I. ambient light
    II. nail polish
    III. the patient's hemodynamics
    IV. patient motion
    a. I
    b. I and II
    c. I, II, and III
    d. I, II, III, and IV

25. The term isosebestic point refers to:
    a. hemoglobin's freezing temperature.
    b. the wavelength where two or more variants have similar absorptions.
    c. the wavelength where all variants have differing absorptions.
    d. the wavelength of light that is not affected by hemoglobin.

26. Pulse oximeters measure hemoglobin saturation:
    I. continuously.
    II. during systole.
    III. during diastole.
    a. I
    b. I and II
    c. I and III
    d. III

27. Which of the following end tidal CO_2 monitors positions the sensor on the patient's airway?
    I. mainstream
    II. sidestream
    III. proximal diverting
    a. I
    b. II
    c. III
    d. II and III

28. Which of the following removes some exhaled gas and measures the CO_2 concentration away from the patient's airway?
    I. mainstream
    II. sidestream
    III. proximal diverting
    a. I
    b. II
    c. III
    d. II and III

29. When is the use of a colormetric CO_2 monitor most useful?
    a. for continuous monitoring
    b. for trending data over time
    c. to detect esophageal intubation
    d. none of the above

30. Impedance plethysmography:
    I. detects expansion and contraction of the chest
    II. is a technique employed by apnea monitors
    III. is a technique employed by home sleep monitors
    IV. uses ECG electrodes as a patient interface
    a. I
    b. I and II
    c. I, II, and III
    d. I, II, III, and IV

Selected Bibliography

Adams, A. P., & Hahn, C. E. W. (1979). Principles and practice of blood-gas analysis. *Franklin Scientific Projects.*

Aloan, C. A. (1987). *Respiratory care of the newborn.* J. B. Lippincott.

American Association for Respiratory Care. (1991). Clinical practice guideline: Pulse oximetry. *Respiratory Care, 36,* 1406–1409.

American Association for Respiratory Care. (1994). Clinical practice guideline: Transcutaneous blood gas monitoring for neonatal & pediatric patients. *Respiratory Care, 39,* 1176–1179.

American Association for Respiratory Care. (2001). Clincical practice guidelines: Blood gas analysis and hemoximetry (Rev.). *Respiratory Care, 46,* 490–505.

American Association for Respiratory Care. (2003). Clinical practice guideline: Capnography/capnometry during mechanical ventilation. *Respiratory Care, 48,* 534–539.

Apria Healthcare. *Instructions: Patient preparation for the edentrace sleep recorder.*

Barnes, T., et al. (1994). *Respiratory care practice* (2nd ed.). Mosby-Yearbook.

BCI International. (1992). *BCI 3301 oximeter operation/service manual.* Waukesha.

Beer, F., & Johnson, R. (1988). *Vector mechanics for engineers* (5th ed.). McGraw-Hill.

Branson, R. D., et al. (1999). Inhaled nitric oxide: Delivery systems and monitoring. *Respiratory Care, 44*(3), 281–307.

Branson, R. D. (1990). The measurement of energy expenditure: Instrumentation, practical considerations, and clinical application. *Respiratory Care, 25*(7), 640–659.

Burton, G., Hodgkin, J., et al. (1997). *Respiration care: A guide to clinical practice* (4th ed.). J. B. Lippincott.

Datex Division Instrumentarium Corporation. (1992). *First steps in CO_2 monitoring.* Helsinki.

East, T. D. (1990). What makes noninvasive monitoring tick? A review of basic engineering principles. *Respiratory Care, 35*(6).

Hess, D. (1990). Capnometry and capnography: Technical aspects, physiologic aspects and clinical applications. *Respiratory Care, 25*(6).

Instrumentation Laboratory, Inc. (1973). *Blood gas quality control.* Lexington.

Kacmarek, R., et al. (1985). *The essentials of respiratory therapy* (2nd ed.). Mosby-Yearbook.

Kinasewitz, G. T. (1982). Use of end-tidal capnography during mechanical ventilation. *Respiratory Care, 82*(27).

Kireg, B. P. (1990). Ventilatory pattern monitoring: Instrumentation and applications. *Respiratory Care, 35*(7), 697–708.

McPherson, S. P., et al. (1995). *Respiratory therapy equipment* (5th ed.). Mosby-Yearbook.

Malviyz, S., et al. (2000). False alarms and sensitivity of conventional pulse oximetry versus the masimo SET technology in the pediatric postanesthesia care unit. *Anesth Analg, 90,* 1336–1340.

Nellcor, Incorporated. (1987). *Measurement of functional and fractional oxygen saturation.* Hayward.

Nellcor, Incorporated. (1991). *Operator's manual Nellcor N-180 pulse oximeter.* Hayward.

Nellcor, Incorporated. (1993). *Ultra Cap™ N-6000 pulse oximeter and capnograph operator's manual.* Hayward.

Nonin Medical. (1992). *Instruction and service manual model 8500 and model 8500M hand held pulse oximeter.* Plymouth.

Novametrix Medical Systems, Inc. (1992). *Capnogard ETCO₂ monitor user's manual.* Wallingford.

Novametrix Medical Systems, Inc. (1992). *Oxypleth pulse oximeter user's manual.* Wallingford.

Novametrix Medical Systems, Inc. (1992). *PtcO₂/PtcCO₂ monitor model 840 user's manual.* Wallingford.

Ohmeda. (1988). *Ohmeda 3740 pulse oximeter operation and maintenance manual.* Louisville.

Portnoy, A. L. *A review of the principles of quality control: A programmed text.* Fisher Diagnostics.

Pulwer, E. & Plaut, D. (1979). *Quality Control.* Miami.

Ruppel, G. (1994). *Manual of pulmonary function testing* (6th ed.). Mosby-Yearbook.

Severinghaus, J. W. (1992). Transcutaneous blood gas analysis. *Respiratory Care, 27*(82).

Sitting, S. E. (2000). Infant home apnea monitoring: Transitional technology from NICU to home. *AARC Times, 24*(9), 37-40.

Welch, J. P., & DeCesare, R. Pulse oximetry: Instrumentation and clinical applications. *Respiratory Care, 35*(6).

White, G. C. (2003). *Basic clinical lab competencies for respiratory care* (4th ed.). Thomson Delmar Learning.

CHAPTER 7

MECHANICAL VENTILATOR THEORY AND CLASSIFICATION

INTRODUCTION

Mechanical ventilators play a very important role in the management of critically ill patients. A wide variety of both newborn and adult ventilators are used in multiple patient care settings.

Despite the variety in ventilators, certain features are common to all. The first section will focus on the common elements of ventilation. A classification system will be developed to help you group ventilators having similar function or operation. You will also learn how gas laws, gas control systems, and flow and pressure measuring devices are applied to a ventilator's design. Once this knowledge is attained, you will understand the advantages and disadvantages of the ventilator control systems in use today.

The next section of the chapter will discuss special ventilatory procedures. These include how to modify or add PEEP, CPAP, or intermittent mandatory ventilation (IMV) to a ventilator not having these mode capabilities. Although the majority of the contemporary adult ventilators incorporate these features, a careful study of an external circuit will facilitate your understanding of a contemporary ventilator's operation.

OBJECTIVES

After completing this chapter, the student will accomplish the following objectives:

- Explain how Poiseuille's law can be applied when mechanically ventilating a patient.
- Explain how strain gauges, vortex sensors, and differential pressure transducers can be used to measure pressure and flow.
- Explain the operation of the following valves:
  - Solenoid valve
  - Proportional solenoid valve
  - Servo-controlled scissor valve
  - Demand valve
- Define work in physical science terms, and apply that definition to pulmonary work.
- Define ventilator support in relation to pulmonary work.
- Explain the ventilator control circuit including:
  - Input power
  - Power conversion or transmission
  - Identify the types of control circuits including:
    - Mechanical

- Pneumatic
- Fluidic
- Electric
- Electronic

- Define the term *control variable* and what conditions must be met for a ventilator to be classified as one of the following:
  - Pressure controller
  - Volume controller
  - Flow controller
  - Time controller
- Define the term *phase variable* and state how that variable may be used during the four phases of ventilation:
  - Limit variable
  - Cycle variable
  - Baseline variable
  - Conditional variable
- Describe the different output waveforms and their characteristics.
- Describe the characteristics of the ventilator/patient circuit including:
  - Single versus double

- Compliance
- Resistance
- Washout time
- Explain the operation of the following PEEP/CPAP devices:
  - Boeringer valve
  - Downs' valve
  - Magnetic valve
  - Emerson water column
  - Water seal
- Explain how PEEP, IMV, and IMV with CPAP may be added externally to a ventilator.

- Explain the purpose of ventilator alarm systems and the types of alarms that are used.
- Describe different types of ventilator alarms:
  - Input power
  - Control circuit
  - Output alarms
- Describe the modes of ventilation and classify them according to Chatburn's ventilator classification system.

KEY TERMS

Assist/control
Boeringer valves
Closed loop control circuit
Coanda effect
Compressible volume
Continuous Positive Airway Pressure (CPAP)
Corrected tidal volume

Demand valves
Differential pressure transducer
Downs' valves
Negative pressure ventilators
Open loop control circuit
Positive pressure ventilator
Proportional scissor valves

Proportional solenoid valves
Servo feedback control
Solenoid valves
Strain gauge pressure transducer
Tubing compliance
Water column

PHYSICS OF MECHANICAL VENTILATORS

GAS LAWS THAT APPLY TO MECHANICAL VENTILATION

Knowing how gas laws apply to mechanical ventilation is important to the understanding of mechanical ventilator operation and airway management (see Chapter 1).

One important concept is the ability to determine **tubing compliance** and **compressible volume**. Compliance, by definition, is a change in volume per unit of pressure.

To calculate these values, the ventilator is adjusted to deliver 200 mL of volume, the patient wye is occluded, and a spirometer is placed at the expiratory limb to measure expiratory volumes. The ventilator is allowed to cycle for 10 to 12 breaths, permitting an accurate determination of expired volume. The peak pressure on the pressure manometer is also recorded. To calculate tubing compliance and compressible volume, complete the following steps.

Measured volume: 200 mL

Measured pressure: 70 cmH$_2$O

$$\text{Compliance} = \text{Volume/Pressure}$$
$$= 200 \text{ mL}/70 \text{ cmH}_2\text{O}$$
$$= 2.86 \text{ mL/cmH}_2\text{O}$$

In this example, the tubing/circuit compliance is 2.86 mL/cmH$_2$O. That is, for every centimeter of water pressure applied to the circuit, the volume of gas delivered to the patient will be decreased by 2.86 mL.

Not all the volume given with each breath is delivered to the patient. Some volume is lost in the circuit due to compression. Calculation of the compressible volume, or tubing loss as it is referred to, may be accomplished by multiplying the tubing compliance by the peak pressure required to deliver a given volume to the patient.

Measured volume: 800 mL

Peak pressure: 25 cmH$_2$O

Tubing compliance: 2.86 mL/cmH$_2$O

Compressible volume

$= \text{Peak pressure} \times \text{Tubing compliance}$

$= 25 \text{ cmH}_2\text{O} \times 2.86 \text{ mL/cmH}_2\text{O}$

$= 71.5 \text{ mL}$

To determine the actual volume delivered to the patient, the compressible volume must be subtracted from the measured volume. This is the **corrected tidal volume**.

Corrected Tidal Volume

Measured volume: 800 mL

Peak pressure: 25 cmH$_2$O

Compressible volume: 72 mL

Corrected Tidal Volume

= Measured Tidal Volume
    – Compressible Volume

= 800 mL – 72 mL

= 728 mL

Poiseuille's Law

Mechanical ventilation involves the bulk movement of gas volumes into and out of the lungs. Therefore, the laws governing the behavior of fluids apply. As you recall, Poiseuille's law relates resistance to gas flow to the radius and length of a tube.

When the diameter of an airway decreases, a significant increase in resistance results. This reduction in diameter can occur because of obstruction from secretions, herniation of the cuff, kinking of the artificial airway, or other causes. If the radius of the airway is reduced by one-half of the original radius, resistance to gas flow increases a full 16 times. Therefore, a higher pressure must be used to deliver a given volume in a given time.

MEASUREMENT OF GAS FLOW AND PRESSURE

Various devices and methods are used by ventilator manufacturers to measure gas flow and pressure. Many devices are relatively simple; others are quite complex. An understanding of the various methods of measurement is important in understanding the characteristics and monitoring abilities of the different ventilators.

Strain Gauge Pressure Transducer

One way to measure pressure and flow is to use a **strain gauge pressure transducer** (Figure 7-1). A strain gauge pressure transducer consists of a diaphragm with a strain gauge attached to it, exposed to the area where pressure measurement is desired. The strain gauge is connected by a set of wires to a Wheatstone bridge circuit that is sensitive to a change in resistance.

Figure 7-1 *A strain gauge pressure transducer.*

Pressure exerted on the diaphragm causes the strain gauge to elongate. As the gauge lengthens, the resistance to electrical current increases. This causes the Wheatstone bridge circuit to produce a change in voltage proportional to the pressure applied to the diaphragm. The pressure may be displayed digitally or by an analog gauge.

A strain gauge flow transducer employs a flexible wire with a flag or flat plate on one end. A strain gauge is mounted to the wire in such a way that it is sensitive to bending of the wire. As gas flows past the flag, pressure against it causes the wire to bend or flex. The strain gauge, in turn, flexes, causing a change in electrical resistance. This change then causes a change in voltage. The voltage change is proportional to the gas flow. This type of mechanism is used in the Servo 900C ventilator to measure flow (Figure 7-2).

Figure 7-2 *A schematic of the strain gauge flowmeter used on the Siemens Medical Systems 900C ventilator. (Courtesy Siemens Life Support Systems, Scheumberg, IL)*

Vortex Sensor

Vortex sensors, as described in Chapter 6, are also used on some ventilators to directly measure flow. These sensors employ the vortex shedding principle previously described, using ultrasonic energy to detect changes in gas flow (Figure 7-3).

Differential Pressure Transducer

A **differential pressure transducer** is a strain gauge–type transducer that compares two pressures by using a diaphragm to separate them (Figure 7-4).

Another means of monitoring pressure changes is to use the principle of magnetism. Movement of a magnetically permeable diaphragm in close proximity to a wire-wound coil will cause changes in reluctance (a measure of magnetic potential difference), by increasing or decreasing the air gap (Figure 7-5). This change in reluctance will alter the induction ratio of an alternating current (AC) bridge circuit. Therefore, a change in magnetic flux causes a change in output voltage from the AC bridge circuit.

Flow may be accurately determined by connecting the pressure inputs of a sensitive differential pressure transducer to a resistive type flow transducer, venturi tube flow transducer, or even by measuring a pressure drop across a flow delivery valve. If sampling time is known, volume also can be measured (volume = flow × time). This type of measuring system, besides being used in ventilators, is also used in pulmonary function equipment to measure flow and volume.

VALVE OPERATION

Valves are used in mechanical ventilators to control or direct gas flow. Valves operate using different control systems and ways of regulating gas direction and flow. Some valves are automated while others allow the operator to control their function. An understanding of the basic types of valves used in mechanical ventilators is important in order to understand the capabilities of mechanical ventilators.

Solenoid Valves

Solenoid valves are often used in mechanical ventilators to direct or control main gas flow to the patient. The solenoid valve operates as a simple on-off switch. Solenoid valves may be automated (controlled by an electric

Figure 7-3 *A schematic of a flowmeter using the vortex shedding principle. (Courtesy Bear Medical Systems, Inc., Riverside, CA)*

Figure 7-4 *A schematic diagram of a differential pressure transducer. Note the two pressure-measuring ports.*

Figure 7-5 *A variable reluctance (magnetic) differential pressure transducer. (Courtesy Validyne Engineering Corporation, Northridge, CA)*

timer or microprocessor), manually activated, pressure activated, or all three (Figure 7-6).

The valve consists of a gate or plunger, valve seat, electromagnet, diaphragm, spring,

Figure 7-6 *A schematic of a solenoid valve.*

and two electrical contacts. The valve is opened when electric current flows through the electromagnet and creates a magnetic field that pulls the plunger open. Conversely, when the current stops, the magnetic field collapses and a spring closes the plunger against its seat.

The current to the electromagnet may be controlled in three different ways. First, an electric timer or microprocessor can send an electric current to the electromagnet, activating it and opening the valve. Second, sub-ambient pressure created by the patient attempting to take a breath will cause the diaphragm to descend, closing an electrical contact, which then opens the valve. Lastly, many ventilators allow the operator to deliver a "manual breath" by pushing a button or closing a switch. This causes current to be delivered to the electromagnet, opening the solenoid valve.

PROPORTIONAL SOLENOID VALVES

Proportional solenoid valves are valves that are able to open in very small increments. The solenoid valve previously described is either fully open or fully closed. Proportional control of gas flow allows ventilator manufacturers to design equipment that better responds to patient needs using microprocessor feedback and control mechanisms.

The term **servo feedback control** is often used to describe the operation of the control systems for these valves. Sensors monitor pressure, flow, and sometimes F_IO_2 inside the ventilator, in the patient circuit, or both. Signals from these sensors are compared to reference values set by the operator who adjusts the controls. Other reference values may be provided by monitoring the patient's respiratory rate, volume, compliance, or other physiological parameters. When the measured values from the sensors differ from the reference values, the microprocessor sends signals opening or closing the valves, adjusting the output to more closely match the reference value. This system of monitoring, comparing, and monitoring again, can be repeated by the microprocessor thousands of times each second and is termed a closed feedback loop control system.

Proportional solenoid valves (PSOLs) are incorporated into the design of the Puritan-Bennett 7200a ventilator. These valves are microprocessor controlled and have several thousand different positions from fully closed to fully open. These valves regulate flow, volume, pressure, F_IO_2, and waveform in the operation of this ventilator. Signals from the feedback control system open or close the valves in response to changes in the measured values.

Proportional Scissor Valves

Proportional scissor valves are incorporated into the design of the Servo Ventilators manufactured by Siemens Medical Systems. Both valves in the 900C use moveable arms that function like a scissors compressing or opening a rubber tube (Figure 7-7).

Signals from the control system cause the stepper motor to open or close the valve in small intervals or steps. The valve opens or closes at a rate of up to 480 steps per second. Each step results in a change in flow of roughly 10%. Photoelectric cells determine whether the valve is fully open or closed. This occurs when a cam obstructs the light path indicating the valve is open in one position and closed in the other.

The expiratory valve illustrated in Figure 7-8 opens by an electromagnet. Signals from the control system cause a fluctuation in current applied to the electromagnet. Depending on the strength of the current, the magnetic field is either strong (fully closing the valve) or weak (partially closing the valve). If no current flows through the magnet, a spring opens the valve. This is a safety feature that will allow the patient to exhale in the event of a power failure.

DEMAND VALVES

Demand valves are specialized valves that respond to a patient's inspiratory efforts (generation of sub-ambient pressures). Unlike solenoid valves that also respond to sub-ambient pressures, demand valves provide a continuous flow of gas to the patient when they open. This continuous flow allows the patient to breathe spontaneously, without ventilator assistance (machine breaths or volumes).

A simplified demand valve is illustrated in Figure 7-9. When sub-ambient pressure is communicated to the chamber of the demand valve, the diaphragm distorts, opening the valve. Gas then flows into the patient circuit until pressure in the chamber moves the diaphragm in the opposite direction, closing the valve.

Many ventilators incorporate demand valves, which allow the ventilator to operate in Synchronized Intermittent Mandatory Ventilation (SIMV) and Continuous Positive Air-

Figure 7-7 *A schematic drawing of the Siemens Medical Systems 900C inspiratory scissor valves. (Courtesy Siemens Life Support Systems, Scheumberg, IL)*

Figure 7-8 *A schematic drawing of the Siemens Medical Systems 900C expiratory scissor valves. (Courtesy Siemens Life Support Systems, Scheumberg, IL)*

Figure 7-9 *A schematic of a demand valve.*

way Pressure (CPAP) modes (refer to the "Modes of Ventilation" section in this chapter). The valves allow the ventilator to deliver gas flow in response to the patient's spontaneous efforts.

VENTILATOR CLASSIFICATION

Ventilator technology has evolved since the introduction of mechanical ventilators over 30 years ago. Since that time, a multitude of manufacturers have produced and marketed ventilators of all sizes, descriptions, and capabilities. Many manufacturers have coined new terms to describe their ventilators and to accentuate how their product is different from the others. Several different ventilator classification systems may be employed to describe mechanical ventilators. The majority of these systems focus on the differences between ventilators rather than on the similarities.

CHATBURN'S CLASSIFICATION SYSTEM

Robert Chatburn has proposed a new way to classify mechanical ventilators based upon related features, physics, and engineering. Chatburn's ventilator classification system has been featured in several articles and textbooks. It allows flexibility, as ventilator technology evolves, in contrast to other systems that employ more narrowly defined design principles, or rely to a greater extent on manufacturer's terms.

As ventilator technology evolves over the next decade or more, the flexibility of Chatburn's classification system will be validated. Unfortunately today, not all practitioners, or educators, have adopted this newer classification system. This author feels the system is important enough that it should be included in this text and others that describe ventilator operational characteristics. A student learning about this classification system should refer to the bibliography at the conclusion of this chapter and read Chatburn's original contributions as well as this textbook.

VENTILATORY WORK

Pulmonary physiologists have described the work ventilatory muscles perform during inspiration and how muscles can actively assist during exhalation. During inspiration, the primary ventilatory muscles cause the size (volume) of the thoracic cage to increase, overcoming the elastic forces of the lungs and thorax, and the resistance of the airways. As the volume of the thoracic cage increases, intrapleural pressure becomes more negative, resulting in lung expansion as the visceral pleura expand with the parietal pleura. Gas flows from the atmosphere and into the lungs as a result of the transairway pressure. During expiration, the muscles of inspiration relax. The elastic forces of the lungs and thorax cause the chest to decrease in volume. Exhalation occurs as a result of the greater pressure at the alveolus when compared to atmospheric pressure. All of this muscle activity, to overcome the elastic and resistance properties of the lungs and thorax, requires energy and work.

The work that the muscles and/or the ventilator must perform is proportional to the pressure required for inspiration multiplied by the tidal volume. The pressure required to deliver the tidal volume is referred to as the "load" either the muscles or the ventilator must work against. There is an elastic load (proportional to volume and inversely proportional to compliance) and a resistance load (proportional to airway resistance and inspiratory flow). These variables are related by the equation of motion for the respiratory system:

Muscle Pressure + Ventilator Pressure = Volume\Compliance + (Resistance)(Flow)

Compliance is defined as a change in volume divided by a change in pressure, which is a measure of the elastic forces of the lungs and thorax. Flow, as defined earlier, is a unit of volume divided by a unit of time. Resistance is the force that must be overcome to move gas through the conducting airways, which is best described by Poiseuille's law.

A mechanical ventilator is simply a machine or device that can fully or partially substitute for the ventilatory work accomplished by the patient's muscles. If the patient's ventilatory muscles contribute no work (sedation, paralysis, etc.), the mechanical ventilator provides full ventilatory support. If the patient's muscles are able to sustain all of the patient's ventilatory requirements, no support is provided by the machine and ventilatory support is zero. Between the two extremes, partial support can be provided by the mechanical ventilator in assisting the ventilatory muscles.

INPUT POWER

Mechanical ventilators may be first classified as to the power source that is utilized to provide the energy required to support the patient's ventilation. As described earlier, ventilation requires work and, therefore, energy.

Pneumatically powered ventilators use compressed gas as an energy source for their operation. Medical gases are anhydrous, and oil-free at a pressure of 50 psi. Examples of ventilators that utilize pneumatic power include the Bennett PR-2, Bird Mark 7, Percussionaire IPV, Monaghan 225/SIMV, and the Percussionaire VDR.

Ventilators may also be electrically powered, utilizing 120 volt, 60 Hz alternating current or 12-volt direct current for a power source. The electrical power can be used to run electric motors to drive pistons, compressors, or other mechanical devices that generate gas flow. An example of an electrically powered ventilator include the, Puritan-Bennett LP-10 and the Bear Medical Systems Bear 33.

A ventilator may also be powered by a combination of both pneumatic and electric power sources. Many third-generation ventilators require both an electrical (for microprocessor control systems) and a pneumatic power source. These ventilators include the Bear 1000, Hamilton Veolar, Puritan-Bennett 7200ae, and many other third-generation ventilators.

DRIVE MECHANISM

The drive mechanism is the system utilized by the ventilator to transmit or convert the input power to useful ventilatory work. The type of drive mechanism determines the characteristic flow and pressure patterns each ventilator produces. The use of microprocessors and proportional solenoid valves allows current generation ventilators to produce a variety of user selected inspiratory flow or pressure patterns. An understanding of the different drive mechanisms will allow you to apply a ventilator more effectively in the clinical environment. Drive mechanisms include pistons, bellows, reducing valves, and pneumatic circuits.

Piston Drive Mechanism

An electrically driven piston, with an inspiratory one-way valve, can be used to generate a pressure gradient to drive a ventilator (Figure 7-10). During the back stroke of the piston, gas enters the cylinder through the one-way valve. When the piston travels in the opposite direction, a second one-way valve opens, delivering the compressed gas to the patient.

Pistons are usually electrically powered. However, they may be rotary or linear driven. Figure 7-11 compares a linear driven and a rotary driven piston. Output waveforms, which are discussed later in this chapter, vary depending upon how the piston is driven.

Bellows Drive Mechanism

Ventilators may also use a bellows to compress the gas for delivery to the patient (Figure 7-12). A bellows may be compressed by a spring, a weight, or by gas pressure if it is in a sealed chamber. A one-way valve admits gas to the bellows, expanding it. When it is compressed, the one-way valve closes, causing gas delivery to the patient.

Figure 7-10 *A schematic diagram of a rotary-driven piston drive mechanism for a mechanical ventilator.*

Figure 7-11 *A comparison between (A) a rotary-driven piston and (B) a linear driven piston drive mechanism for a mechanical ventilator.*

Figure 7-12 *A schematic diagram of a bellows drive mechanism for a mechanical ventilator.*

Reducing Valve Drive Mechanism

A reducing valve may be used to drive a ventilator providing enough of a pressure gradient to cause ventilation. The Bennett PR-2 is one example of a ventilator that uses a reducing valve. (The PR-2 and its drive mechanism were discussed in Chapter 3.)

Microprocessor-Controlled Pneumatic Drive Mechanisms

Although, technically speaking, both pistons and bellows are pneumatic systems, a separate classification is required for the newer ventilators, which use proportional solenoid valves and microprocessor controls.

Current generation ventilators use programmed algorithms in the microprocessors to open and close the solenoid valves to mimic virtually any flow or pressure wave pattern. Furthermore, with advances in clinical medicine, the microprocessors can be reprogrammed to deliver new patterns that may not yet be described in the literature. Ventilator manufacturers, using microprocessors and the associated proportional solenoid valves, have a greater flexibility in designing and updating ventilator technology.

CONTROL CIRCUIT

The control circuit is the system that governs, or controls, the ventilator drive mechanism or output control valve. The control circuit is the system that is responsible for the characteristic output waveforms, which will be discussed later in this chapter. Control circuits may be classified as open or closed loop control circuits, mechanical, pneumatic, fluidic, electric, and electronic.

An **open loop control circuit** is one where the desired output is selected and the ventilator achieves the desired output without any further input from the clinician or the ventilator itself.

A **closed loop control circuit** is one where the desired output is selected and then the ventilator measures a specific parameter or variable (flow, pressure, or volume) continuously. The input is constantly adjusted to match the desired output. This type of control circuit may also be referred to as servo controlled.

Mechanical

Mechanical control circuits employ simple machines such as levers, pulleys, or cams to control the drive mechanism. Early mechanical ventilators utilized these systems to control their outputs. Being mechanical, some of these control systems were very durable but lacked flexibility by being an open loop–type control system.

Pneumatic

Pneumatic devices can be utilized as control circuits. These devices include valves, nozzles, ducted ejectors, and diaphragms. The IPPB ventilators and the Percussionaire IPV and VDR ventilators all utilize pneumatic control circuits.

FLUIDICS

Fluidics is the application of gas flow and pressure to control the direction of other gas flows and to perform logic functions. As you will learn, moving gases can be used to alter the direction of another gas flow. The logic functions of fluidics have their origin in digital electronics. Fluidic elements, just like digital electronic gates, control their outputs according to the inputs received. By combining fluidic elements in a specific way, a ventilator can be designed that operates in ways similar to other ventilators that are electronically controlled. The Monaghan 225 is an example of a ventilator that is purely pneumatically powered and pneumatically controlled.

Functional Characteristics of Fluidic Elements

Although control and logic operations differ among fluidic elements, all elements have certain similarities. These similarities include the **Coanda effect**, that the element is either mono- or bi-stable, and the way that the output may be described using a truth table.

Coanda Effect

If gas exits a jet at a high velocity adjacent to a wall (Figure 7-13), the gas flow will attach to one of the adjacent walls. This occurs because of the formation of a separation bubble. An area of reduced lateral pressure is formed around the fast moving gas. The separation bubble forms between the wall and the gas stream. Until the flow is interrupted or other forces cause it to be deflected, it will remain attached to the wall.

Fluidic elements use a flow splitter located beside adjacent walls to control the direction of flow and to perform logic functions (Figure 7-14). An element may either be mono-stable

(attaching to one specific wall, unless acted upon) or bi-stable (having no preference for either wall).

The phenomenon of beam deflection occurs as a result of a control input. If a control signal (pressure) is applied at port C1 (Figure 7-15), the gas jet or beam will be deflected to the opposite channel or port 02. This of course will result in a change in the output of the device. If the device is bi-stable, the flow will remain attached to the new wall. If it is mono-stable, when the control signal is removed, it will reattach to the original wall.

Figure 7-14 *A schematic diagram illustrating a fluidic flow splitter.*

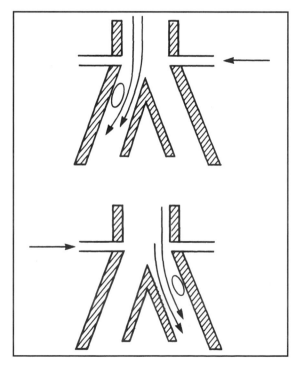

Figure 7-15 *A schematic diagram illustrating beam deflection as a result of a control input.*

Figure 7-13 *A schematic illustrating the Coanda effect.*

Fluidic Nomenclature

As stated earlier, the nomenclature used to describe fluid elements has its roots in digital electronics. The terms used to describe a fluidic element and its truth table have a corresponding element with equivalent logic in an electrical component. The names may seem unusual for medical devices, but the technology first began with early work in digital electronics, specifically computer technology.

Truth tables are based on the fact that an electronic component has essentially two functions or positions. Like a lightbulb it is either on or it is off. Electronic inputs control the output of these devices, turning them on or off. If a digital element is on, it is assigned a value of one in the truth table. If it is off, it is assigned a value of zero. Similar truth tables are constructed to describe the operation of fluidic elements. Boolean algebra and binary, hexadecimal, and octal codes are used by engineers to combine elements to perform a useful function.

Operation and Logic of Fluidic Elements

In this section the operation of the fluidic elements, their truth tables, and the application of the element in ventilator design will be discussed. The elements include the flip-flop, and/nand, or/nor, back pressure switch, Schmidt trigger, and the proportional amplifier.

Flip-Flop

The flip-flop element is a bi-stable device that may be applied as a control valve to control the phase of ventilation (inspiration or

expiration). Figure 7-16 is a schematic of a flip-flop valve. Notice that the valve has two control inputs (C1 and C2). Application of a jet of gas to either port will cause the gas flow or beam to be deflected to the other opposite wall, causing a change of output to 01 or 02. Depending upon the control input, C1 or C2 will have a logic value of one. This is shown in the following truth table (Table 7-1). Since the element is bi-stable, it is said to have a memory. It will remain in the attached position (output 01 or 02), until a control input changes its position.

And/Nand Gate

The and/nand gate is a mono-stable element with two control ports (Figure 7-17). The stable position or output for this element is 02. An application of a control signal to port C1 or C2 will not cause beam deflection. This is because the control signal simply exits the other control port. If a control signal is applied at both C1 and C2, then beam deflection will occur, resulting in the logic value of one at 01. The Monaghan ventilator uses these elements

TABLE 7-1 Flip-Flop Truth Table

Control Ports		Output	
C1	**C2**	**01**	**02**
1	0	1	0
0	0	1	0
0	1	0	1
0	0	0	1

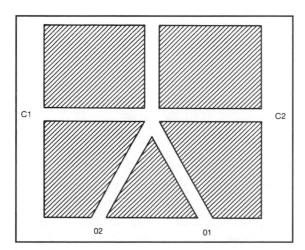

Figure 7-16 *A schematic diagram of a flip-flop fluidic element.*

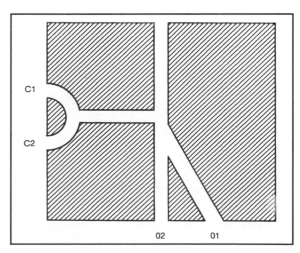

Figure 7-17 *A schematic diagram of an and/nand fluidic element.*

TABLE 7-2 And/Nand Truth Table

Control Ports		Output	
C1	C2	01	02
0	0	0	1
1	0	0	1
0	1	0	1
1	1	1	0

TABLE 7-3 Or/Nor Truth Table

Control Ports		Output	
C1	C2	01	02
0	0	0	1
0	1	1	0
1	0	1	0
1	1	1	0

to power the mushroom exhalation valve in the ventilator circuit.

The truth table for the and/nand gate is shown in Table 7-2. As you can see by studying the truth table, a control input at both C1 and C2 is required to cause a change in the output logic from 02 to 01.

Or/Nor Gate

Like the and/nand gate, the or/nor gate is a mono-stable device. Unlike the and/nand gate, application of a control input at either C1 or C2 will cause beam deflection (Figure 7-18). In the Monaghan 225, the or/nor logic is combined with other element outputs to control the exhalation valve in concert with the flip-flop element.

The truth table for an or/nor gate with two control inputs is shown in Table 7-3. As the table illustrates, application of a control signal at either control port or both results in a change from the mono-stable condition (output 02) to the output 01.

Back Pressure Switch

The back pressure switch is a mono-stable element that requires the diversion of some of the main gas flow powering it to cause the logic to change. A restriction distal to the control port channel causes some of the flow to be diverted (Figure 7-19). If the control port C1 is blocked, pressure builds because of a restriction between the outlet of the control port and the point where the beam is deflected. This restriction acts to amplify the diverted flow. When enough pressure builds, beam deflection occurs, changing the output to 01. Blockage of the control port is usually electronically controlled rather than pneumatically controlled. The logic for this element is shown in Table 7-4.

By studying the table, you can see that only if the control port is blocked will the logic change from 02 to 01. Once the control port is opened again, the element resumes its output at 02.

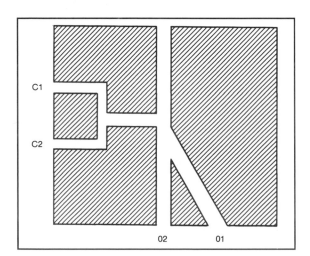

Figure 7-18 *A schematic diagram of an or/nor fluidic element.*

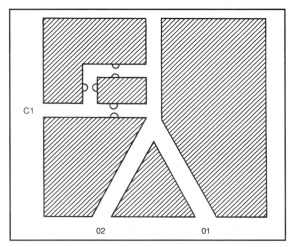

Figure 7-19 *A schematic diagram of a back-pressure switch fluidic element.*

TABLE 7-4 Truth Table for the Back Pressure Switch

Control Port	Output	
C1	01	02
0	0	1
1	1	0

Proportional Amplifier

A proportional amplifier is a device with two opposing control ports, C1 and C2 (Figure 7-20). Gas can exit the element through both outputs 01 and 02 simultaneously. The signal strength from each control port determines where and how strong the output is. If the signal from C1 is greater than that from C2, 01 will have the greater portion of the flow passing through it. An advantage of the proportional amplifier is its ability to boost the control signal gain or level. Typically these devices will boost the signal strength by a factor between five to seven times. If these devices are connected in series, signal strength may be amplified dramatically. For example, if three proportional amplifiers are connected in series, each having a gain of 5, total signal strength will be boosted 125 times ($5 \times 5 \times 5$)!

Schmidt Trigger

The Schmidt trigger is an element that is commonly used to sense negative or positive pressure changes. Although only one element is shown in Figure 7-21, it is actually composed of three proportional amplifiers and two flip-flop elements. If the inputs from the control ports C1 and C2 are equal, equal amounts of gas exit both 01 and 02. If the C2 signal becomes greater than the C1 signal, the logic changes to the 02 output and vice versa. If the C1 signal becomes greater than the C2 signal, the logic changes to the 01 output and vice versa. The total output from the element is considered to be the difference between 01 and 02. The proportional amplifiers incorporated in this fluidically integrated circuit allow small pressure changes to be sensed and cause the original small signal to change the logic of the device.

Electric

Electric control circuits utilize simple switches to control the drive mechanism. Some home care ventilators control tidal volume delivery using electric switches to control the travel limit of the piston that drives the ventilator. The Emerson 3-MV ventilator uses two microswitches to control the inspiratory and expiratory time.

Electronic

Electronic devices such as resistors, diodes, transistors, integrated circuits, and microprocessors can be used to provide sophisticated levels of control over the drive mechanisms of contemporary ventilators. Electronic control systems provide greater flexibility but often at the expense of complexity.

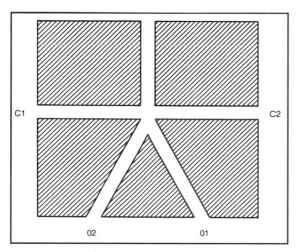

Figure 7-20 *A schematic diagram of a proportional amplifier fluidic element.*

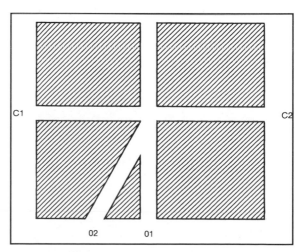

Figure 7-21 *A schematic diagram illustrating a Schmidt trigger fluidic element.*

CONTROL VARIABLES

When providing ventilatory support, the mechanical ventilator can control four primary variables during inspiration. These four variables are volume, pressure, flow, and time. Figure 7-22 illustrates an algorithm that can be applied to determine which variable the ventilator is controlling.

Pressure Controller

A ventilator is classified as a pressure controller if the ventilator controls the trans-respiratory system pressure (airway pressure minus body surface pressure). Further classification of a ventilator, as a positive or negative pressure ventilator, depends upon whether the airway pressure rises above baseline (positive) or body surface pressure is lowered below baseline (negative).

A **positive pressure ventilator** applies pressure inside the chest to expand it. This type of ventilator requires the use of a tight-fitting mask, or more commonly, an artificial airway. A pressure greater than atmospheric pressure is applied to the lungs, causing them to expand (Figure 7-23). Once positive pressure is no longer applied, the patient is allowed to exhale passively to ambient pressure. Exhalation occurs because of the pressure differential between the lungs and the atmosphere and through the elastic recoil of the lungs and thorax. This is the type of ventilator most commonly used today.

Negative pressure ventilators apply sub-atmospheric pressure outside of the chest to inflate the lungs. The negative pressure causes the chest wall to expand, and the pressure difference between the lungs and the atmosphere causes air to flow into the lungs (Figure 7-24). Once negative pressure is no longer applied, the patient is allowed to exhale passively to ambient pressure. Positive pressure may also

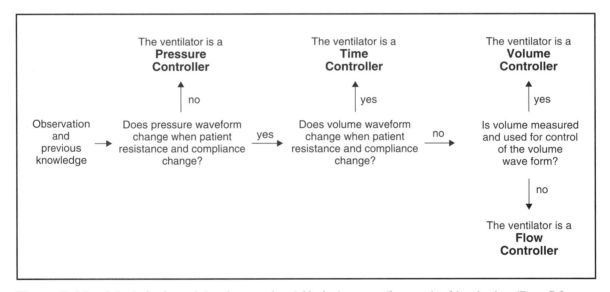

Figure 7-22 *Criteria for determining the control variable during a ventilator-assisted inspiration. (From R.L. Chatburn, 1991. Respiratory Care, 36, copyright 1991. Reprinted with permission.)*

Figure 7-23 *A schematic diagram illustrating positive pressure ventilation.*

Figure 7-24 *A schematic diagram illustrating negative pressure ventilation.*

be applied to further assist the patient during exhalation.

Regardless of whether a ventilator is classified as positive or negative pressure, the lungs expand as a result of the positive transrespiratory system pressures generated. It is the transrespiratory pressure gradient that largely determines the depth or volume of inspiration. An ideal pressure controller is unaffected by changes in the patient's compliance or resistance. That is, the pressure level which is delivered to the patient will not vary in spite of changes in patient compliance or resistance.

Volume Controller

To be classified as a volume controller, volume must be measured and used as a feedback signal to control the output (volume) delivered. A volume controller allows pressure to vary with changes in resistance and compliance, while volume delivery remains constant.

Volume controllers can measure volume by the displacement of the piston, or bellows, which serves as the ventilator's drive mechanism. If the displacement of the bellows, or piston, is controlled, volume therefore is also controlled. An example of this type of ventilator is the Monaghan 225 SIMV discussed later in the text. Another way to control volume is to measure flow and turn it into a volume signal electronically.

Flow Controllers

Flow controllers allow pressure to vary with changes in the patient's compliance and resistance while directly measuring and controlling flow. Flow may be measured by vortex sensors, heated wire grids, venturi pneumotachometers, strain gauge flow sensors, and other devices. What is important is that the ventilator directly measures flow and uses the flow signal as a feedback signal to control its output.

Many ventilators are incorrectly classified as "volume ventilators." Even though a tidal volume is set or displayed, many ventilators measure flow and then derive volume from the flow measurement (volume = flow × time). However, if a ventilator is operated in pressure support, or pressure control mode, the ventilator then becomes a pressure controller, since pressure is the variable which is measured and controlled.

Time Controllers

Time controllers are ventilators that measure and control inspiratory and expiratory time. These ventilators allow pressure and volume to vary with changes in pulmonary compliance and resistance. Since neither pressure nor volume is directly measured or used as a control signal, time (inspiratory, expiratory, or both) remains the only variable that may be controlled.

PHASE VARIABLES

A ventilator-supported breath may be divided into four distinct phases; (1) the change from expiration to inspiration, (2) inspiration, (3) the change from inspiration to expiration, and (4) expiration. More detail can be learned by studying what occurs to the four variables (pressure, volume, flow, and time) during these phases. When the variable is examined during a particular phase, it is termed a phase variable.

Trigger Variable

The trigger variable is the variable that determines the start of inspiration (Figure 7-25). Pressure, volume, flow, or time may be measured by the ventilator and used as a variable to initiate inspiration. Most ventilators use time or pressure as trigger variables.

Figure 7-25 *Criteria for determining the phase variables during a ventilator-assisted breath. (From R.L. Chatburn, Respiratory Care, 36, No. 10, copyright 1991. Reprinted with permission.)*

Some third-generation ventilators measure flow. When the patient's inspiratory flow reaches a specific value, a ventilator-supported breath is delivered. Flow triggering has been shown to be more sensitive and responsive to a patient's efforts than pressure triggering.

One infant ventilator (Sechrist IV-100B and 200) uses inductive plethysmography to initiate a ventilator supported breath. When the infant's chest expands, a small electrical signal is generated between two chest leads, which is commonly used to monitor the infant's respiratory rate. The ventilator is interfaced to the respiratory rate monitor, and inspiratory triggering occurs when the signal is detected by the ventilator. This type of triggering is much faster and more responsive than pressure or flow triggering, since it directly measures the infant's inspiratory efforts or excursions.

How hard the patient must work to initiate, or trigger, a breath is termed the ventilator sensitivity. If the ventilator is made more sensitive to the patient's efforts (pressure, flow, or volume), it is easier for the patient to trigger a breath. The converse, is also true.

Limit Variables

During a ventilator-supported breath, volume, pressure, and flow all rise above their respective baseline values. Inspiratory time is defined as the time interval between the start of inspiratory flow and the beginning of expiratory flow. If one or more variables (pressure, flow, or volume) is not allowed to rise above a preset value during the inspiratory time, it is termed a limit variable. Note that in this definition, inspiration does not end when the variable reaches its preset value. The breath delivery continues, but the variable is held at the fixed, preset value. Figure 7-25 provides a useful algorithm for determining the limit variable during the inspiratory phase.

Cycle Variable

Inspiration ends when a specific variable (pressure, flow, volume, or time) is reached. This variable must be measured by the ventilator and used as a feedback signal to end inspiratory flow delivery, which then allows exhalation to begin (Figure 7-25).

Again it is easy to make false assumptions regarding many ventilators by classifying them as volume-cycled. Most newer ventilators measure flow, and are flow controllers. Since flow is measured and used as a feedback signal for gas delivery, volume becomes a function of flow and time (volume = flow × time). Therefore, these ventilators are really time-cycled, rather than "volume-cycled." Inspiration ends because a preset time interval has passed, and volume has not been directly measured.

Baseline Variable

Expiratory time is defined as the interval between the start of expiratory flow and the beginning of inspiratory flow. This is also termed the expiratory phase. The variable, which is controlled during the expiratory phase or expiratory time, is termed the baseline variable. Most commonly, pressure is controlled during the expiratory phase.

Applications of Positive End Expiratory Pressure (PEEP) and Continuous Positive Airway Pressure (CPAP) are used to increase the Functional Residual Capacity (FRC), to improve gas distribution and oxygenation. These pressures, when applied during exhalation, maintain the lungs in a partially inflated state. This helps to prevent alveolar collapse, recruit previously collapsed alveoli, and distend those alveoli which are already patent. PEEP and CPAP pressures must be titrated carefully, monitoring hemodynamic functions, blood gases or oximetry, and compliance, to achieve the greatest benefit with the least amount of detrimental side effects.

Conditional Variable

Conditional variables are defined as patterns of variables that are controlled by the ventilator during the ventilatory cycle. Early ventilators, such as the Puritan-Bennett MA-1, used relatively simple conditional variables (volume-cycled, pressure-limited, pressure-triggered, and PEEP). Newer third-generation microprocessor controlled ventilators, such as the Puritan-Bennett 7200ae, are capable of delivering complex ventilatory patterns. Figure 7-26 summarizes the ventilator classification system as described to this point.

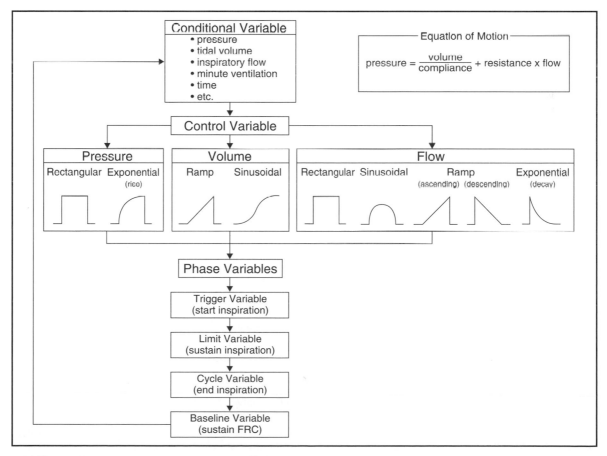

Figure 7-26 *A summary of the ventilator classification system as described by Robert L. Chatburn. (From R.L. Chatburn,* Respiratory Care, *37, No. 9, copyright 1992. Reprinted with permission.)*

OUTPUT WAVEFORMS

Output waveforms are graphical representations of the control or phase variables in relation to time. Output waveforms are typically presented in the order of pressure, volume, and flow. The ventilator determines the shape of the control variable, while the other two are dependent upon the patient's compliance and resistance. Convention dictates that flow values above the horizontal axis are inspiratory, while flow below the horizontal axis is expiratory. This corresponds to pressure and flow values rising above the horizontal axis for inspiration and falling back to the baseline during expiration. The ideal waveforms are represented in Figure 7-27.

Careful observation and assessment of waveforms during mechanical ventilation can provide useful information for the clinician. Waveforms can assist the clinician in the detection of inadvertent PEEP, the patient's ventilatory work, resistance, and compliance changes as well as many other events or changes. Some ventilators are able to present pressure versus volume waveforms to assist in minimizing the patient's work of breathing. Still other manufacturers can present flow versus volume waveforms to aid in the assessment of bronchodilator therapy during mechanical ventilation and the assessment of airway obstruction. As waveforms become widely used, their usefulness will approach that of the electrocardiogram (ECG) tracing in the assessment of the heart.

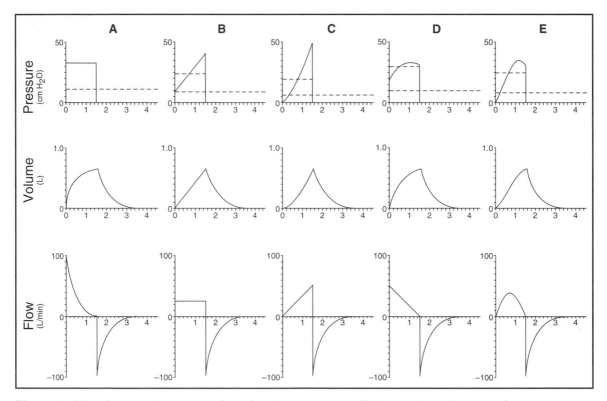

Figure 7-27 *Theoretical output waveforms for (A) pressure-controlled inspiration with rectangular pressure waveform, identical to flow-controlled inspiration with an exponential-decay flow waveform; (B) flow-controlled inspiration with rectangular flow waveform, identical to volume-controlled inspiration with an ascending-ramp flow waveform; (C) flow-controlled inspiration with an ascending-ramp flow waveform; (D) flow-controlled inspiration with a descending-ramp flow waveform; and (E) flow-controlled inspiration with a sinusoidal flow waveform. The short dashed lines represent mean inspiration pressure, while the longer dashed lines denote mean airway pressure (assuming zero end-expiratory pressure). For the rectangular pressure waveform in (A), the mean inspiratory pressure is the same as the peak inspiratory pressure. These output waveforms were created by (1) defining the control waveform (e.g., an ascending-ramp flow waveform is specified as flow = constant 3 time) and specifying that tidal volume equals 644 mL (about 9 mL/kg for a normal adult); (2) specifying the desired values for resistance and compliance (for these waveforms, compliance = 20 mL/cm H_2O and resistance = 20 cm H_2O/L/sec, according to ANSI recommendations); (3) substituting the above information into the equation of motion; and (4) using a computer to solve the equation for pressure, volume, and flow and plotting the results against time. (From R.L. Chatburn, Respiratory Care, 36, No. 10, copyright 1991. Reprinted with permission.)*

Pressure Waveforms

Pressure waveforms include rectangular, exponential, sinusoidal, and oscillating (Figure 7-28). Each of these waveforms would have these characteristic shapes, providing that pressure is the control variable. The descriptor used to describe each waveform is based upon its respective shape.

The rectangular waveform is characterized by a near instantaneous rise to a peak pressure value, which is held to the start of exhalation. During expiration, the pressure rapidly drops to baseline.

The exponential waveform is depicted by a more gradual increase in pressure when compared with the rectangular waveform. This type of waveform is common in some infant ventilators and has become an option on some adult ventilators. Ventilator settings such as flow and inspiratory time regulate how steep the waveform rises toward peak inspiratory pressure.

The sinusoidal waveform resembles one-half of a sine wave (the positive portion.).

Sinusoidal waveforms are characteristically produced by ventilators having a rotary-driven piston drive mechanism (Figure 7-29). Ventilators using this drive mechanism include the Emerson 3-MV, Respironics PLV-100, Bear 33, and the Puritan-Bennett LP-10.

The oscillating waveform is usually produced by a high frequency ventilator, such as the Infrasonics Star. The waveform is unique, in that negative (sub-ambient) pressures may be generated if the average pressure, or mean pressure, is near zero (ambient).

Volume Waveforms

Volume waveforms can be classified into two types, (1) ascending ramp and (2) sinusoidal. The ascending ramp waveform is produced by a constant (i.e., rectangular) inspiratory flow pattern. The shape is characterized by a linear rise to the peak inspiratory pressure value. Sinusoidal volume waveforms are produced by ventilators that have a rotary-driven piston drive mechanism

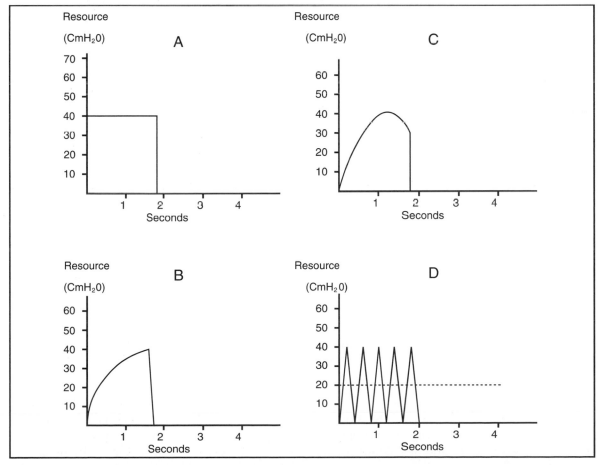

Figure 7-28 *The four types of pressure waveforms: (A) rectangular, (B) exponential, (C) sinusoidal, and (D) oscillating.*

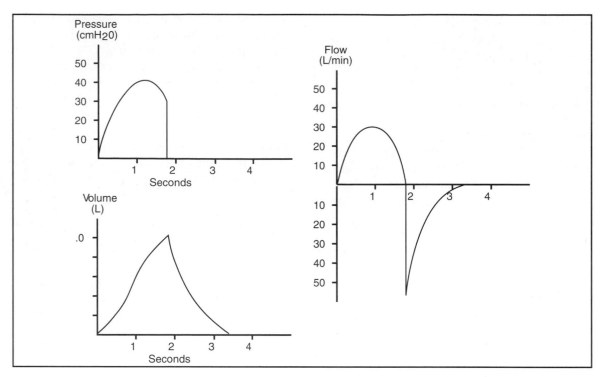

Figure 7-29 *The sinusoidal pressure waveform illustrated with the corresponding volume and flow waveforms. This type of pattern is typical of a rotary-driven piston drive mechanism.*

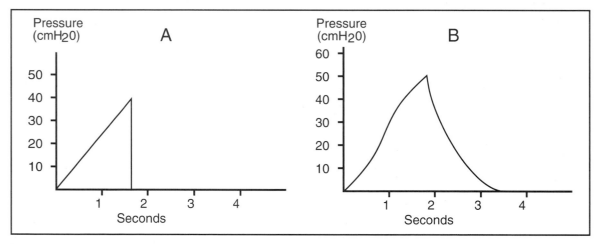

Figure 7-30 *The two types of volume waveforms: (A) ascending ramp and (B) sinusoidal.*

(Figure 7-30). Ventilators using this drive mechanism include the Emerson 3-MV, Respironics PLV-100, Bear 33, and Puritan-Bennett LP-10.

Flow Waveforms

The types of flow waveforms are shown in Figure 7-31. The waveforms include rectangular, ramp (ascending and descending), and sinusoidal.

The rectangular waveform is produced when volume is the control variable and the output is an ascending ramp. The flow waveform (a derivative of the volume waveform with respect to time) assumes the characteristic rectangular shape.

The ramp waveform can either be ascending or descending (Figure 7-31). If flow rises as the breath is delivered, it is termed ascending ramp. If flow falls during the ventilator supported breath, it is called descending ramp.

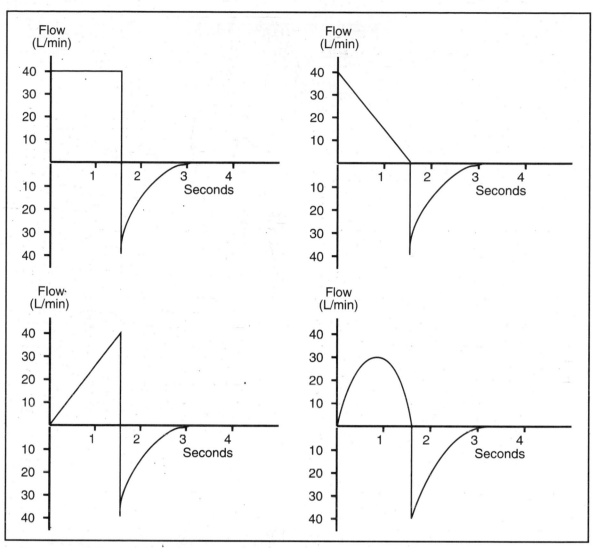

Figure 7-31 *The four types of flow waveforms: (A) rectangular, (B) ascending ramp, (C) descending ramp, and (D) sinusoidal.*

The sinusoidal waveform, as described earlier and illustrated in Figure 7-30B, resembles the positive portion of a sine wave. It is generated by a rotary-driven piston drive mechanism. ·

PATIENT CIRCUIT

The ventilator circuit may be classified as a single or double circuit. A single circuit is one in which the gas that drives the ventilator is the same gas that is delivered to the patient (Figure 7-32A). A double circuit uses an independent gas source in the drive mechanism, while a separate gas source is delivered to the patient (Figure 7-32B).

The patient's ventilator circuit also has an effect on the output of the ventilator during supported breaths. The circuit (tubing) has its own characteristic compliance, and the gas, as it flows through the circuit, becomes compressed. Therefore, if one were to measure control or phase variables, or waveforms, at the airway, they would be different than if measured at the ventilator.

The volume delivered to the patient may be calculated from the following equation:

Volume delivery =

$$\frac{1}{1 + \dfrac{C_{pc}}{C_{rs}}} \text{ (volume setting on ventilator)}$$

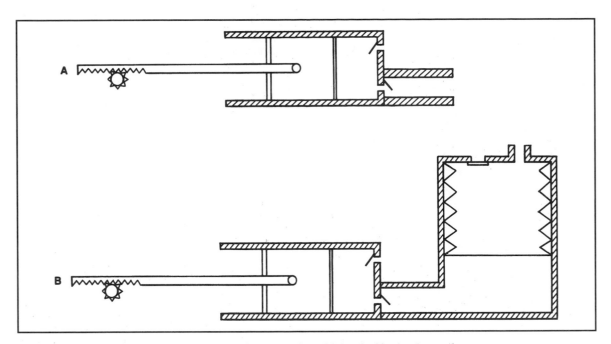

Figure 7-32 *A schematic representation of (A) a single and (B) a double circuit ventilator.*

where C_{pc} is the compliance of the patient circuit (tubing compliance) and C_{rs} is the compliance of the patient's lungs and thorax. As the compliance of the ventilator circuit increases when compared to the patient, volume delivery to the patient decreases.

Tubing compliance may be calculated using the following formula:

$$C_{pc} = \frac{V_{T\text{-set}}}{P_{plateau} - EEP}$$

where $V_{T\text{-set}}$ is the set tidal volume delivered through the ventilator circuit, $P_{plateau}$ is the plateau pressure, and EEP is the end expiratory pressure.

Washout time refers to the time necessary for a change in F_IO_2 to stabilize at the patient's airway. For example, if a patient is being ventilated at an F_IO_2 of 0.30 and you change the F_IO_2 to 1.0 in order to hyperoxygenate before suctioning, it may take several minutes before 100% oxygen is delivered to the airway. Washout time depends upon the ventilator settings (rate and tidal volume), length of the ventilator circuit, and whether or not the ventilator has a large internal volume (reservoir, accumulator, bellows, etc.).

Positive End Expiratory Pressure (PEEP)

As you recall from earlier in this chapter, PEEP is the application of positive pressure during the expiratory phase. Before ventilators were designed that incorporated PEEP systems into their circuitry, PEEP was added by placing a device on the expiratory limb of the patient circuit. These devices include water seals, water columns, Boeringer valves, Downs' valves, and magnetic valves.

Water Column

A **water column** is the simplest and most easily understood PEEP device (Figure 7-33). A water seal consists of a large jar filled with water.

Figure 7-33 *A photograph of an underwater seal PEEP system.*

The expiratory limb of the circuit is immersed into the water to the desired level of PEEP. If 10 cmH$_2$O of PEEP is the clinical goal, the expiratory limb is submerged 10 cm below the level of the water. The patient, when exhaling, must first overcome the positive pressure from the water.

The advantages of this system are (1) simplicity and (2) cost. Disadvantages include (1) PEEP changes with evaporation, (2) personnel may spill the water, and (3) rapidly flowing gas splashes the water and creates a mess.

Water-Weighted Diaphragm

The Emerson water column is illustrated in Figure 7-34. The exhaled gas from the patient's circuit is directed against a diaphragm at the base of a water column. Water above the diaphragm provides the positive end expiratory pressure.

Advantages of this system include its smaller size and the fact that exhaled gas passing through it does not cause water to splash. Problems due to evaporation are less due to the smaller surface area of the water column.

The water column also may be mounted on the ventilator, so the likelihood of water spills is lessened.

Boeringer Valves

Boeringer valves are specially designed valves with a weighted ball (Figure 7-35). The weight of the ball determines the PEEP level. When the valve is placed on the expiratory limb, the patient's exhaled gas must overcome the pressure exerted by gravity's attraction on the ball, creating the PEEP level.

Advantages include the lack of problems associated with a water-type system and its compact size. The disadvantage is that PEEP pressures may be less than desired, or even lost entirely, if the valve is not absolutely vertical.

Downs' Valves

Downs' valves are one example of spring-loaded PEEP valves. The Downs' valve is a fixed value PEEP valve. Other spring-type valves are adjustable. Figure 7-36 is an illustration of a Downs' valve. Exhaled gas passing the diaphragm must overcome spring tension, thus creating the PEEP. The Downs' valve has the advantage of being small, inexpensive, and capable of being used in any position without altering PEEP levels.

Figure 7-34 *A functional diagram of the Emerson Water Column PEEP/CPAP generator.*

Figure 7-35 *A schematic drawing of a Boeringer valve PEEP/CPAP generation device.*

Figure 7-36 *A schematic of a Downs' CPAP/PEEP valve.*

Magnetic Valves

Magnetic valves utilize a permanent magnet and a ferrous metal diaphragm (Figure 7-37). The threaded barrel of the valve allows the position of the magnet to change in relation to the diaphragm, varying the amount of magnetic attraction between them. As magnet attraction increases, more pressure must be generated to overcome it, increasing the positive pressure within the circuit, thereby creating PEEP.

Intermittent Mandatory Ventilation (IMV) Systems

Long before current-generation ventilators offered SIMV as a feature, these systems were added externally to the ventilator circuits. The disadvantage of external IMV systems is that, since they are not synchronized with the patient, it is possible to deliver a mandatory

Figure 7-37 *A schematic drawing of a magnetic CPAP/PEEP valve.*

breath following the patient's spontaneous breath (breath stacking). IMV systems may be divided into open and closed IMV systems.

Open IMV System

In this system, a blender or oxygen mixer powers a heated nebulizer (Figure 7-38). Gas from the nebulizer flows to an aerosol T (Brigg's adapter) and a reservoir of large-bore tubing open to the atmosphere (hence the open system name). Gas is then conducted to a one-way valve attached to the inspiratory limb of the patient circuit. When the patient inhales, the one-way valve opens in response to the pressure change and gas flows to the patient's lungs. During a mandatory breath, positive pressure closes the one-way valve, causing the breath to be delivered to the patient. Occasionally, you may be required to construct this type of circuit for home care ventilators that do not have IMV built into their control functions.

Closed IMV System

A closed IMV system is shown in Figure 7-39. This may also be referred to as an IMV "H" valve. An oxygen blender mixes air and oxygen to the desired F_IO_2 and the gas is conducted to a nipple that supplies flow to a 4- to

Figure 7-38 *An open IMV system.*

5-liter reservoir bag. Gas flows from the reservoir bag through a one-way valve to the ventilator's humidifier. The humidifier warms and humidifies the inspired gas going to the patient. When the patient initiates an inspiratory effort, the one-way valve opens in response to the pressure change, delivering gas. During a mandatory breath, the positive pressure in the ventilator circuit closes the one-way valve, causing gas from the ventilator to be delivered to the patient. Occasionally, you may be required to construct this type of circuit for home care ventilators that do not have IMV built into their control functions.

Continuous Positive Airway Pressure (CPAP) Systems

CPAP systems may be freestanding or incorporated into the new generation's ventilator systems. A freestanding CPAP system is shown in Figure 7-40. The oxygen blender mixes the gases to the desired F_1O_2. Gas is then conducted through a humidifier (others may be substituted for the Cascade shown), which warms and humidifies it. The gas then is

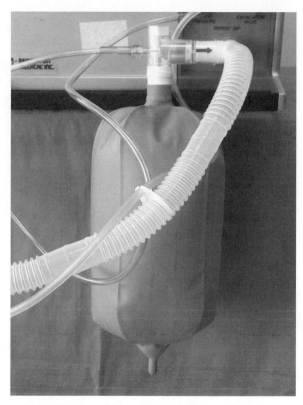

Figure 7-39 *A closed IMV system.*

Figure 7-40 *A CPAP system.*

Figure 7-41 *A one-way valve assembly for a CPAP system.*

directed to two places: a reservoir bag and positive pressure device, and the patient. The reservoir bag typically has a 3- to 5-liter capacity and provides a large reserve in the event the patient has an instantaneously high flow or volume demand. The positive pressure device may be any of the PEEP devices described earlier. The patient limb of the circuit consists of a Rudolph valve (Figure 7-41), which is a unidirectional valve composed of two one-way valves in series and another positive pressure PEEP device. It is important to note that the pressures of both PEEP devices must be equal; otherwise, a pressure differential will exist, resulting in undesirable gas flow.

CPAP with IMV

A circuit may be constructed to provide CPAP during the spontaneous ventilation portion of IMV and PEEP during the mandatory breaths (Figure 7-42). The CPAP side functions identically to the CPAP system described above. The gas from the CPAP system is delivered to the inspiratory limb of the patient circuit through a one-way valve. The ventilator circuit incorporates a PEEP device on the expiratory limb of the circuit. Both the PEEP device and the CPAP pressure device must be of equal value.

When the patient inhales spontaneously, gas is drawn from the CPAP system at a pressure greater than ambient. During exhalation, the one-way valve closes, and the exhaled gas passes through the PEEP valve on the expiratory limb, maintaining positive pressure. During the mandatory portion of the IMV, the system functions identically to a ventilator with a PEEP device added to the expiratory limb of the circuit.

ALARM SYSTEMS

Alarm systems are designed to alert the clinician to events. Day and MacIntyre have defined an event as any condition that requires clinician awareness or action. As the complexity of mechanical ventilators has increased, so have the number and complexity of the alarm systems. Technical events are those events limited to the performance of the ventilator, while patient events are those relating to the patient's condition. Alarms can be visual, audible, or both, depending upon the seriousness of the event.

Input Power Alarms

Input power alarms can be further classified as to loss of electrical or pneumatic power.

Loss of electrical power usually results in the ventilator activating a backup alarm, which is battery powered. Most battery backup alarms are powered by rechargeable nickel cadmium batteries, which are recharged when alternating current power is available. When commercial power is lost, the backup batteries activate audible and visual alarms.

Loss of either air or oxygen pneumatic sources will result in a technical event alarm. If either input pressure falls below a specified value from 50 psi, the alarm will result. Some alarms are electronic (BEAR 1000, BEAR I, II, and III, Puritan-Bennett 7200ae), while others are pneumatic reed alarms, such as those employed in oxygen blenders.

Control Circuit Alarms

Control circuit alarms alert the clinician to settings or parameters that are not within acceptable ranges or specifications, or indicate that the ventilator has failed some part of a self-diagnostic test. In the event of an incompatible setting or parameter, the clinician is allowed the opportunity to change the input to one that is compatible. A failure of a ventilator self-diagnostic test may render the ventilator inoperative, with a message displayed to the clinician indicating that failure has occurred.

Output Alarms

Output alarms can be further subdivided into pressure, volume, flow, time, inspiratory, and expiratory gas.

Pressure alarms include high/low peak, mean, and baseline airway pressures. High and low values may be set for each of these output parameters, to alert the clinician to changes in the patient's physiological status.

Additionally, an alarm may be provided to detect failure of the airway pressure to return to the baseline valve. This could be caused by airway obstructions, circuit obstructions, or ventilator malfunctions.

Volume alarms include high/low exhaled tidal volumes for both ventilator-supported breaths and spontaneous breaths. Low volumes may result from sedation (spontaneous volumes), disconnection, or apnea (spontaneous volumes).

Flow alarms are limited to exhaled minute volume. High and low values may be set on some ventilators to alert the clinician to changes in the patient's minute ventilation.

Time alarms include high/low frequency or rate, excessive or inadequate inspiratory time, and excessive or inadequate expiratory time. High/low ventilatory rate alarms alert the clinician to changes in the patient's venti-

Figure 7-42 *A circuit that provides CPAP with IMV.*

latory rate. Inspiratory and expiratory time alarms may alert the practitioner to circuit obstructions or malfunctions, changes in gas distribution, or inappropriate ventilator settings.

Inspired gas alarms alert the clinician to changes in oxygen concentration or gas temperature. Some ventilators incorporate an oxygen analyzer to detect changes in F_IO_2. High/low alarms alert the clinician to these changes. Inspired gas temperature may be controlled by a servo-controlled humidifier or monitored by an independent ventilator temperature alarm. High/low temperature alarms can alert the clinician to changes in the inspiratory gas temperature.

Exhaled oxygen tension or end tidal carbon dioxide tension can be monitored and high/low alarms can be servoed to the exhaled gas monitoring system. These monitors can assist the clinician in determining the V_D/V_T, gas exchange and the respiratory exchange ratio (R).

MODES OF VENTILATION

Ventilators operate in different ways to provide support to patients in respiratory failure. Not all patients require full ventilatory support. The availability of different modes of ventilation allows the practitioner to adjust the level of support to meet a given patient's needs. The next section of this chapter will describe the various modes of mechanical ventilation and classify them according to the system described by Robert Chatburn.

Continuous Mandatory Ventilation (CMV)

As the name implies, continuous mandatory ventilation (CMV) supports a patient in respiratory failure (Figure 7-43). The ventilator determines when and how much gas is given.

The ventilator initiates inspiration and the inspiratory phase is terminated based on volume, pressure, time, or flow. In CMV, the patient is unable to initiate inspiration. All the patient's spontaneous efforts are ignored by the ventilator. This mode should only be used if a patient is apneic or if ventilation is suppressed by the use of drugs such as Pavulon. Any attempt to use control mode on a patient with spontaneous ventilator efforts may result in asynchronous ventilation and an increase in the work of breathing.

CMV is only classified according to what occurs during the mandatory breaths, since no spontaneous ventilation is permitted. The control variables may be pressure, volume, or flow; the trigger variable is time; the limit variable may be pressure, volume, or flow; the cycle variable may be time, pressure, volume, or flow; and there are no conditional variables. Table 7-5 compares CMV with the other ventilator modes currently available.

Assist/Control

The **assist/control** allows the patient to initiate a breath (Figure 7-44). These ventilators have a sensitivity or assist system that will respond to the patient's inspiratory effort by opening the main solenoid valve, delivering a breath. If the patient fails to initiate a breath, the ventilator functions automatically, as in CMV, and ventilates the patient. This backup rate guarantees that the patient will receive an adequate minute ventilation to support their physiological needs. Note that when pressure falls below baseline pressure, the ventilator initiates inspiration. Besides being pressure triggered as shown in Figure 7-44, this mode may also be volume or flow triggered, depending upon what ventilator is being used (manufacturer specific).

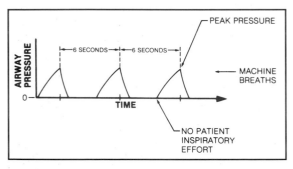

Figure 7-43 *A graphical representation of Continuous Mandatory Ventilation (CMV).*

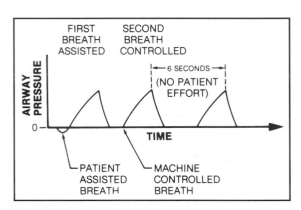

Figure 7-44 *A graphical representation of Assist/Control ventilation.*

TABLE 7-5 Expanded Classification of Modes of Ventilator Operation

| Mode | Mandatory Breath | | | | Spontaneous Breath | | | | | Control Logic | |
	Control	Trigger	Limit	Cycle	Control	Trigger	Limit	Cycle	Supported	Conditional Variable	Action
CMV*	Pressure, volume, or flow	Time	Pressure, volume, or flow	Time, pressure, volume, or flow	—	—	—	—	—	—	—
A/C	Pressure, volume, or flow	Time, pressure, volume, or flow	Pressure, volume, or flow	Time, pressure, volume, or flow	—	—	—	—	—	Time or patient effort	Machine-to-patient triggered
AMV	Pressure, volume, or flow	Pressure, volume, or flow	Pressure, volume, or flow	Time, pressure, volume, or flow	—	—	—	—	—	—	—
IMV	Pressure, volume, or flow	Time	Pressure, volume, or flow	Time, pressure, volume, or flow	Pressure	Pressure, volume, or flow	Pressure	Pressure	No	—	—
SIMV	Pressure, volume, or flow	Time, pressure, volume, or flow	Pressure, volume, or flow	Time, pressure, volume, or flow	Pressure	Pressure, volume, or flow	Pressure	Pressure	No	Time or patient effort	Machine-to-patient triggered
CPAP	—	—	—	—	Pressure	Pressure, volume, or flow	Pressure	Pressure	No	—	—
PCV	Pressure	Time	Pressure	Time	—	—	—	—	—	—	—
PC-IMV	Pressure	Time	Pressure	Time	Pressure	Pressure, volume, or flow	Pressure	Pressure	No	—	—

(continues)

TABLE 7-5 Expanded Classification of Modes of Ventilator Operation *(continued)*

Mode	Mandatory Breath				Spontaneous Breath					Control Logic	
	Control	Trigger	Limit	Cycle	Control	Trigger	Limit	Cycle	Supported	Conditional Variable	Action
PC-SIMV	Pressure	Time, pressure, volume, or flow	Pressure	Time	Pressure	Pressure, volume, or flow	Pressure	Pressure	No	Time or patient effort	Machine-to-patient triggered
PCIRV	Pressure	Time	Pressure	Time	Pressure						
APRV	Pressure	Time or pressure	Pressure	Time	Pressure	Pressure, volume, or flow	Pressure	Pressure	No	Time or patient effort	Machine-to-patient triggered
PSV	—	—	—	—	Pressure	Pressure, volume, or flow	Pressure	Volume	Yes		
MMV	Volume or flow	Time	Volume or flow	Time, volume, or flow	Pressure	Pressure, volume, or flow	Pressure	Pressure or volume	Yes*	Minute ventilation, time	Spontaneous-to-mandatory breath
VAPS	Flow	Time or pressure	Flow	Time or volume	Pressure	Pressure or flow	Pressure	Flow	Yes*	Tidal volume	Pressure-to-volume control
BiPAP	Pressure	Time	Pressure	Time	Pressure	Pressure	Pressure	Pressure	No	—	—

*CMV = continuous mandatory ventilation; NA = not applicable; A/C = assist/control; AMV = assisted mechanical ventilation; IMV = intermittent mandatory ventilation; SIMV = synchronized intermittent mandatory ventilation; CPAP = continuous positive airway pressure; PCV = pressure-controlled ventilation; PC-IMV = pressure-controlled IMV; PCIRV = PC inverse-ratio ventilation; APRV = airway pressure release ventilation; PSV = pressure support ventilation; MMV = mandatory minute ventilation; VAPS = volume-assisted pressure support; BiPAP = bilevel positive airway pressure.

Source: "Technical description and classification of modes of ventilator operation" by R. D. Branson and R. L. Chatburn, Respiratory Care, September 1992, Vol. 37, No. 9, p. 1029. (Copyright 1992 Daedalus Enterprises, Inc. Adapted with permission.)

This mode of ventilation is only classified during mandatory portion, since spontaneous breathing without ventilatory support is not permitted. Control variables may be pressure, volume, or flow. Trigger variables may be time, pressure, volume, or flow. Limit variables may be pressure, volume, or flow. Cycle variables may be time, pressure, volume, or flow. Table 7-5 compares assist/control with other mechanical ventilation modes.

Assisted Mechanical Ventilation (AMV)

Assisted mechanical ventilation is a variation of assist/control in which there is no set respiratory rate. All breaths are patient-triggered, with pressure, flow, and volume as the trigger variables. Since no breaths are guaranteed as in assist/control, the patient's respiratory drive must be intact or hypoventilation and hypercarbia will result.

This mode is classified in the following way. Control variables may be pressure, volume, or flow. Trigger variables may be pressure, volume, or flow. Cycle variables may be time, pressure, volume, or flow. Table 7-5 compares the AMV classification with other ventilator modes.

Intermittent Mandatory Ventilation (IMV) and Synchronized Intermittent Mandatory Ventilation (SIMV)

IMV and SIMV will be considered together even though slight differences exist in the way each functions. Both IMV and SIMV modes allow the patient to breathe spontaneously between ventilator breaths (mandatory breaths). When spontaneously breathing, the patient determines his or her own rate and tidal volume (Figure 7-45). The ventilator rate or mandatory rate ensures that, should the patient fail to breathe enough, the ventilator will provide the ventilatory support needed.

Figure 7-45 *A graphical representation of SIMV ventilation.*

Most newer models of ventilators functioning in the SIMV modes rely on demand valve systems to provide the gas flow required by the patient. The patient's spontaneous efforts open the demand valve, and gas flows into the circuit to the patient.

When IMV was first described and used on adults, the circuit was added externally to the ventilator (this will be described later in the "Special Ventilatory Procedures" section). In this configuration, it is possible for the ventilator to deliver a breath after the patient has just taken one spontaneously. This is referred to as stacking breaths. Breath stacking results in unusually large tidal volumes and higher than normal peak airway pressures. However, research showed that most patients synchronized themselves with the ventilator.

SIMV eliminates breath stacking by synchronizing the mandatory breaths so that they are not delivered on top of a spontaneous breath. This is typically accomplished through the sensitivity controls of the ventilator. When a spontaneous effort is first sensed, the ventilator will deliver a mandatory breath.

Continuous Positive Airway Pressure (CPAP)

Continuous Positive Airway Pressure (CPAP) is the application of continuous positive pressure during both inspiration and expiration during spontaneous ventilation. The patient breathes at his or her own rate, tidal volume, and frequency. CPAP pressures increase the patient's FRC, improving gas exchange. No ventilator (machine) support is provided in terms of guaranteed tidal volumes or respiratory rates. During CPAP, baseline pressure is always greater than ambient pressure (Figure 7-46).

Since CPAP is purely a spontaneous mode, only that portion is classified. The control variable is pressure (set CPAP pressure above ambient pressure). The trigger variable may be pressure, volume, or flow. The limit variable and the cycle variable are both pressure (Table 7-5).

Pressure Controlled Ventilation (PCV)

Pressure Controlled Ventilation (PCV) is a form of continuous mandatory ventilation in which all breaths are pressure limited and time cycled. All ventilation is provided by the mechanical ventilator.

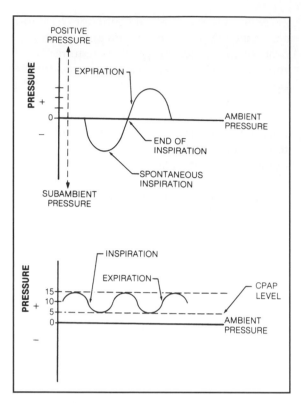

Figure 7-46 *A graphical representation of CPAP.*

Pressure controlled ventilation may be provided during CMV as described above or also utilized in conjunction with IMV or SIMV. When employed in conjunction with these modes, the mandatory breaths (machine) are all pressure controlled, time triggered, pressure limited, and time cycled. The spontaneous breaths are pressure controlled, pressure volume or flow triggered, pressure limited, and pressure cycled. Table 7-5 compares the classification of PCV-IMV and PCV-SIMV with the other modes of ventilation.

Pressure Regulated Volume Control (PRVC) Ventilation

In pressure regulated volume control (PRVC) ventilation, tidal volume or minute volume is set to deliver a constant value (per breath or per minute's time interval). A mandatory rate is also set for the patient. Pressure during inspiration is limited to a maximum value of 5 cmH_2O below the level set for the pressure limit. The breaths can be patient or time triggered.

The ventilator delivers a sequence of test breaths beginning at 5 cmH_2O and then compares the volume/pressure value for the previous breath. Pressure can change +3 cmH_2O from one breath to the next. If the measured

volume (tidal or minute volume) is too high, pressure will be reduced. If it is too low, pressure will be increased. The pressure delivery is automatically regulated between the PEEP level set and 5 cmH_2O below the pressure limit setting.

Inverse Ratio Ventilation

Pressure Controlled, Inverse Ratio Ventilation (PCIRV)

Pressure Controlled, Inverse Ratio Ventilation (PCIRV) is a form of PCV in which no patient triggered breaths are permitted. Additionally, the inspiratory time is longer than the expiratory time (inverse ratio), resulting in I:E ratios varying between 4:1 and 1:1.1. The inverse I:E ratio results in gas trapping, which causes an increase in the baseline pressure above ambient pressure.

PCIRV is classified as a pressure controlled, time triggered, pressure limited, time cycled mode of ventilation (Table 7-5). The feature that distinguishes it from PCV is the inverse I:E ratio.

Volume Controlled Inverse Ratio Ventilation (VCIRV)

Volume controlled inverse ratio ventilation, like PCIRV, is a mode in which the inspiratory phase is longer than the expiratory phase (inverse ratio). In VCIRV, inspiratory time is extended directly (some ventilators allow this) or indirectly by reducing flow rates, use of descending ramp waveforms, and/or use of an inspiratory pause. However inspiration is extended, volume rather than pressure is the control variable.

Airway Pressure Release Ventilation (APRV)

Airway Pressure Release Ventilation (APRV) combines two separate levels of CPAP pressures. The patient may breathe spontaneously from both CPAP levels. The higher CPAP level provides for volume augmentation during the patient's spontaneous breathing. Periodically, pressure is dropped to the lower CPAP level, reducing mean airway pressure. The expiratory time is kept short to minimize the loss of FRC. Often, the I:E ratio is inverse as in PCIRV. The time spent at each different CPAP level is adjustable. In this mode, the mandatory (machine) breaths are those in which the pressure rises to the higher CPAP level.

Mandatory breaths in APRV are classified as pressure controlled, time or pressure triggered, pressure limited, and time cycled. The spontaneous breaths (lower CPAP level) are classified as pressured controlled, pressure, volume or flow triggered, pressure limited, and pressure cycled (Table 7-5).

BiPAP® (Bilevel Positive Airway Pressure)

BiPAP® is a trademark of Respironics, Inc. BiPAP® is another form of APRV except that pressure support (described later in this section) can be provided concurrently with the spontaneous ventilation. The clinician sets two pressure levels for BiPAP®, one pressure for inspiration—Inspiratory Positive Airway Pressure (IPAP)—and one for expiration—Expiratory Positive Airway Pressure (EPAP). If pressure support is delivered (mandatory breaths), they are time triggered and pressure limited.

BiPAP®'s mandatory breaths are classified as pressure controlled, time triggered, pressure limited, and time cycled. The spontaneous breaths are pressure controlled, pressure triggered, pressure limited, and pressure cycled (Table 7-5).

Pressure Support Ventilation (PSV)

Pressure support ventilation provides pressure augmentation during spontaneous breathing. The breath may be pressure, flow, or volume triggered. Once triggered, a set pressure is delivered above baseline to augment the patient's spontaneous tidal volume. The breath ends when the delivered flow drops to a percentage of the peak inspiratory flow (typically 25%). The patient then determines their rate, inspiratory time, and volume.

Pressure support is classified as pressure controlled, pressure, volume or flow triggered, pressure limited, and volume cycled. Table 7-5 compares pressure support with other modes of ventilation.

Mandatory Minute Ventilation (MMV)

Mandatory Minute Ventilation (MMV) automatically adjusts minute ventilation based upon the patient's spontaneous ventilation. The practitioner selects the minute ventilation that is desired for the patient and adjusts the ventilator's tidal volume and flow to accom-plish it. If the patient's spontaneous ventilation meets or exceeds the set mandatory ventilation, no supported breaths are delivered. If the patient's spontaneous ventilation falls below the set mandatory ventilation level, supported breaths are given by the ventilator to ensure that the desired minute ventilation is met (at the set tidal volume and flow rate). Some ventilators accomplish the MMV minute volume using pressure support rather than mandatory breaths. This mode is helpful during weaning, when a patient may become fatigued and not breathe enough spontaneously to sustain physiological needs.

MMV's mandatory breaths are classified as volume or flow controlled, time triggered, volume, or flow limited, and time, volume or flow cycled. The spontaneous breaths are pressure controlled, pressure, volume or flow triggered, pressure limited, and volume cycled. Table 7-5 compares MMV with the other modes of ventilation.

Volume Assured Pressure Support (VAPS)

Volume Assured Pressure Support (VAPS) is a form of pressure support that assures that the patient will receive a specific tidal volume during pressure supported breaths. If the patient's pressure supported volume falls below minimum tidal volume desired by the clinician, flow is held constant, allowing pressure to rise until the desired volume has been delivered.

With VAPS, a given breath may be either a flow-controlled, mandatory breath (i.e., flow limited and volume cycled) or a pressure-controlled, spontaneous breath (i.e., pressure limited, flow cycled) depending on the relative values of the ventilator settings (i.e., pressure limit, flow limit, and tidal volume) and patient effort. Table 7-5 compares VAPS with the other modes of ventilation.

Proportional Assist Ventilation (PAV)

Proportional assist ventilation (PAV) is a mode of ventilation in which airway pressures are increased or decreased in proportion to the patient's effort. As the patient's demand (effort) increases or decreases, the ventilator's support (pressure) responds by increasing or decreasing as well. PAV is thought to improve ventilator synchrony. Since the ventilator is responding to patient effort on a breath-by-breath basis, a more physiologic breathing pattern may result. PAV is based upon the equation of motion, previously described in this chapter.

Adaptive Support Ventilation (ASV)

Adaptive support ventilation (ASV), like PAV, is a means of adapting or adjusting the ventilator's output on a breath-by-breath basis. The goal of ASV is to provide a preset minute ventilation, while at the same time minimizing the work of breathing.

The practitioner sets ASV mode by entering the patient's ideal body weight (kg) and the % minute volume (25–350%) to account for variations in the patient's dead space volume. The maximum pressure limit is set along with the pressure or flow trigger level. Rise time on the ascending ramp waveform is also adjusted.

If the patient is apneic, breaths are time triggered, pressure targeted, and time cycled. As the patient initiates spontaneous ventilation, the ventilator adjusts its support level based upon the amount of ventilatory work the patient is able to provide. Tidal volume and rate delivery are targeted to be maintained automatically at a calculated ideal value.

CLINICAL CORNER

Flow and Pressure Measurement Equipment

1. You are called to check a patient on a BEAR 2 ventilator. The low tidal volume alarm intermittently sounds while you are monitoring the patient. What could you check or do to correct the situation?

PEEP/CPAP and IMV Equipment

1. The ventilator your home care company uses does not have provisions for PEEP. How can you set up the ventilator to provide the 10-cmH$_2$O PEEP the patient needs?

2. You need to supply PEEP for an intubated patient with a self-inflating manual resuscitator while you transport the patient from CT to the ICU. How will you do this using a manual resuscitator?

3. You need to provide IMV for a patient's home care ventilator. The ventilator does not have IMV as a built-in feature. How can you provide it?

Self-Assessment Quiz

1. Poiseuille's law is significant in mechanical ventilation and affects:
   I. gas flow through artificial airways.
   II. gas flow through patient circuits.
   III. driving pressure.
   IV. resistance.
   a. I only
   b. I and II
   c. I, II, and III
   d. I, II, III, and IV

2. Strain gauge pressure transducers may be used to measure:
   I. circuit pressures.
   II. blood pressure.
   III. central venous pressure.
   IV. intracranial pressure.
   a. I only
   b. I and II
   c. I, II, and III
   d. I, II, III, and IV

3. A vortex shedding spirometer measures flow by using:
   a. a differential pressure transducer.
   b. a strain gauge.
   c. a venturi tube.
   d. ultrasonic waves.

4. In contrast to a solenoid valve, a proportional solenoid valve:
   I. is either open or closed.
   II. easily responds to patient effort.
   III. opens in discrete intervals.
   IV. is often under microprocessor control.
   a. I only
   b. I and II
   c. II and III
   d. II, III, and IV

5. Ventilator drive mechanism refers to:
   a. the power source for the ventilator.
   b. the system used to convert the input power to ventilatory work.
   c. the system used to control rate and tidal volume.
   d. the gas pressure powering the ventilator.

6. Physics defines work as force times distance. The equivalent ventilatory work performed by the muscles of inspiration is:
   a. volume divided by compliance plus resistance times flow.
   b. pressure times compliance.
   c. pressure times volume.
   d. resistance times compliance.

7. If a ventilator is a volume controller
   I. a constant volume is delivered each breath.
   II. volume must be measured.
   III. flow is measured and used to control flow waveform.
   IV. the breath ends when a preset time is reached.
   a. I
   b. I and II
   c. I and III
   d. III and IV

8. A cycling variable is:
   a. the variable measured and used to begin inspiration.
   b. the variable measured and used to end inspiration.
   c. the variable measured and used to control inspiration.
   d. the variable measured and used during expiration.

9. A trigger variable is:
   a. the variable measured and used to begin inspiration.
   b. the variable measured and used to end inspiration.
   c. the variable measured and used to control inspiration.
   d. the variable measured and used during expiration.

10. Which of the following can be control variables?
    I. pressure
    II. volume
    III. flow
    IV. time
    a. I
    b. I and II
    c. I, II, and III
    d. I, II, III, and IV

11. Which of the following can be trigger variables?
    I. pressure
    II. volume
    III. flow
    IV. time
    a. I
    b. I and II
    c. I, II, and III
    d. I, II, III, and IV

12. The difference between a limit variable and a cycle variable is:
    I. inspiration does not end when the limit is met.
    II. the limit variable is not allowed to rise above a preset level.
    III. inspiration ends and an alarm sounds.
    IV. the variable is only measured during expiration.
    a. I
    b. I and II
    c. II and III
    d. III and IV

13. Expiratory time is defined as:
    a. the time between the start of inspiratory flow to the start of expiratory flow.
    b. the time between the start of expiratory flow and the start of inspiratory flow.
    c. the ratio of inspiratory to expiratory time.
    d. the time when baseline pressure is zero.

14. Types of pressure waveforms include:
    I. rectangular.
    II. exponential.
    III. sinusoidal.
    IV. oscillating.
    a. I
    b. I and II
    c. I, II, and III
    d. I, II, III, and IV

15. Types of flow waveforms include:
    I. rectangular.
    II. ramp.
    III. sinusoidal.
    IV. oscillating.
    a. I
    b. I and II
    c. I, II, and III
    d. I, II, III, and IV

16. Ventilator washout time refers to:
    a. the time required clean the ventilator following use.
    b. the time it takes gas to flow through the circuit..
    c. the amount of time before an F_IO_2 change reaches a stable value.
    d. the time necessary to exhale the tidal volume.

17. A single circuit ventilator:
    a. has one gas source, which drives the ventilator and is delivered to the patient.
    b. has only one tube from the ventialtor to the patient.
    c. uses one exhalation valve.
    d. takes less time to clean than a double circuit ventilator.

18. Which of the following are PEEP devices?
    I. Downs' valve
    II. water column

III. magnetic valve
IV. Boeringer valve
a. I
b. I and II
c. I, II, and III
d. I, II, III, and IV

19. Input power alarms include:
I. loss of electrical power.
II. failure of a self-diagnostic test.
III. loss of pneumatic power.
IV. low delivered tidal volume.
a. I and II
b. I and III
c. II and III
d. III and IV

20. Output alarms include:
I. failure of self-diagnostic test.
II. low delivered tidal volume.
III. loss of pneumatic power.
IV. flow alarms.
a. I and II
b. II and III
c. II and IV
d. III and IV

21. Which of the following are true regarding Pressure Controlled Ventilation (PCV)?
I. It can be employed during CMV, IMV or SIMV.
II. Pressure is the control variable.
III. Pressure is the limit variable.
IV. Volume or flow may be the trigger variable.
a. I
b. I and II
c. I, II, and III
d. I, II, III, and IV

22. Which of the following are true regarding CPAP?
I. Pressure is the control variable.
II. Pressure or flow may be the trigger variable.
III. Pressure is the limit variable.
IV. Pressure is the cycle variable.
a. I
b. I and II
c. I, II, and III
d. I, II, III, and IV

23. A mode of ventilation that allows spontaneous breathing but guarantees a minimum minute ventilation is:
a. assist/control.
b. SIMV.
c. pressure support.
d. MMV.

24. A mode of ventilation that augments spontaneous ventilation with a constant positive pressure is:
a. assist/control.
b. SIMV.
c. pressure support.
d. MMV.

25. A mode of ventilation that delivers mandatory breaths irrespective of patient effort is:
    a. CMV.
    b. assist/control.
    c. SIMV.
    d. MMV.

26. Fluidic logic operates using:
    a. Bernoulli's principle.
    b. Venturi's principle.
    c. the Coanda effect.
    d. electronic elements.

27. A fluidic element commonly used to control the cycling of a ventilator between inspiration and expiration is:
    a. a back pressure switch.
    b. a flip-flop.
    c. an or/nor.
    d. an and/nand.

28. A fluidic element often used to sense a patient's inspiratory effort is:
    a. a back pressure switch.
    b. a flip-flop.
    c. a Schmidt trigger.
    d. an or/nor.

29. Truth tables are used to:
    a. describe the logic of the fluidic element.
    b. determine when it is off.
    c. combine one element with another.
    d. all of the above.

30. What fluidic element does the Sechrist IV-100B use to initiate inspiration?
    a. a back pressure switch
    b. a flip-flop
    c. a Schmidt trigger
    d. an or/nor

Selected Bibliography

Aequitron Medical, Inc. (1987). *LP-6 volume ventilator reference manual.* Minneapolis.

Albert, R. K. (1988). Non-respiratory effects of positive end-expiratory pressure. *Respiratory Care, 33*(6), 464–471.

Banner, M. J. (1987). Expiratory positive-pressure valves: Flow resistance and work of breathing. *Respiratory Care, 32*(6), 431–439.

Bear Medical Systems. (1977). *Instruction manual, Bourns adult volume ventilator (Bear I), part number 5000-10500.* Riverside.

Bear Medical Systems. (1983). *Instruction manual, Bear 5, part number 50000-10700.* Riverside.

Bear Medical Systems. (1984). *Bear 33 volume ventilator clinical instruction manual, part number 50000-10133.* Riverside.

Bear Medical Systems. (1974). *Instruction manual, Bourns infant pressure ventilator (Model BP200), part number 50000-10200.* Riverside.

Bird Products Corporation. (1991). *VIP Bird infant-pediatric ventilator instruction manual, part number L1194.* Palm Springs.

Branson, R. D., et al. (2002). Closed-loop mechanical ventilation. *Respiratory Care, 47,* 427–453.

Branson, R. D., & Chatburn, R. L. (1992). Technical description and classification of modes of ventilator operation. *Respiratory Care, 37*(9), 1026–1044.

Chatburn, R. L. (1991). A new system for understanding mechanical ventilators. *Respiratory Care, 36*(10), 1123–1155.

Chatburn, R. L. (1992). Classification of mechanical ventilators. *Respiratory Care, 37*(9), 1009–1025.

Nellcor Puritan-Bennett. (1999). *840 operator's and technical reference manual*. Carlsbad.

Siemens. *Servo[i] ventilator system user's manual*. Danvers.

CHAPTER 8

ADULT ACUTE CARE VENTILATORS: VENTILATORS HAVING VOLUME AS A CONTROL VARIABLE

INTRODUCTION

Chapter 7 described the ventilator classification system developed by Robert Chatburn. According to the classification system, ventilators can be classified according to their input power, drive mechanism (power conversion or transmission), control scheme, output, and alarm systems. In this chapter and the remaining chapters, the control variable has been chosen as a means to distinguish ventilators from one another as well as to group ventilators with common traits together.

Use of the input power and drive mechanism can be quite broad and all encompassing. Using these criteria for classification would include too many ventilators in one particular group and not allow sufficient differences to distinguish one from another. The same would be true by using output or alarm systems as a means to classify the various ventilators.

Classifying ventilators by their control variable will group smaller numbers of ventilators together while allowing sufficient detail to be added to the phase variables, output, and alarm systems to distinguish one ventilator from another's capabilities and control circuitry.

OBJECTIVES

After completing this chapter, the student will be able to accomplish the following objectives:

- Explain what is meant by the control variable and how specifically a ventilator can be classified as having volume as a control variable.
- For the ventilators described in this chapter, apply Chatburn's classification system and classify them according to:

    — Input power
    — Drive mechanism
    — Control scheme
    — Output
    — Alarm systems

- Describe how to assemble and trouble-shoot the Monaghan 225/SIMV ventilator.

THE CONTROL VARIABLE

During a ventilator-supported breath, a mechanical ventilator can control one of the following variables: pressure, volume, flow, or time. In order for a ventilator to be classified as controlling one of these variables, two con-ditions must be met. First that variable must be measured, and second it must be used as feedback to control the ventilator's output. Therefore, for a ventilator to be classified as a volume controller, volume must be measured and used as feedback to control the ventilator's output.

MONAGHAN 225/SIMV VENTILATOR

Input Power

The Monaghan 225/SIMV ventilator is a pneumatically powered and fluidically controlled ventilator (Figure 8-1A and B). The power sources required to operate the ventilator are a 50-psi air and oxygen medical gas source.

Drive Mechanism

The drive mechanism of the 225/SIMV ventilator is the 50-psi gas source. The incoming gas passes through a fluid amplifier (Figure 8-2) and then is directed through the flow rate control and into the bellows canister. The gas admitted to the bellows canister pressurizes it, causing the contents of the bellows to be emptied, delivering gas to the patient.

Control Scheme

Control Circuit

The Monaghan 225/SIMV ventilator is unique in that it is entirely fluid controlled. Various fluidic elements are used for regulation of control, phase, and output variables as well

Figure 8-1 *(A) The Monaghan 225/SIMV volume ventilator (B) The Monaghan 225/SIMV control panel.*

Figure 8-2 *A schematic of the Monaghan 225/SIMV pneumatic system. (Courtesy Monaghan Medical Corporation, Plattsburgh, NY.)*

as alarm systems. Each control system and its components will be discussed as the classification of the ventilator is further developed.

Control Variable

The control variable for the 225/SIMV is volume. Tidal volume is controlled by turning a crank at the base of the bellows canister, which causes the bottom of the bellows to rise or fall. The outside of the bellows canister is calibrated in liters, indicating the volume contained in the bellows. The volume of the bellows contents determines tidal volume delivery. When the bellows reaches the top of the canister, a control port is occluded, sending a control signal to the master flip-flop, terminating the inspiratory phase. Volume is adjustable from 0 to 3,000 mL.

Phase Variables

Trigger Variables

The trigger variables of the 225/SIMV are pressure, time, and manual triggering. The trigger sensitivity control establishes the effort required by the patient to initiate inspiration during assist/control and SIMV modes. Sensitivity may be adjusted from autocycling to a

−10 cmH$_2$O. The sensitivity system employs a Schmidt trigger in its operation (Figure 8-2).

Although a Schmidt trigger is represented schematically with one symbol, it is, in reality, a series of fluidic elements. The Schmidt trigger in the Monaghan 225/SIMV is composed of three proportional amplifiers and three flip-flop gates. The Schmidt trigger senses patient effort, amplifies it, and ultimately sends a control signal to initiate inspiration.

Sub-ambient pressure from the patient circuit is applied to the control-port of the patient trigger circuit (Figure 8-2). If enough sub-ambient pressure is generated, the patient trigger switches output from 4R to 2R. The new output is used as a control input for the master flip-flop, changing from expiration to inspiration.

Adjustment of the sensitivity control causes a needle valve to be opened or closed. Flow through the needle valve provides a reference signal to the second element in the patient trigger system. Flow from the needle valve is directed just opposite, from the sub-ambient pressure input from the patient. Increased flow, from the sensitivity control, causes beam deflection toward the sub-ambient input, therefore making it easier for the patient to initiate a breath.

In the absence of any spontaneous effort, the ventilator is time triggered. The rate control determines the frequency of ventilator-assisted breaths. The rate control determines the length of expiratory time. (This is discussed in the section on the cycle variable.)

The ventilator may also be manually triggered by depressing the manual inspiration button on the control panel. When depressed, a control signal is applied to the master flip-flop, initiating inspiration.

Limit Variable

Flow is the limit variable for the 225/SIMV ventilator. The flow rate control at the base of the bellows canister is a needle valve. Adjustment of the control regulates the flow of gas into the bellows canister. Flow rates are adjustable between near zero to 100 L/min.

Cycle Variable

There are several cycling variables for the Monaghan 225/SIMV ventilator. These include pressure, volume, and time.

Pressure. The ventilator is pressure cycled when the inspiratory pressure reaches the pressure set on the pressure limit control. The pressure limit control operates during CMV, assist/control, and the mandatory breaths during SIMV. When the pressure limit is reached, inspiration is terminated.

This control operates using a device similar to the sensitivity control. A control signal

(pressure from the patient circuit) provides a control input to a Schmidt trigger (Figure 8-3). If sufficient pressure is generated in the circuit, output changes, resulting in a control input to the master flip-flop. Output from the master flip-flop changes from 5L to 6R, ending inspiration.

Adjustment of the pressure limit control changes the position of a needle valve. Flow from the needle valve is directed opposite the control input signal (pressure in the patient circuit). Since in this case flow opposes the pressure signal, an increase in flow from the pressure limit control causes the ventilator to pressure limit (lower pressure) sooner.

Volume. Volume cycling occurs when the volume of the bellows is adjusted using the tidal volume control (crank) at the base of the bellows. This system was discussed earlier in the control variable section on this ventilator.

Time. The ventilator can be time cycled if inspiration is completed before the bellows reaches its control port at the top of the bellows canister. This is accomplished through a pneumatic timing device.

During inspiration, a small bellows (right-hand bellows, Figure 8-4) is filled by the output of the flip-flop gate to the right of the master flip-flop. Flow into the bellows chamber occurs at a constant rate since gas is admitted through a fixed orifice. Inspiratory time becomes a function of the distance the bellows travels before contacting the control port at the top of the bellows compartment. Adjustment

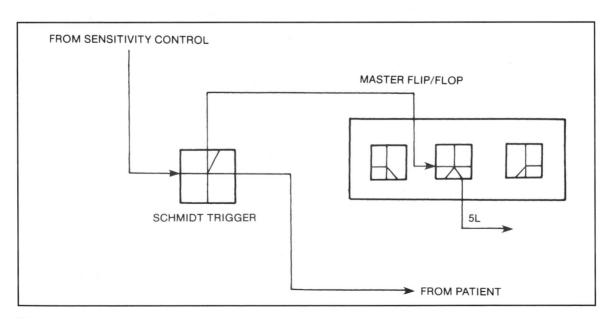

Figure 8-3 *A schematic of the Monaghan 225/SIMV assist/sensitivity system.*

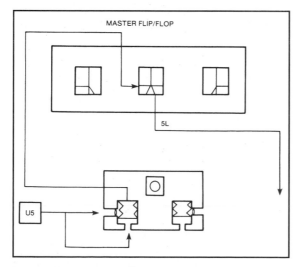

Figure 8-4 *Once the touch sensor closes contact, a signal is sent to the fluidic amplifier A2. The output from the fluidic amplifier changes the output of the master flip-flop from 5L to 5R, terminating inspiration.*

of the rate control causes the control port sensor to be moved closer to or farther from the bellows, increasing or decreasing inspiratory time.

The length of the expiratory time is controlled in a similar way. The small, left-hand bellows (Figure 8-5) is filled by gas from the U5 or/nor gate. Gas from the or/nor gate fills the bellows·through a fixed orifice, similar to the right-hand bellows described earlier. When the bellows contacts its control port, a signal is sent to the master flip-flop changing the output to 5L, beginning inspiration. Adjustment of the control port is also accomplished by adjustment of the rate control.

Figure 8-5 *A schematic of the Monaghan 225/SIMV timing mechanism during the expiratory phase.*

Baseline Variable

The baseline variable the ventilator controls is pressure (PEEP). Baseline pressure is adjustable from 0 to 20 cmH2O. The PEEP control is a needle valve. The PEEP control is supplied with gas pressure between 5 and 7 psi. Gas pressure is applied to a four-way crossover valve and to a resistance element that vents most of the pressure to the atmosphere (Figure 8-2). Output from the resistive element is conducted to the sensitivity system (to reference the sensitivity to PEEP pressure) and to the exhalation valve to achieve the desired PEEP level. Functionally, as the needle valve is opened, more gas flow goes to the exhalation valve, increasing its pressure, and increasing the PEEP pressure above ambient pressure.

Conditional Variables

Two conditional variables are employed during SIMV ventilation: pressure and time. During spontaneous ventilation, the exhalation valve is not pressurized, so gas is delivered to the patient in a flow-by fashion. Sub-ambient pressure, generated by the patient through the assist system, causes gas to be delivered from the bellows. Since gas is delivered under a slight pressure, the patient will not draw room air in through the patient circuit from the exhalation valve. Once the left-hand exhalation time bellows reaches its touch sensor, the next patient effort (pressure) will trigger a mandatory breath. The variable between mandatory breaths is time, which is determined by the rate control adjusting the position of the control port on the expiration time bellows.

Output
Output Waveforms

The Monaghan 225/SIMV delivers a rectangular flow and exponential pressure waveform. These waveforms were discussed in Chapter 7 and are illustrated in Figures 7-27 and 7-28, pp. 396-397.

Output Monitors

The ventilator has several output monitors including pressure, pressure cycle, time cycle, and tidal volume. The pressure in the patient circuit is displayed on an analog pressure gauge on the front panel of the ventilator. When the ventilator pressure cycles, a pressure cycle visual indicator changes color. (A colored lid covers the indicator window when pressure is applied to it.) The time cycle indicator changes color when the ventilator is time cycled and not volume cycled. It is an indicator similar in design to the pressure cycle indicator. The tidal volume is monitored by viewing the position of the bellows in relation to the calibration marks on the bellows canister.

Alarm Systems

The Monaghan 225/SIMV does not incorporate any audible alarms in its monitoring/alarm systems. The visual monitors were discussed in the previous section. An external pressure disconnect alarm is frequently added to alert the practitioner to any patient disconnect situations.

Modes of Ventilation

With the 225/SIMV ventilator, when operating in the CMV mode (Control), all breaths are time triggered, volume cycled, and pressure limited. If the inspiratory pressure reaches the setting on the pressure limit control prior to delivery of the full tidal volume, the breath is then time triggered and pressure cycled. The ventilator supported breath may also be time cycled if the inspiratory time ends prior to the delivery of the set tidal volume, as described earlier.

During assist/control all breaths are pressure or time triggered, pressure limited, and volume cycled. Similar circumstances, as described above, could result in either pressure or time cycling in lieu of volume cycling.

During SIMV, the mandatory breaths are pressure triggered, pressure limited, and volume cycled. The spontaneous breaths are pressure triggered, pressure limited, and pressure cycled.

Control Interactions

A significant control interaction is the relationship of the flow rate, tidal volume, and the respiratory rate on the inspiratory time. While inverse ratios are not possible, ratios as low as 1:1 may occur. When delivering large volumes, it is important to increase the flow rate to prevent the ventilator from time cycling.

Although the sensitivity system attempts to compensate for PEEP levels, full compensation does not occur. At high levels of PEEP

($20 \, cmH_2O$), the patient may need to generate inspiratory pressure of up to $4 \, cmH_2O$ below PEEP to initiate inspiration. Careful observation of the manometer is important to minimize the work of breathing when using higher levels of PEEP. Table 8-1 summarizes the capabilities of the Monaghan 225/SIMV.

The classification and operation of the Monaghan 225/SIMV was covered in this section. Table 8-2 illustrates the complete classification of this ventilator.

TABLE 8-1 Monaghan 225/SIMV Ventilator

Tidal Volume	0–3000 mL
Respiratory Rate	6–60 Breaths/minute
Expiratory Time	0.5–7.5 Seconds
Flow Rate	0.0–100 L/minute
Maximum Pressure	100 cmH_2O
PEEP	0.0–25 cmH_2O
Sensitivity	Autocycling–10.0 cmH_2O
Oxygen (F_IO_2)	.21–1.00
Modes	CMV, Assist/Control, SIMV

TABLE 8-2 Classification of Volume Controllers

Ventilator: Monaghan 225/SIMV

Input Power	Pneumatic
Circuit	Double
Drive Mechanism	Bellows
Control Mechanism	Fluidic
Control Variable	V
Trigger Variable	P/T/M
Limit Variable	F
Cycling Variable	P/V/T
Alarms	P/V/T

P — Pressure, T — Time, F — Flow,
V — Volume, M — Manual.

ASSEMBLY AND TROUBLESHOOTING

Assembly—Monaghan 225/SIMV

To assemble the Monaghan 225/ SIMV for use, follow the suggested assembly guide.

1. Connect the high pressure gas lines to 50-psi oxygen and air sources.

2. Assemble and fill the humidifier. Since various humidifiers may be used, specific assembly instructions will not be included here.

3. Connect a bacteria filter to the ventilator outlet using an appropriate adapter.

4. Connect the humidifier inlet to the bacteria filter using a length of large-bore tubing.

5. Connect the inspiratory limb of the patient circuit to the outlet of the humidifier.

6. Connect the exhalation valve tubing to the exhalation valve nipple on the ventilator.

7. If the use of an in-line nebulizer is desired, connect its drive line to the nebulizer nipple on the ventilator.

8. Pressure test the ventilator circuit.

Troubleshooting

ALG 8-1 illustrates a flowchart for troubleshooting the Monaghan 225/SIMV ventilator.

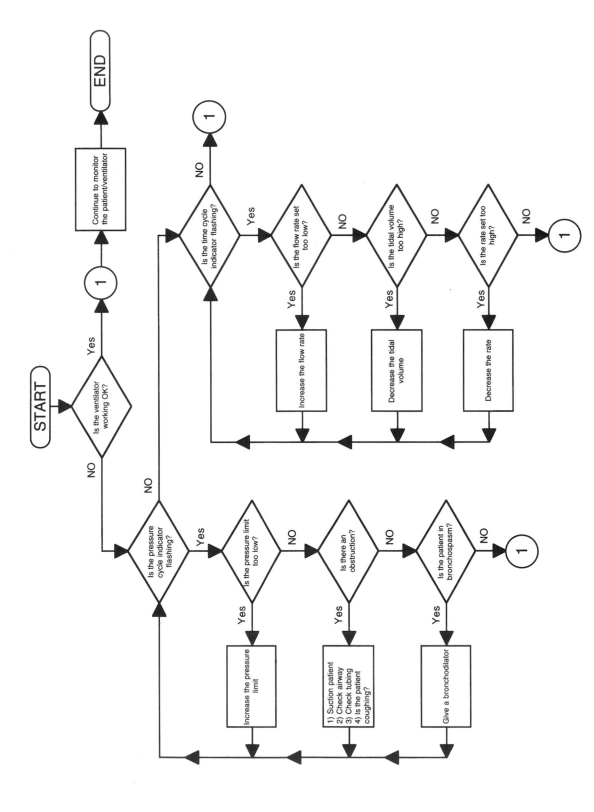

ALG 8-1 *A troubleshooting flowchart for the Monaghan 225/SIMV volume ventilator.*

Self-Assessment Quiz

1. What is the input power for the Monaghan 225/SIMV ventilator?
   a. electrical
   b. pneumatic
   c. mechanical
   d. a and b

2. The drive mechanism for the Monaghan 225/SIMV consists of:
   a. a bellows.
   b. a fluidic circuit.
   c. a rotary-driven piston.
   d. a venturi ejector.

3. The control circuit of the Monaghan 225/SIMV consists of:
   I. electrical.
   II. mechanical.
   III. pneumatic.
   IV. fluidic.
   a. I
   b. I and II
   c. I and IV
   d. III and IV

4. The control variable of the Monaghan 225/SIMV is:
   a. pressure.
   b. volume.
   c. flow.
   d. time.

5. The limit variable for the Monaghan 225/SIMV is:
   a. pressure.
   b. volume.
   c. flow.
   d. time.

6. The cycling variables for the Monaghan 225/SIMV are:
   I. pressure.
   II. volume.
   III. flow.
   IV. time.
   a. I and II
   b. I, II, and IV
   c. III and IV
   d. II and IV

7. Conditional variables for the Monaghan 225/SIMV include:
   I. pressure.
   II. volume.
   III. flow.
   IV. time.
   a. I
   b. I and IV
   c. I and II
   d. II and IV

8. The output waveforms for the Monaghan 225/SIMV are:
   I. sinusoidal pressure, volume, and flow waveform.
   II. rectangular flow waveform.
   III. rectangular volume waveform.
   IV. exponential pressure waveform.

  a. I
  b. II
  c. II and IV
  d. III and IV

9. Modes of ventilation for the Monaghan 225/SIMV include:
   I. CMV.
   II. assist/control.
   III. SIMV.
   IV. pressure support.
   a. I
   b. I and II
   c. I, II, and III
   d. I, II, III, and IV

10. Output monitors for the Monaghan 225/SIMV ventilator include:
    I. pressure.
    II. pressure cycle.
    III. time cycle.
    IV. tidal volume.
    a. I
    b. I and II
    c. I, II, and III
    d. I, II, III, and IV

Selected Bibliography

Branson, R. D., & Chatburn, R. L. (1992). Technical description and classification of modes of ventilator operation. *Respiratory Care, 37*(9), 1026–1044.

Chatburn, R. L. (1991). A new system for understanding mechanical ventilators. *Respiratory Care, 36*(10), 1123–1155.

Chatburn, R. L. (1992). Classification of mechanical ventilators. *Respiratory Care, 27*(9), 1009–1025.

Corning Fluidic Products. (1971). *Fluidic industrial control modules, part number EPD EBR-3.* Corning.

Dupis, Y. (1992). *Ventilators: Theory and clinical application* (2nd ed.). Mosby-Yearbook.

Floyd, T. L. (1986). *Digital fundamentals* (3rd ed.). Charles E. Merrill.

Monaghan. (1975). *Monaghan 225 volume ventilator operator's manual: Questions and answers, form 13929-01 5m.* Littleton.

Monaghan. (1976). *Fluidics and Monaghan volume ventilators, form part number 66007-02.* Littleton.

Pierson, D. J. (1986). Maximum ventilator capabilities of four current-generation mechanical ventilators. *Respiratory Care, 31*(11), 1054–1058.

Smith, R. K. (1973). Respiratory applications of fluidics. *Respiratory Therapy, (3)*3, 29–32.

CHAPTER 9

ADULT ACUTE CARE VENTILATORS: VENTILATORS HAVING FLOW AND PRESSURE CONTROL VARIABLES

INTRODUCTION

Chapter 8 described the adult acute care ventilators employing volume as a control variable. This chapter will describe the adult acute care ventilators that utilize flow and pressure as the control variables.

As discussed in Chapter 7, for a variable (pressure, volume, flow, or time) to be classified as a control variable, certain conditions must be met. Those conditions are that (1) the variable must be measured, and (2) the variable must be used as a feedback signal to control the ventilator's output. The group of ventilators discussed in this chapter directly measure the delivered flow or pressure and use this signal to modify and control the ventilator's output. Pressure becomes a control variable when the ventilators are operated in the CPAP or pressure support modes.

OBJECTIVES

After completing this chapter, the student will accomplish the following objectives:

- Explain what is meant by the term *control variable* and how a specific ventilator may be classified as having flow or pressure as a control variable.
- For the ventilators described in this chapter, apply Chatburn's classification system and classify them according to:
  - Power input
  - Drive mechanism
  - Control scheme
  - Output
  - Alarm systems
- Describe how to assemble and trouble-shoot the following ventilators:

- Bear Medical Systems, Inc., Bear 1, 2, 3, 5, and 1000
- Bird Products Corporation, 8400ST®*i*
- Bird Products Corporation, TBird® AVS
- Dräger, Evita 4
- Hamilton Galileo
- Hamilton Medical, Veolar
- Infrasonics, Adult Star
- Newport Medical Instruments, Wave
- Puritan-Bennett Corporation, 7200ae
- Nellcor Puritan-Bennett, 840
- Siemens-Elema Servo 900C, Servo 300, and Servo*i*
- Viasys Vela

THE CONTROL VARIABLE

During a ventilator-supported breath, a mechanical ventilator can control one of the following variables: pressure, volume, flow, or time. In order for a ventilator to be classified as controlling one of these variables, two conditions must be met. First, that variable must be measured, and second it must be used as feedback to control the ventilator's output. Therefore, for a ventilator to be classified as a flow or pressure controller, flow or pressure must be measured and used as a signal to control the output from the ventilator. The ventilators discussed in this chapter meet these criteria and are classified as either a flow or pressure controller.

BEAR MEDICAL SYSTEMS, BEAR 1, 2, AND 3

The Bear 1, 2, and 3 ventilators are similar to one another and therefore will be discussed together (Figures 9-1A, 9-1B, 9-2A, 9-2B, 9-3A, and 9-3B). When differences occur, they will be presented and compared.

Figure 9-1A *A photograph of the Bear 1 volume ventilator.*

Figure 9-1B *A photograph showing the control panel of the Bear 1 ventilator.*

Figure 9-2A *A photograph of the Bear 2 volume ventilator.*

Input Power

The Bear ventilators are both pneumatically powered and electronically controlled. Alternating electric current at 120 volts, 60 Hz, is utilized to control the electronic control circuitry. The ventilator also relies on a pneumatic gas source (30 to 100 psi) for oxygen and air. If compressed medical air is not available, an internal compressor will provide air (10 to 11.2 psi) to the blender.

Drive Mechanism

The pneumatic drive mechanism reduces the line pressure of the incoming gas to between 10 and 11 psi. Once the incoming pressure has been reduced, air and oxygen are mixed in the blender to the desired F_IO_2. Gas exiting the blender is reduced in pressure once again to between 1 and 3 psi by the waveform control and the peak flow control.

The waveform control is a variable orifice distal to the main solenoid valve. When set at the square wave position, 3.2 psi is provided

Figure 9-2B *A photograph showing the control panel of the Bear 2 ventilator.*

Figure 9-3A *A photograph of the Bear 3 volume ventilator.*

to the inlet of the variable orifice when the main solenoid valve has opened. Depending upon the patient's airway resistance and compliance, a pressure drop occurs across the waveform control valve. If the airway resistance is low and compliance is high, a higher flow will result through the valve since the pressure drop is low. Conversely, if the patient's airway resistance is high and compliance is low, a greater pressure drop will result and flow through the valve will be decreased. In the square wave setting, the drop in peak flow can be as high as 20% if the back pressure in the circuit reaches 100 cmH$_2$O.

Adjustment of the waveform control valve to the tapered position results in a further reduction in the delivered flow, tapering it. In the taper position, drive pressure through the variable orifice valve is reduced to 1.8 psi. At this lower drive pressure, changes in resistance and compliance (circuit back pressure) will cause a more dramatic reduction in delivered flow. The waveform control on the Bear 1 is infinitely variable between the square and tapered settings. The Bear 1 and 3 waveform controls are two-position switches (50% taper or square).

Figure 9-3B *A photograph showing the control panel of the Bear 3 ventilator.*

The flow rate control determines the peak flow delivered during a ventilator-supported breath (Control, Assist/Control, and the mandatory portion of SIMV). It is also a variable orifice operating in tandem with the waveform control valve. Adjustment of the waveform control valve opens or closes the peak flow control valve to maintain the desired peak inspiratory flow rate.

Control Circuit

The Bear 1, 2, and 3 utilize pneumatic and electronic devices in their control circuitry. During spontaneous modes of ventilation (SIMV and CPAP), a pneumatic demand valve (Figure 9-4) opens in response to a pressure drop in the patient circuit (below PEEP). Once fully opened, flow rates of up to 100 L/min can be provided to meet the patient's inspiratory needs.

The assist transducer is a thermistor that measures flow output from the demand valve. A constant current is applied to the small thermistor bead, heating it to a constant temperature. When gas flows across the thermistor, cooling it, a voltage drop occurs. During the

mandatory portion of SIMV, when a voltage drop is sensed by the assist transducer, a signal is sent to the main solenoid valve, delivering a mandatory breath, synchronizing the mandatory breath with the patient's spontaneous efforts. The assist transducer is also used during SIMV and CPAP to detect spontaneous breaths. When a voltage drop occurs, the ventilators activate the spontaneous light, and the breath rate reflects the combined ventilatory rate (ventilator and patient).

During Assist/Control operation, the assist sensitivity can be set by adjusting the flow threshold of the assist transducer. In its most sensitive position, approximately 10 mL, or -1 cmH$_2$O below PEEP, must be generated to trigger a mandatory breath. In its least sensitive position, 70 mL, or -5 cmH$_2$O below PEEP, is required to trigger a mandatory breath.

During control mode, an electronic solenoid locks out the demand valve (lockout solenoid). Once locked out, gas flow to the patient circuit is solely controlled by the main solenoid valve and the electronic timing circuitry (rate control).

Volume delivery is controlled by a flow transducer located at the output of the ventilator. The delivered volume is determined by the integration of flow during the inspiratory time. Hence, volume is determined indirectly as a function of flow, and these ventilators are classified as flow controllers. The measured volume is compared to a reference signal (tidal volume control), and when the signals match, the main solenoid closes, ceasing mandatory gas delivery from the ventilator.

Pressure is measured by a pressure transducer near the ventilator outlet (Bear 1). The Bear 2 and 3 measure pressure using the proximal airway line. The pressure transducer converts gas pressure to an electronic signal, which is utilized in the alarm system and the pressure limit systems for normal and sigh breath delivery.

PEEP pressure is controlled by the application of pressure to the exhalation valve in the patient circuit and the demand valve. Pressure is generated by a venturi inside the ventilator. Pressure from the venturi is conducted to the reference side of the demand valve (so that application of PEEP will not affect the sensitivity) and to the exhalation valve (Figure 9-4). The pressure applied to the exhalation valve closes it slightly during the expiratory phase, which maintains pressure in the circuit and the patient's lungs.

Figure 9-4 *A schematic drawing illustrating the Bear demand valve. (Courtesy Bear Medical Systems, Inc., Riverside, CA)*

Control Variables

As described earlier, during Assist/Control, Control, and the mandatory portion of SIMV, the Bear 1, 2, and 3 function as flow controllers. Flow is measured by a vortex shedding transducer located near the outlet of the ventilator. Its signal is compared to a reference setting (tidal volume or sigh volume controls) and used to control the ventilator's output. Volume is measured directly as a function of flow over time.

During CPAP (Bear 1, 2, and 3) and Pressure Support (Bear 3), pressure is measured and used as a feedback signal to control the ventilator output via the demand valve. During these modes, inspiratory flow varies to maintain the set CPAP or pressure support level.

Phase Variables

Trigger Variables

The trigger variables for the Bear 1, 2, and 3 can be pressure/flow, time, or manual. The assist transducer senses flow as a result of the opening of the demand valve (pressure). Therefore, the ventilator is neither purely pressure or purely flow triggered, but rather a combination of both.

Time triggering occurs when inspiration begins following a set time interval (rate control). This may occur during Control, Assist/Control, and SIMV modes.

Manual triggering can occur with all three ventilators by depressing the single breath control or manual sigh control, delivering a single mandatory breath (normal or sigh).

Limit Variables

The limit variables for the Bear ventilators include pressure, volume, and flow. The ventilators become pressure limited when they are operated in the spontaneous modes (SIMV, CPAP, and pressure support). The demand valve in these modes limits inspiratory pressures to the settings adjusted on the PEEP/CPAP control or the pressure support control. The demand valve maintains the pressure level by varying flow and is capable of providing up to 100 L/min (Bear 1), and 120 L/min (Bear 2 and 3).

Volume becomes a limit variable when the inspiratory pause control is set to a value greater than zero. Under these conditions, the inspired volume is held until the pause time has elapsed. Inspiratory pause is adjustable between 0 and 2 seconds. Once the inspiratory pause time has elapsed, the ventilator ends inspiration. Therefore, volume becomes the limit variable (volume is not allowed to exceed a preset value, and inspiration has not been terminated).

The ventilators become flow limited when operated in the rectangular waveform. When the waveform control is set in this position, inspiratory flow is limited to the value set on the peak flow control (adjustable between 20 and 120 L/min).

Cycle Variables

The cycle variables for the Bear ventilators include pressure, flow (Bear 3), and time. Pressure becomes a cycling variable if the pressure limit, or sigh pressure limit controls are set below the peak inspiratory pressure level during mandatory breaths (Control, Assist/Control, or mandatory portion of SIMV). The ventilators are also pressure cycled during SIMV and CPAP when the demand valve opens and closes in response to pressure gradients. The Bear 3 becomes flow cycled during pressure support. In this mode, inspiratory flow is measured and monitored. When the inspiratory flow drops to 25% of the peak flow value, the pressure-supported breath is terminated.

Baseline Variable

The baseline variable for the Bear ventilators is pressure. Pressure is controlled during CPAP and PEEP to maintain a positive pressure in the airway. CPAP/PEEP pressures are controlled by adjusting a needle valve, which regulates flow through a venturi. The output from the venturi is applied to the exhalation valve in the patient circuit and also to the demand valve, so that the demand valve is pressure compensated for CPAP/PEEP pressures. Baseline pressure is adjustable from zero to 30 cmH$_2$O (Bear 1) and zero to 50 cmH$_2$O (Bear 2 and 3).

Conditional Variables

Time

Time becomes a conditional variable during sigh delivery. During normal tidal volume delivery, the ventilator breaths flow controlled, pressure, time, or manually triggered, and pressure or time cycled. During sigh delivery, each hour may be divided into windows lasting between 1 and 30 minutes. That is, every 1 to 30 minutes, the ventilator switches to sigh mode and the sigh controls become active. Once activated, the ventilator will deliver between one and three breaths. Under these circumstances, the conditional variable is time.

Time and Pressure

Time and pressure become conditional variables during SIMV mode. The rate control determines the frequency of mandatory breath delivery during SIMV mode. The rate control is essentially an electronic timer, delivering a breath at specified time intervals. Between mandatory breath deliveries, the patient opens and closes the demand valve as a result of pressure fluctuations in the patient circuit. As the spontaneous breathing window closes, the ventilator senses the next inspiration (assist transducer) and activates the main solenoid valve, delivering a mandatory breath.

Output Waveforms

The Bear ventilators can deliver either a rectangular or descending ramp flow waveform output. In the rectangular position under conditions of low resistance and high compliance, the output waveform is rectangular. As resistance increases and compliance decreases, the flow waveform can taper as much as 20%.

When set in the descending ramp waveform position, less driving pressure is available (1.8 psi), resulting in a more drastic tapering of the rectangular flow waveform output due to changes in the patient's resistance or compliance.

The Bear 1 is infinitely variable between the rectangular and the descending ramp flow waveform positions. The Bear 2 and 3 can be selected between each setting, but an adjustable output is not possible.

Control Interactions

The tidal volume and flow rate controls can have a profound effect upon inspiratory time. As tidal volume is increased, inspiratory time is also increased (unless compensated for by increasing the peak flow). A decrease in the peak flow rate control will have the same effect. If I:E ratios of 1:2 or greater are desired, adjustment of the tidal volume, rate, and peak flows must be manipulated correctly.

If inverse I:E ratio ventilation is desired, the Bear ventilators can be adjusted to provide it. To ventilate a patient using inverse ratios, the 1:1 ratio limit control must be turned off and the controls adjusted to achieve an I:E ratio greater than 1:1.

Monitoring and Alarm Systems

Monitoring Systems

Several monitors are available to assist the practitioner in patient management. Three Bear monitors are described in Table 9-1.

Alarm Systems

Input Power

The Bear ventilators have three input power alarms: for loss of electrical power, loss of oxygen pressure, and loss of air pressure. In the event air pressure is lost, a built-in compressor will be activated, and it will supply the pneumatic pressure required to operate the blender and other systems. These alarms are both visual and audible. The loss of electric power alarm is battery powered and operates from a bank of rechargeable nickel cadmium batteries.

TABLE 9-1 Bear Ventilator Monitors

	Bear 1	Bear 2	Bear 3
Exhaled Volume	X	X	X
Rate	X	X	X
Status Indication	X	X	X
Mode Display	X	X	X
Pressure Manometer	X	X	X
Spontaneous Breath Monitor	X	X	X
Assisted Breath Monitor	X	X	X
Controlled Breath Monitor	X	X	X
Sigh Breath Monitor	X	X	X
Alert Display	X	X	X
Alarm Display	X	X	X
1:1 Limit Off Display	X		
I:E Ratio	X	X	X
Temperature		X	X

Control Circuit Alarms

Inverse I:E Ratio. The I:E ratio limit control, when activated, prevents patient ventilation at a ratio of greater than 1:1. It works by monitoring the inspiratory and expiratory time. In the control mode, if the inspiratory time equals 50% of the total ventilatory cycle, the main solenoid closes, ending inspiration. If inspiration is terminated, the ventilator then functions as a time-cycled ventilator.

If the control is off, a light illuminates on the control panel and inverse I:E ratio ventilation is possible. Each time a breath is delivered at an inverse I:E ratio, an indicator light will illuminate.

Ventilator Inoperative. The ventilator inoperative alarm will be activated on the Bear ventilators during conditions of adequate power and gas pressure if an internal malfunction in the volume control circuitry is detected. If electric power and gas pressure are adequate and the alarm is activated, the ventilator must be removed from use and alternative ventilation for the patient must be provided.

Output Alarms

Pressure. High peak pressure alarms are available on the Bear ventilators. These alarms may be adjusted between 0 and 100 cmH_2O (Bear 1) and 0 and 120 cmH_2O (Bear 2 and 3). When pressure in the patient circuit reaches the reference setting on the normal pressure limit or sigh pressure limit controls, inspiration is terminated and visual and audible alarms are activated. Pressure is measured by a pressure transducer near the outlet of the ventilator (Bear 1, referenced to machine pressure) or at the proximal airway (Bear 2 and 3). To adjust the alarm, it is necessary to depress the proximal/machine pressure switch to measure the machine pressure and properly reference the alarm (Bear 1).

Low inspiratory pressure alarms are also available on the Bear ventilators. They function in a similar way to the high peak pressure alarms. Settings are adjustable between 0 and 50 cmH2O (Bear 1) and 0 and 75 cmH2O (Bear 2 and 3).

ASSEMBLY AND TROUBLESHOOTING

Assembly—Bear 1, Bear 2, Bear 3

The following is a suggested guide for the assembly of the Bear 1, Bear 2, and Bear 3 ventilators:

1. Using a universal rubber adapter, connect the bacterial filter to the ventilator outlet.

2. Humidifier assembly:
   a. Assemble the humidifier and connect it to its heating element on the front of the ventilator. Since many popular humidifiers may be adapted for use on this ventilator, specific instructions are not included here.
   b. Attach a short piece of large-bore tubing between the bacteria filter and the humidifier inlet.

3. Assemble the circuit as shown in Figure 9-5. The Bear circuit requires that the temperature probe be placed close to the proximal airway.

4. Attach the inspiratory limb of the circuit to the humidifier outlet.

5. Attach the ¼-inch diameter proximal airway line to the external condenser assembly (Bear 1) or proximal line filter (Bear 2 and 3).

6. Attach the exhalation valve drive line to the exhalation valve nipple on the front of the ventilator.

7. Attach the vortex sensing tube to the expiratory limb of the circuit at the manifold, distal to the exhalation valve.

8. Connect the air (if available) and oxygen inlets to 50-psi medical gas sources.

9. Connect the power cord to a 120 volt, 60 Hz power source.

10. Pressure test the ventilator in accordance with the manufacturer's recommendations.

Troubleshooting

Refer to the troubleshooting algorithms found at the end of this chapter.

A—ATTACHMENT POINT FOR SUPPORT ARM
B—ATTACH TO HUMIDIFIER OUTLET
C—FLOW SENSOR ASSEMBLY
D—EXHALATION VALVE DRIVE LINE
E—PATIENT ELBOW
F—PROXIMAL AIRWAY PRESSURE PORT
G—TEMPERATURE MONITORING PORT
H—PROXIMAL AIRWAY LINE (BEAR I)

Figure 9-5 *The Bear Medical Systems Bear 1 volume ventilator circuit.*

Baseline pressure alarms are available to alert the practitioner to loss of baseline (PEEP/CPAP) pressures. The alarm is adjustable to between 0 and 30 cmH$_2$O (Bear 1) and 0 and 50 cmH$_2$O (Bear 2 and 3).

Volume. Low tidal volume alarms are included on the Bear ventilators. Exhaled tidal volume is measured by an external flow sensor located on the patient circuit's expiratory limb. The alarm is adjustable between 0 and 2 liters. If the exhaled volume falls below the threshold set on the alarm for three consecutive breaths, both visual and audible alarms are activated.

Apnea. The apnea alarm alerts the practitioner to absence of ventilation (spontaneous or mechanical). The alarm is activated if no breaths are sensed over a 20-second interval.

The Bear 2 and 3 have an adjustable apneic period alarm (the same function as the apnea alarm). The alarm is adjustable between a 2- and a 20-second interval.

High Ventilatory Rate. The Bear 2 and 3 ventilators have a high ventilatory rate alarm to alert the practitioner of high ventilatory rates. The alarm is adjustable between 10 and 80 breaths per minute.

Table 9-2 compares the alarm systems of the Bear 1, 2, and 3 ventilators, and Table 9-3 compares their capabilities.

TABLE 9-2 Bear 1, 2, and 3 Alarm Systems

	Bear 1	Bear 2	Bear 3
Input Power			
Oxygen Pressure	X	X	X
Air Pressure	X	X	X
Electric Power	X	X	X
Control Circuit			
Inverse I:E ratio	X	X	X
Ventilator Inop.	X	X	X
Output			
High Pressure	X	X	X
Low Pressure	X	X	X
Low Baseline Pressure	X	X	X
Low Tidal Volume	X	X	X
Apnea	X	X	X
High Ventilatory Rate		X	X

TABLE 9-3 Bear 1, 2, and 3 Ventilator Capabilities

	Bear 1	**Bear 2**	**Bear 3**
Modes	CMV, Assist CMV, SIMV, CPAP	CMV Assist CMV, SIMV, CPAP	CMV, Assist CMV, SIMV, CPAP, Pressure Support
Volume	0–2200 mL	0–2200 mL	0–2200 mL
Pressure	0–100 cmH2O	0–120 cmH2O	0–120 cmH2O
Rate	0–60	0–60	0–60
Peak Flow	0–120 L/min	0–120 L/min	0–120 L/min
PEEP/CPAP	0–30 cmH$_2$O	0–50 cmH2O	0–50 cmH2O
Sigh Volume	150–3000 mL	150–3000 mL	150–3000 mL
Insp. Pause	0–2 seconds	0–2 seconds	0–2 seconds
F$_I$O$_2$	.21–1.0	.21–1.0	.21–1.0

BEAR MEDICAL SYSTEMS, BEAR 5

The Bear Medical Systems Bear 5 is a microprocessor-controlled pediatric and adult ventilator. The microprocessor controller and the Cathode Ray Tube (CRT) display/monitor provide a flexible machine capable of ventilating a variety of patients (Figures 9-6 and 9-7).

The Bear 5 is classified as a flow and pressure controller. Flow is measured and used as a feedback signal to control the stepper motor valves to regulate volume delivery. The ventilator operates as a pressure controller during CPAP and pressure support modes.

Input Power

Power to run the microprocessor control circuitry and the stepper motor control system is provided by 115 volt, 60 Hz electrical power. The pneumatic system is powered by 50-psi air and oxygen. If 50-psi medical air is not available, the built-in compressor may be used to supply the gas needed to operate the ventilator.

Drive Mechanism

The pneumatic drive mechanism (Figure 9-8) reduces the line pressure of the incoming gas to 18.2 psi (±.1 psi) by means of the air regulator and the O$_2$ relay. The gas pressures and temperatures are closely matched to enhance the accuracy of the blending system.

Gas flows from these pressure-controlling elements to the oxygen blender.

The oxygen blender is a type of proportioning valve that mixes the oxygen and air. Signals from the microprocessor control a stepper motor that controls the position of the

Figure 9-6 *A photograph of the Bear 5 volume ventilator.*

Figure 9-7 *A photograph showing the control panel of the Bear 5 ventilator.*

proportioning valve. Gas then exits the blender to an accumulator.

The accumulator is a reservoir with a volume of 3.6 liters. The accumulator helps to minimize instantaneous flow demands from the blender. It also functions as a mixing chamber enhancing oxygen stability and enables the ventilator to meet instantaneous flow demands of up to 150 L/min.

Control Circuit

The Bear 5 ventilator uses a microprocessor and a stepper motor–controlled flow control valve to regulate flow output from the ventilator. This system, operating in conjunction with an internal vortex flow transducer, regulates gas flow during bias flow, continuous flow, demand flow, and during ventilator-supported breaths. The vortex flow sensor measures flow and uses it as a feedback signal to the microprocessor, controlling the position of the stepper motor and regulating the output from the flow control valve. A temperature sensor located proximal to the vortex flow sensor measures temperature, allowing the ventilator to deliver gas at BTPS, assuming the gas is

100% saturated with water vapor when delivered to the patient.

This system also allows delivery of tidal volumes, which are compensated for the volume compressed in the patient circuit. The circuit compliance factor may be entered into the microprocessor, which will automatically compensate the delivered volume, correcting for volume lost due to compression in the patient circuit.

Output waveforms include rectangular, ascending and descending ramp, and sinusoidal waveforms. All of these waveforms are possible through microprocessor control of the stepper motor in the flow control valve.

Pressure is controlled by the pilot pressure control/exhalation valve system. The pilot pressure control valve is also controlled by a stepper motor receiving signals from the microprocessor. Pressure is sensed by a proximal pressure transducer and is used to provide a feedback signal to the microprocessor. Output from the pilot pressure control valve is directed to the exhalation valve diaphragm, which controls the pressure in the patient circuit. The application of PEEP/CPAP is also controlled through this system.

Figure 9-8 *A schematic diagram of the Bear 5 pneumatic system. (Courtesy Bear Medical Systems, Inc., Riverside, CA)* *(continues)*

Bear Medical Systems, Inc.

Figure 9-8 *(continued)*

Control Variables

As described earlier, during CMV (Control), Assist CMV (Assist/Control), and the mandatory portions of SIMV, the ventilator operates as a flow controller. Flow is measured by a vortex sensor downstream from the flow control valve. Its output is used as a feedback signal to the microprocessor, controlling the operation of the flow control valve. The tidal volume setting and sigh volume setting provide a reference signal and are used to servo the flow control valve. Volume delivery is determined directly as a function of flow and time by the microprocessor.

During CPAP and pressure support and time-cycled ventilation, inspiratory pressure is regulated by the flow control valve described earlier. Pressure sensed by the proximal pressure transducer is used as feedback to adjust flow to the circuit to maintain the desired pressure. Any excess pressure is vented through the exhalation valve. When operated in these modes, the ventilator becomes a pressure controller.

Phase Variables

Trigger Variables

Inspiration may be pressure, time, or manually triggered. The ventilator is pressure triggered when the pressure in the patient circuit drops to the level set on the assist sensitivity control. Pressure in the patient circuit will fall below baseline pressure when the patient initiates a breath. Sensitivity levels between 0.5 and 5.0 cmH$_2$O subbaseline may be selected. Pressure is sensed by the proximal pressure transducer, located in the ventilator.

The ventilator is time triggered when no patient effort is sensed by the microprocessor through the Assist/Sensitivity system or when operating in CMV mode. The setting on the normal rate control determines the time interval (respiratory rate) for ventilator assisted breaths. Rate may be set between 0.5 and 150 breaths per minute. After the set time interval has passed, a ventilator-supported breath will be initiated.

The ventilator may also be manually cycled by the practitioner by depressing the manual breath or sigh control.

Limit Variables

The Bear 5 may be pressure, volume, or flow limited. The ventilator is pressure limited during the spontaneous breaths in the pres-

sure support and CPAP modes. The flow control valve, operating in conjunction with the pilot pressure control valve, will maintain the desired pressure in the patient circuit. During pressure support, pressure support levels may be adjusted between 0 and 72 cmH$_2$O. During PEEP and CPAP, pressures are adjustable between 0 and 50 cmH$_2$O.

The ventilator becomes volume limited any time the inspiratory pause control is set for a time greater than zero. Under these conditions, the inspired volume is held until the pause time has elapsed. Inspiratory pause is adjustable between 0 and 2 seconds. Once the inspiratory pause time has elapsed, the ventilator ends inspiration. Therefore, volume becomes the limit variable (volume is not allowed to exceed a preset value and inspiration has not been terminated). Under these conditions, volume becomes the limit variable since the delivered volume is always reached prior to the termination of the breath.

The ventilator is flow limited during flow-controlled breaths. Under these circumstances, flow is limited to the setting on the peak flow control. Peak inspiratory flow is adjustable between 5 and 150 L/min.

Cycle Variables

The Bear 5 ventilator can be pressure, flow, or time cycled. The ventilator becomes pressure cycled if the proximal airway pressure exceeds the value set on the high peak normal or sigh pressure alarm setting. If this pressure level is reached prior to delivery of the mandatory breath, both an audible and visual alarm will sound and inspiration will be terminated.

The ventilator becomes flow cycled during pressure support mode. During pressure support, the ventilator-assisted breath is terminated when inspiratory flow falls to a value less than 25% of the peak inspiratory flow required to maintain the pressure support level.

Time cycling occurs when the ventilator is time cycled and pressure controlled. Inspiration ends when the inspiratory time has elapsed. Inspiratory times are adjustable between 0.1 and 3.0 seconds. Time is also a cycling variable when the inspiratory pause control is adjusted greater than zero. Inspiration is terminated following the set inspiratory pause (time).

Baseline Variable

The baseline variable for the Bear 5 is pressure. Baseline pressure may be adjusted during PEEP and CPAP between 0 and 50 cmH$_2$O.

Conditional Variables

Time

Time becomes a conditional variable during sigh delivery. Normal ventilator-supported breaths are flow controlled, pressure triggered, and pressure or time cycled. During sigh delivery, each hour may be divided into windows lasting between 1 and 30 minutes. That is, every 1 to 30 minutes, the ventilator switches to sigh mode and the sigh controls become active. Once activated, the ventilator will deliver between one and three breaths. Under these circumstances, the conditional variable is time.

Time and Pressure

Time and pressure become conditional variables during SIMV mode. The rate control determines the frequency of mandatory breath delivery during SIMV mode. The rate control is essentially an electronic timer, delivering a breath at specified time intervals. Between mandatory breath delivery, the patient breathes through the flow/volume/demand control subsystem. The ventilator measures proximal airway pressure to determine if the patient is attempting to initiate a breath. In response to the pressure change, the patient is able to draw gas spontaneously through the flow control valve to meet their inspiratory needs. Flow may be provided on a demand basis or by a continuous flow of gas of between 5 and 40 L/min baseline flow.

Time and Volume

Time and volume become conditional variables during AMV ventilation. A set minimum exhaled volume is established by the practitioner. Should the patient fail to meet this minute volume, the ventilator will deliver breaths at a rate equal to the minimum minute volume setting divided by the set tidal volume. Apnea results in time-triggered ventilation. Flow becomes the conditional variable because the Bear 5 measures flow and determines volume directly as a function of flow and time.

Output Waveforms

Pressure

The Bear 5 can deliver a rectangular pressure waveform when operated using time-cycled or pressure-supported ventilation. Under these circumstances, pressure rises rapidly to a constant value where it remains

through the delivery of the breath. At the termination of inspiration, pressure falls to the baseline value.

Flow

The flow output waveform capabilities of the Bear 5 include rectangular, ascending and descending ramp, and sinusoidal. As described earlier, these waveforms can be accurately reproduced by the feedback system between the internal vortex flow transducer, the microprocessor, and the stepper motor-driven flow control valve.

Alarms

Input Power Alarms

The input power alarms include loss of electrical and loss of pneumatic power. In the event of a loss of electrical power, a battery powered alarm will be activated both visually and audibly. During a loss of electrical power, the power LED on the upper left corner of the control panel will not be illuminated.

If the oxygen line pressure falls below 27 psi, an audible and visual alarm will be activated. In the event that air pressure falls below 27 psi and electric power is still available, the compressor will be activated to compensate for the loss of air pressure. The compressor's power switch must be in the ON position, and the compressor must be connected to a 115 volt, 60 Hz electrical outlet for the compressor to act as a backup system for the piped medical air system.

Control Circuit Alarms

The control circuit alarms include ventilator inoperative settings, incompatible settings, and inverse I:E ratio alarms. The ventilator inoperative alarm may indicate the following correctable situations: (1) the patient circuit has become kinked (expiratory limb or proximal airway line), (2) the temperature control chamber door is open (TCC Door Open/TCC Temp Low), or (3) an improperly installed external flow sensor (Ext. Flow Sensor). The practitioner should attempt to correct these conditions and disable the ventilator inoperative alarm. If the alarm cannot be silenced or cannot be traced to these situations, an internal problem has been detected and the ventilator should be removed from service.

An alarm will alert the practitioner to settings which are not compatible. For example,

ASSEMBLY AND TROUBLESHOOTING

Assembly—Bear 5

Although the Bear 5 is a complex ventilator, circuit assembly is very easy. The following is a suggested assembly guide:

1. Attach the high pressure hoses to an oxygen and air source. If no source of 50-psi air is available and the ventilator is equipped with the optional compressor, no air supply is required.

2. Verify that the exhalation valve assembly is well secured to its slide mount. Screw the collection jar into place and tighten it.

3. Place the vortex flow tube into its holder in the temperature control chamber and connect the external flow sensors to the flow tube.

4. Attach the crossover flow tube between the vortex sensor and the exhalation valve. Then close the door to the temperature control chamber.

5. Attach the collector vial to the exhalation valve filter and close its door.

6. Assemble and fill the humidifier and attach it to the front of the ventilator. Many different humidifiers may be adapted to the Bear 5, so specific assembly instructions will not be included here.

7. Assemble the adult circuit, verifying the integrity of connections at the proximal airway port, patient wye, and temperature probe ports.

8. Connect the main flow bacteria filter between the ventilator outlet and the humidifier. Attach the adult circuit to the outlet of the humidifier and the exhalation limb to the collection jar proximal to the temperature control chamber.

9. Connect the power cord to a suitable 120 volt, 60 Hz outlet.

Troubleshooting

Refer to the troubleshooting algorithms found at the end of this chapter.

---

if a tidal volume of 3000 is entered, an "E" will appear at the left of the keypad display and "Available Range 50 to 2000" will appear on the CRT display.

The inverse I:E ratio alarm is enabled if the 1:1 ratio limit is activated by the practitioner. If activated, the ventilator will terminate inspiration if the I:E ratio reaches 1:1. If the ratio limit is overridden, I:E ratios of less than 1:1 may be used up to a maximum of a 3:1 I:E ratio.

Output Alarms

Pressure. Pressure output alarms include high and low peak, high and low baseline, and high and low mean pressures. The high and low peak airway pressure alarms are adjustable between 0.0 and 140 cmH_2O except during time-cycled ventilation, when it is adjustable between 0.0 and 80 cmH_2O. Mean airway pressure alarms are adjustable between 0.0 and 75 cmH_2O. Baseline pressure alarms may be set between 0.0 and 55 cmH_2O.

Volume. A low exhaled tidal volume is available for both mandatory breaths and spontaneous breaths. The alarm parameters are adjustable between 30 and 2000 mL for both mandatory and spontaneous alarms.

Flow. A low exhaled minute volume alarm may be adjusted between 0.3 and 40.0 L/min. A high exhaled minute volume alarm can be adjusted between 1.0 and 80.0 L/min.

Time. A high and low ventilatory rate alarm can be set between 3 and 155 breaths per minute. During time-cycled ventilation, the alarm is adjustable between 0.0 and 155 breaths per minute.

A high and low inspiratory time alarm is available when operating the Bear 5 in time-cycled ventilation. The low inspiratory time is adjustable between 0.05 and 3.00 seconds and the high inspiratory time alarm is adjustable between 0.10 and 3.2 seconds.

Table 9-4 illustrates the Bear 5 alarm systems and Table 9-5 illustrates its capabilities.

TABLE 9-4 Bear 5 Alarm Systems

Alarm	Condition/Settings
Input Power	
Oxygen Pressure	<27 psi
Air Pressure	<27 psi
Electric Power	Loss of 115 volt, 60 Hz power
Control Circuit	

Ventilator Inoperative	Correctable:
	   Kinked patient circuit
	   Temperature Control Chamber door open
	   External Flow Sensor installed wrong
	Not Correctable:
	   Internal malfunction detected

Incompatible Settings	Practitioner selected settings not compatible with the ventilator's capabilities
I:E Ratio	I:E ratio less than 1:1 if the ratio limit is enabled
Output Alarms	
High Airway Pressure	0.0–140 cmH$_2$O
Low Airway Pressure	0.0–140 cmH$_2$O
High Baseline Pressure	0.0–55 cmH$_2$O
Low Baseline Pressure	0.0–55 cmH$_2$O
High Mean Airway Pres.	0.0–75 cmH$_2$O
Low Mean Airway Pres.	0.0–75 cmH$_2$O
Low Exhaled Tidal Vol.	30–2000 mL
(Spontaneous)	30–2000 mL
High Minute Volume	1.0–80 L/min
Low Minute Volume	0.3–40 L/min
High Breath Rate	3–155 breaths per minute (BPM)
(Time Cycled Vent.)	0–155 BPM
High Insp. Time	0.10–3.2 seconds
Low Insp. Time	0.01–3.0 seconds

BEAR MEDICAL SYSTEMS, BEAR 1000

The Bear Medical Systems Bear 1000 is a microprocessor-controlled pediatric and adult ventilator (Figures 9-9 and 9-10). The microprocessor controller allows operator flexibility and the ability to upgrade the ventilator to meet future needs.

The Bear 1000 is classified as a pressure controller. During volume delivery (Assist CMV and the mandatory portion of SIMV), pressure is measured and used as a feedback signal controlling the ventilator's output. Flow and volume are determined indirectly as a function of pressure (differential pressure across the flow control valve). During CPAP,

TABLE 9-5 Bear 5 Ventilator Capabilities

Modes	CMV, Assist CMV, SIMV/IMV, CPAP, AMV (MMV), Time Cycle, Pressure Support
Volume	50–2000 mL
Pressure	0.0–150 cmH$_2$O
Rate	0.0–150 BPM
Peak Flow	5–150 L/min
PEEP/CPAP	0.0–50 cmH$_2$O
Sigh Volume	65–3000 mL
Insp. Pause	0.0–2.0 seconds
F$_I$O$_2$	0.21–1.00

Figure 9-9 *A photograph of the Bear 1000 volume ventilator. (Courtesy Bear Medical Systems, Inc., Riverside, CA)*

pressure control, and pressure support, pressure is also measured and used to control the output of the flow control valve.

Input Power

Power to run the microprocessor control circuitry and the stepper motor control system is provided by 120 volt, 60 Hz electrical power. The pneumatic system is powered by 50-psi air and oxygen. If 50-psi medical air is not available, a built-in compressor may be used to supply the gas needed to operate the ventilator.

Drive Mechanism

The pneumatic drive mechanism (Figure 9-11) reduces the line pressure of the incoming gas to 18.0 psi (±.1 psi) by means of the air regulator and the O$_2$ relay. The gas pressures and temperatures are closely matched to enhance the accuracy of the blending system. In the event medical air or oxygen pressure is lost (<27.5 psi), a crossover solenoid opens, diverting the remaining high pressure gas to the air regulator. Under these circumstances, the F$_I$O$_2$ delivered is 1.0 or 0.21, depending upon which gas was lost. Gas flows from these pressure controlling elements to the oxygen blender.

The oxygen blender is a type of proportioning valve that mixes the oxygen and air. Signals from the microprocessor control a stepper motor that regulates the opening and closing of the proportioning valve. Gas then exits the blender to an accumulator.

The accumulator is a reservoir with a volume of 3.5 liters at 10.0 to 18.0 psi, depending upon flow demands. The accumulator is a reservoir with a volume of 3.5 liters at 10.0 to 18.0 psi, depending upon flow demands. The accumulator helps to minimize instantaneous flow demands from the blender. The accumulator also functions as a mixing chamber enhancing oxygen stability. The accumulator also enables the ventilator to meet instantaneous flow demands of over 200 L/min.

Figure 9-10 *A photograph showing the control panel of the Bear 1000 ventilator.*

Figure 9-11 *A schematic diagram of the Bear 1000 ventilator's pneumatic system. (Courtesy Bear Medical Systems, Inc., Riverside, CA)*

Control Circuit

The Bear 1000 ventilator uses a microprocessor and a stepper motor–driven flow control valve to regulate flow output from the ventilator. This system operates in conjunction with two pressure transducers, one located at the inlet and the other located at the outlet of the flow control valve. When the valve is open, a pressure difference will exist between the flow control valve inlet and outlet. This pressure is proportional to flow at the present position of the flow control valve. The microprocessor logic uses reference values established by the tidal volume, peak flow, and waveform control settings to establish an initial flow signal to the flow control valve. Once the valve is opened, signals from the pressure transducers are used to ensure that flow delivery matches the ventilator settings for tidal volume delivery. Tidal volume delivery becomes a function of time and flow, with flow being determined as a function of the pressure differential across the flow control valve and the valve's position. Technically, the ventilator is really a pressure controller when delivering mandatory breaths, since pressure is measured and used as a signal to regulate the output from the flow control valve.

This system also allows delivery of tidal volumes, which are compensated for the volume compressed in the patient circuit. The circuit compliance factor may be entered into the microprocessor, which will automatically compensate the delivered volume, correcting for volume lost due to compression in the patient circuit.

Output waveforms include rectangular, descending ramp, and sinusoidal waveforms. All of these waveforms are possible through microprocessor control of the stepper motor in the flow control valve.

Pressure must be measured and controlled during pressure-controlled ventilation, pressure support, and pressure augmentation. Pressure in the patient circuit is regulated by the feedback from the proximal pressure transducer via adjustment of flow from the flow control valve and the low pressure control system regulating the exhalation valve. Reference signals from the pressure support/inspiratory pressure, inspiratory time, and the PEEP controls are used as inputs to the microprocessor. The flow control valve is opened providing sufficient flow to maintain the proximal airway pressure established by these controls.

Pressure-controlled breath delivery ceases based upon the inspiratory time set by the practitioner. PEEP regulation is accomplished through the low pressure control system. Gas supplied from the PEEP control needle valve and the jet pump are directed through the exhalation solenoid valve to the exhalation diaphragm, regulating PEEP pressure in the patient circuit.

Control Variables

As described earlier, the control variable used by the Bear 1000 ventilator is pressure. Differential pressure measured across the flow control valve is used to regulate the valve during tidal volume delivery during mandatory breaths. Pressure is also the control variable during PEEP/CPAP, pressure controlled ventilation, pressure support, and pressure augmentation.

Phase Variables

Trigger Variables

The trigger variables for the Bear 1000 include pressure, flow, time, and manual variables. When inspiratory pressure falls below the threshold established by the assist sensitivity control, the ventilator will initiate a breath. The assist sensitivity may be set between 0.2 and 5.0 cmH$_2$O below baseline pressure by the practitioner.

Flow becomes a trigger variable when flow triggering is established by adjusting base flow and flow trigger (sensitivity) levels. Base flow is adjustable between 5 and 20 L/min. The flow trigger may be set between 1 and 15 L/min. When the flow transducer senses that flow has dropped below the trigger level, a breath is given.

Time becomes a trigger variable during assist CMV, SIMV, and pressure control if no inspiratory effort (pressure drop) is sensed by the ventilator. If the patient does not trigger a breath, the ventilator will deliver a mandatory breath at the set breath rate. This is also true during pressure-control ventilation.

The ventilator may be manually triggered by the practitioner depressing the manual breath key on the control panel. When depressed, the ventilator will deliver a volume-controlled breath (assist/CMV, SIMV, and CPAP) or a pressure-controlled breath during pressure control mode.

Limit Variables

The limit variables of the Bear 1000 include pressure, volume, and flow. Pressure becomes a limit variable during SIMV (with PEEP applied), CPAP, pressure support, pressure augmentation, and pressure control ventilation. Under these conditions, the ventilator will augment flow to maintain the desired pressure level. PEEP/CPAP pressures are adjustable between 0.0 and 50.0 cmH$_2$O. Pressure support is adjustable between 0.0 and 80.0 cmH$_2$O.

Volume becomes a limit variable when the inspiratory pause control is adjusted greater than zero. Inspiratory pause may be adjusted between 0.0 and 2.0 seconds. When activated, a volume breath is delivered and held until the set inspiratory pause time period has elapsed.

Flow becomes a limit variable when the rectangular waveform output is selected during assist/CMV or during sigh breath delivery. When selected, the rectangular waveform output limits flow during inspiration to the setting established on the peak flow control. Peak flow is adjustable between 10 and 150 L/min.

Cycle Variables

Cycle variables for the Bear 1000 include pressure, volume, flow, and time. Pressure becomes a cycle variable if the inspiratory pressure reaches the setting on the peak inspiratory pressure control. Peak inspiratory pressure may be adjusted between 0 and 120 cmH$_2$O. When the pressure limit is reached, inspiration is terminated and both audible and visual alarms are activated.

Volume becomes a cycle variable during sigh breath delivery. When selected, a sigh breath will be given every 100th breath. The sigh volume delivered will be 150% of the normal tidal volume setting. Sigh breath delivery cannot be used during pressure-control ventilation. During assist CMV and the mandatory portion of SIMV, the ventilator is also volume cycled. The control circuit uses the pressure drop across the flow control valve and its position to determine volume. The breath ends once the volume delivery is complete.

Flow becomes a cycle variable during pressure support ventilation. Inspiration is terminated when inspiratory flow falls to approximately 30% of the peak inspiratory flow. Once flow decays to this point, pressure falls to the baseline value. During pressure augmentation if the patient requires additional gas flow beyond the set tidal volume, the ventilator also becomes flow cycled.

Time becomes a cycle variable during pressure control ventilation. In this mode, a constant pressure is applied until the time set on the inspiratory time control has been reached. The trigger variable during pressure control is also time, which is established by the rate control. Time is also a cycle variable when the inspiratory pause control is set greater than zero. Inspiration is terminated after the inspiratory pause time has elapsed (0.0 to 2.0 seconds).

Baseline Variable

PEEP/CPAP pressures are adjustable between 0 and 50 cmH2O. Baseline pressures are increased above ambient by the exhalation solenoid partially closing the exhalation valve.

Conditional Variables

Time. Time becomes a conditional variable during sigh delivery. During normal ventilator supported breaths, they are pressure controlled, pressure triggered, pressure or time cycled. During sigh delivery, a sigh breath will be given every 100th breath.

Time and Pressure. Time and pressure become conditional variables during SIMV mode. The rate control determines the frequency of mandatory breath delivery during SIMV mode. The rate control is essentially an electronic timer, delivering a breath at specified time intervals. Between mandatory breath delivery, the patient breathes through the flow control valve subsystem. The ventilator measures proximal airway pressure to determine if the patient is attempting to initiate a breath. In response to the pressure change, the patient is able to draw gas spontaneously through the flow control valve to meet inspiratory needs.

Time and Volume. Time and volume become conditional variables during MMV (Mandatory Minute Ventilation). A set minimum exhaled volume is established by the practitioner. Should the patient fail to meet this minute volume, the ventilator will deliver breaths at a rate equal to the minimum minute volume setting divided by the set tidal volume. Apnea results in time-triggered ventilation. Flow becomes the conditional variable because the Bear 1000 measures flow and determines volume indirectly as a function of flow and time.

ASSEMBLY AND TROUBLESHOOTING

Assembly—Bear 1000

To prepare the Bear 1000 for use, follow this suggested assembly guide:

1. Attach the high pressure hoses to an oxygen and air source. If no source of 50-psi air is available and the ventilator is equipped with the optional compressor, no air supply is required.

2. Exhalation valve assembly:
   a. Insert the small end of the exhalation valve into the exhalation valve diaphragm and secure it by turning the retaining nut until it stops over the end of the diaphragm.
   b. Pull out on the diaphragm inflating it.
   c. Occlude the end of the exhalation valve and press on the diaphragm to ensure it remains inflated and is secured properly.

3. Insert the assembled exhalation valve into its seat on the ventilator and attach the condensate jar to the exhalation valve by inserting it over the valve and rotating the assembly counterclockwise.

4. Install the external flow sensor assembly to the outlet of the condensate jar and attach its coiled cable to it.

5. Assemble and fill the humidifier, and attach it to the front of the ventilator. Many different humidifiers may be adapted to the Bear 1000, so specific assembly instructions will not be included here.

6. Assemble the adult circuit, verifying the integrity of connections at the proximal airway port, patient wye, and temperature probe ports.

7. Connect the main flow bacteria filter between the ventilator outlet and the humidifier. Attach the adult circuit to the outlet of the humidifier and the exhalation limb to the condensate jar.

8. Connect the power cord to a suitable 115 volt, 60 Hz outlet.

Troubleshooting

Refer to the troubleshooting algorithms found at the end of this chapter.

Output Waveforms

Pressure

The pressure output of the Bear 1000 ventilator may be rectangular or adjustable. The rectangular waveform output occurs when the ventilator is operating in the pressure support and pressure control modes. In these modes, pressure rises sharply to the level set on the pressure support/inspiratory pressure control.

The pressure waveform may be adjusted by using the pressure slope control. When employed, the pressure can be adjusted to rise slowly or quickly to its peak value.

Volume

Volume output is an ascending ramp when the ventilator is operated with the flow output in the rectangular waveform setting. Under these conditions, the volume gradually increases in a linear fashion as pressure increases.

Flow

The flow output of the Bear 1000 may be adjusted between rectangular, descending ramp, and sinusoidal outputs. The stepper motor–driven flow control valve, in combination with the microprocessor and pressure feed back system, enables the ventilator to accurately reproduce these flow output waveforms.

Alarms

Input Power

Input power alarms on the Bear 1000 include loss of electrical and pneumatic power. When electrical power is lost, the failed-to-cycle alarm will be activated for a minimum of 5 minutes or until power is restored. A nickel cadmium battery pack powers the audible and visual alarm, independent of the 115 volts, 60 Hz power for the ventilator.

If air or oxygen pressure falls below 27.5 psi, the gas supply failure alarm will be activated. Both audible and visual alarms will be activated when this condition exists.

Control Circuit Alarms

Control circuit alarms on the Bear 1000 include failure to cycle and time/I:E limit. The failed-to-cycle alarm is activated when power is lost or an internal fault is found when the microprocessor conducts its diagnostics routine. The time/I:E limit alarm is activated if the practitioner has set an improper tidal volume, rate and peak flow, and inspiratory pause settings. The alarm will also activate if the inspiratory time exceeds 5 seconds plus pause time or if the I:E ratio exceeds the set limit.

Output Alarms

Pressure. The Bear 1000 incorporates high and low peak pressure and high and low base-line pressure alarms. The high peak pressure alarm is adjustable between 0.0 and 120 cmH$_2$O and the low peak pressure alarm is adjustable between 3 and 99 cmH$_2$O. The high and low baseline pressure alarms are adjustable between 0.0 and 50 cmH$_2$O.

Flow. High and low minute volume alarms are incorporated into the Bear 1000. The low minute volume alarm is adjustable between 0.0 and 50 L/min. The high minute volume alarm is adjustable between 0.0 and 80 L/min.

Time. Adjustable high and low breath rate alarms are also incorporated into the Bear 1000 ventilator. The low breath rate alarm is adjustable between 3 and 99 breaths per minute. The high breath rate alarm can be adjusted between 0 and 155 breaths per minute.

Table 9-6 summarizes the Bear 1000 ventilator alarm systems, and Table 9-7 summarizes its capabilities.

BIRD PRODUCTS CORPORATION, 8400ST®*i*

The Bird Products Corporation's 8400ST®*i* volume ventilator is a pneumatically powered, microprocessor-controlled ventilator which is capable of ventilating a wide spectrum of

TABLE 9-6 Bear 1000 Alarms

Alarm	Condition/Settings
Input Power	
Oxygen Pressure	< 27.5 psi
Air Pressure	< 27.5 psi
Electric Power	Loss of 120 volt, 60 Hz power
Control Circuit	
Failed to Cycle	Internal Faults Detected
Time/I:E Limit	Inspiratory time exceeds 5 seconds plus inspiratory pause or I:E ratio exceeds the limit set.
Output Alarms	
High Airway Pressure	0.0–120 cmH$_2$O
Low Airway Pressure	3.0–99 cmH$_2$O
High Baseline Pressure	0.0–50 cmH$_2$O
Low Baseline Pressure	0.0–50 cmH$_2$O
High Minute Volume	0.0–80 L/min
Low Minute Volume	0.0–50 L/min
High Breath Rate	0–155 BPM
Low Breath Rate	3–90 BPM

TABLE 9-7 BEAR 1000 Ventilator Capabilities

Modes	Assist CMV, SIMV/CPAP, Pressure Support, MMV, Pressure Control, and Pressure Augmentation
Volume	10–2,000 mL
Min. Minute Volume	0.0–50 L/min
Pressure	0.0–120 cmH$_2$O
Press. Support	0.0–80 cmH$_2$O
Rate	0.0–120 BPM
Peak Flow	5–150 L/min
PEEP/CPAP	0.0–50 cmH$_2$O
Sigh Volume	150% of Tidal Volume
Insp. Pause	0.0–2.0 seconds
Insp. Time	0.1–5.0 seconds
F$_I$O$_2$	0.21–1.0

patients (Figures 9-12, 9-13). The microprocessor, in conjunction with the flow control valve and electronically controlled exhalation valve, gives the ventilator a high degree of flexibility.

Input Power

Power to run the microprocessor control circuitry and the stepper motor control system is provided by alternating 120 volt, 60 Hz electrical power or 16-volt DC power. The pneumatic system is powered by 50 psi air and oxygen. The oxygen and air must be mixed using an external blender such as the Bird 3800™ MicroBlender.

Control Circuit

Gas from the blender enters the ventilator and passes though a coalescing filter which removes both liquid and solid particles from the compressed gas source (Figure 9-14). The gas then passes through a relief valve (100 psi) and into a 1.1-liter accumulator. The accumulator functions as a reservoir to provide gas to

meet high instantaneous flow demands. From the accumulator, the gas is reduced in pressure to 20 psi by a reducing valve (regulator).

The 8400ST®i ventilator uses a microprocessor and a stepper motor–driven flow control valve to regulate flow output from the ventilator. The valve is supplied with gas at a pressure of 20 psi from the reducing valve. Between the reducing valve and the flow control valve is a 200-mL pulsation dampener. Since the valve can instantaneously demand more gas flow, the pulsation dampener helps to reduce pressure fluctuations and acts as a buffer between the reducing valve and the flow control valve.

The way the 8400ST®i determines flow from the flow control valve is based upon valve position. An optical sensor detects the valve's position. Gas flow exiting the valve is sonic up to a back pressure of 210 cmH$_2$O (3 psi). Mass flow from the flow control valve is unchanged up to back pressures of 210 cmH$_2$O downstream (patient circuit). Therefore, flow from the valve is directly proportional to how far the valve has opened. The

Figure 9-12 *A photograph of the Bird Medical Products Corporation 8400ST volume ventilator. (Courtesy Bird Products Corporation, Palm Springs, CA)*

Figure 9-13 *A drawing showing the control panel of the Bird 8400ST ventilator. (Courtesy Bird Products Corporation, Palm Springs, CA)*

microprocessor uses an algorithm to determine flow based upon the feedback from the optical sensor, which senses valve position. Although flow is not directly measured, valve position is directly proportional to flow. Output from the flow control valve varies from 0.0

to 120 L/min in 1-L/min increments, or steps, of resolution.

Pressure must be measured and controlled during pressure control, pressure support, and PEEP/CPAP. Pressure in the patient circuit is regulated by the dynamic exhalation valve,

Figure 9-14 *A schematic drawing showing the Bird 8400ST ventilator's pneumatic system. (Courtesy Bird Products Corporation, Palm Springs, CA)*

flow control valve, and the airway pressure transducer. Feedback from the transducer determines the output (flow) from the flow control valve required to maintain a given level of pressure support during inspiration. The exhalation valve changes position, partially closing, and when provided with flow from the flow control valve can maintain the desired level of PEEP/CPAP, acting as a threshold resister.

Control Variables

The control variables for the 8400ST®*i* are flow and pressure. Flow is the control variable during volume breath delivery (Control, Assist/Control, and SIMV). When a volume breath is delivered, volume is determined as a function of flow and time. As stated earlier, flow is not directly measured but is a linear function of valve position.

Pressure becomes the control variable during pressure control, CPAP, and pressure support. Pressure is measured by the airway pressure transducer and is used by the microprocessor to determine output from the flow control valve and position of the exhalation valve.

Phase Variables

Trigger Variables

The trigger variables of the 8400ST®*i* include pressure, flow, time, and manual. Pressure becomes a trigger variable when the patient inhales, reducing pressure in the circuit below the reference level set on the sensitivity control. Sensitivity may be adjusted between 1.0 and 20 cmH2O below baseline pressure. Pressure operates as a trigger variable for mandatory breaths during assist control, SIMV, and pressure support.

Flow is a trigger variable when the special flow triggering flow sensor has been installed. Once installed, a bias flow of 10 L/min flows through the patient circuit. Sensitivity levels of between 1 and 10 L/min threshold may be set using the sensitivity control. Once the flow threshold has been detected, inspiration is triggered.

Time is a trigger variable during control, assist control, and SIMV when no spontaneous breaths occur. Breath delivery is based upon the rate control (time) and is adjustable between 0 and 80 breaths per minute.

The ventilator may also be manually triggered by depressing the manual breath button.

When depressed, the ventilator initiates a controlled breath at the tidal volume, waveform and peak flow or inspiratory pressure, and inspiratory time (for pressure control breaths) set on the control panel.

Limit Variables

The limit variables include pressure, volume, and flow. Pressure becomes the limit variable during SIMV (with PEEP/CPAP), CPAP, pressure control, and pressure support modes. The demand flow system (flow control valve, exhalation valve, and airway pressure transducer) maintains pressure in the patient circuit at the desired level. PEEP/CPAP is adjustable between 0.0 and 30 cmH2O. Pressure support may be adjusted between 0.0 and 50 cmH$_2$O.

Volume becomes a limit variable when the inspiratory hold button is depressed. When depressed, inspiration will be held following breath delivery until the button is released or 6 seconds have elapsed. The inspiratory hold button facilitates the measurement of static inspiratory pressure in the patient circuit, since both the flow control valve and the exhalation valve are held in the closed position.

Flow is the limit variable when the rectangular inspiratory flow waveform is selected. Flow is adjustable between 10 and 120 L/min. The flow delivery is limited to the value set on the peak flow control.

Cycle Variables

The cycle variables include pressure, flow, and time. Pressure becomes the cycle variable when inspiratory pressure reaches the pressure set on the high peak pressure control. The high peak pressure is adjustable between 1 and 140 cmH$_2$O. When the pressure limit is reached, inspiratory flow is stopped and both audible and visual alarms are activated.

Flow becomes the cycle variable during pressure support. When inspiratory flow decays to 25% of the peak inspiratory flow, breath delivery stops. When the ventilator is flow triggered in CPAP mode (flow support), inspiration is also flow cycled.

Time becomes the cycle variable during mandatory breath delivery. The microprocessor determines volume as a function of flow and inspiratory time. Once the appropriate inspiratory time has been reached, based upon peak flow and tidal volume settings or inspiratory time setting (pressure control), breath delivery ceases.

Baseline Variable

PEEP/CPAP pressures are adjustable between 0.0 and 30 cmH2O. As described earlier, the dynamic exhalation valve acts as a threshold resistor, creating the PEEP/CPAP pressure.

Conditional Variables

Time

Time becomes a conditional variable during sigh delivery. During normal ventilator supported breaths, they are flow controlled, pressure or flow triggered, or pressure flow or time cycled. During sigh delivery, a sigh breath will be given every 100th breath equal to 150% of the tidal volume set on the tidal volume control. Sigh breath delivery is available during all modes of ventilation except pressure control.

Time and Pressure

Time and pressure become conditional variables during SIMV mode. The rate control determines the frequency of mandatory breath delivery during SIMV mode. The rate control is essentially an electronic timer, delivering a breath at specified time intervals. Between mandatory breath delivery the patient breathes through the flow control valve demand system. The ventilator measures proximal airway pressure to determine if the patient is attempting to initiate a breath. In response to the pressure change, the patient is able to draw gas spontaneously through the flow control valve to meet their inspiratory needs.

Output Waveforms

Pressure

Pressure waveform output is rectangular. This waveform occurs during pressure support and pressure control. During pressure support, pressure rises rapidly to the pressure support level and is maintained there until flow decays to 25% of the peak inspiratory flow value. During pressure control, pressure rises rapidly to the inspiratory pressure level and is maintained there until the inspiratory time has elapsed.

Flow

The flow output may be selected between rectangular and decelerating ramp waveforms. The waveform is selected using the mode control switch.

Alarms

Input Power

In the event of electrical power failure, the "Ventilator Inoperative" LED will be illuminated and an audible warning will be activated. This alarm is battery powered and operates independently from the 120 volt, 60 Hz electrical power.

The low inlet gas alarm is activated whenever system gas pressure drops below 16 psi for 1 second. The alarm is both audible and visual. Loss of system pressure can occur from loss of supply pressure, a clogged inlet filter, or a reducing valve malfunction.

Control Circuit Alarms

Control circuit alarms include ventilator inoperative, sensor disconnect, and I:E alarms. The ventilator inoperative alarm will be activated in the event that an internal system failure has been detected by the microprocessor.

The sensor disconnect alarm is both an audible and a visual alarm. This alarm is activated if the flow sensor becomes disconnected during ventilator operation.

The I:E ratio LED will flash every time a breath is delivered in an inverse I:E ratio. The flashing will stop once settings are adjusted such that inverse I:E ratio ventilation has ceased.

Output Alarms

Pressure. High and low peak pressure alarms are available on the 8400ST®*i* ventilator. The high peak pressure alarm is adjustable between 1 and 140 cmH$_2$O. The low peak pressure alarm is adjustable between 2 and 140 cmH$_2$O.

A low baseline pressure alarm will alert the practitioner to loss of PEEP/CPAP pressures. The alarm is adjustable between –20 and 30 cmH$_2$O. The sub-ambient pressure setting may be used to detect inspiratory efforts on a patient who was previously being ventilated in the control mode.

Flow. A low minute ventilation alarm may be set between 0.0 and 60.0 L/min. The alarm may be used for all modes of ventilation, alerting the practitioner to hypoventilation.

Time. A high breath rate alarm may be set to alert the practitioner to tachypnea. The alarm is adjustable between 3 and 150 breaths per minute.

ASSEMBLY AND TROUBLESHOOTING

Assembly—Bird 8400ST®*i*

1. Attach a 90° elbow adapter to the outlet of the ventilator and connect the ventilator outlet to a bacteria filter with a short length of large-bore tubing.

2. Connect the opposite end of the bacteria filter to the humidifier.

3. Since various humidifiers may be used with the 8400ST®*i*, specific assembly instructions will not be included here.

4. Exhalation valve assembly:
   a. Install the exhalation valve diaphragm by inserting it onto its seat on the ventilator.
   b. Install the exhalation valve body onto the ventilator.

5. Connect the inspiratory limb of patient circuit to the outlet of the humidifier and the expiratory limb to the exhalation valve assembly.

6. Connect the flow transducer assembly to the outlet of the exhalation valve, and connect the male end into the female receptacle on the lower right front of the ventilator.

7. Check all tubing connections and pressure test the ventilator circuit.

8. Connect the power cord to a 120 volt, 60 Hz source.

Troubleshooting

Refer to the troubleshooting algorithms found at the end of this chapter.

An apnea interval alarm may be adjusted between 10 and 60 seconds, alerting the practitioner to periods of patient apnea.

Table 9-8 illustrates the Bird 8400ST®*i* alarms, and Table 9-9 illustrates its capabilities.

TABLE 9-8 8400ST®*i* Alarms

Alarm	Condition/Settings
Input Power	
System Pressure	< 16 psi for one minute
Electric Power	Loss of 120 volt, 60 Hz power
Control Circuit	
Ventilator Inoperative	System failure detected
I:E ratio	Inverse ratio ventilation
Output Alarms	
High Airway Pressure	1.0–140 cmH$_2$O
Low Airway Pressure	2.0–140 cmH$_2$O
Low Baseline Pressure	–20–30 cmH$_2$O
Low Minute Volume	0.0–60.0 L/min
High Breath Rate	3–150 BPM
Apnea	10–60 seconds

TABLE 9-9 8400ST®*i* Ventilator Capabilities

Modes	Control, Assist/Control, SIMV, Flow Support (flow triggering), Pressure Support, Volume Assured Pressure Support, Pressure Control, CPAP, SIGH
Volume	50–2,000 mL
Pressure	0.5–100 cmH2O
Press. Support	0.0–50 cmH2O
Rate	0–80 BPM
Insp. Time	0.1–9.8 seconds
Peak Flow	5–120 L/min
PEEP/CPAP	0.0–30 cmH$_2$O
Sigh Volume	150% of Tidal Volume
Insp. Hold	up to 6 seconds
Insp. Pause	0.0–2.0 seconds
F$_I$O$_2$	0.21–1.0

BIRD PRODUCTS CORPORATION, TBIRD® AVS VENTILATOR

The Bird Products Corporation's TBird® Advanced Ventilatory System (AVS) ventilator is designed to meet the needs of acute care patients (Figure 9-15). The TBird® AVS is an electrically and pneumatically powered ventilator, which is microprocessor controlled. The ventilator's microprocessor control system, when combined with its pressure and flow sensors, provides a flexible system capable of caring for a wide variety of patients.

Input Power

Electrical power supplies the microprocessor control system, the drive mechanism, and the various pressure and flow sensors of the TBird® AVS ventilator. Power is selectable between 120 v, 60 Hz AC and 220 v, 60 Hz AC; internal battery; or external 48V DC battery. Power may be selected by means of a switch located on the rear of the ventilator.

Pneumatic power for the ventilator is supplied by an oxygen source between 40 and 60 psi. Two DISS fittings on the rear of the ventilator are provided for the attachment of oxygen sources. In the event a clinician wishes to transfer from piped wall oxygen to a cylinder, the cylinder may be connected before

Figure 9-15 *A photograph of the TBird® ventilator. (Courtesy Bird Products Corporation, Palm Springs, CA)*

interruption of the wall oxygen, thus providing a seamless transition between the two sources.

Drive Mechanism

Once gas enters the ventilator, it passes through check valves and into the blender system (Figure 9-16). The blender consists of five solenoids with a fixed orifice at each output. The microprocessor determines which and how many solenoids are required to be opened to add the required oxygen to the accumulator/diffuser.

Ambient air passes through a filter (Figure 9-16) and into the accumulator/diffuser. The accumulator/diffuser functions to initially mix the two gases (oxygen and air) and acts as a baffling device to muffle the noise of the high-speed turbine.

The drive mechanism of the TBird® AVS is a small pneumatic turbine capable of providing near-instantaneous flows with a rapid response time. Gas from the accumulator/diffuser passes through a filter silencer to the turbine. The turbine rapidly compresses the blended gas and provides the instantaneous flow demands needed by the patient. The turbine further homogenates the mixture of air and oxygen through its operation. Gas exiting the turbine passes through another silencer, which muffles the turbine noise.

Control Circuit

The control circuit of the TBird® AVS ventilator consists of a turbine differential pressure transducer, an exhalation differential pressure transducer, an electrodynamic exhalation valve, and the microprocessor.

The turbine differential pressure transducer monitors the pressure drop across the turbine (Figure 9-16). The differential pressure, combined with the speed of the turbine, is used by the microprocessor to precisely regulate the turbine's output. An optical sensor detects the turbine's speed, providing feedback to the microprocessor.

The exhalation differential pressure transducer provides a flow signal to the microprocessor, which reflects what is being exhaled by the patient (Figure 9-16). The body of the expiratory flow transducer has a variable orifice element in the center. The flexible element bends as flow increases, creating a pressure drop across the two ports, which is sensed by the pressure transducer.

Figure 9-16 *A schematic drawing showing the TBird® ventilator's pneumatic system. (Courtesy Bird Products Corporation, Palm Springs, CA)*

The electrodynamic exhalation valve is used to regulate PEEP/CPAP pressures, and it closes during mandatory breaths. The valve consists of a high-energy permanent magnet with a suspended coil, which is energized with current. As current is applied to the coil, it is drawn into the core of the valve, closing it.

Control Variable

The control variable for the TBird® AVS is pressure. Differential pressure is detected across the turbine and is used to regulate its output. The microprocessor integrates turbine speed (optically sensed) and the pressure differential to precisely regulate the flow and pressure provided by the turbine drive mechanism.

Phase Variables

Trigger Variables

The trigger variables of the TBird® AVS are flow, time, and manual triggering. During flow-triggered operation, the clinician sets a base flow through the patient circuit. Base flows are adjustable between 10 and 20 L/min. The flow sensitivity is then set; and it is adjustable between 1 and 8 L/min.

Time triggering occurs during mandatory breaths and is a function of the breath rate control, which may be set between 2 and 80 breaths per minute (BPM). When the appropriate time interval has passed, the exhalation valve closes and the ventilator provides a mandatory breath.

The TBird® AVS may be manually triggered by the clinician depressing the manual breath button located at the lower left of the control panel. Depressing this button delivers a volume or pressure-controlled breath, depending upon the breath type selected.

Limit Variables

The limit variables of the TBird® AVS include pressure, volume, and flow. Pressure becomes the limit variable during SIMV (with PEEP/CPAP, CPAP, pressure control, and pressure support ventilation. When the TBird® AVS is operating in these modes, pressure is measured and maintained at a consistent level during breath delivery. PEEP/CPAP pressure may be adjusted between 0 and 30 cmH$_2$O. Pressure control and pressure support may be adjusted between 1 to 100 cmH$_2$O and 1 to 60 cmH$_2$O, respectively.

Volume becomes a limit variable when inspiratory pause is selected. Inspiratory pause may be adjusted between 0 and 2.0 seconds. When inspiratory pause is selected, the inspiratory hold valve closes in conjunction with the exhalation valve, holding the breath in the patient's lungs for the set time interval (Figure 9-16). Under these conditions, volume becomes limited during the inspiratory phase.

Flow becomes a limit variable when the Square Waveform button is depressed and the ventilator is set for volume-controlled ventilation (rate, tidal volume, and peak flow). Peak flow is adjustable between 10 and 140 L/min. The inspiratory flow limit becomes the value selected using the peak flow control.

Cycle Variables

The cycle variables for the TBird® AVS include pressure, flow, and time. Pressure becomes a cycle variable when inspiratory pressure reaches the value set on the high pressure limit control. This control is adjustable between 5 and 120 cmH$_2$O. When the high pressure limit is reached, inspiration is terminated and exhalation begins, and both audible and visual alarms are activated.

Flow is the cycling variable during pressure support. When inspiratory flow decays to 25% of the peak inspiratory flow value, the breath is terminated and the patient is allowed to exhale. If the flow is slow to decay during inspiration, the breath will be terminated after 3 seconds or breath periods, whichever occurs first.

Time is a cycle variable during mandatory breath delivery. The microprocessor determines volume as a function of flow and inspiratory time. Once the desired time has been met, the breath is terminated.

Conditional Variables

Time

Time becomes a conditional variable during sigh breath delivery. During sigh breath delivery, a sigh breath is delivered every 100 breaths, which is equal to 150% of the set tidal volume. Sigh breaths may be used in all modes of ventilation.

Time and Pressure

Time and pressure become conditional variables during SIMV mode. The rate control determines the frequency of mandatory breath delivery during SIMV move. The rate control is essentially an electronic timer, delivering a breath at specified time intervals. Between periods of mandatory breath delivery the patient can obtain spontaneous breaths (pressure support or pure spontaneous) through the ventilator's gas delivery system.

Output Waveforms

Pressure

Pressure waveform output is rectangular. This output waveform occurs during pressure support and pressure control. During these modes, pressure rises rapidly and plateaus at the set pressure level until exhalation begins.

Flow

The flow waveform may be toggled between rectangular (square) and decelerating during volume-controlled breath delivery. This is accomplished by selecting or not selecting the Square Waveform button on the lower left of the control panel.

Alarms

Input Power

The input power alarms consist of electrical power and gas pressure alarms. In the event that AC power is interrupted, the ventilator switches to battery backup power without interrupting ventilation and an audible alarm sounds, while simultaneously the internal battery indicator is illuminated. In the event that the internal or external batteries are low on power, both audible and visual alarms will result.

When the oxygen inlet pressure is less than 35 psi and the oxygen percentage control is set to greater than 21%, both audible and visual alarms will be activated. Remember, the TBird® AVS may be powered by two independent oxygen sources, and when thus connected, one source can serve as a backup for the other.

Control Circuit

The control circuit alarm consists of internal operations, circuit fault, and EEPROM failure alert. All of these alarms are part of the ventilator's self-testing and troubleshooting systems. In the event these alarms are triggered, you should discontinue use of the ventilator and contact a certified Bird service technician or have the unit checked by a suitable biomedical repair facility.

ASSEMBLY AND TROUBLESHOOTING

Assembly—TBird® AVS

1. Exhalation valve assembly: Install the exhalation valve diaphragm and the exhalation valve body into the ventilator. When correctly installed, you will hear a click as it seats into the correct position.

2. Attach a 90° elbow adapter to the ventilator outlet and secure a bacteria filter to it. Connect the ventilator to a heated humidifier using a short length of 22-mm diameter, large-bore tubing.

3. Connect the inspiratory limb from the outlet of the humidifier to the patient wye and the expiratory limb of the circuit to the exhalation valve assembly. The use of water traps in both the inspiratory and expiratory limbs of the circuit is recommended.

4. Connect the ventilator to a 50-psi oxygen source.

5. Connect the power cord to a suitable AC power outlet.

Troubleshooting

Refer to the troubleshooting algorithm found at the end of this chapter.

The flow sensor alarm will sound if a flow sensor is not detected by the ventilator. In this case, check to ensure that the exhalation valve body is correctly seated in its receptacle or replace it with a new one.

Output Alarms

Pressure

Pressure alarms consist of high and low pressure alarms. The high pressure limit alarm may be set at between 5 and 120 cmH$_2$O. The low pressure alarm alerts the practitioner to decreased inspiratory pressures and is adjustable between 2 and 60 cmH$_2$O.

Flow

A low minute ventilation alarm may be set between 0.1 and 99.9 mL. The alarm may be used in all modes to alert the clinician to hypoventilation.

Time

The ventilator incorporates a high breath rate and an apnea alarm. The high breath rate alarm is adjustable between 2 and 150 breaths per minute.

The apnea alarm alerts the clinician to apneic periods. The alarm interval may be adjusted from 10 to 60 seconds. If a breath is not detected within the set time window, the ventilator will automatically switch to backup ventilation. Table 9-10 illustrates the Bird Products Corporation TBird® AVS alarm, and Table 9-11 illustrates its capabilities.

TABLE 9-10 TBird® AVS Alarms

Alarm	Condition
Input Power	
Battery On	AC power failure
Low Battery	Internal battery power is low
Ext Battery	External battery power is low
Control Circuit	
Circuit Fault	Kinked or occluded breathing circuit
EEPROM Fault	EEPROM fails to accept a new value
Vent Inop.	Internal ventilator fault has been detected
Output Alarms	
High Pressure	5–120 cmH$_2$O
Low Pressure	2–60 cmH$_2$O
Low Minute Volume	0.1–99.9 mL/min
High Breath Rate	3–150 breaths per minute
Apnea	10–60 seconds

TABLE 9-11 TBird® AVS Ventilator Capabilities

Modes	Volume control, pressure control, assist/control, SIMV, plus Pressure Support, CPAP, SIGH
Volume	50–2,000 mL
Pressure	5–100 cmH$_2$O
Pressure support	1–60 cmH$_2$O
Rate	2–80 breaths per minute
Inspiratory time	0.3–10 seconds
Peak flow	10–140 L/min
Sigh volume	150% of tidal volume
Inspiratory pause	0.0–2.0 seconds
F$_I$O$_2$	0.21–1.00

DRÄGER, EVITA 4 INTENSIVE CARE VENTILATOR

The Dräger, Inc., Evita 4 intensive care ventilator is a microprocessor-controlled ventilator intended for intensive care use for adults and pediatric patients having a body weight of at least 3 kg (Figure 9-17). The ventilator is very flexible, having both pressure and volume-controlled ventilation with a good monitoring and alarm package to facilitate its application in the care of critically ill patients.

Input Power

The Evita 4 requires both electrical and pneumatic power for its operation. Electric power may be provided by 120 v, 60 Hz or 220 v, 60 Hz AC power, or the unit may be powered by a 12- or 24-V DC external battery. Electrical power is used for the microprocessor control system and the various pressure and flow monitoring and display systems.

Both air and oxygen supplies are required for the Evita 4 ventilator. DISS fittings are located on the rear of the ventilator and gas pressures should range between 43.5 and 87 psi (maximum), with the standard of 50 psi being the preferred pressure.

Gases enter the rear of the ventilator, and each type (air and oxygen) passes through a filter and into the mixing unit (Figure 9-18). A gauge pressure transducer monitors the incoming line pressure before the gas line pressure before the gas enters solenoid valves, which accurately blend the air and oxygen to the desired percentage.

Figure 9-17 *A photograph of the Dräger Evita 4 ventilator. (Courtesy Dräger, Inc., Telford, PA)*

Control Circuit

The control circuit consists of the microprocessor, the flow control valve, a differential pressure transducer, and the exhalation valve (Figure 9-18). Differential pressure measured across the flow control valve is proportional to the flow-out of the ventilator. The microprocessor integrates flow over time to determine the delivered volume.

The exhalation valve is used to regulate pressure during the PEEP/CPAP and pressure ventilation modes. Partial closure of the valve creates pressure in the circuit and a pressure transducer provides a feedback signal to the microprocessor, which then regulates the output of the flow control valve.

In the event of gas supply or electrical power failure, ambient air may be drawn in through a port and filter to provide gas to the patient. The check valve prevents gas from the ventilator's pneumatic system from escaping to ambient pressure.

Control Variables

The control variables for the Evita 4 ventilator are flow and pressure. Flow is a control variable during the volume control modes. As described earlier, the ventilator integrates flow over time to determine volume delivery.

Pressure is the control variable during pressure-controlled ventilation, pressure support, and PEEP/CPAP. The exhalation valve partially closes the patient circuit, which permits pressure to build and be regulated by the microprocessor and flow control valve system.

Phase Variables

Trigger Variables

Trigger variables for the Evita 4 ventilator include flow, time, and manual triggering. Flow is the trigger variable for the Evita 4 ventilator. Flow triggering is adjustable between 1 and 15 L/min and is available during all breath modes.

Figure 9-18 *A schematic drawing showing the Evita 4 ventilator's pneumatic system. (Courtesy Dräger, Inc., Telford, PA)*

Time triggering occurs during mandatory breath delivery in the absence of a patient-initiated breath. When the ventilator is time triggered, breath delivery is governed by the breath rate control, which may be adjusted from 0 to 100 breaths per minute.

Manual triggering occurs when the clinician depresses the manual breath button. When selected, a manual breath is delivered in all modes except for CPAP without pressure support.

Limit Variables

The limit variables for the Evita 4 ventilator include pressure and flow. Pressure becomes a limit variable during CPAP, pressure control, and pressure support modes of ventilation. The inspiration unit (gas flow delivery system) maintains an appropriate flow to provide the constant pressure required in the circuit.

Flow becomes a limit variable during volume-controlled breaths when the ventilator is delivering a square wave flow pattern. Inspiratory flow is adjustable between 6 and 120 L/min.

Cycle Variables

The cycle variables for the ventilator include pressure, flow, and time. Pressure becomes the cycling variable when inspiratory pressure reaches the level set on the inspiratory pressure limit control. The peak pressure limit may be adjusted between 0 and 100 cmH$_2$O. When the pressure limit is reached, inspiration is terminated and both audible and visual alarms result.

Flow is a cycling variable during pressure support, during which, if inspiratory flow tapers to 25% of the peak inspiratory flow value, the inspiratory phase is terminated. If the flow is slow to decay, the breath will automatically end after 4 seconds have elapsed.

Time is a cycle variable during mandatory breath delivery. The microprocessor determines what inspiratory time is required for a specific volume to be delivered, or ends the breath based upon the inspiratory time setting (during pressure-controlled ventilation).

Baseline Variable

The baseline variable for the Evita 4 ventilator is pressure. PEEP/CPAP pressures may be adjusted between 0 and 35 cmH$_2$O. As described earlier, the exhalation valve functions as a threshold resistor, creating pressure in the circuit.

Conditional Variables

Time and Flow

Time and flow become conditional variables during SIMV mode. The rate control determines the frequency of mandatory breath delivery. The rate control is essentially an electronic timer, which determines mandatory breaths at specific time intervals. Between mandatory breaths, the ventilator monitors flow to determine whether the patient is initiating a spontaneous breath. The gas delivery system responds to the patient's efforts, providing gas for spontaneous ventilation and synchronizing mandatory breaths.

Output Waveforms

Pressure

The pressure output is rectangular during pressure support and pressure control ventilation modes. During these modes, pressure rises rapidly to the set pressure value and is held there until exhalation begins.

Flow

Flow output can be rectangular (square), during volume breath delivery, or decelerating, during pressure-controlled breath delivery.

Alarms

Input Power

The input power alarms include electrical power failure and gas supply failure (air and oxygen). In the event that AC electrical power is lost, audible and visual alarms will sound. The Evita 4 ventilator can operate for about 10 minutes on internal battery power if the optional 12/24-V DC battery pack is installed. In the event of either gas or air pressure loss, both audible and visual alarms will result. If the line pressure falls below 43.5 psi (air or oxygen), the alarm will be triggered.

Control Circuit

The Evita 4 ventilator control circuit alarms include Check Settings, Device Failure, Expiratory Valve Inop (inoperative), Fan Failure, Flow Measurement Inop, Flow Sensor, Failure to Cycle, and Loss of Data. The ventilator, through the microprocessor, constantly evaluates and verifies the function of many key components required for safety during ventilator operation. The Check Settings alarm occurs if there is a power interruption while alarms or settings are being entered. To correct the alarm, check the settings and then reset the alarm.

A device failure alarm is triggered if the microprocessor detects the failure of a critical internal component. When this occurs, disconnect the ventilator, provide an alternate means of ventilatory support for the patient, and remove the unit from service.

The Expiratory Valve Inop alarm occurs if the valve is not properly seated, the flow sensor is defective or not calibrated, or the expiratory valve is defective. Make sure the valve is correctly installed, calibrate the flow sensor, and/or replace the exhalation valve to correct the alarm.

A Fan Failure alarm occurs if the internal fan ceases to function. Discontinue using the ventilator, provide an alternate means of supporting the patient, and remove the unit from service.

The Flow Measurement Inop alarm occurs if the ventilator fails to detect flow through the flow sensor. Usually this occurs with a flow sensor failure. Discontinue using the ventilator, provide an alternate means of supporting the patient, and remove the unit from service.

The Flow Sensor alarm occurs if the sensor is not seated properly. Disconnect the sensor and reinstall it, making certain it is fully inserted in the rubber tip of the exhalation valve.

A Failure to Cycle alarm can occur if the ventilator fails to deliver a breath or the microprocessor detects a critical fault in the control system. If this alarm occurs, first check the peak pressure settings to verify that they are correct. If the alarm persists, discontinue use of the ventilator and remove it from service.

If the internal lithium battery becomes fully discharged, a Loss of Data alarm will result. Discontinue using the ventilator, provide an alternate means of supporting the patient, and remove the unit from service.

Output Alarms

Pressure

The Evita 4 ventilator pressure alarms include High and Low Airway Pressure and High PEEP or Baseline Pressure. The High Airway Pressure alarm is adjustable between 10 and 100 cmH_2O.

The Low Airway Pressure alarm is linked to the PEEP control setting. In the event of a circuit or cuff leak that drops the baseline pressure, the Low Airway Pressure alarm will sound to alert the clinician of the event. The High PEEP alarm is also nonadjustable and is linked to the PEEP control setting. In the event the expiratory circuit or exhalation valve becomes obstructed, raising the baseline pressure, this alarm will alert the clinician to the event.

Volume

The Evita 4 ventilator includes an adjustable High Tidal Volume alarm and a nonadjustable Low Tidal Volume alarm. The High Tidal Volume alarm is adjustable between 30 and 4000 ml. The Low Tidal Volume alarm is linked to the tidal volume setting and, like the Low PEEP alarm, it alerts the clinician to cuff or circuit leaks.

Flow

Both High- and Low-Minute Ventilation alarms are available on the Evita 4 ventilator. The High-Minute Ventilation alarm may be set between 0.5 and 41 L/min, and the Low-Minute alarm, between 0 and 40 L/min. These alarms may be used in all modes.

Time

The High Rate alarm is adjustable between 5 and 120 breaths per minute. The High Rate alarm serves to alert the clinician to tachypneic events. An Apnea alarm also alerts the clinician to apneic events. The Apnea alarm is adjustable between 15 and 60 seconds.

Inspired Gas

The inspired gas alarm consists of High and Low F_IO_2 alarms. The alarm limits are not adjustable but are based upon the F_IO_2 settings. If the F_IO_2 is 0.60 or less, the alarm will automatically be set for ±4%, and if the F_IO_2 is greater than 0.60, the limits will automatically be set for ±6%.

Expired Gas

The Evita 4 ventilator also incorporates an Exhaled CO_2 monitor and alarm. Alarm limits are available for both Upper and Lower $PetCO_2$. The upper limit is adjustable between 0 and 100 mmHg, while the lower limit is adjustable between 0 and 99 mmHg.

Table 9-12 summarizes the Dräger Evita 4 alarms, and Table 9-13 summarizes its capabilities.

TABLE 9-12 Dräger Evita 4 Alarms

Alarm	Condition/Settings
Input Power	
Air supply low	Air pressure less than 43.5 psi
Oxygen supply low	Oxygen pressure less than 43.5 psi
Electrical power failure	Loss of AC power
Control Circuit	
Check settings	Power interruption during entry
Device failure	Internal fault/system failure detected
Exp valve inop	Valve not seated, flow sensor not calibrated or expiratory valve failure
Fan failure	Failure of internal fan
Flow measurement inop	Flow sensor defective or flow measurement defect
Flow sensor	Flow sensor not seated correctly
Failure to cycle	Incorrect peak pressure settings or internal failure
Loss of data	Lithium battery fully discharged
Output Alarms	
High airway pressure	10–100 cmH$_2$O
Low airway pressure	Automatic
High baseline pressure	Automatic
Low baseline pressure	Automatic
High tidal volume	30–4,000 mL
Low tidal volume	Automatic
High breath rate	5–120 BPM
Apnea	15–60 seconds
Inspired Gas	
Oxygen	±4% or ±6%, depending on FIO2 setting
Expired Gas	
High PetCO$_2$	0–100 mmHg
Low PetCO$_2$	0–99 mmHg

TABLE 9-13 Dräger Evita 4 Ventilator Capabilities

Modes	Volume controlled, pressure controlled, SIMV, MMV, pressure support/ CPAP, APRV, MMV
Volume	.02–2.0 liters
Pressure	0–80 cmH$_2$O
Pressure support	0–80 cmH$_2$O
Rate	0–100 / min
Insp. time	0.1–10 seconds
Peak flow	6–120 L/min
PEEP/CPAP	0–35 cmH$_2$O
Insp. hold	15 seconds
F$_I$O$_2$	0.21–1.0

ASSEMBLY AND TROUBLESHOOTING

Assembly—Dräger Evita 4

1. Install the exhalation valve:
   a. Tilt the control panel upward for better access to the valve set and flow sensor fittings.
   b. Push the valve assembly into its receptacle. Check to ensure it is seated by gently pulling on the exhalation port.
   c. Connect a flow sensor by pushing it into place, ensuring that it is seated on the rubber lip of the exhalation valve.

2. Install an O_2 sensor capsule:
   a. Turn the exhalation port to the left.
   b. Use a coin or a large screw driver to remove the protective cover.
   c. Loosen the two thumbscrews and open the sensor chamber.
   d. Install a new sensor capsule and replace the chamber cover and protective plate.

3. Turn the ventilator outlet port to the right and install a bacteria filter.

4. Assemble the patient circuit:
   a. Connect the bacteria filter to a heated humidifier with a short length of 22-mm, large-diameter tubing.
   b. Connect the inspiratory limb of the patient circuit to the outlet of the humidifier, and the opposite end to the patient wye.
   c. Connect the expiratory limb to the exhalation port.
   d. It is recommended that water traps be used on both the inspiratory and expiratory limbs of the circuit.
   e. Connect the humidifier temperature probe to the port on the airway.
   f. If PetCO$_2$ monitoring is desired, install the sensor between the patient wye and the patient's airway.

5. Connect 50-psi air and oxygen supplies to their respective DISS fittings on the rear of the ventilator.

6. Connect the electrical supply cord to an appropriate AC outlet.

Troubleshooting

Refer to the troubleshooting algorithms found at the end of this chapter.

HAMILTON MEDICAL, GALILEO

Hamilton Medical, Inc. markets the Galileo ventilator, which is a pneumatically powered, microprocessor-controlled flow controller (Figures 9-19 and 9-20). The ventilator requires 50-psi air and oxygen, however an optional compressor can be purchased if compressed air is not available. The microprocessor in conjunction with the ventilator's flow and pressure sensors provides a very flexible platform allowing for a variety of ventilation modes and extensive monitoring capability.

Input Power

The microprocessor control system is powered by 120 v, 60 Hz electrical power (the main power is switchable to 240 v, 60 Hz as well). The pneumatic system requires 50-psi air and oxygen sources. If 50-psi air is not available, an optional compressor will mount on the rear of the ventilator's stand to provide the compressed air to operate the pneumatic system.

Drive Mechanism

The 50-psi air and oxygen enter the rear of the ventilator through DISS fittings. Internally, the 50-psi pressure is reduced to 22 psi by means of two reducing valves. The gases each enter a separate mixer valve that proportionally matches oxygen and air to the desired oxygen concentration. Unlike a blender, each gas is metered separately before being joined together at the inlet to a reducing valve.

After leaving the mixer valves, the metered gas enters another reducing valve where the pressure is reduced to 350 cmH$_2$O. The gas, now blended to the desired oxygen concentration, then is conducted into a large reservoir

Figure 9-19 *A photograph of the Hamilton Galileo volume ventilator. (Courtesy Hamilton Medical, Reno, NV)*

Figure 9-20 *A photograph showing the Galileo ventilator's control panel. (Courtesy Hamilton Medical, Reno, NV)*

that holds up to 8 liters. The reservoir helps the ventilator to meet high instantaneous flow demands, and further helps to homogenize the gas concentration. A safety popoff valve set at 400 cmH$_2$O provides a safety margin if excessive pressures build in the pneumatic circuit, protecting the patient.

Control Circuit

The Galileo uses a microprocessor and an electrodynamic flow control valve to regulate flow output from the ventilator (Figure 9-21). The flow control valve is a plunger type valve, which is electromagnetically controlled and is a modified version of the valve used in the Hamilton Veolar ventilator. A potentiometer measures the actual valve opening, ensuring precise and virtual instantaneous control. This system operates in conjunction with a differential pressure transducer. When the valve is open, a pressure difference will exist between the flow control valve inlet and outlet. This

pressure differential is proportional to flow. The microprocessor has programmed into its memory the resistance the valve has at various positions. This resistance will cause a pressure drop that is proportional to gas flow. Volume delivery becomes a function of inspiratory flow and time. Technically, the ventilator is really a pressure controller when delivering mandatory breaths, since pressure is measured and used as a signal to regulate the output from the flow control valve.

Flow output waveforms include rectangular, descending ramp, 50% descending ramp, and sinusoidal waveforms. All of these waveforms are possible through microprocessor control of the flow control valve.

The exhalation valve is an electronically controlled valve. The dynamic motor is actually an electromagnetic device and is a modified version of the valve used on the Hamilton Veolar ventilator. During inspiration, the plunger valve closes, causing gas to flow into the patient circuit and into the patient's lungs. During expiration, the motor opens the exhalation valve and the patient exhales. The valve also determines PEEP levels, partially closing to maintain pressure in the patient circuit.

Control Variables

As described earlier, the control variable used by the Hamilton Galileo ventilator is pressure. Differential pressure, measured across the flow control valve, is used to regulate the valve during tidal volume delivery during mandatory breaths. Pressure is also the control variable during PEEP/CPAP and pressure support.

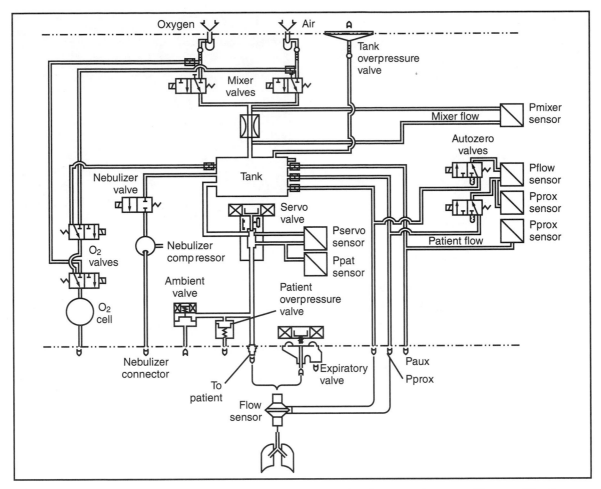

Figure 9-21 *A schematic drawing of the Hamilton Galileo ventilator's pneumatic system. (Courtesy Hamilton Medical, Reno, NV)*

Phase Variables

Trigger Variables

The trigger variables for the Hamilton Galileo include pressure, flow, time, and manual variables. Pressure is used as a trigger variable for demand breaths during assist/CMV, SIMV, and pressure support. When inspiratory pressure falls below the threshold established by the trigger sensitivity control, the ventilator will initiate a breath. The trigger sensitivity may be set between 0.5 and 10.0 cmH2O (adult) and 0.5 to 5 cmH$_2$O (infant) below baseline pressure by the practitioner.

The Hamilton Galileo can be flow triggered as well. Flow sensitivity may be set from 0.5 to 15 L/min (adult or pediatric) and 0.5 to 5 L/min (infant). Base flow is automatically set between 4 and 30 L/min, depending upon what the practitioner has set for the trigger level. Inspiratory flow is monitored at the proximal airway via a small differential pressure transducer positioned at the patient's airway. Both adult and neonatal flow sensors are available, allowing the ventilator to accommodate all patients.

Time becomes a trigger variable during assist CMV if no inspiratory effort (pressure drop or flow change) is sensed by the ventilator. If the patient does not trigger a breath, the ventilator will deliver a mandatory breath at the set tidal volume and rate. Respiratory rates are adjustable between 5 and 120 breaths per minute (CMV) or 1 and 60 breaths per minute (SIMV).

The ventilator may be manually triggered by the practitioner depressing the manual breath key on the control panel. When depressed, the ventilator will deliver a volume-controlled breath (Assist/CMV, SIMV, and CPAP).

Limit Variables

The limit variables of the Hamilton Galileo include pressure, volume, and flow. Pressure becomes a limit variable during pressure control modes, SIMV (with PEEP applied), MMV, CPAP, and pressure support. Under these conditions, the ventilator will augment flow to maintain the desired pressure level. Pressure during pressure control mode may be adjusted between 5 and 100 cmH$_2$O (adult/pediatric) and 5 to 50 cmH$_2$O (infant). PEEP/CPAP pressures are adjustable between 0.0 and 50.0 cmH$_2$O. Pressure support is adjustable between 5 and 100 cmH$_2$O (adult/pediatric) and 5 to 50 cmH$_2$O (infant).

Volume becomes a limit variable when the inspiratory pause time is adjusted to greater than zero. Inspiratory pause time may be set between 0 to 70 % of the cycle time (adult/ pediatric). When activated, a volume breath is delivered and held until the set inspiratory pause time period has elapsed.

Flow becomes a limit variable during mandatory volume breath delivery. During start-up of the ventilator, by pressing the M knob (monitor leftmost knob) the practitioner can control the timing of breath delivery during volume control modes. By selecting Peak Flow, the inspiratory flow is determined by the setting on the peak flow setting. When this option has been configured, flow is limited to the maximum value set by the peak flow setting.

If T$_I$ (inspiratory time) or I:E ratio are selected during start-up, flow rate is a function of the tidal volume, respiratory rate and inspiratory time percent, and waveform control settings. Flow is variable between 1 and 180 L/min.

Cycle Variables

Cycle variables for the Hamilton Galileo include pressure, flow, and time. Pressure becomes a cycle variable if the inspiratory pressure reaches the setting on the maximum inspiratory pressure control. Peak inspiratory pressure may be adjusted between 10 and 120 cmH$_2$O. When the pressure limit is reached, inspiration is terminated and both audible and visual alarms are activated. As a practitioner, you should set the upper pressure limit to 5 to 10 cmH$_2$O greater than the peak ventilating pressure during pressure or volume-controlled modes.

Flow becomes a cycle variable during pressure support ventilation. Inspiration is terminated when inspiratory flow falls to 25% (adults) or 15% (pediatrics) of the peak inspiratory flow (pre-programmed values). Once inspiratory flow reaches this point, pressure falls to the baseline value. This value for percentage of peak flow for breath termination in pressure support is adjustable by the practitioner between 10% and 40% (expiratory trigger sensitivity). For example, if the peak flow is set at 90 L/min and the expiratory trigger sensitivity is set at 30%, the breath will be terminated when flow reaches 27 L/min.

Time becomes a cycle variable when inspiratory pause has been set or when being used in pressure control modes. Inspiratory pause may be activated when the pause time has been set to greater than zero. Pause times may be adjusted between 0 and 70 % of the cycle time. If inspiratory pause has been activated, inspiration will be terminated when the set pause time has elapsed.

During pressure control modes of ventilation (P-A/C, P-SIMV or P-A/C + APV) the practitioner sets the inspiratory pressure limit, the inspiratory time (cycle variable), and the trigger variable (pressure or flow). Time is the cycling variable and is determined by the setting for the TI value, and is adjustable between 0.1 to 3 seconds.

Baseline Variable

PEEP/CPAP pressure is generated by the electrodynamic exhalation valve partially closing during exhalation, creating the PEEP/ CPAP pressure. PEEP/CPAP pressures are adjustable between 0.0 and 50 cmH$_2$O (adult/ pediatric) and 0 to 25 cmH$_2$O (infant).

Output Waveforms

Pressure

The Hamilton Galileo can deliver a rectangular pressure waveform during volume control modes and also during pressure support (SIMV or spontaneous modes). Under these conditions, pressure rises rapidly and is held until inspiration is terminated.

Flow

The flow output waveform capabilities of the Galileo include rectangular, descending ramp, 50% descending ramp, and sinusoidal

---

ASSEMBLY AND TROUBLESHOOTING

Assembly—Hamilton Galileo Ventilator

To assemble the Hamilton Galileo, follow this suggested assembly guide.

1. Connect high pressure hoses to a 50-psi medical air and oxygen source.

2. Connect the power cord to a 120 volt, 60 Hz outlet.

3. Attach a bacteria filter to the ventilator outlet.

4. Connect the humidifier inlet to the bacteria filter using large-bore tubing.

Since a variety of humidifiers may be used with this ventilator, specific instructions will not be included here.

5. Connect the inspiratory limb of the circuit to the outlet of the humidifier. Attach the expiratory limb to the exhalation valve fitting.

6. Connect the proximal airway line to the proximal airway fitting on the ventilator.

Troubleshooting

Refer to the troubleshooting algorithms found at the end of this chapter.

---

waveforms. As described earlier, these waveforms can be accurately reproduced by the feedback system between the internal differential pressure transducer, the microprocessor, and the electrodynamic flow control valve.

Alarms

Input Power

In the event of electrical power failure, the "Power" LED will be illuminated and an audible warning will be activated. This alarm is powered by a rechargeable battery and operates independently from the 120 volts, 60 Hz electrical power.

The low inlet gas alarm is activated whenever system gas pressure drops below 29 psi. The alarm is both audible and visual. An alarm will also alert the practitioner if the reservoir pressure falls below 200 cmH$_2$O.

Control Circuit Alarms

Control circuit alarms include ventilator inoperative and check settings (incompatible settings) problems. The ventilator inoperative alarm will be activated in the event that an internal system failure has been detected by the microprocessor.

The check settings (incompatible settings) alarm will be activated if the practitioner adjusts the controls such that they are out of range for the ventilator.

Output Alarms

Pressure. High and low peak pressure alarms are available on the Galileo ventilator. The high peak pressure alarm is adjustable between 10 and 120 cmH$_2$O. The loss of PEEP pressure alarm is not adjustable and activates when pressure falls 3 cmH$_2$O below the set baseline pressure for a time period of 10 seconds.

Flow. A low and high minute ventilation alarm may be set between 1 and 50 L/min (adult) and 0 to 10 L/min (pediatric/infant). The alarm may be used for all modes of ventilation, alerting the practitioner to hypoventilation or hyperventilation.

Time. A low/high breath rate alarm may be set to alert the practitioner to bradypnea or tachypnea. The alarm is adjustable between 0 to 130 breaths per minute.

An apnea interval alarm alerts the practitioner to periods of patient apnea. The alarm is adjustable between a time interval of 15 to 60 seconds (adult/pediatric) and 10 to 60 seconds (infant). The alarm becomes active when no flow has been detected through the flow sensor during the time interval set.

Inspired Gas. An oxygen alarm is incorporated into the ventilator to facilitate patient management. If the oxygen concentration is lower or higher than the adjusted oxygen concentration (range of 18 to 103%), a high/low

TABLE 9-14 Hamilton Galileo Alarms

Alarm	Condition/Settings
Input Power	
Gas Supply Pressure	< 28 psi
Power	Loss of 120 volt, 60 Hz power, Battery
Control Circuit	
Technical Fault	System failure detected
Check Settings	Incompatible settings
Output Alarms	
High Airway Pressure	10–120 cmH$_2$O
Loss of PEEP	3.0 cmH$_2$O below baseline for > 10 seconds
Low Minute Volume	1–50 L/min (adult), 0–10 L/min (pediatric/infant)
High Breath Rate	0–130 BPM
Apnea	15–60 seconds
Inspired Gas	High/Low Oxygen Tension (18–103%)

TABLE 9-15 Hamilton Galileo Ventilator Capabilities

Modes	CMV, Spontaneous (CPAP), SIMV, Pressure Control, MMV, Pressure Support
Volume	100–2,000 mL (adult), 20–300 mL (pediatric)
Pressure	5–100 cmH$_2$O (adult/pediatric), 5–50 cmH$_2$O (infant)
Press. Support	0.0–100 cmH$_2$O (adult), 0–50 cmH$_2$O (infant)
Rate	5–120 BPM (adult/pediatric), 10–120 (infant)
I:E	1:4 to 4:1
Peak Flow	Up to 180 L/min (not adjustable)
PEEP/CPAP	0.0–50 cmH$_2$O (adult/pediatric), 0–25 cmH$_2$0 (infant)
Insp. Pause	0 to 70% of the cycle time
F$_I$O$_2$	0.21–1.0

oxygen alarm will alert the practitioner to the condition.

Table 9-14 illustrates the Hamilton Galileo alarms, and Table 9-15 illustrates its capabilities.

HAMILTON MEDICAL, VEOLAR

Hamilton Medical, Inc., markets the Veolar ventilator, which is another example of a pneumatically powered, microprocessor-controlled flow controller (Figures 9-22 and 9-23). The microprocessor, when combined with appropriate flow and pressure sensors, can provide a flexible feedback control system allowing a variety of modes, monitors, and alarms.

Input Power

Power to run the microprocessor control circuitry is provided by 115 volt, 60 Hz electrical power. The pneumatic system is powered by 50-psi source of medical air and oxygen.

Figure 9-22 *A photograph of the Hamilton Veolar volume ventilator. (Courtesy Hamilton Medical, Reno, NV)*

Figure 9-23 *A photograph showing the Veolar ventilator's control panel. (Courtesy Hamilton Medical, Reno, NV)*

Drive Mechanism

The pneumatic drive mechanism (Figure 9-24) reduces the line pressure of the incoming gas to 22 psi by means of the air and oxygen reducing valves. The gas pressures are closely matched to enhance the accuracy of the blending system. Gas flows from these pressure controlling elements to the oxygen blender.

The oxygen blender is a type of proportioning valve that mixes the oxygen and air. Gas then exits the blender to another reducing valve, which holds a constant pressure of 350 cmH$_2$O. The gas flows from the second reducing valve to a tank or reservoir. When pressurized to 350 cmH$_2$O, the reservoir volume is close to 8 liters. The large reservoir serves as a buffer when high flow demands are made on the ventilator. A safety popoff valve set at 400 cmH$_2$O provides a margin of safety if excessive pressures build in the pneumatic circuit, protecting the patient.

If rapid changes in F$_I$O$_2$ are required, the flush control button may be depressed and held. When held down, 60 L/min of gas flows through the reservoir, quickly expelling the gas and facilitating a more rapid change in oxygen concentration.

Control Circuit

The Veolar uses a microprocessor and an electrodynamic flow control valve to regulate flow output from the ventilator. The flow control valve is a plunger-type valve, which is electromagnetically controlled. A potentiometer measures the actual valve opening, ensuring precise and virtually instantaneous control. This system operates in conjunction with a differential pressure transducer. When the valve is open, a pressure difference will exist between the flow control valve inlet and outlet. This pressure differential is proportional to flow. The microprocessor has programmed into its memory the resistance the valve has at various positions. This resistance will cause a pressure drop that is proportional to gas flow. Volume delivery becomes a function of inspiratory flow and time. Technically, the ventilator is really a pressure controller when delivering mandatory breaths, since pressure is measured and used as a signal to regulate the output from the flow control valve.

Flow output waveforms include rectangular, ascending and descending ramp, and sinusoidal waveforms. All of these waveforms are possible through microprocessor control of the flow control valve.

The exhalation valve is an electronically controlled valve. The dynamic motor is actually an electromagnetic device. During inspiration, the plunger valve closes, causing gas to flow into the patient circuit and into the patient's lungs. During expiration, the motor opens the exhalation valve and the patient exhales. The valve also determines PEEP levels, partially closing to maintain pressure in the patient circuit.

Control Variable

As described earlier, the control variable used by the Hamilton Veolar ventilator is pressure. Differential pressure, measured across the flow control valve, is used to regulate the valve during tidal volume delivery during mandatory breaths. Pressure is also the control variable during PEEP/CPAP and pressure support.

Phase Variables

Trigger Variables

The trigger variables for the Hamilton Veolar include pressure, time, and manual variables. Pressure is used as a trigger variable for demand breaths during assist/CMV, SIMV, and pressure support. When inspiratory pressure falls below the threshold established by the trigger sensitivity control, the ventilator will initiate a breath. The trigger sensitivity may be

Figure 9-24 *A schematic drawing of the Hamilton Veolar ventilator's pneumatic system. (Courtesy Hamilton Medical, Reno, NV)*

set between 1.0 and 15.0 cmH$_2$O below baseline pressure by the practitioner or turned off.

Time becomes a trigger variable during assist CMV if no inspiratory effort (pressure drop) is sensed by the ventilator. If the patient does not trigger a breath, the ventilator will deliver a mandatory breath at the set tidal volume and rate. Respiratory rates are adjustable

between 5 and 60 breaths per minute (CMV) or 0.5 and 30 breaths per minute (SIMV).

The ventilator may be manually triggered by the practitioner depressing the mandatory breath key on the control panel. When depressed, the ventilator will deliver a volume-controlled breath (Assist/CMV, SIMV, and CPAP).

Limit Variables

The limit variables of the Hamilton Veolar include pressure, volume, and flow. Pressure becomes a limit variable during SIMV (with PEEP applied), MMV, CPAP, and pressure support. Under these conditions, the ventilator will augment flow to maintain the desired pressure level. PEEP/CPAP pressures are adjustable between 0.0 and 50.0 cmH$_2$O. Pressure support is adjustable between 0.0 and 100 cmH$_2$O.

Volume becomes a limit variable when the inspiratory pause is adjusted to greater than zero. Inspiratory pause may be activated when the inspiratory and expiratory time controls are separated. The difference between them becomes the inspiratory pause. When activated, a volume breath is delivered and held until the set inspiratory pause time period has elapsed.

Flow becomes a limit variable during mandatory breaths. Flow rate is a function of the tidal volume, respiratory rate and inspiratory time percent, and waveform control settings. Flow is variable between 0 and 180 L/min.

Cycle Variables

Cycle variables for the Hamilton Veolar include pressure, flow, and time. Pressure becomes a cycle variable if the inspiratory pressure reaches the setting on the maximum inspiratory pressure control. Peak inspiratory pressure may be adjusted between 10 and 110 cmH$_2$O. When the pressure limit is reached, inspiration is terminated and both audible and visual alarms are activated.

Flow becomes a cycle variable during pressure support ventilation. Inspiration is terminated when inspiratory flow falls to approximately 25% of the peak inspiratory flow. Once flow decays to this point, pressure falls to the baseline value.

Time becomes a cycle variable when inspiratory pause has been adjusted. Inspiratory pause may be activated when the inspiratory and expiratory time controls are separated. If inspiratory pause has been activated, inspiration will be terminated when the pause time has elapsed.

Baseline Variable

PEEP/CPAP pressure is generated by the electrodynamic exhalation valve partially closing during inspiration, creating the PEEP/CPAP pressure. PEEP/CPAP pressures are adjustable between 0.0 and 50 cmH$_2$O.

Output Waveforms

Pressure

The Hamilton Veolar can deliver a rectangular pressure waveform during MMV mode and also during pressure support (SIMV or spontaneous modes). Under these conditions, pressure rises rapidly and is held until inspiration is terminated.

Flow

The flow output waveform capabilities of the Veolar include rectangular, ascending and descending ramp, and sinusoidal. As described earlier, these waveforms can be accurately reproduced by the feedback system between the internal differential pressure transducer, the microprocessor, and the electrodynamic flow control valve.

ASSEMBLY AND TROUBLESHOOTING

Assembly—Hamilton Veolar Ventilator

To assemble the Hamilton Veolar, follow this suggested assembly guide:

1. Connect high-pressure hoses to a 50-psi medical air and oxygen source.

2. Connect the power cord to a 120 volt, 60 Hz outlet.

3. Attach a bacteria filter to the ventilator outlet.

4. Connect the humidifier inlet to the bacteria filter using large-bore tubing.

Since a variety of humidifiers may be used with this ventilator, specific instructions will not be included here.

5. Connect the inspiratory limb of the circuit to the outlet of the humidifier. Attach the expiratory limb to the exhalation valve fitting.

6. Connect the proximal airway line to the proximal airway fitting on the ventilator.

Troubleshooting

Refer to the troubleshooting algorithms found at the end of this chapter.

Alarms

Input Power

In the event of electrical power failure, the "Power" LED will be illuminated and an audible warning will be activated. This alarm is powered by a rechargeable battery and operates independently from the 120 volts, 60 Hz electrical power.

The low inlet gas alarm is activated whenever system gas pressure drops below 29 psi. The alarm is both audible and visual. An alarm will also alert the practitioner if the reservoir pressure falls below 200 cmH₂O.

Control Circuit Alarms

Control circuit alarms include ventilator malfunction and user (incompatible settings) problems. The ventilator malfunction alarm will be activated in the event that an internal system failure has been detected by the microprocessor.

The user (incompatible settings) alarm will be activated if the practitioner adjusts the controls such that they are out of range for the ventilator.

Output Alarms

Pressure. High and low peak pressure alarms are available on the Veolar ventilator. The high peak pressure alarm is adjustable between 10 and 120 cmH₂O. The loss of PEEP pressure alarm is not adjustable and activates when pressure falls 3 cmH₂O below the set baseline pressure.

Flow. A low minute ventilation alarm may be set between 0.2 and 50 L/min. The alarm may be used for all modes of ventilation, alerting the practitioner to hypoventilation.

Time. A high breath rate alarm may be set to alert the practitioner to tachypnea. The alarm is adjustable between 10 to 70 breaths per minute.

An apnea interval alarm alerts the practitioner to periods of patient apnea. The alarm is not adjustable and becomes active when no flow has been detected through the flow sensor during the past 15 seconds. A failure-to-cycle alarm is activated if no flow has been detected through the flow control valve over the past 20 seconds.

Inspired Gas. An oxygen alarm is incorporated into the ventilator to facilitate patient management. If the oxygen concentration is lower or higher than the adjusted oxygen concentration (range of 18 to 103%), a high/low oxygen alarm will alert the practitioner to the condition.

Table 9-16 illustrates the Hamilton Veolar alarms, and Table 9-17 illustrates its capabilities.

TABLE 9-16 Hamilton Veolar Alarms

Alarm	Condition/Settings
Input Power	
Gas Supply Pressure	< 29 psi
Power	Loss of 120 volt, 60 Hz power
Control Circuit	
Dysfunction	System failure detected
User	Incompatible settings
Output Alarms	
High Airway Pressure	10.0–120 cmH₂O
Loss of PEEP	3.0 cmH₂O below baseline for > 10 seconds
Low Minute Volume	0.2–50 L/min
High Breath Rate	10–70 BPM
Apnea	15–20 seconds
Inspired Gas	High/Low Oxygen Tension (18–103%)

TABLE 9-17 Hamilton Veolar Ventilator Capabilities

Modes	CMV, Spontaneous (CPAP), SIMV, Pressure Control, MMV, Pressure Support
Volume	20–2,000 mL
Pressure	0.0–120 cmH₂O
Press. Support	0.0–100 cmH₂O
Rate	5–60 BPM
I:E	1:4 to 4:1
Peak Flow	Up to 180 L/min (not adjustable)
PEEP/CPAP	0.0–50 cmH₂O
MMV	1–25 L/min
Insp. Pause	Difference between Insp. and Exp. Time (0.0–3.0 seconds)
F₁O₂	0.21–1.0

INFRASONICS, ADULT STAR

The Adult Star, marketed by Infrasonics, Inc., is another example of a pneumatically powered, microprocessor-controlled flow controller (Figures 9-25 and 9-26). The microprocessor system, when combined with appropriate flow and pressure sensors, can provide a flexible feedback control system allowing a variety of modes, monitors, and alarms. The Adult Star incorporates the use of five microprocessors in the control system design architecture.

Input Power

Power to run the microprocessor control circuitry is provided by an internal 12-volt battery which is continually charged by 120 volt, 60 Hz electrical power. The pneumatic system is powered by 50-psi source of medical air and oxygen. If 50-psi medical air is not available, an internal compressor can provide the air source to power the ventilator.

Drive Mechanism

Two reducing valves (air and oxygen) reduce the 50-psi line pressure to between 6.5 and 7.5 psi (Figure 9-27). The gas pressures are closely matched to enhance the accuracy of the blending system. Gas flows from these pressure controlling elements to paired proportional flow control valves.

These flow control valves control the inspiratory waveform, oxygen concentration, volume, and inspiratory flow. The flow control valves are microprocessor-controlled solenoid valves capable of opening and closing in dis-

Figure 9-25 *A photograph of Infrasonics, Inc., Adult Star ventilator. (Courtesy Infrasonics, Inc., San Diego, CA)*

crete steps in response to the signals from the microprocessor.

From the flow control valves, gas flows through a screen-type pneumotachometer, which measures the inspiratory flow provid-

Figure 9-26 *A drawing showing the Adult Star control panel. (Courtesy Infrasonics, Inc., San Diego, CA)*

ing feedback to the microprocessor. Pressure drop across the screen elements is proportional to flow through the pneumotachometer. Gas flows from the pneumotachometer into the patient circuit.

A small internal compressor can be used to power a small-volume nebulizer in the patient circuit. Gas powering the compressor is removed from the patient circuit just distal to the flow control valves and is then added back into the circuit through the nebulizer. This system prevents variation of tidal volume and changes in F_IO_2 when the nebulizer is operated.

Control Circuit

As described earlier, the Adult Star uses two microprocessors and two proportional flow control valves to regulate output from the ventilator. This system operates in conjunction with a screen pneumotachometer and a differential pressure transducer to measure flow. When the flow control valves are open, a pressure difference will exist across the individual control valve orifice. This pressure differential is proportional to flow. The two microprocessors (one for each valve) use the flow signal as a feedback system to control the proportional solenoid valves regulating oxygen concentration, inspiratory waveforms, flow rates, and volume delivery. Flow output is verified by a screen pneumotachometer.

Flow output waveforms include rectangular, ascending and descending ramp, and sinusoidal waveforms. All of these waveforms are possible through microprocessor control of the flow control valves.

The exhalation valve is a large-surface diaphragm valve, which is pneumatically controlled. During inspiration, the valve closes, causing gas to flow into the patient circuit and into the patient's lungs. During expiration, the valve opens and the patient exhales. The valve also determines PEEP levels, partially closing to maintain pressure in the patient circuit. Distal to the exhalation valve is an expiratory flow pneumotachometer, similar to the inspiratory flow pneumotachometer. This flow system senses expiratory flow rates and indirectly determines exhaled volumes for the display and alarm systems.

Control Variable

As described earlier, the control variable used by the Adult Star ventilator is flow. Differential pressure, measured across the individual flow control valves, is used to regulate the position of the flow control valves regulating tidal volume delivery during mandatory breaths. Proximal airway pressure is also the control variable during PEEP/CPAP and pressure support.

Phase Variables

Trigger Variables

The trigger variables for the Infrasonics Adult Star include pressure, time, and manual variables. Pressure is used as a trigger variable for demand breaths during assist/CMV, SIMV, and pressure support. When inspiratory pressure falls below the threshold established by the sensitivity control, the ventilator will initiate a breath. The sensitivity may be set between 0.5 and 20.0 cmH$_2$O below baseline pressure by the practitioner.

Time becomes a trigger variable during assist CMV if no inspiratory effort (pressure drop) is sensed by the ventilator. If the patient does not trigger a breath, the ventilator will deliver a mandatory breath at the set tidal volume, peak flow, and rate established by the practitioner.

The ventilator may be manually triggered by the practitioner depressing the manual breath button on the control panel. When depressed, the ventilator will deliver a volume-controlled breath (assist/CMV, SIMV, and CPAP). When in pressure-controlled ventilation, a pressure-controlled breath is delivered when the manual breath button is depressed.

Limit Variables

The limit variables of the Adult Star include pressure, volume, and flow. Pressure becomes a limit variable during SIMV (with PEEP applied), CPAP, pressure support, and pressure control. Under these conditions, the ventilator will augment flow to maintain the desired pressure level. PEEP/CPAP pressures are adjustable between 0.0 and 30.0 cmH$_2$O. The Adult Star is available with 0 to 50 cmH$_2$O of PEEP/CPAP as an option. Pressure support is adjustable between 0.0 and 70 cmH$_2$O.

Volume becomes a limit variable when the inspiratory pause is adjusted greater than zero. Inspiratory pause may be adjusted between 0.0 and 2.0 seconds. When activated, a volume breath is delivered and held until the set inspiratory pause time period has elapsed.

Flow becomes a limit variable when the rectangular waveform output is selected dur-

Figure 9-27 *A schematic drawing showing the Adult Star ventilator's pneumatic system. (Courtesy Infrasonics, Inc., San Diego, CA)* **(continues)**

ing assist/CMV. When selected, the rectangular waveform output limits flow during inspiration to the flow rate set on the peak flow control. Peak inspiratory flow is adjustable between 10 and 120 L/min.

Cycle Variables

Cycle variables for the Adult Star include pressure, flow, and time. Pressure becomes a cycle variable if the inspiratory pressure reaches the setting on the high inspiratory

Figure 9-27 *(continued)*

pressure control. Inspiratory pressure limits may be adjusted between 10 and 120 cmH$_2$O. When the pressure limit is reached, inspiration is terminated and both audible and visual alarms are activated.

Flow becomes a cycle variable during pressure support ventilation. Inspiration is terminated when inspiratory flow falls to 4 L/min. Once flow decays to this point, pressure falls to the baseline value. Inspiration is also termi-

ASSEMBLY AND TROUBLESHOOTING

Assembly—Infrasonics Adult Star

To assemble the Infrasonics Adult Star, follow this suggested assembly guide:

1. Connect high-pressure hoses to a 50-psi medical air and oxygen source.

2. Connect the power cord to a 120 volt, 60 Hz outlet.

3. Attach an inspiratory and expiratory bacteria filter into their respective receptacles.

4. Connect the humidifier inlet to the inspiratory bacteria filter using large-bore tubing. Since a variety of humidifiers may be used with this ventilator, specific instructions will not be included here.

5. Connect the inspiratory limb of the circuit to the outlet of the humidifier. Attach the expiratory limb to the exhalation water trap and expiratory bacterial filter fitting.

6. Connect the proximal airway line to the proximal airway fitting on the ventilator.

Troubleshooting

Refer to the troubleshooting algorithms found at the end of this chapter.

---

nated during pressure support ventilation if pressure reaches 3 cmH$_2$O greater than the pressure support setting plus PEEP or if 3.5 seconds of inspiratory time has elapsed.

Time becomes a cycle variable when inspiratory pause has been adjusted. If inspiratory pause has been activated, inspiration will be terminated when the pause time has elapsed.

Baseline Variable

The baseline variable for the Adult Star is pressure. Baseline pressure is adjustable between 0 and 30 cmH$_2$O or optionally available between 0 and 50 cmH$_2$O. As described earlier, PEEP/CPAP pressure is generated by the exhalation valve partially closing during expiration.

Output Waveforms

Pressure

The Infrasonics Adult Star can deliver a rectangular pressure waveform when the flow to the ventilator is operated in pressure support and pressure control ventilation. Under these circumstances, pressure rises rapidly to a constant value where it remains through the delivery of the breath. At the termination of inspiration, pressure falls to the baseline value.

Flow

The flow output waveform capabilities of the ventilator include rectangular, ascending and descending ramp, and sinusoidal. As described earlier, these waveforms can be accurately reproduced by the feedback system between the internal flow transducer, the microprocessor, and the proportional flow control valves.

Alarms

Input Power Alarms

The input power alarms include loss of electrical and loss of pneumatic power. In the event of a loss of electrical power, a red LED will be illuminated, and the ventilator will continue to operate since it is powered by the battery at all times. The battery backup will operate the ventilator for up to 30 minutes without AC power. If the internal battery voltage drops to 10.9 volts for more than 15 seconds, the low battery alarm will be activated. If voltage drops further to 10.0 volts for 5 seconds, a ventilator inoperative condition will result.

If the oxygen line pressure falls below 26 psi, an audible and visual alarm will be activated. In the event that air pressure falls below 26 psi and electric power is still available, the compressor will be activated to compensate for the loss of air pressure. Should the air compressor fail to deliver at least 16 psi, a low air pressure result will occur, and the ventilator will automatically switch to 100% oxygen.

Control Circuit Alarms

The control circuit alarms include ventilator inoperative, insufficient inspiration, and exhalation time. The ventilator inoperative alarm may indicate the following situations: detection of an internal malfunction, and loss of electrical power (with an internal battery charge of less than 10.0 volts).

An alarm will alert the practitioner if inspiratory or expiratory times are not sufficient. If inspiratory time is less than 0.24 seconds, the insufficient inspiration time alarm will be activated. If expiratory time is less than 0.20 seconds, or 0.26 seconds for pressure support, the insufficient exhalation time alarm will be activated.

Output Alarms

Pressure. Pressure output alarms include high and low peak and low baseline. The high inspiratory pressure alarm is adjustable between 10.0 and 120 cmH$_2$O. Low inspiratory pressure may be set between 3 and 60 cmH$_2$O. Baseline pressure alarms may be set between 0.0 and 30 cmH$_2$O (0 to 50 cmH$_2$O optionally).

Volume. Low mechanical volume and low spontaneous volume alarms are available for both mandatory breaths and spontaneous breaths. The mechanical volume alarm parameters are adjustable between 0.0 and 2,500 mL for both mandatory and spontaneous alarms.

Flow. A low exhaled minute volume alarm may be adjusted between 0.0 and 60.0 L/min. In the event that the patient's exhaled minute volume falls below the threshold parameter, audible and visual alarm will be activated.

Time. A high ventilatory rate alarm can be set between 0 and 90 breaths per minute. In the event that the patient's respiratory rate exceeds the established threshold, both an audible and visual alarm will result.

Table 9-18 illustrates the Infrasonics Adult Star alarm systems, and Table 9-19 illustrates its capabilities.

TABLE 9-18 Adult Star Alarm Systems

Alarm	Condition/Settings
Input Power	
Oxygen Pressure	< 26 psi
Air Pressure	< 26 psi or < 16 psi from compressor
Electric Power	Loss of 120 volt, 60 Hz power; Battery power less than 10.0 volts
Control Circuit	
Ventilator Inoperative	Internal malfunction detected
Insuf. Insp. Time	Insp. time less than 0.250 seconds
Insuf. Exp. Time	Exp. time less than 0.20 seconds
Output Alarms	
High Airway Pressure	10.0–120 cmH$_2$O
Low Airway Pressure	3.0–60 cmH$_2$O
Low Baseline Pressure	0.0–30 cmH$_2$O
Low Exhaled Tidal Vol.	0.0–2,500 mL
(Spontaneous)	0.0–2,500 mL
Low Minute Volume	0.0–60 L/min
High Breath Rate	0–90 BPM

TABLE 9-19 Adult Star Ventilator Capabilities

Modes	Assist/Control, SIMV, Pressure Support, Pressure Control, CPAP
Volume	100–2,500 mL (50–2,500 mL with optional pediatric ventilation)
Pressure	0.0–120 cmH$_2$O
Press. Support	0.0–70 cmH$_2$O
Rate	0.5–80 BPM (0.5 to 120 BPM with optional pediatric ventilation)
Peak Flow	10–120 L/min (machine); 10–160 L/min Spontaneous, Pressure Support, and Pressure Control
PEEP/CPAP	0.0–30 cmH$_2$O
Sigh Volume	100–2,500 mL (50–2,500 mL with pediatric ventilation option)
Sigh Rate	0 to 20 sighs per hour (SPH)
Multiple Sighs	1 to 3 sighs
Insp. Pause	0.0 to 2.0 seconds
Sensitivity	0.5 to 20 below baseline pressure
F$_I$O$_2$	0.21 to 1.0

NEWPORT MEDICAL INSTRUMENTS, WAVE

Newport Medical Instruments, Inc., manufactures and distributes the Newport Wave ventilator (Figures 9-28 and 9-29). The ventilator is a pneumatically powered and microprocessor-controlled flow and pressure controller. Flow is utilized by the microprocessor to control the ventilator's output.

Input Power

Power to run the microprocessor control circuitry is provided by 120 volt, 60 Hz (220 volt, 60 Hz switchable) electrical power. The pneumatic system is powered by 50-psi source of medical air and oxygen.

Drive Mechanism

The 50-psi air and oxygen source gas enters the ventilator's blender where the two

Figure 9-28 *A photograph of Newport Medical Instruments E200 Wave ventilator. (Courtesy Newport Medical Instruments, Inc., Costa Mesa, CA)*

Figure 9-29 *A photograph of the E200 Wave ventilator's control panel. (Courtesy Newport Medical Instruments, Inc., Costa Mesa, CA)*

gases are mixed to the desired F_IO_2 level (Figure 9-30). Gas exits the blender at 28 psi, where it flows to an accumulator tank. The accumulator functions as a reservoir to meet high patient flow demands and also as a mixing chamber to further stabilize the oxygen concentration. The volume of the accumulator tank is 1 liter at a pressure of 2 atmospheres.

Control Circuit

Gas exits the accumulator through a filter and into a servoid metering valve. The servoid valve is an electrodynamic valve, which is controlled by the microprocessor. Gas flowing from the servoid valve passes through a laminar flow element with pressure taps proximal and distal to it. Feedback signals from a differential pressure transducer provide flow information to the microprocessor to regulate inspiratory flow. Hence, the ventilator is a flow controller. The flow output waveform for the Wave ventilator is a rectangular waveform. During pressure control ventilation, proximal airway pressure is used as a feedback signal to the microprocessor, which adjusts flow output to regulate the pressure.

The exhalation valve diaphragm is pneumatically actuated. During inspiration the valve closes, causing gas to flow into the patient circuit and into the patient's lungs. During expiration the valve opens and the patient exhales. The valve also determines PEEP levels, partially closing to maintain pressure in the patient circuit.

Control Variables

The control variables used by the Newport Wave ventilator are flow and pressure. Flow becomes the control variable during mandatory volume delivery, volume-controlled assist/control, and SIMV ventilation. During pressure-controlled assist/control and pressure support, pressure becomes the control variable.

Phase Variables

Trigger Variables

The trigger variables for the Newport Wave ventilator include pressure, time, and manual variables. Pressure is used as a trigger variable for demand breaths during volume-controlled assist/control, SIMV, sigh breath delivery, pressure control, and pressure support. When inspiratory pressure falls below the threshold established by the assist sensitiv-

ity control, the ventilator will initiate a breath. The sensitivity may be set between 0.0 and 5.0 cmH$_2$O below baseline pressure by the practitioner.

Time becomes a trigger variable if no inspiratory effort (pressure drop) is sensed by the ventilator (volume- or pressure-controlled ventilation). If the patient does not trigger a breath, the ventilator will deliver a mandatory breath at the established rate, inspiratory time and peak flow, and pressure (pressure-control ventilation).

The ventilator may be manually triggered by the practitioner by depressing the manual breath button on the control panel. When depressed, a mandatory breath will be delivered (volume- or pressure-controlled).

Limit Variables

The limit variables of the Newport Wave include pressure, volume, and flow. Pressure becomes a limit variable during pressure-controlled ventilation. During pressure control, inspiratory pressure reaches a preset limit and is held there until the inspiratory time has passed. During volume-controlled ventilation, it is also possible to pressure limit the ventilator. This is accomplished by setting the pneumatic pressure relief valve to a level that is lower than the peak inspiratory pressure. Peak inspiratory pressure is a function of inspiratory time and flow rate settings. The pneumatic pressure relief valve is adjustable between 0.0 and 120 cmH$_2$O.

Volume becomes a limit variable when the inspiratory pause control is active. Inspiratory pause may be adjusted between 10, 20, or 30% of the cycle time. When activated, a volume breath is delivered and held until the set inspiratory pause time period has elapsed. This is only available during volume-controlled assist/control and the mandatory portions of SIMV.

Flow becomes a limit variable during volume-controlled assist/control, the mandatory portion of volume controlled SIMV, or during sigh breath delivery. When a rectangular waveform output is delivered, flow during inspiration is limited to the setting established on the peak flow control. Peak flow is adjustable between 1 and 100 L/min.

Cycle Variables

Cycle variables for the Newport Wave ventilator include pressure, flow, and time. Pressure becomes a cycle variable if the inspiratory

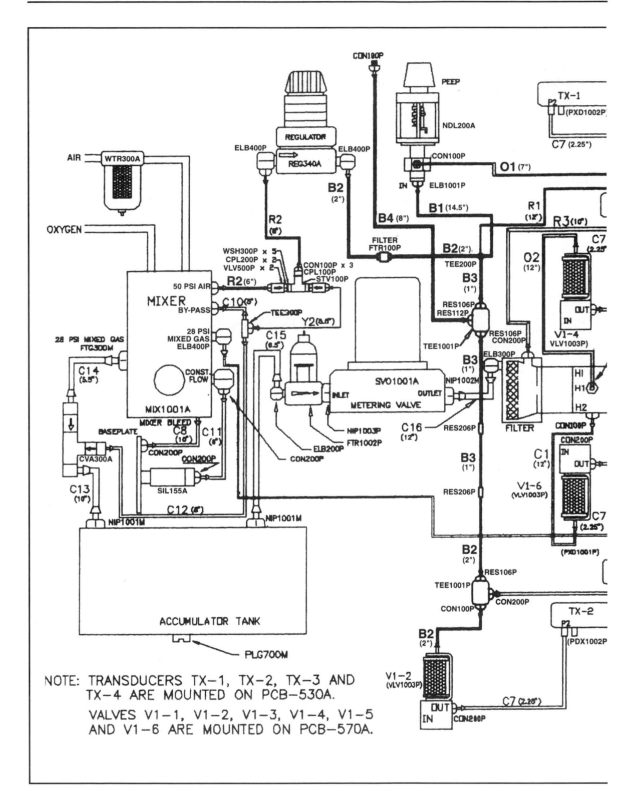

Figure 9-30 *A schematic drawing of the E200 Wave ventilator's pneumatic system. (Courtesy Newport Medical Instruments, Inc., Costa Mesa, CA)* **(continues)**

Figure 9-30 *(continued)*

pressure reaches the setting on the high pressure alarm control or the automatic high pressure alarm during pressure-controlled or pressure-support ventilation. The peak inspiratory pressure alarm may be adjusted between 10 and 120 cmH$_2$O. When the pressure limit is reached, inspiration is terminated and both audible and visual alarms are activated.

Flow becomes a cycle variable during pressure support ventilation. Inspiration is terminated when inspiratory flow falls to a value determined by the following formula: K × Peak Flow$^{0.6}$ × Elapsed Time, where K equals a constant. A pressure-supported breath is also terminated when tidal volume exceeds 4 L, when peak pressure reaches 2 cmH$_2$O over pressure support level, or when inspiratory time exceeds 3 seconds.

Time becomes a cycle variable during pressure control ventilation. In this mode, a constant pressure is applied until the time set on the inspiratory time control has been reached. Inspiratory times are adjustable between 0.1 and 3.0 seconds. Time may also be a cycle variable in pressure support if the inspiratory time exceeds 3 seconds.

Baseline Variable

The ventilator is capable of delivering PEEP/CPAP pressures. PEEP/CPAP pressures are adjustable between 0 and 45 cmH$_2$O. Baseline pressures are elevated in the patient circuit by the exhalation valve partially closing, acting as a threshold resistor.

Conditional Variables

Time. Time becomes a conditional variable during sigh delivery. During normal ventilator-supported breaths, they are flow or pressure controlled; pressure or time triggered; pressure, volume, or flow limited; or pressure, time, or flow cycled. During a sigh delivery, a sigh breath will be given every 100th breath. A sigh volume of 150% of the tidal volume is delivered by extending the inspiratory time by 1.5 times the chosen setting.

Time and Pressure. Time and pressure become conditional variables during SIMV mode. The rate control determines the frequency of mandatory breath delivery during SIMV mode. The rate control is essentially an electronic timer, delivering a breath at specified time intervals. Between mandatory breath deliveries, the patient breathes through the flow control valve. The ventilator measures proximal airway pressure, or distal endotracheal tube pressure, to determine if the patient is attempting to initiate a breath. In response to the pressure change, the patient is able to draw gas spontaneously through the flow control valve to meet inspiratory needs.

Output Waveforms

Pressure

During pressure-controlled ventilation, the pressure waveform is a combination of rectangular and exponential. The waveform diminishes (ramps) as the pressure in the airway approaches the pressure control level. If inspiratory time is short, inspiratory pressure may never reach the pressure control level.

Flow

The flow wave for output of the ventilator is a rectangular waveform output during volume-controlled ventilation. This occurs providing that the peak inspiratory pressure is less than the setting on the pressure control adjustment.

During pressure-controlled ventilation, the flow waveform is a descending ramp. With the exhalation valve closed during inspiration, the ramped flow pattern prevents pressure from increasing above the set pressure limit.

Alarms

Input Power Alarms

The input power alarms include loss of electrical and loss of pneumatic power. In the event of a loss of electrical power, an audible alarm will be activated for a minimum of 10 minutes.

If the oxygen or air line pressure falls below 32 psi, an audible alarm will be activated.

Control Circuit Alarms

The control circuit alarms include ventilator inoperative and inverse I:E ratio. The ventilator inoperative alarm indicates detection of an internal malfunction.

ASSEMBLY AND TROUBLESHOOTING

Assembly—Newport Wave Ventilator

To assemble the Newport Wave ventilator, follow this suggested assembly guide.

1. Connect high-pressure hoses to a 50-psi medical air and oxygen source.

2. Connect the power cord to a 120 volt, 60 Hz (220 volt, 60 Hz selectable) outlet.

3. Attach an inspiratory bacteria filter to the ventilator outlet.

4. Connect the humidifier inlet to the inspiratory bacteria filter using large-bore tubing (adult) or pediatric tubing. Since a variety of humidifiers may be used with this ventilator, specific instructions will not be included here.

5. Connect the inspiratory limb of the circuit to the outlet of the humidifier. Attach the expiratory limb to the exhalation valve fitting.

6. Connect the exhalation valve to the exhalation valve nipple on the front of the ventilator.

7. Connect the proximal airway line to the proximal airway fitting on the ventilator.

Troubleshooting

Refer to the troubleshooting algorithms found at the end of this chapter.

An I:E ratio alarm is available to alert the practitioner to long inspiratory times. The alarm is selectable between two positions, 1:1 and 3:1. The ventilator is capable of delivering inverse I:E ratios of up to 3:1 if the alarm is set at the 3:1 position. Once inspiratory time exceeds 75% of the ventilatory cycle, the ventilator will automatically terminate inspiration. If the ratio limit alarm is limited to an I:E ratio of 1:1 and the inspiratory time exceeds 50% of the ventilatory cycle, the alarm condition will result, terminating inspiration.

Output Alarms

Pressure. Pressure output alarms include high and low peak pressure alarms. The high inspiratory pressure alarm is adjustable between 5.0 and 120 cmH$_2$O. Low inspiratory pressure may be set between 0.3 and 110 cmH$_2$O.

Flow. A high and low inspiratory minute volume alarm is available on the Newport Wave. The high inspiratory minute volume alarm is adjustable between 0 to 50 and 0 to 5 L/min. The low inspiratory minute volume alarm is adjustable between 0.0 and 49 L/min.

Table 9-20 illustrates the Newport Wave ventilator's alarm systems, and Table 9-21 illustrates its capabilities.

TABLE 9-20 Newport Wave Ventilator Alarm Systems

Alarm	Condition/Settings
Input Power	
Oxygen Pressure	< 32 psi
Air Pressure	< 32 psi
Electric Power	Loss of 120 volt, 60 Hz (220 volt, 60 Hz) power
Control Circuit	
Ventilator Inoperative	Internal malfunction detected
I:E Ratio	Insp. time > 75% of cycle time (3:1)
	Insp. time > 50% of cycle time (1:1)
Output Alarms	
High Airway Pressure	10.0–120 cmH$_2$O
Low Airway Pressure	3.0–99 cmH$_2$O
Low Minute Volume	0.0–49 L/min
High Minute Volume	0.0–50 L/min BPM

TABLE 9-21 Newport Wave Ventilator Capabilities

Modes	Volume Controlled Ventilation
	Assist/Control (with or without bias flow)
	SIMV (with or without bias flow or pressure support)
	Pressure Controlled Ventilation
	Assist/Control (with or without bias flow)
	SIMV (with or without pressure support or bias flow)
	Spontaneous Modes
	Pressure support (with or without bias flow)
Volume	10–2,000 mL
Pressure	0.0–120 cmH$_2$O
Press. Support	0.0–60 cmH$_2$O
Press. Control	0.0–80 cmH$_2$O
Rate	0–100 BPM
Peak Flow	1 to 100 L/min (Machine); 1 to 160 L/min (Spontaneous)
Bias Flow	0.0–30 L/min
Insp. Time	0.1–3.0 seconds
PEEP/CPAP	0.0–45 cmH$_2$O
Sigh Volume	150% of tidal volume
Sigh Rate	Every 100th breath
Insp. Pause	10, 20, or 30%
Sensitivity	0.0 to 5 cmH$_2$O below baseline pressure
F$_I$O$_2$	0.21 to 1.0

PURITAN-BENNETT CORPORATION, 7200AE

The Puritan-Bennett 7200ae is a pneumatically driven, electrically powered, microprocessor-controlled ventilator (Figure 9-31 and 9-32). A single pneumatic circuit drives the ventilator while microprocessor control provides control, assist/control, SIMV, PEEP/CPAP, pressure support, and pressure control in either assist/control or SIMV. All breath types may be pressure or flow triggered.

Input Power

Power to run the microprocessor control circuitry is provided by 120 volt, 60 Hz electrical power. The pneumatic system is powered by 35- to 100-psi source of medical air and

Figure 9-31 *A photograph of the Puritan-Bennett 7200ae ventilator. (Courtesy Puritan-Bennett Corporation, Carlsbad, CA, Puritan-Bennett® and the 7200® series ventilatory system)*

Figure 9-32 *A photograph of the Puritan-Bennett 7200ae control panel. (Courtesy Puritan-Bennett Corporation, Carlsbad, CA. Puritan-Bennett® and the 7200® series ventilatory system)*

oxygen. If compressed medical air is not available, an optional internal compressor in the pedestal will provide an air source to power the pneumatic system.

Drive Mechanism

The pneumatic drive mechanism (Figure 9-33) reduces the line pressure of the incoming gas to 10 psi by means of the air and oxygen reducing valves. A crossover solenoid connects the air and oxygen supply so, in the event air pressure is lost, the ventilator will still operate using oxygen. Gases are conducted through flow and temperature transducers before they reach the proportional solenoid valves (PSOLs were discussed in Chapter 7.).

Control Circuit

The 7200ae uses a microprocessor, two flow transducers, two temperature transducers, a pressure transducer, and two PSOL valves to regulate flow output from the ventilator. The PSOLs regulate F_IO_2, inspiratory flow, pressure, and volume delivery.

Gases are conducted through flow and temperature transducers before they reach the PSOLs. The purpose of the flow and tempera-

ture transducers is to provide feedback to the microprocessor. The microprocessor constantly monitors the flow and temperature transducers (air and oxygen) during the inspiratory phase. The opening of the PSOLs is adjusted to establish the exact volume, flow, F_IO_2, flow pattern, and mode, as set by the practitioner using the keyboard.

Gas flows from the PSOLs to the patient outlet, passing through a safety check valve. Output from the PSOLs also is conducted to an absolute pressure transducer. This transducer provides feedback to the microprocessor, monitoring ambient pressures to correct for varying gas densities.

The exhalation valve is powered by diversion of some of the gas pressure from the patient circuit. When the solenoid is open, the exhalation valve diaphragm is pressurized, closing it. Gas flow from the PSOLs is then directed into the patient's lungs. The exhalation valve also plays an important role in the regulation of PEEP/CPAP pressures.

Activation of the PEEP/CPAP control knob causes gas to be delivered from the PEEP/CPAP solenoid to the PEEP/CPAP regulator (control adjustment). Pressure from the regulator powers a venturi. Flow from the venturi is directed against the exhalation valve diaphragm, pressurizing it. The partially pressurized diaphragm maintains pressure within the circuit equal to the pressure applied to it. PEEP/CPAP may be adjusted between 0 and 45 cmH_2O.

During the expiratory phase, the microprocessor sends signals to the PSOLs, closing them. When the PSOLs have closed, all gas flow to the patient ceases. Simultaneously, a signal is sent to the exhalation pilot control solenoid, which switches to the output position and allows the exhalation valve to depressurize. Gas behind the exhalation valve exits the ventilator and the valve opens.

The patient's exhaled air passes through a heated bacteria filter before entering the expiratory flow sensor. This removes contaminant from the exhaled air and warms it to above body temperature. Particulate water is removed; only water vapor will pass through the filter system. The exhaled gas then flows through a temperature and flow transducer that measures exhaled gas temperature and flow. The exhaled gas is then allowed to vent to the atmosphere.

Flow output waveforms include rectangular, descending ramp, and sinusoidal waveforms. All of these waveforms are possible through microprocessor control of the pneumatic system.

Figure 9-33 *A schematic diagram of the Puritan Bennett 7200ae ventilator pneumatic system. (Courtesy Puritan-Bennett Corporation, Carlsbad, CA)* *(continues)*

Control Variables

The control variable for the 7200ae can be either flow or pressure. Inspiratory flow is measured by the two flow transducers proximal to the air and oxygen PSOLs. Flow is used as a control variable during control, assist/control, and the mandatory portions of SIMV for volume delivered breaths. In these modes volume becomes a derivative of flow (flow multiplied by inspiratory time). Pressure is also the control variable during the inspiratory phase of PEEP/CPAP, pressure support, and pressure control delivery. Pressure is monitored by the expiratory pressure transducer, and flow output from the PSOLs is adjusted to maintain the desired pressure levels.

Phase Variables
Trigger Variables

The trigger variables of the Puritan-Bennett 7200ae include pressure, flow, time, and manual. Pressure becomes a trigger variable when the patient inhales, reducing pressure in the circuit below the reference level set on the sensitivity control. Sensitivity may be adjusted between 0.5 and 20 cmH2O below baseline pressure. Pressure operates as a trigger variable for all breaths during control assist/control, SIMV, pressure support, and pressure control modes.

Flow becomes a trigger variable when flow-by has been selected (Option 50). When selected the practitioner enters the desired

Figure 9-33 *(continued)*

base flow (bias flow) between 5 and 20 L/min. Following base flow entry, the practitioner must enter the flow sensitivity, which is adjustable between 1 and 15 L/min. This flow sensitivity is the drop in returned flow to the expiratory sensor, used as a threshold to detect a breath. Once the established flow threshold (flow sensitivity) has been sensed by the microprocessor, the PSOLs open to deliver a breath.

Time is a trigger variable during control, assist/control, and SIMV, when no spontaneous efforts occur. Breath delivery is based upon the respiratory rate setting (time).

The ventilator may also be manually triggered by depressing the manual inspiration key. When depressed, the ventilator initiates a controlled breath at the tidal volume, waveform, and peak flow set in volume-controlled ventilation or at the pressure level and inspiratory time in pressure-controlled ventilation.

Limit Variables

The limit variables include pressure, volume, and flow. Pressure becomes the limit variable during the spontaneous breaths when in SIMV (with PEEP/CPAP added), CPAP, pressure control, and pressure support modes. The pneumatic system will maintain the desired pressure in the patient circuit as adjusted by the practitioner. PEEP/CPAP is adjustable between 0.0 and 45 cmH_2O, pressure support may be adjusted between 0.0 and

70 cmH$_2$O, and pressure control may be set between 5 and 100 cmH$_2$O.

Volume becomes a limit variable when inspiratory hold has been selected by the practitioner. When selected, inspiratory hold may be adjusted between 0.0 and 2.0 seconds. The ventilator will deliver a breath and it will be held following breath delivery until the set time interval has elapsed.

Flow is the limit variable when the ventilator delivers mandatory flow-controlled breaths. Flow is adjustable between 10 and 120 L/min. The flow delivery is limited to the value set on the peak flow control.

Cycle Variables

The cycle variables include pressure, flow, and time. Pressure becomes the cycle variable when inspiratory pressure reaches the pressure set on the high pressure limit alarm. The high pressure limit is adjustable between 10 and 120 cmH$_2$O. When the pressure limit is reached, inspiratory flow is stopped and both audible and visual alarms are activated.

Flow becomes the cycle variable during pressure support. When inspiratory flow decays to 5 L/min, or inspiratory pressure falls to 1.5 cmH$_2$O above the set pressure, breath delivery stops.

Time becomes the cycle variable during mandatory breath delivery. The microprocessor determines volume as a function of flow and inspiratory time. Once the appropriate inspiratory time has been reached, based upon peak flow, flow waveform, and tidal volume settings, breath delivery ceases. If pressure support fails to cycle off (in the event of a leak), the breath will terminate after 5 seconds.

Baseline Variables

The baseline variable for the Puritan-Bennett 7200ae is pressure. PEEP/CPAP pressures are adjustable between 0 and 45 cmH$_2$O. As described earlier, baseline pressure is created by the exhalation valve partially closing during exhalation.

Conditional Variables

Time. Time becomes a conditional variable during sigh delivery. During normal ventilator-supported breaths, they are flow or pressure controlled; pressure or flow triggered; or pressure, flow, or time cycled. During sigh delivery, sigh volumes may be adjusted between 10 and 2,500 mL at a rate of 1 to 15 sighs per hour,

with sigh multiples between 1 and 3. The sigh breaths have their own high pressure limit, which is adjustable between 10 and 120 cmH$_2$O.

Time and Pressure or Time and Flow. Time and pressure become conditional variables during the SIMV mode. The rate control determines the frequency of mandatory breath delivery during SIMV mode. The rate control is essentially an electronic timer, allowing time window for the patient to trigger a breath or delivering a breath at specified time intervals if no efforts are detected. Between mandatory breath delivery, the patient breathes through the ventilator's pneumatic system. The ventilator measures pressure to determine if the patient is attempting to initiate a breath. In response to the pressure change, the patient is able to draw gas spontaneously through the pneumatic system to meet inspiratory needs.

Time and flow become conditional variables during SIMV when flow-by has been selected. The microprocessor senses inspiratory effort using flow rather than pressure. In response to a patient effort, the PSOLs open, attempting to maintain the desired PEEP/CPAP pressure established by the practitioner.

Output Waveforms

Pressure

The pressure output of the 7200ae ventilator is rectangular when the ventilator is operating in the pressure support and pressure control modes. In these modes, pressure rises sharply to the level set by the practitioner. Pressure is maintained until flow reaches approximately 5 L/min, or in pressure control when the set inspiratory time has lapsed.

Flow

The flow output of the 7200ae may be adjusted between rectangular, descending ramp, and sinusoidal outputs in volume control ventilation. The PSOL valves, in combination with the microprocessor and feedback control system, enable the ventilator to accurately reproduce these flow output waveforms.

Alarms

Input Power

Input power alarms on the 7200ae include loss of electrical and pneumatic power. When electrical power is lost, an audible alarm will sound and the safety valve will open. A nicad battery pack powers the audible and visual alarm, independent of the 120 volt, 60 Hz power for the ventilator. If power is restored or the On/Off switch is turned off, the alarm will cease.

If air or oxygen pressure falls below 35 psi, the low air or O_2 pressure alarm will be activated. Both audible and visual alarms will be activated when this condition exists.

Control Circuit Alarms

Control circuit alarms on the 7200ae include ventilator inoperative, incompatible settings, and I:E limit. The ventilator inoperative alarm is activated when the microprocessor conducts its diagnostics routine and an internal fault is found in the pneumatic delivery section. If the fault is in the microprocessor alone, the "Back Up Ventilator" alarm sounds and the patient is ventilated with an analog circuit at factory preset parameters. The incompatible settings alarm occurs when the practitioner attempts to enter a value falling outside of established parameters for that control. It is an audible alarm in which four short beep tones are given to alert the practitioner. The visual-only I:E limit alert is activated if the practitioner has set a tidal volume, rate and peak flow, and inspiratory pause settings which result in an inspiratory time exceeding 50% of the cycle time.

Output Alarms

Pressure. The 7200ae incorporates high and low inspiratory pressure alarms and a low baseline pressure alarm. The high peak pressure alarm is adjustable between 10.0 and 120 cmH$_2$O and the low peak pressure alarm is adjustable between 3 and 99 cmH$_2$O. The low baseline (PEEP/CPAP) pressure alarm is adjustable between 0.0 and 45 cmH$_2$O.

Volume. A low tidal volume alarm alerts the practitioner to events resulting in the low volume threshold not being met. These could include leaks, patient disconnects, and other problems. The low tidal volume alarm is adjustable between 0 and 2,500 mL.

Flow. A low minute volume alarm is incorporated into the 7200ae. The low minute volume alarm is adjustable between 0.0 and 60 L/min.

Time. An adjustable high respiratory rate alarm is also incorporated into the 7200ae ventilator. The high breath rate alarm can be adjusted between 0 and 70 breaths per minute.

Emergency Modes of Ventilation

There are four emergency modes of ventilation that may become active in the event of gas pressure or other systems failures. These modes include apnea ventilation, disconnect ventilation, backup ventilator, and safety valve open.

ASSEMBLY AND TROUBLESHOOTING

Assembly—7200ae

To assemble the 7200ae ventilator for use, complete the following suggested assembly guide:

1. Rotate the filter clamp away from the ventilator housing and install an exhalation bacteria filter into its compartment. Rotate the clamp toward the ventilator, locking the filter into place. Attach a water collection vial to the inlet of the expiratory bacterial filter.

2. Install a bacteria filter to the ventilator's outlet by opening the filter compartment door to the right of the control panel.

3. Assemble the humidifier and connect the humidifier inlet to the bacteria filter with a length of large-bore tubing.

4. Attach the patient circuit to the support arm. Connect the inspiratory limb to the outlet of the humidifier. Attach the expiratory limb to the collection vial connected to the expiratory bacteria filter.

5. Connect the nebulizer in the patient circuit to the nebulizer nipple on the front of the ventilator housing.

6. If a servo controlled humidifier is used, connect the temperature probe to the inlet side of the patient wye.

7. Connect the air and oxygen DISS fittings to 50-psi sources.

8. Connect the power cord to a suitable 120 volt, 60 Hz outlet.

Troubleshooting

Refer to the troubleshooting algorithms found at the end of this chapter.

Apnea Ventilation

If, during an operator set time interval, the expiratory flow sensor fails to detect a volume greater than 50 mL, the apnea alarm will be activated.

Apnea ventilation is operator selectable, and the parameters are listed in Table 9-22. If the operator fails to adjust the apnea parameters, the following parameters are the default values: apnea interval, 20 seconds; tidal volume, .5 L; respiratory rate, 12 breaths/min; peak flow, 45 L/min; oxygen concentration, 100%. The ventilator will revert to apnea ventilation whenever apnea is detected.

If the patient takes two consecutive breaths and exhales to or greater than one-half of the delivered tidal volume, the ventilator will reset itself to the previous state of operation.

Disconnect Ventilation

If the proximal airway pressure line (Model 7200) becomes disconnected, if the patient circuit becomes occluded, or if the expiratory pressure transducer fails, disconnect ventilation is declared. Disconnect ventilation results in the ventilator reverting to the settings established for apnea ventilation. Sensitivity is not recognized by the feedback control system during disconnect ventilation.

Backup Ventilator (BUV)

The backup ventilator is a backup system that operates independently from the microprocessor. The PSOLs are controlled by analog circuits rather than by the digital microprocessor. In the event of a microprocessor failure, patient ventilation is still possible.

If the microprocessor or the electrical system fails, the backup ventilation emergency mode is activated. Backup ventilator settings are the same as the default values listed under apnea ventilation (the operator may not select the settings), except that the alarm silence and alarm reset are both inoperative, and the pres-

sure limit is 30 cmH$_2$O, guaranteeing appropriately small volumes for pediatric patients.

Safety Valve Open

The safety valve circuit opens to allow the patient to breathe unassisted from ambient air. No PEEP/CPAP is applied, so the patient is also breathing at ambient pressures.

This system is activated if any of the following conditions are met:

- Both air and oxygen supplies are lost.
- The POST (Power On Self-Test) is running.
- A system fault has been detected, resulting in an inability of the the Backup Ventilator circuit to run the pneumatic system.
- Power to the ventilator has been disrupted.

Table 9-23 summarizes the Puritan-Bennett 7200ae alarms, and Table 9-24 summarizes its capabilities.

TABLE 9-23 Puritan-Bennett 7200ae Ventilator Alarm Systems

Alarm	Condition/Settings
Input Power	
Oxygen Pressure	< 35 psi
Air Pressure	< 35 psi
Electric Power	Loss of 120 volt, 60 Hz power
Control Circuit	
Ventilator Inoperative	Internal malfunction detected
Incompatible Settings	Four "beeps" alerting practitioner to parameters that are out of range
I:E Ratio	Insp. time > 50% of cycle time
Output Alarms	
High Pressure Limit	10.0–120 cmH$_2$O
Low Inspiratory Pressure	3.0–99 cmH$_2$O
Low PEEP/CPAP Pressure	0.0–45 cmH$_2$O
Low Exhaled Minute Vol.	0.0–2.5 L
Low Minute Volume	0.0–60 L/min
High Resp. Rate	0–70 BPM

TABLE 9-22 Operator Selectable Apnea Parameters

Apnea interval	10–60 seconds
Tidal volume	.1–2.5 L
Respiratory rate	.5–70 breaths/min
Peak flow	10–120 L/min
F$_I$O$_2$	.21–1.00

TABLE 9-24 Puritan Bennett 7200ae Ventilator Capabilities

Modes	CMV (volume controlled), CMV (pressure controlled), SIMV, CPAP, Pressure Support, Flow-By (Flow triggering)
Volume	10–2,500 mL
Pressure	0.0–120 cmH$_2$O
Press. Support	0.0–70 cmH$_2$O
Press. Control	5.0–100 cmH$_2$O
Rate	0.5–70 BPM
Peak Flow	10–120 L/min
Base Flow	5–20 L/min
Flow Sens.	1–15 L/min
Insp. Time	0.2–5.0 seconds
PEEP/CPAP	0.0–45 cmH$_2$O
Sigh Volume	0.10 to 2.5 L
Sigh Rate	1–15/hr
Sigh Multiple	1–3
Insp. Pause	0.0 to 2.0 seconds
Sensitivity	0.5 to 20 cmH$_2$O below baseline pressure
F$_I$O$_2$	0.21 to 1.0

Figure 9-34A *The Nellcor Puritan-Bennett 840 Ventilator.*

NELLCOR PURITAN-BENNETT, 840 VENTILATOR

The Nellcor Puritan-Bennett 840 ventilator is a pneumatically driven, electrically powered, microprocessor-controlled ventilator (Figures 9-34A and 9-34B). A single pneumatic circuit drives the ventilator, while microprocessor control provides control, assist/control, SIMV, and pressure support in both volume and pressure controlled ventilation. Breaths may be either time, manual, pressure, or flow triggered.

Input Power

Power for the microprocessor control system is provided by AC power, which may be either 120 volts, 60 Hz or 220 volts, 60 Hz AC power. The pneumatic system requires medical-grade air and oxygen between 35 and 100 psi. If medical-grade compressed air is not available, an optional compressor in the pedestal will provide an air source to power the pneumatic system.

Figure 9-34B *The control panel of the 840.*

Drive Mechanism

Air and oxygen enter the ventilator through DISS fittings on the rear of the ventilator and pass through their respective filters (Figures 9-35A and 9-35B, pp. 497–498). Line pressure is reduced to 10 psi by means of the air- and oxygen-reducing valves. A crossover solenoid connects the air and oxygen supply so that in the event gas pressure is lost, the remaining gas pressure (air or oxygen) can continue to power the pneumatic system. From the regulators, gas enters the inspiratory module.

Control Circuit

The 840 ventilator uses a microprocessor and the inspiratory control module to regulate flow output from the ventilator (Figures 9-35A and 9-35B). The inspiratory module consists of two parallel elements, one for air and the other for oxygen. The inspiratory module consists of two proportional solenoid valves (PSOL valves were discussed in Chapter 7), flow sensors, and pressure sensors. The inspiratory modules regulate F_IO_2, inspiratory flow, pressure, and volume delivery. Inspiratory flow and temperature transducers provide feedback to the microprocessor, which precisely regulates the PSOLs, delivering the exact volume, flow, pressure, and F_IO_2 desired by the clinician. Gas flows from the inspiratory modules through a bacteria filter and check valve to the patient circuit.

PEEP/CPAP pressures are regulated by the active electrodynamic exhalation valve. When positive expiratory pressures are desired, the exhalation valve partially closes, creating a threshold resistor, generating the positive pressure.

Control Variables

The control variables for the Nellcor Puritan-Bennett 840 ventilator include flow and pressure. Flow is measured by the two inspiratory flow transducers (air and oxygen) in the inspiratory modules and is used as a feedback signal during volume-controlled breaths for the control, assist/control, and the mandatory portions of SIMV. In these modes, volume delivery is equal to the inspiratory flow multiplied by the inspiratory time.

Pressure is a control variable during PEEP/CPAP, pressure support, and pressure-controlled ventilation. Pressure is monitored by the expiratory pressure transducer and used as a feedback signal through the micro-

processor, whereby it controls the PSOLs outputs and thus maintains the desired pressure levels.

Phase Variables

Trigger Variables

The Nellcor Puritan-Bennett 840 ventilator trigger variables include pressure, flow, time, and manual triggering. Pressure triggering may be set between 0.1 and 20 cmH_2O below baseline pressure. During inspiration, when the patient inhales, pressure falls in the circuit. When the pressure drop in the circuit equals the sensitivity level, the inspiratory phase begins and gas is delivered to the patient.

Flow triggering may be established by selecting Flow-by™. Flow sensitivity is adjustable between 0.5 and 20 L/min. Base flow and bias flow are not adjustable, but are fixed at a value of 1.5 times the flow sensitivity. For example, if a flow sensitivity of 3 L/min is selected, base flow is automatically set at 4.5 L/min. Once a flow sensitivity is established, when the patient's inspiratory (spontaneous) flow equals the sensitivity value, the inspiratory phase begins and gas is delivered to the patient.

Time triggering occurs during control, assist/control, and SIMV provided no spontaneous efforts occur. Breath delivery is based upon the ventilatory rate setting established by the clinician. The rate may be adjusted between 1 and 100 breaths per minute.

Manual trigger may be accomplished by depressing the manual inspiration soft key. When depressed, a manual breath is delivered according to the mandatory settings. The breath may be volume controlled (set tidal volume, inspiratory flow, and F_IO_2) or pressure controlled (set inspiratory pressure, inspiratory time, and F_IO_2).

Limit Variables

The limit variables for the 840 ventilator include pressure, volume, and flow. Pressure becomes a limit variable during the spontaneous breaths when in SIMV (with PEEP/CPAP added), CPAP, pressure control, and pressure support modes. In these modes, the pneumatic system will maintain the desired pressure in the circuit as adjusted by the practitioner. PEEP/CPAP pressures may be adjusted between 0.0 and 45 cmH_2O. Pressure control levels are adjustable between 5 and 90

Figure 9-35A *The Nellcor Puritan-Bennett, 840 Ventilator pneumatic circuit.* **(continues)**

Reference designator	Component	Description
	Inspiratory module	
—	Fitting, inlet	Connects external oxygen and air sources to ventilator via hoses. Fittings include diameter index system standard (DISS) (male or female), noninterchangeable screw thread (NIST), Air Liquide, and Sleeved Index System (SIS).
—	Manifold, PSOL/SV	Houses proportional solenoid valves (PSOL1 and PSOL2) and safety valve (SV).
—	Port, inspiratory pressure relief	Bypasses inspiratory check valve to release pressure when an occlusion is present in exhalation circuit while safety valve is open.
CV2 CV4	Check valve, air/compressor	CV2 opens to admit external compressed air and CV4 closes to isolate compressor module. When CV4 opens to allow compressor-supplied compressed air, CV2 closes to prevent compressed air (compressor source) from venting through external air-conditioning components.
CV3	Check valve, inspiratory	Opens to supply inspiratory gas and prevents exhalation flow in reverse direction.
F1	Filter, oxygen impact	Traps particles larger than 65 to 110 m (microns).
F3 F2	Filter, inlet, oxygen/air	Filters matter greater than 0.3 μm (micron). These filters are part of REG1 or REG2.
F5 F4	Filter, screen, oxygen/air impact	Filters large debris from REG1 and REG2.
F7 F6	Filter, pneumatic noise, oxygen/air	Increases frequency of turbulence to prevent flow sensor tracking. These filters are part of the flow sensor manifold (2 each gas).
OS	Sensor, oxygen (percentage)	Measures partial pressure of oxygen in inspired gas. Range is 21 to 100% O_2.
PA	Pressure transducer, absolute	Measures atmospheric pressure (psia). Located on inspiration PCB.
PI	Pressure transducer, inspiratory	Measures pressure (psig) at outlet manifold. Located on inspiration PCB.
PS1 PS2	Pressure switch, oxygen/air	Opens when pressure is less than 17 psig (117.2 kPa) nominal. Closes when pressure is greater than 30 psig (206.9 kPa) nominal.
PSOL1 PSOL2	Proportional solenoid valve, oxygen/air	0 to 200 L/min BTPS output (intermittent) or 0 to 180 L/min BTPS output (steady state)
Q1 Q2	Sensor, flow, oxygen/air	Measures oxygen or air flow before PSOL.
REG1 REG2	Regulator, oxygen/air	Reduces input supply pressure (35 to 100 psi, flow up to 200 L/min BTPS) to output pressure (10.5 psi minimum to 11.5 psi maximum).
SOL1	Solenoid, autozero, inspiratory pressure transducer	+6 V, three-way solenoid. Energized (common to normally closed) when transducer is autozeroed. De-energized (common to normally open) all other times.
SV	Safety valve	+24 V actuator. Commanded open (de-energized) at 100 cmH$_2$O, during power on self test (POST), loss of both source gases, or due to ventilator inoperative condition. Energized (closed) all other times.
TP1 TP2	Pressure valve, oxygen/air	Allows measurement of REG1 and REG2 output
WT1	Water trap, air	Houses air inlet filter (F2) and includes a manual drain.
	Patient system	
—	Humidification device (optional)	Humidifies inspired gas.
—	Wye	Connects inspiration and expiration tubing, forming a closed circuit.
F8	Filter, inspiratory (main flow)	Filters matter greater than 0.3 μm (micron) (nominal) at 100 L/min flow.
WT	Trap, water	Collects excessive water.

Figure 9-35B *Abbreviations for the drawing shown in Figure 9-35A.* **(continues)**

Reference designator	Component	Description
Exhalation module		
—	Port, sample, metabolic monitor	Provides a sample port for Nellcor Puritan Bennett 7250 Metabolic Monitor. Future option.
CV5	Check valve, exhalation	Opens during exhalation to let exhaled gas into exhalation system. Prevents rebreathing when safety valve is open.
ECV	Collection vial	Collects water (up to 250 mL) due to condensation in patient circuit.
EV	Exhalation valve	Electronically controlled, electrically operated valve that opens during exhalation, as required to maintain positive end expiratory pressure (PEEP)/continuous positive airway pressure (CPAP). Closed during inspiration.
F9	Filter, expiratory	Filters matter greater than 0.3 μm (micron) (nominal) at 100 L/min flow.
HTR	Heater, exhalation	16 W heater that maintains gas temperature above condensation level.
PE	Pressure transducer, expiratory	Measures pressure (psig) at a port on exhalation PCB.
Q3	Sensor, exhalation flow	Measures exhalation flow.
SOL2	Solenoid valve, autozero	+6 V, three-way solenoid valve. Energized (common to normally closed) when transducer is autozeroed. De-energized (common to normally open) all other times.
Compressor module		
A/HE	Accumulator/heat exchanger	Stores and cools compressed air generated by compressor.
CV1	Check valve, compressor accumulator	Prevents accumulator compressed air from venting back through compressor when SOL3 energizes or the compressor is turned off during stand-by operation. Opens to admit compressor output into accumulator to charge or recharge accumulator.
D1	Diffuser, SOL4	Prevents spraying of water when SOL4 is de-energized.
F10	Filter, compressor outlet	Filters matter greater than 0.3 μm (micron).
F11	Filter, compressor pressure transducer.	Protects this pressure transducer.
FS1	Filter, inlet silencer	Acts as silencer for compressor air intake. Provides filtering for compressor air intake.
HE	Heat exchanger	Transfers heat from the motor compressor output gas flow to the accumulator/heat exchanger output gas flow.
HTR	Heater, water evaporative tray	Speeds evaporation of water in WET.
MC	Motor compressor	Compresses gas up to 25 psi.
RV	Relief valve	Opens when accumulator pressure is greater than 30 psi. Protects system from overpressurization if unloading solenoid valve (SOL3) fails.
PC	Pressure transducer, compressor	Measures pressure of accumulator/heat exchanger. Located on compressor PCB.
PD	Pressure damper	Dampens pressure fluctuations from motor compressor.
R1	Restrictor, damper	Dampens pressure to PC.
S1	Silencer	Reduces the sound of venting gas from SOL3.
SOL4	Solenoid valve, drain, compressor	+12 V, three-way solenoid valve. When de-energized, drains accumulator condensate from accumulator/heat exchanger.
SOL3	Solenoid valve, unloading, compressor	+12 V, two-way solenoid valve. When energized, ensures compressor does not start against back pressure in the circuit Also, when energized, vents excessive compressor output.
WET	Water evaporative tray	Holds water due to condensation from the accumulator/heat exchanger.

Figure 9-35B *(continued)*

cmH$_2$O. Pressure control levels are adjustable between 5 and 90 cmH$_2$O. Pressure support may be adjusted between 0.0 and 70 cmH$_2$O.

Volume becomes a limit variable when an inspiratory hold has been selected by the practitioner. Inspiratory hold is adjustable between 0.0 and 2.0 seconds. When selected, the ventilator will deliver a breath, which will be held following breath delivery until the set time interval has lapsed.

Flow is a limit variable when the ventilator delivers mandatory flow-controlled breaths.

Flow is adjustable between 3 and 150 L/min. If the peak flow delivered is less than that set by the inspiratory flow rate, flow becomes the limit variable.

Cycle Variables

Cycle variables for the 840 ventilator include pressure, flow, and time. Pressure becomes a cycle variable when inspiratory pressure exceeds the value set by the high circuit pressure alarm. High pressure limits are adjustable between 7 and 100 cmH$_2$O. When the pressure limit is reached, inspiration is terminated and the expiratory phase begins.

Flow is a cycle variable during spontaneous breaths (with or without pressure support). When inspiratory flow decays to the following value:

$$\text{End-Inspiratory Flow} = \frac{\text{Peak Flow(Expiratory Sensitivity)}}{100}$$

inspiration ends and the expiratory phase begins. Expiratory sensitivity is adjustable between 1 and 45%.

Time becomes a cycle variable during mandatory breath delivery. The microprocessor determines volume as a function of flow and inspiratory time. Once the appropriate inspiratory time has been reached, breath delivery ceases. During pressure-controlled ventilation, inspiratory time becomes a cycle variable and is adjustable between 0.2 and 8.0 seconds.

Baseline Variable

The baseline variable for the Nellcor Puritan-Bennett 840 ventilator is pressure. PEEP/CPAP pressures are adjustable between 0 and 45 cmH$_2$O. The ventilator creates baseline pressure by partially closing the electrodynamic exhalation valve during the expiratory phase.

Conditional Variables

Time and Pressure or Time and Flow

Time and pressure or time and flow become conditional variables during the SIMV mode. The rate control determines the frequency of mandatory breath delivery during the SIMV mode. The rate control is an electronic timer, allowing a time window for the patient to trigger a breath or delivering a breath at specified time intervals if no efforts are detected. Between mandatory breath delivery, the patient breathes through the ventilator's pneumatic system. The ventilator measures pressure or flow to determine if the patient is attempting to initiate a breath. In response to the trigger variable's change, the patient is able to draw gas spontaneously through the pneumatic system to meet his or her inspiratory needs.

Output Waveforms

Pressure

The pressure output waveform of the 840 ventilator is rectangular when the ventilator is operating in the pressure support and pressure control modes. In these modes, pressure rises sharply to the present value and is then maintained at that value until the inspiratory phase ends.

Flow

The flow output may be adjusted between rectangular and descending ramp waveforms. The PSOLs, in combination with the microprocessor and feedback control system, enable the ventilator to accurately reproduce these output waveforms.

Alarms

Input Power

Input power alarms include AC power loss, low battery, no air supply, and no oxygen supply alarms. The AC power loss alarm is activated when AC power is interrupted or not available. During this time, the ventilator is powered by the backup power source (BPS), which is an internal DC battery. When this occurs, the clinician should check the AC power source and prepare for alternate ventilation.

The low battery alarm is activated when the BPS has less than 2 minutes of operational time remaining. If AC power is lost and the ventilator is operating on BPS, an alternative means of ventilation should be established.

Air and oxygen alarms are activated if air or oxygen pressure falls to less than 35 psi. Should this occur, an alternate gas source should be established. A compressor inoperative alarm will also alert the user to compressor failure in the event the optional air compressor fails to supply sufficient pressure to power the ventilator.

Control Circuit

Control circuit alarms include device alert and procedure error. The device alert alarm is activated when the ventilator's microprocessor detects an error during a background or POST test. When this condition occurs, an alternate means of ventilation for the patient should be provided.

The procedure error alarm will occur if the patient is connected to the ventilator circuit prior to completion of the start-up procedure. You should wait until the POST test is complete before attaching the patient to the circuit.

Output Alarms

Pressure. The 840 ventilator includes high circuit and internal pressure alarms. If the circuit pressure is equal to or greater than the set limit, the high circuit pressure alarm will be activated. When this alarm is activated, the inspiratory phase is terminated and exhalation begins. The high circuit pressure is adjustable between 7 and 100 cmH$_2$O.

When operating the ventilator in volume controlled ventilation, the high internal pressure alarm will be activated if pressure exceeds 100 cmH$_2$O. When this occurs, inspiration is terminated and exhalation begins.

Volume. In the event that the patient's exhaled tidal volumes exceed the upper or lower limits, an alarm will alert the practitioner to the event. The high exhaled tidal volume alarm may be set between 50 and 3000 mL or not used at all (off). A low exhaled tidal volume may be set for both mandatory and spontaneous breaths. These alarms are adjustable between 5 and 2,500 mL.

Flow. The 840 ventilator incorporates high and low minute volume alarms. The low minute volume alarm may be set between 0.05

and 60.0 L/min, while the high minute volume alarm may be set between 0.1 and 99.9 L/min. When the patient exceeds the value set on the alarm, the ventilator will alert the practitioner.

Time. A high respiratory rate alarm is provided to alert the practitioner when the patient has a high ventilatory rate. This alarm is adjustable between 10 and 110 breaths per minute. When the patient exceeds the value set, the alarm condition will result.

Emergency Modes of Ventilation

Apnea Ventilation

If the 840 ventilator fails to detect inspiratory flow during the time interval set by the practitioner, apnea ventilation will be invoked by the ventilator and an apnea alarm will result. Apnea intervals may be selected between 10 and 60 seconds. The clinician may select breath type (pressure or volume-controlled), flow pattern and rate, inspiratory pressure, respiratory rate, tidal volume, oxygen percentage, and I:E ratio within the same limits as for nonapnea ventilator settings. If the patient triggers two consecutive breaths and the exhaled volume is at least 50% of the delivered volume, the ventilator will reset itself into the nonapnea ventilation mode.

Safety Ventilation

In the event the practitioner connects the patient prior to completion of the start-up procedure, the procedure error alarm will be activated and safety ventilation will be invoked. Safety ventilation is not clinician adjustable and will result in pressure-controlled ventilation using the settings in Table 9-25.

TABLE 9-25 Safety Ventilation Settings

Mode	Pressure controlled, A/C
Inspiratory pressure	10 cmH$_2$O
Inspiratory time	1.0 seconds
Respiratory rate	16/minute
PEEP	3.0 cmH$_2$O
Pressure triggered	–2 cmH$_2$O
Flow acceleration	50%
Oxygen percentage	100%

Safety Valve Open

In the event the ventilator detects system faults (which will not prevent it from providing reliable ventilatory support), the ventilator will alarm and enter the safety valve open (SVO) emergency state. During SVO, the safety, exhalation, and inspiratory valves are opened, allowing the patient to breath spontaneously from room air. Check valves on both the inspiratory and expiratory circuits minimize the rebreathing of exhaled gas by the patient. The ventilator will display the elapsed time of SVO; it will not display patient data (including waveforms) or detect circuit occlusion or patient disconnect conditions.

Table 9-26 summarizes the Nellcor Puritan-Bennett 840 ventilator alarms, and Table 9-27 summarizes its capabilities.

TABLE 9-27 Nellcor Puritan-Bennett 840 Ventilator Capabilities

Modes	CMV (volume or pressure controlled), SIMV, CPAP, Pressure Support, Spontaneous
Volume	25–2,500 ml
Pressure	5–90 cmH$_2$O
Pressure support	0.0–70 cmH$_2$O
Rate	1.0–100 BPM
Peak flow	3–150 L/min
Flow sensitivity	0.5–20 L/min
Pressure sensitivity	0.1–20 cmH$_2$O below baseline
Inspiratory time	0.2–8.0 seconds
PEEP/CPAP	0.0–45 cmH$_2$O
Insp. pause	0.0–2.0 seconds
F$_I$O$_2$	0.21–1.0

TABLE 9-26 Nellcor Puritan Bennett 840 Ventilator Alarms

Alarm	Condition/Settings
Input Power	
Oxygen	<35 psi
Air	<35 psi
AC Power	Loss of AC power
Low Battery	Less than 2 minutes of operation time remaining
Control Circuit	
Device Alert	A failure of a background or POST test has been detected
Procedure Error	The patient was connected before completion of startup
Output Alarms	
High Insp Pressure	5–90 cmH$_2$O
High Circuit Pressure	7–100 cmH$_2$O
High Internal Pressure	100 cmH$_2$O
High Exhaled Tidal Volume	50–3,000 mL
Low Exhaled Spont. Tidal Vol	5–2,500 mL
Low Exhaled Mandatory Vol	5–2,500 mL
High Minute Volume	0.1–99.9 L/min
Low Minute Volume	0.05–60.0 L/min
High Frequency	10–110 BPM

SIEMENS-ELEMA SERVO 900C

The Siemens-Elema Servo 900C ventilator is a pneumatically powered, electronically-controlled single circuit ventilator (Figures 9-36 and 9-37). It can function in volume control, volume control + sigh, SIMV, SIMV + Pressure Support, CPAP, pressure control, and pressure support modes. It can operate as a pressure or flow controller.

Drive Mechanism

The Servo 900C requires 120 volts, 60 Hz electrical power to run the microprocessor control system. The electrical cord and power switch are both located on the rear of the ventilator.

The Servo 900C does not have an oxygen blender built into its design. Air and oxygen must be mixed externally before entering the

ASSEMBLY AND TROUBLESHOOTING

Assembly—Nellcor Puritan-Bennett 840 Ventilator

To assemble the 840 ventilator for use, complete the following suggested assembly guide:

1. Connect the ventilator to an appropriate AC power source (120 volts, 60 Hz, or 200 volts, 60 Hz).

2. Connect the ventilator to 50-psi air and oxygen supplies. If compressed air is not available, the optional air compressor may be used.

3. Lift the exhalation filter latch into the up position, and install the exhalation filter into position. Once positioned, push the latch down.

4. Connect the ventilator outlet to an inspiratory bacteria filter and then connect the outlet of the filter to a heated humidifier using a short length of 22-mm diameter tubing.

5. Connect the inspiratory limb of the circuit to the outlet of the humidifier and the expiratory limb to the exhalation filter assembly.

6. Complete an extended self-test (EST) prior to use.

Troubleshooting

Refer to the troubleshooting algorithms found at the end of this chapter.

---

ventilator. Currently the manufacturer recommends either the model 960 or 965 blender.

Gas enters the ventilator via a quick-connect fitting. The gas passes through a non-return valve (one-way valve) to an oxygen-sensing cell (Figure 9-38). The oxygen-sensing cell is a polarographic cell forming part of the oxygen-analyzing system. From the sensing cell, the gas passes through a bacteria filter and into the spring-loaded bellows.

The drive mechanism is the pneumatic gas source (50-psi air and oxygen) and the spring-loaded bellows. Spring tension on the bellows may be adjusted between 10 and 120 cmH$_2$O.

Figure 9-36 *A photograph of the Siemens Elema Servo 900C ventilator.*

Figure 9-37 *A photograph of the Siemens Medical Systems, Inc., Servo 900C control panel.*

Figure 9-38 *A schematic diagram of the Servo 900C ventilator's pneumatic system. (Courtesy Siemens Medical Systems, Danvers, MA)*

The gas supply and the spring tension maintain a uniform pressure within the bellows (working pressure). The working pressure is displayed on a manometer directly above and between the expired minute volume and airway pressure displays.

Control Circuit

Gas from the bellows flows through a safety valve. The safety valve vents gas from the bellows to the ambient air if pressure exceeds 120 cmH$_2$O or if the bellows overfills.

Gas then flows to a flow transducer and on to the inspiratory proportional scissor valve. The flow transducer consists of a flag in the inspired gas flow that bends or distorts a strain gauge. The strain sensed by the strain gauge becomes proportional to flow, as described earlier in this section.

The inspiratory proportional valve opens and closes in response to control signals from the electronic control system. The feedback control system consists of the inspiratory flow transducer and a pressure transducer exposed to the inspiratory flow (Figure 9-38). A stepper motor moves in discrete steps or positions in response to signals from the control circuit, opening or closing the valve to match the flow or pressure to the control settings established by the practitioner.

Gas flows from the patient circuit, through an expiratory flow transducer, to an expiratory pressure transducer, and on to the expiratory valve.

The Servo 900C does not have an exhalation valve incorporated into the patient circuit. The expiratory valve is a servo-controlled electromagnetic valve. The control circuit varies the amount of electrical current applied to the valve and therefore controls its opening and closing. (A complete description of the expiratory valve was included in Chapter 7.)

From the expiratory valve, the exhaled gas flows through a one-way flapper valve into the ambient air. The flapper valve is required to prevent backflow into the circuit so that the trigger sensitivity can operate correctly.

PEEP/CPAP pressure is regulated by the expiratory valve. The expiratory valve will remain partially closed during exhalation, maintaining the desired pressure in the circuit as it acts as a threshold resistor. PEEP/CPAP pressures are adjustable between 0.0 and 50 cmH$_2$O.

Control Variables

As described earlier, the control variable used by the Servo 900C ventilator is flow or pressure. Flow becomes the control variable during mandatory volume delivery, during volume control, volume control + sigh, and the mandatory portion of SIMV ventilation. During these modes of operation, flow is measured and used as a feedback signal to regulate volume delivery (flow multiplied by inspiratory time).

During pressure control and pressure support, pressure becomes the control variable. Pressure is measured and used as a feedback signal to maintain the desired pressure in the patient circuit.

Phase Variables

Trigger Variables

Trigger variables for the Servo 900C include pressure and time triggering. Pressure may be a trigger variable in all modes of ventilation. The trigger threshold is adjusted using the trigger sensitivity control. The sensitivity may be adjusted between 0.0 and 20 cmH$_2$O below baseline pressure.

Time becomes a trigger variable during volume control, the mandatory portions of SIMV, and pressure control if no inspiratory effort (pressure drop) is sensed by the ventilator. The time interval for triggering is established by the breath rate control. Rates are adjustable between 5 and 120 breaths per minute (volume control and pressure control modes) and .4 to 4 or 4 to 40 breaths per minute in SIMV mode. If the patient does not trigger a breath, the ventilator will deliver a mandatory breath at the established inspiratory time percent and minute volume settings.

Limit Variables

The limit variables of the Servo 900C include pressure, volume, and flow. Pressure becomes a limit variable during SIMV (with PEEP applied), CPAP, pressure support, and pressure control ventilation. Under these conditions, the ventilator will augment flow to maintain the desired pressure level. PEEP/CPAP pressures are adjustable between 0.0 and 50.0 cmH$_2$O. Pressure levels for pressure support and pressure control are adjustable between 0.0 and 100.0 cmH$_2$O.

Volume becomes a limit variable when the inspiratory pause time percent control is active. Inspiratory pause time percent control may be adjusted between 0 and 30% of the cycle time in increments of 5% (0 to 10% pause time) and 10% (10 to 30% pause time). When activated, a volume breath is delivered and held, until the set inspiratory pause time period has elapsed. This is only available during volume control, pressure control, and the mandatory portions of SIMV.

Flow becomes a limit when the rectangular output waveform has been selected. When a rectangular waveform output is delivered, flow during inspiration is limited by the settings established on the minute volume and inspiratory time percent controls.

The inspiratory flow rate is not adjustable on the Servo 900C. Inspiratory flow becomes a function of minute volume and the inspiratory time percent. The ventilator adjusts flow to maintain the desired inspiratory time percent. The inspiratory flow rate may be calculated by multiplying the minute volume by a factor based on the inspiratory time percent. The factors are shown in Table 9-28.

Assume the minute volume is 10 liters per minute and the inspiratory time percent is 25%. The peak inspiratory flow will be 40 liters per minute (4×10 L/min).

Alternatively, minute volume may be divided by the inspiratory time percent to calculate the average flow rate. For example, if the minute volume is 12 liters per minute and the inspiratory time percent is 25%, the average flow will be 48 liters per minute.

Cycle Variables

Cycle variables for the Servo 900C ventilator include pressure, flow, and time. Pressure becomes a cycle variable if the inspiratory pressure reaches the setting on the upper pressure limit control. Peak inspiratory pressure may be adjusted between 16 and 120 cmH$_2$O. When the pressure limit is reached, inspiration is terminated, and both audible and visual alarms are activated.

Volume becomes a cycle variable during sigh breath delivery. When selected, a sigh breath will be given every 100th breath. The sigh volume delivered will be 200% of the tidal volume (minute volume divided by the

TABLE 9-28 Flow Rate Calculation Factors

Inspiratory Time (Percent)	Factor
20%	5
25%	4
33%	3
50%	2
67%	1.5
80%	1.25

breath rate). Sigh breath delivery cannot be used during pressure control ventilation.

Flow becomes a cycle variable during pressure support ventilation. Inspiration is terminated when inspiratory flow falls to approximately 25% of the peak inspiratory flow. When inspiratory flow drops to this value, inspiratory pressure support is terminated.

Time becomes a cycle variable during pressure control ventilation. In this mode, a constant pressure is applied until the time set on the inspiratory time percent control has been reached.

Baseline Variable

PEEP/CPAP pressures may be adjusted between 0.0 and 50 cmH$_2$O. The Servo 900 ventilator creates PEEP/CPAP pressure by partially closing the exhalation valve.

Conditional Variables

Time

Time becomes a conditional variable during sigh delivery. During normal ventilator supported breaths, they are pressure controlled, pressure triggered, pressure or time cycled. During sigh delivery, a sigh breath will be given every 100th breath.

Time and Pressure

Time and pressure become conditional variables during SIMV mode. The rate control determines the frequency of mandatory breath delivery during SIMV mode. The rate control is essentially an electronic timer, delivering a breath at specified time intervals. Between mandatory breath delivery, the patient breathes through the flow control valve subsystem. The ventilator measures proximal airway pressure to determine if the patient is attempting to initiate a breath. In response to the pressure change, the patient is able to draw gas spontaneously through the flow control valve to meet inspiratory needs.

Output Waveforms

Pressure

Pressure waveform output is rectangular during pressure control and pressure support. During pressure control and pressure support, pressure rises rapidly to the inspiratory pressure level and is maintained there until the inspiratory time percent value has been reached.

Flow

The flow output may be selected between rectangular and sinusoidal waveforms. The waveform is selected using the waveform toggle switch.

Alarms

Input Power

Input power alarms include gas supply and power failure. The gas supply alarm is activated in the event that gas supply is lost or disconnected. This alarm is inactivated if the respiratory rate is greater than 80 BPM and the inspiratory time percent is 20 or 25. The alarm is both visual and audible.

A power failure alarm will sound if the external 120 volt, 60 Hz source fails, and the green power light will go off. The alarm is battery powered and will function for 5 to 10 minutes.

Output Alarms

Pressure. The Servo 900C has an upper pressure limit alarm. The upper pressure limit alarm is adjustable between 16.0 and 120 cmH$_2$O. When the pressure limit is reached, inspiration is terminated and both audible and visual alarms are activated.

Flow. The Servo 900C incorporates both high and low minute ventilation alarms, which rely on the expiratory flow transducer signal to the control system. Lower limits range from 0.0 to 4.0 liters per minute (infants), while the upper limits ranges from 0 to 40 liters per minute (adults).

Time. If no inspiratory pressure drop has been sensed for 15 seconds, this alarm will be activated. The alarm alerts the practitioner to the patient's absence of inspiratory efforts.

Inspired Gas. The Servo 900C has a built-in oxygen analyzer. Alarm limits may be set above and below the desired F_IO_2. If those parameters are exceeded, the alarm will be activated.

Table 9-29 summarizes the Servo 900C alarms, and Table 9-30 summarizes its capabilities.

TABLE 9-29 Servo 900C Ventilator Alarm Systems

Alarm	Condition/Settings
Input Power	
Gas Supply	Loss of gas supply pressure
Electric Power	Loss of 120 volt, 60 Hz power
Output Alarms	
High Pressure Limit	16.0–120 cmH$_2$O
Low Exhaled Minute Vol.	0.0–4.0 L/min
Low Minute Volume	0.0–40 L/min
Apnea	No pressure trigger or mandatory breath for 15 seconds
Inspired Gas Oxygen Percentage	20–100% oxygen

TABLE 9-30 Servo 900C Ventilator Capabilities

Modes	Volume Control, Volume Control + Sigh, SIMV, SIMV + Pressure Support, Pressure Control, Pressure Support, CPAP
Minute Volume	0.5–40 L/min
Pressure	0.0–120 cmH$_2$O
Press. Support	0.0–100 cmH$_2$O
Press. Control	0.0–100 cmH$_2$O
Rate	5–120 BPM
Insp. Time %	20, 25, 33, 50, 67, or 80%
PEEP/CPAP	0.0–50 cmH$_2$O
Sigh Volume	200% of tidal volume
Sigh Rate	Every 100th breath
Insp. Pause	0, 5, 10, 20, or 30%
Sensitivity	0.0 to 20 cmH$_2$O below baseline pressure
F_IO_2	0.21 to 1.0

ASSEMBLY AND TROUBLESHOOTING

Assembly—Servo 900C

To assemble the Siemens-Elema Servo 900C for use, complete this suggested assembly guide.

1. Assemble the humidifier and attach it to the side of the ventilator. Fill it with water and connect the inlet of the humidifier to the ventilator outlet. Since many humidifiers may be adapted to this ventilator, assembly instructions will not be included here.

2. Assemble the patient circuit and attach the inspiratory limb to the humidifier outlet and the expiratory limb to the expiration inlet channel.

3. Connect the ventilator to an oxygen blender and the blender supply lines to 50-psi air and oxygen sources.

4. Connect the power cord to a 120 volt, 60 Hz outlet.

5. Adjust the working pressure control to 60 cmH$_2$O.

6. Perform a leak test using the inspiratory pause hold control.

Troubleshooting

The comprehensive monitors and alarms simplify ventilator troubleshooting. Careful assembly and pressure testing will readily identify leaks in the patient circuit.

Other leaks may occur internally. Sources include the valve assemblies (incorrect installation) or the bellows itself. If performance seem sluggish or erratic, check the silicone rubber pinch valves to ensure they were not twisted upon assembly. Also check the exhalation flow transducer screen for obstruction by contamination or condensation from the expiratory limb of the patient circuit.

Refer to the troubleshooting algorithms found at the end of this chapter for further troubleshooting assistance.

SIEMENS-ELEMA SERVO 300

The Siemens-Elema Servo 300 ventilator is a pneumatically powered, electronically-controlled single circuit ventilator (Figures 9-39 and 9-40). It can function in pressure control, volume control, pressure regulated volume control, volume support, SIMV (pressure control or volume control) + pressure support, and CPAP + pressure support. The ventilator can operate as a pressure or flow controller.

Figure 9-39 *A photograph of the Siemens Medical Systems, Inc., Servo 300 ventilator. (Courtesy Siemens Medical Systems, Inc., Electromedical Group, Danvers, MA)*

Figure 9-40 *A photograph of the Siemens Medical Systems, Inc., Servo 300 control panel. (Courtesy Siemens Medical Systems, Inc., Electromedical Group, Danvers, MA)*

Drive Mechanism

Power to run the microprocessor control circuitry is provided by 120 volt, 60 Hz electrical power. The pneumatic system is powered by 50-psi source of medical air and oxygen.

The pneumatic drive mechanism (Figure 9-41) consists of two servo control valves, one for air and the other for oxygen. Oxygen and air may enter the servo valves between 29 and

Figure 9-41 *A schematic diagram showing the Servo 300 ventilator's pneumatic system. (Courtesy Siemens Medical Systems, Inc., Electromedical Group, Danvers, MA)*

94 psi (2–6.5 bar). However, the valves are designed to operate the most efficiently and accurately at the standard line pressures of 50 psi.

Control Circuit

The Servo 300 utilizes six microprocessors, two servo control valves, two differential pressure transducers, and a flow transducer to regulate the output from the ventilator. These components are all contained within the gas control modules (one each for air and oxygen). The ventilator determines flow output from the servo valves based upon valve position (how far it has opened), control settings, and signals from the two differential pressure transducers. Valve position is determined by an optical sensor contained within each gas control module. The two servo valves regulate flow, pressure, volume (flow multiplied by time), and F_IO_2.

Control Variables

The control variable for the Servo 300 is both flow and pressure. Inspiratory flow is measured by the flow transducer and differential pressure transducers contained within the gas control modules. Flow is used as a control variable during control and the mandatory portions of SIMV. In these modes volume becomes a derivative of flow (flow multiplied by inspiratory time).

Pressure is used as the control variable during PEEP/CPAP, pressure support, and pressure control delivery and pressure regulated volume control and volume support. Pressure is monitored by two pressure transducers, one on the inspiratory side and one on the expiratory side. Flow output from the gas control modules is adjusted by the feedback control system to maintain the desired pressure levels.

Phase Variables
Trigger Variables

The trigger variables of the Servo 300 include pressure, flow, time, and manual. Pressure becomes a trigger variable when the patient inhales, reducing pressure in the circuit below the reference level set on the trigger sensitivity control. Trigger sensitivity may be adjusted between 0.0 and 17 cmH$_2$O below baseline pressure. Pressure operates as a trigger variable in all modes.

Flow becomes a trigger variable when the trigger sensitivity control has been adjusted into the area marked in "green" or "red." Flow triggering may be set for the following types of patients: adult (0.7 to 2.0 L/min), pediatric (0.3 to 1.0 L/min), and infant (0.17 to 0.5 L/min). Once the established flow threshold (flow sensitivity) has been sensed by the microprocessor, the flow control valves open, delivering flow to the patient circuit. Flow triggering may be used in all breath types and all modes.

Time is a trigger variable during volume control, pressure regulated volume control, pressure control, and SIMV when no spontaneous breaths occur. Breath delivery is based upon the respiratory rate setting (time).

The ventilator may also be manually triggered by rotating the start breath control. When rotated into this position, the ventilator initiates a controlled breath at the tidal volume, inspiratory time percent, pause time, rise time percent, and F_IO_2 set on the control panel.

Limit Variables

The limit variables include pressure, volume, and flow. Pressure becomes the limit variable during the spontaneous breaths when in SIMV (with PEEP/CPAP added), CPAP, pressure control, and pressure support modes. The pneumatic system will maintain the desired pressure control and pressure support modes. The pneumatic system will maintain the desired pressure in the patient circuit as adjusted by the practitioner. PEEP/CPAP is adjustable between 0.0 and 50 cmH$_2$O, pressure support may be adjusted between 0.0 and 100 cmH$_2$O above PEEP, and pressure control may be set between 0.0 and 100 cmH$_2$O above PEEP.

Volume becomes a limit variable when inspiratory pause time percent has been selected by the practitioner. When selected, inspiratory pause time percent may be adjusted between 0 and 30% of the ventilatory cycle. The ventilator will deliver a breath and it will be held following breath delivery until the set time interval has elapsed.

Flow is the limit variable during volume-controlled ventilation. The flow delivery is limited to the values set on the tidal volume and inspiratory time percent controls. Inspiratory flow is equal to the minute volume divided by the inspiratory time fraction. This is only true in the volume control, volume control + SIMV, and pressure support modes.

Cycle Variables

The cycle variables include pressure, flow, and time. Pressure becomes the cycle variable when inspiratory pressure reaches the pressure set on the upper pressure limit control. The upper pressure limit is adjustable between 16 and 120 cmH$_2$O. When the pressure limit is reached, inspiratory flow is stopped and both audible and visual alarms are activated and the patient is allowed to exhale.

Flow becomes the cycle variable during pressure support. When inspiratory flow decays to 5% of the peak inspiratory flow or 80% of the patient breath cycle time has been reached, breath delivery stops.

Time becomes the cycle variable during mandatory breath delivery. The microprocessor determines volume as a function of flow and inspiratory time percent. Once the appropriate inspiratory time has been reached, breath delivery ceases.

Baseline Variable

PEEP/CPAP pressures may be adjusted between 0.0 and 50 cmH$_2$O. The Servo 300 ventilator creates PEEP/CPAP pressure by partially closing the exhalation valve.

Output Waveforms

Pressure

The pressure output of the Servo 300 ventilator may be rectangular, exponential, or adjustable. The rectangular waveform output occurs when the ventilator is operated with the inspiratory rise time percent control set at the zero position. In this setting, pressure rises sharply to the level set on the pressure support/insp pressure control. Pressure is maintained until the criteria for breath termination has been met.

Pressure output becomes exponential when the flow output is rectangular. When the flow output is rectangular, pressure output becomes exponential.

Pressure output becomes adjustable when the ventilator is operated in pressure regulated volume control. The basic waveform morphology, however, remains rectangular with the rise time set at zero. The pressure output is variable, depending upon the patient's compliance and resistance. Each delivered breath is compared to the previous breath, and pressure is adjusted between 0 and 3 cmH$_2$O, until the tidal volume delivery corresponds to the settings on the control panel when it becomes constant. If excess volume is delivered, pressure decreases in incremental values until the desired volume delivery has been met.

Volume

Volume output is an ascending ramp when the ventilator is operated with the inspiratory rise time percent control set at zero. Under these conditions, the volume gradually increases in a linear fashion as pressure increases.

Flow

The flow output of the Servo 300 is rectangular. The flow waveform may be modified by use of the inspiratory rise time percent control. This control determines how quickly the flow rises to its limit value. The rise time percent is adjustable between 0 and 10% of the ventilatory cycle.

Alarms

Input Power Alarms

The input power alarms include loss of electrical and loss of pneumatic power. In the event of a loss of electrical power, an audible and visual alarm will be activated. The ventilator will automatically switch to internal battery operation. If sufficient capacity is left in the battery, the alarm can be silenced and a visual caution indicator will be illuminated.

If the oxygen or air lines become disconnected, or if either gas control module becomes disconnected, an audible and visual alarm will be activated.

Control Circuit Alarms

The control circuit alarms are included in the technical alarms section of the control panel. Some of these alarms may be corrected by the practitioner, while others require the attention of a qualified biomedical service technician. The alarm conditions that can be checked by the practitioner include circuit leakage, check tubings (internal pressure transducer tubing on the inspiratory and expiratory sides), and over range (control settings out of range for the maximum flow or volume capability for the patient range).

Output Alarms

Pressure. The pressure output alarm is the upper pressure limit control. The upper pressure limit is adjustable between 16 and 120 cmH_2O. There is also a high continuous pressure alarm which will be activated if the airway pressure exceeds the PEEP/CPAP level by 15 cmH_2O for greater than 15 seconds.

Flow. The Servo 300 incorporates both high and low minute ventilation alarms which rely on the expiratory flow transducer signal to the microprocessor. Lower limits range from 0.06 to 60 L/min (adult) or 0.0 to 0.6 L/min (neonatal), while the upper limits range from 0.3 to 40 L/min (adult) or 0.06 to 4 L/min (neonatal).

Time. An apnea alarm may be set between 10 and 20 seconds. If a breath has not been detected within this time window, both audible and visual alarms will be activated.

Inspired Gas. The Servo 300 has a built-in oxygen analyzer. Alarm limits are set at 6%

ASSEMBLY AND TROUBLESHOOTING

Assembly—Servo 300

To assemble the Siemens Medical Systems Servo 300 for use, complete this suggested assembly guide.

1. Assemble the humidifier and attach it to the side of the ventilator using the supplied rail system. Fill it with water and connect the inlet of the humidifier to the ventilator outlet. Since various humidifiers may be adapted to this ventilator, assembly instructions will not be included here.

2. Assemble the patient circuit and attach the inspiratory limb to the humidifier outlet and the expiratory limb to the expiration channel.

3. Connect the ventilator supply lines to 50-psi air and oxygen sources.

4. Connect the power cord to a 120 volt, 60 Hz outlet.

5. Perform a leak test using the inspiratory pause hold control.

Troubleshooting

The comprehensive monitors and alarms simplify ventilator troubleshooting. Careful assembly and pressure testing will readily identify leaks in the patient circuit.

above and below the desired F_IO_2. If those parameters are exceeded, the alarm will be activated.

Table 9-31 summarizes the Servo 300 alarms, and Table 9-32 summarizes its capabilities.

TABLE 9-31 Servo 300 Ventilator Alarm Systems

Alarm	Condition/Settings
Input Power	
Gas Supply	Loss of air or oxygen supply or disconnection of gas control modules
Electric Power	Loss of 120 volt, 60 Hz power or insufficient internal battery power
Output Alarms	
High Pressure Limit	16.0–120 cmH₂O
Low Exhaled Minute Vol.	0.06–40 L/min
High Minute Volume	0.0–60 L/min
Apnea	No pressure trigger for 10–20 seconds
Inspired Gas	
Oxygen Percentage	20–100% oxygen

TABLE 9-32 Servo 300 Ventilator Capabilities

Modes	Volume Control, Pressure Control, Pressure Regulated Volume Control, Volume Support, SIMV (Volume Control) + Pressure Support, SIMV (Pressure Control) + Pressure Support, Pressure Support/CPAP
Volume	0.0–4,000 mL
PEEP/CPAP	0.0–50 cmH₂O
Press. Support	0.0–100 cmH₂O above PEEP
Press. Control	0.0–100 cmH₂O above PEEP
Rate (control)	5–150 BPM
Rate (SIMV)	0.5 to 40 BPM
Insp. Time %	10 to 80%
Pause Time %	0.0 to 30%
PEEP/CPAP	0.0–50 cmH₂O
Sensitivity	0.0–17 cmH₂O below baseline pressure
Flow Triggering	0.7–2.0 L/min (adult); 0.3–1.0 L/min (pediatric); 0.17–0.5 L/min (neonatal)
F_IO_2	0.21–1.0

SIEMENS SERVO^i VENTILATOR

The Seimens Servo^i ventilator is a flexible universal platform; when equipped with the appropriate options it is capable of ventilating adult, pediatric, and newborn patients (Figure 9-42). The ventilator is manufactured by Siemens-Elema AB, Electromedical Systems Division (Solna, Sweden). The ventilator consists of two primary units: the patient unit where gases are mixed and delivered to the patient, and the user interface where all settings are made and the ventilator is monitored.

The user interface utilizes a combination of a touch screen, rotary dials, and touch pads to make adjustments (Figure 9-43). Data is displayed in graphical as well as numerical form with the alarm limits displayed adjacent to the measured value.

The modes of ventilation include pressure regulated volume control, volume control, pressure control, volume targeted pressure support, pressure support, CPAP, SIMV, and Automode.

Drive Mechanism

Power to run the microprocessor control circuitry is provided by 100–120 volt, 60 Hz or 220–240 volt 60 Hz electrical power. The ventilator also contains an internal 12-volt DC battery that can provide backup power of up to 3 hours. The pneumatic system is powered by 50-psi source of medical air and oxygen.

Figure 9-42 *A photograph of the Siemens Elema AB, Servo^i ventilator.*

Figure 9-43 *A photograph of the Siemens Elema AB, Servo^i ventilator's control panel.*

The pneumatic drive mechanism (Figure 9-44) consists of two servo control valves, one for air and the other for oxygen. Oxygen and air may enter the servo valves between 29 and 94 psi (2–6.5 KPa). However, the valves are designed to operate the most efficiently and accurately at the standard line pressures of 50 psi.

Control Circuit

The Servo^i utilizes six microprocessors, two servo control valves, two differential pressure transducers, and an ultrasonic flow transducer (expiratory limb only) to regulate the output from the ventilator. These components are all contained within the gas control modules (one each for air and oxygen). The ventilator determines flow output from the servo valves based upon valve position (how far it has opened), control settings, and signals from the two differential pressure transducers. Valve position is determined by an optical sensor contained within each gas control module. The two servo valves regulate flow, pressure, volume (flow multiplied by time), and F_IO_2.

Control Variables

The control variables for the Servo^i are both flow and pressure. Inspiratory flow is measured by the flow transducer and differential pressure transducers contained within the gas control modules. Flow is used as a control variable during volume control and the mandatory portions of SIMV. In these modes volume becomes a derivative of flow (flow multiplied by inspiratory time).

Pressure is used as the control variable during PEEP/CPAP, pressure support, and pressure control delivery and pressure regulated volume control and volume support. Pressure is monitored by two pressure transducers, one on the inspiratory side and one on the expiratory side. Flow output from the gas control modules is adjusted by the feedback control system to maintain the desired pressure levels.

Phase Variables

Trigger Variables

The trigger variables of the Servo^i include pressure, flow, time, and manual. Pressure becomes a trigger variable when the patient inhales, reducing pressure in the circuit below the reference level set on the trigger sensitivity control. Trigger sensitivity may be adjusted between 0.0 and 20 cmH_2O below baseline pressure. Correct adjustment of pressure triggering is indicated in reference to the yellow area on the trigger bar (baseline pressure). Pressure operates as a trigger variable in all modes.

Flow becomes a trigger variable when the trigger sensitivity control has been adjusted

SVX-080_EN

Figure 9-44   *A schematic diagram showing the Servo^i ventilator's pneumatic system. (Courtesy Siemens Medical Systems, Inc., Electromedical Group, Danvers, MA)*

into the area marked in "green" or "red." Flow triggering may be set for the following types of patients: adult (0.7 to 2.0 L/min), pediatric (0.3 to 1.0 L/min), and infant (0.17 to 0.5 L/min). Once the established flow threshold (flow sensitivity) has been sensed by the microprocessor, the flow control valves open, delivering flow to the patient circuit. Flow triggering may be used in all breath types and all modes.

Time is a trigger variable during volume control, pressure regulated volume control, pressure control, and SIMV when no spontaneous breaths occur. Breath delivery is based upon the respiratory rate setting (time).

The ventilator may also be manually triggered by pressing the "start breath" soft key on the lower right part of the user interface panel. When depressed, the ventilator initiates a controlled breath at the tidal volume, inspiratory time percent, pause time, rise time percent, and F_1O_2 set on the control panel.

Limit Variables

The limit variables include pressure, volume, and flow. Pressure becomes the limit variable during the spontaneous breaths when in SIMV (with PEEP/CPAP added), CPAP, pressure control, and pressure support modes. The pneumatic system will maintain the desired

pressure as adjusted in pressure control and pressure support modes. PEEP/CPAP is adjustable between 0.0 and 50 cmH$_2$O, pressure support may be adjusted between 0.0 and 100 cmH$_2$O above PEEP, and pressure control may be set between 0.0 and 100 cmH$_2$O above PEEP.

Volume becomes a limit variable when inspiratory pause time percent has been selected by the practitioner. When selected, inspiratory pause time percent may be adjusted between 0 and 30% of the ventilatory cycle. The ventilator will deliver a breath and it will be held following breath delivery until the set time interval has elapsed.

Flow is the limit variable during volume-controlled ventilation. The flow delivery is limited to the values set on the tidal volume and inspiratory time percent controls. Inspiratory flow is equal to the minute volume divided by the inspiratory time fraction. This is only true in the volume control, volume control + SIMV, and pressure support modes.

Cycle Variables

The cycle variables include pressure, flow, and time. Pressure becomes the cycle variable when inspiratory pressure reaches the pressure set on the upper pressure limit control.

The upper pressure limit is adjustable between 16 and 120 cmH2O. When the pressure limit is reached, inspiratory flow is stopped and both audible and visual alarms are activated and the patient is allowed to exhale.

Flow becomes the cycle variable during pressure support. Termination of inspiration during pressure support is adjustable on the Servo^i. The point of exhalation is determined by adjusting the inspiratory cycle-off setting. This setting is adjustable between a range of 1% to 40% of the peak inspiratory flow. Rather than the manufacturer arbitrarily choosing a flow rate based upon a fixed percentage of peek flow, the practitioner can adjust the point at which inspiration begins within parameter's range. It is important for patient comfort to make the setting adjustment high enough to allow for exhalation prior to the delivery of the next breath.

Time becomes the cycle variable during mandatory breath delivery. The microprocessor determines volume as a function of flow and inspiratory time percent. Once the appropriate inspiratory time has been reached, breath delivery ceases. Time is also a cycle variable during pressure control.

Baseline Variable

PEEP/CPAP pressures may be adjusted between 0.0 and 50 cmH$_2$O. The Servo^i ventilator creates PEEP/CPAP pressure by partially closing the exhalation valve.

Output Waveforms

Pressure

The pressure output of the Servo^i ventilator may be rectangular, exponential, or adjustable. The rectangular waveform output occurs when the ventilator is operated with the inspiratory rise time percent control set at the zero position. In this setting, pressure rises sharply to the level set on the pressure support/insp pressure control. Pressure is maintained until the criteria for breath termination has been met.

Pressure output becomes exponential when the flow output is rectangular. When the flow output is rectangular, pressure output becomes exponential.

Pressure output becomes adjustable when the ventilator is operated in pressure regulated volume control. The basic waveform morphology, however, remains rectangular with the rise time set at zero. The pressure output is variable, depending upon the patient's compliance and resistance. Each delivered breath is compared to the previous breath, and pressure is adjusted between 0 and 3 cmH$_2$O, until the tidal volume delivery corresponds to the settings on the control panel when it becomes constant. If excess volume is delivered, pressure decreases in incremental values until the desired volume delivery has been met.

Volume

Volume output is an ascending ramp when the ventilator is operated with the inspiratory rise time percent control set at zero. Under these conditions, the volume gradually increases in a linear fashion as pressure increases.

Flow

The flow output of the Servo^i is rectangular. The flow waveform may be modified by use of the inspiratory rise time percent control. This control determines how quickly the flow rises to its limit value. The rise time percent is adjustable between 0 and 10% of the ventilatory cycle.

Alarms

Input Power Alarms

The input power alarms include loss of electrical and loss of pneumatic power. In the event of a loss of electrical power, an audible and visual alarm will be activated. The ventilator will automatically switch to internal battery operation. If sufficient capacity is left in the battery, the alarm can be silenced and a visual caution indicator will be illuminated.

If the oxygen or air lines become disconnected, or if either gas control module becomes disconnected, an audible and visual alarm will be activated.

Control Circuit Alarms

The control circuit alarms are included in the technical alarms section of the control panel. Some of these alarms may be corrected by the practitioner, while others require the attention of a qualified biomedical service technician. The alarm conditions that can be checked by the practitioner include circuit leakage, check tubings (internal pressure transducer tubing on the inspiratory and expiratory sides), and over range (control settings out of range for the maximum flow or volume capability for the patient range).

Output Alarms

Pressure. The pressure output alarm is the upper pressure limit control. The upper pressure limit is adjustable between 16 and 120 cmH$_2$O. There is also a high continuous pressure alarm, which will be activated if the airway pressure exceeds the PEEP/CPAP level by 15 cmH$_2$O for greater than 15 seconds.

Flow. The Servo^i incorporates both high and low minute ventilation alarms, which rely on the expiratory flow transducer signal to the microprocessor. Lower limits range from 0.5 to 40 L/min (adult) or 0.1 to 20 L/min (neonatal), while the upper limits range from 0.5 to 60 L/min (adult) or 0.1 to 20 L/min (neonatal).

Time. An apnea alarm may be set between 15 and 45 seconds for adults and between 5 and 15 seconds for neonates. If a breath has not been detected within this time window, both audible and visual alarms will be activated.

Inspired Gas. The Servo^i has a built-in oxygen analyzer. Alarm limits are set at 6% above and below the desired F$_I$O$_2$. If those parameters are exceeded, the alarm will be activated.

Table 9-33 summarizes the Servoi alarms, and Table 9-34 summarizes its capabilities.

TABLE 9-33 Siemans Elema AB, Servo^i Ventilator Alarm Systems

Alarm	Condition/Settings
Input Power	
Gas Supply	Loss of air or oxygen supply or disconnection of gas control modules
Electric Power	Loss of 120 volt, 60 Hz power or insufficient internal battery power
Output Alarms	
High Pressure Limit	16.0–120 cmH$_2$O (adult); 16–90 cmH$_2$O (neonatal)
Low Exhaled Minute Vol.	0.05–40 L/min (adult); 0.1–20 L/min (neonatal)
High Minute Volume	0.05–60 L/min (adult); 0.1–30 L/min (neonatal)
Apnea	No patient trigger for 15–45 seconds (adult); 5–15 seconds (neonatal)
Inspired Gas	
Oxygen Percentage	20–100% oxygen

TABLE 9-34 Siemans Elema AB, Servo^i Ventilator Capabilities

Modes	Volume Control, Pressure Control, Pressure Regulated Volume Control, Volume Support, SIMV (Volume Control) + Pressure Support, SIMV (Pressure Control) + Pressure Support, Pressure Support/CPAP, Automode
Volume	0.0–4,000 mL (adult); 5–350 mL (neonatal)
PEEP/CPAP	0.0–50 cmH$_2$O (adult and neonatal)
Press. Support	0.0–120 cmH$_2$O–PEEP (adult); 0.0–80–PEEP (neonatal)
Press. Control	0.0–120 cmH$_2$O–PEEP (adult); 0.0–80–PEEP (neonatal)
Rate (control)	4–100 BPM (adult); 4–150 BPM (neonatal)
Rate (SIMV)	1 to 40 BPM (adult and neonatal)
Insp. Time %	10 to 80%
Pause Time %	0.0 to 30%
PEEP/CPAP	0.0–50 cmH$_2$O
Sensitivity	0.0–20 cmH$_2$O below baseline pressure
Flow Triggering	0.7–2.0 L/min (adult); 0.3–1.0 L/min (pediatric); 0.17–0.5 L/min (neonatal)
F$_I$O$_2$	0.21–1.0

ASSEMBLY AND TROUBLESHOOTING

Assembly—Servo[i]

To assemble the Siemens Elema, AB Servo[i] for use, complete this suggested assembly guide.

1. Assemble the humidifier and attach it to the side of the ventilator using the supplied rail system. Fill it with water and connect the inlet of the humidifier to the ventilator outlet. Since various humidifiers may be adapted to this ventilator, assembly instructions will not be included here.

2. Assemble the patient circuit and attach the inspiratory limb to the humidifier outlet and the expiratory limb to the expiration channel.

3. Connect the ventilator supply lines to 50-psi air and oxygen sources.

4. Connect the power cord to a 120 volt, 60 Hz outlet.

5. Perform a leak test using the inspiratory pause hold control.

Troubleshooting

The comprehensive monitors and alarms simplify ventilator troubleshooting. Careful assembly and pressure testing will readily identify leaks in the patient circuit.

VIASYS VELA VENTILATOR

Viasys Critical Care, Palm Springs, CA is manufacturing and marketing the Vela ventilator. The Vela is an electrically and pneumatically powered ventilator, which is microprocessor controlled. The ventilator's microprocessor control system, when combined with its pressure and flow sensors, provides a flexible system capable of caring for a wide variety of patients from infants to adults (Figure 9-45). Modes of ventilation include A/C, SIMV, CPAP/PSV, volume control and pressure control, and airway pressure release ventilation (APRV). Figure 9-46 is a photograph illustrating the Vela ventilator's control panel.

Figure 9-45 *A photograph of the Viasys Vela ventilator.*

Input Power

Electrical power supplies the microprocessor-controlled system, the drive mechanism, and the various pressure and flow sensors of the Avea ventilator. Power is selectable between 100–120 v, 60 Hz AC and 220–240 v, 60 Hz AC; internal battery; or external 48-V DC battery. Power may be selected by means of a switch located on the rear of the ventilator.

Pneumatic power for the ventilator is supplied by an oxygen source between 40 and 85 psi. Two DISS fittings on the rear of the ventilator are provided for the attachment of oxygen sources. In the event a clinician wishes to transfer from piped wall oxygen to a cylinder, the cylinder may be connected before interruption of the wall oxygen, thus providing a seamless transition between the two sources.

Drive Mechanism

Once gas enters the ventilator, it passes through check valves and into the blender system (Figure 9-47). The blender consists of five solenoids with a fixed orifice at each output. The microprocessor determines which and how many solenoids are required to be opened to add the required oxygen to the accumulator/diffuser.

Ambient air passes through a filter (Figure 9-47) and into the accumulator/diffuser. The accumulator/diffuser functions to initially mix the two gases (oxygen and air), and acts as a baffling device to muffle the noise of the high-speed turbine.

Figure 9-46 *A photograph of the Viasys Vela ventilator's control panel.*

The drive mechanism of the Vela is a small pneumatic turbine capable of providing near-instantaneous flows with a rapid response time. Gas from the accumulator/diffuser passes through a filter silencer to the turbine. The turbine (axial compressor) rapidly compresses the blended gas and provides the instantaneous flow demands needed by the patient. The turbine further homogenates the mixture of air and oxygen through its operation. Gas exiting the turbine passes through another silencer, which muffles the turbine noise.

Control Circuit

The control circuit of the Vela ventilator consists of a turbine differential pressure

Figure 9-47 *A schematic drawing showing the Vela ventilator's pneumatic system.*

transducer, an exhalation differential pressure transducer, an electrodynamic exhalation valve, and the microprocessor.

The turbine differential pressure transducer monitors the pressure drop across the turbine (Figure 9-47). The differential pressure, combined with the speed of the turbine, is used by the microprocessor to precisely regulate the turbine's output. An optical sensor detects the turbine's speed, providing feedback to the microprocessor.

The exhalation differential pressure transducer provides a flow signal to the microprocessor, which reflects what is being exhaled by the patient (Figure 9-47). The body of the expiratory flow transducer has a variable orifice element in the center. The flexible element bends as flow increases, creating a pressure drop across the two ports, which is sensed by the pressure transducer.

The electrodynamic exhalation valve is used to regulate PEEP/CPAP pressures, and it closes during mandatory breaths. The valve consists of a high-energy permanent magnet with a suspended coil, which is energized with current. As current is applied to the coil, it is drawn into the core of the valve, closing it.

Control Variable

The control variable for the Vela is pressure. Differential pressure is detected across the turbine and is used to regulate its output. The microprocessor integrates turbine speed (optically sensed) and the pressure differential to precisely regulate the flow and pressure provided by the turbine drive mechanism.

Phase Variables

Trigger Variables

The trigger variables of the Vela are flow, pressure, time, and manual triggering. During flow-triggered operation, the clinician sets a base flow through the patient circuit. Bias flows are adjustable between 0.4 to 5 L/min. The flow sensitivity is then set; and it is adjustable between 0.1 and 20 L/min.

Pressure is a trigger variable when pressure triggering has been selected. Pressure trigger levels of between 0.1 and 20 cmH_2O may be set. The ventilator will initiate inspiration when the patient's inspiratory effort reaches the value set for the pressure trigger level.

Time triggering occurs during mandatory breaths and is a function of the breath rate control, which may be set between 1–120 breaths per minute (BPM) adult and 1–150 BPM in neonatal mode. When the appropriate time interval has passed, the exhalation valve closes and the ventilator provides a mandatory breath.

The Vela may be manually triggered by the clinician by depressing the manual breath button located at the right side of the control panel. Depressing this button delivers a volume or pressure controlled breath, depending upon the breath type selected.

Limit Variables

The limit variables of the Vela include pressure, volume, and flow. Pressure becomes the limit variable during SIMV (with PEEP/CPAP, CPAP, pressure control, and pressure support ventilation. When the Vela is operating in these modes, pressure is measured and maintained at a consistent level during breath delivery. PEEP/CPAP pressure may be adjusted between 0 and 50 cmH_2O. Pressure control and pressure support may be adjusted between 1 and 90 cmH_2O.

Volume becomes a limit variable when inspiratory pause is selected. Inspiratory pause may be adjusted between 0 and 3.0 seconds. When inspiratory pause is selected, the inspiratory hold valve closes in conjunction with the exhalation valve, holding the breath in the patient's lungs for the set time interval. Under these conditions, volume becomes limited during the inspiratory phase.

Flow becomes a limit variable when the square waveform pattern is selected and the ventilator is set for volume-controlled ventilation (rate, tidal volume, and peak flow). Peak flow is adjustable between 0.4 and 150 L/min. The inspiratory flow limit becomes the value selected using the peak flow control.

Cycle Variables

The cycle variables for the Vela ventilator includes pressure, flow, and time. Pressure becomes a cycle variable when inspiratory pressure reaches the value set on the high pressure limit control. This control is adjustable between 5 and 90 cmH_2O. When the high pressure limit is reached, inspiration is terminated and exhalation begins, and both audible and visual alarms are activated.

Flow is the cycling variable during pressure support. When inspiratory flow decays to 0 to 45% of the peak inspiratory flow value, the breath is terminated and the patient is allowed to exhale. The flow cycling level is adjustable by the practitioner. It is important to adjust the flow cycling (% of peak flow) to a value that allows sufficient time for exhalation. If the flow is slow to decay during inspiration, the breath will be terminated after 3 seconds.

Time is a cycle variable during mandatory breath delivery. The microprocessor determines volume as a function of flow and inspiratory time. Once the desired time has been met, the breath is terminated. Time is also a cycle variable during pressure control ventilation when an inspiratory time determines the end of inspiration.

Conditional Variables

Time

Time becomes a conditional variable during sigh breath delivery. During sigh breath delivery, a sigh breath is delivered every 100 breaths, which is equal to 150% of the set tidal volume. Sigh breaths may be used in all modes of ventilation.

Time and Pressure

Time and pressure become conditional variables during SIMV mode. The rate control determines the frequency of mandatory breath delivery during SIMV mode. The rate control is essentially an electronic timer, delivering a breath at a specified time interval. Between periods of mandatory breath delivery, the patient can obtain spontaneous breaths (pressure support or pure spontaneous) through the ventilator's gas delivery system.

Output Waveforms

Pressure

Pressure waveform output is rectangular. This output waveform occurs during pressure support and pressure control. During these modes, pressure rises rapidly and plateaus at the set pressure level until exhalation begins.

Flow

The flow waveform may be toggled between rectangular (square) and decelerating during volume-controlled breath delivery. This is accomplished by selecting the desired waveform through the user interface.

Alarms

Input Power Alarms

The input power alarms consist of electrical power and gas pressure alarms. In the event that AC power is interrupted, the ventilator switches to battery backup power without interrupting ventilation and an audible alarm sounds, while simultaneously the internal battery indicator is illuminated. In the event that the internal or external batteries are low on power, both audible and visual alarms will result.

When the oxygen inlet pressure is less than 35 psi and the oxygen percentage control is set to greater than 21%, both audible and visual alarms will be activated. Remember, the Vela may be powered by two independent oxygen sources, and when thus connected, one source can serve as a backup for the other.

ASSEMBLY AND TROUBLESHOOTING

Assembly—Viasys Vela Ventilator

1. Exhalation valve assembly: Install the exhalation valve diaphragm and the exhalation valve body into the ventilator. When correctly installed, you will hear a click as it seats into the correct position.

2. Attach a 90° elbow adapter to the ventilator outlet and secure a bacteria filter to it. Connect the ventilator to a heated humidifier using a short length of 22-mm diameter, large-bore tubing.

3. Connect the inspiratory limb from the outlet of the humidifier to the patient wye and the expiratory limb of the circuit to the exhalation valve assembly. The use of water traps in both the inspiratory and expiratory limbs of the circuit is recommended.

4. Connect the ventilator to a 50-psi oxygen source.

5. Connect the power cord to a suitable AC power outlet.

Troubleshooting

Refer to the troubleshooting algorithm found at the end of this chapter.

Control Circuit Alarms

The control circuit alarm consists of internal operations, circuit fault, and EEPROM failure alert. All of these alarms are part of the ventilator's self-testing and troubleshooting systems. In the event these alarms are triggered, you should discontinue use of the ventilator and contact a certified service technician or have the unit checked by a suitable biomedical repair facility.

The flow sensor alarm will sound if a flow sensor is not detected by the ventilator. In this case, check to ensure that the exhalation valve body is correctly seated in its receptacle or replace it with a new one.

Output Alarms

Pressure. Pressure alarms consist of high and low pressure alarms. The high pressure limit alarm may be set at between 5 and 90 cmH_2O. The low pressure alarm alerts the practitioner to decreased inspiratory pressures and is adjustable between 0 and 45 cmH_2O.

Flow. A low minute ventilation alarm may be set between 0.1 and 99.9 mL. The alarm may be used in all modes to alert the clinician to hypoventilation.

Time. The ventilator incorporates a high breath rate and an apnea alarm. The high breath rate alarm is adjustable between 2 and 150 breaths per minute.

The apnea alarm alerts the clinician to apneic periods. The alarm interval may be adjusted from 0.2 to 30 seconds. If a breath is not detected within the set time window, the ventilator will automatically switch to backup ventilation.

Table 9-35 illustrates the Viasys Critical Care Corporation's Vela alarms, and Table 9-36 illustrates its capabilities.

CHAPTER SUMMARY

Several ventilators have been presented in this chapter that are classified as flow and pressure controllers. These ventilators all have a common characteristic in that flow or pressure is measured and used as a feedback control signal to regulate the ventilator's output. Table 9-37 may help you to learn the similarities and differences between the ventilators presented in this chapter.

To assist you in troubleshooting, refer to the algorithms ALG 9-1, 9-2, and 9-3.

TABLE 9-35 Viasys Healthcare Vela Ventilator Alarm Systems

Alarm	Condition/Settings
Input Power	
Battery On	AC power failure
Low Battery	Internal battery power is low
Ext. Battery	External battery power is low
Control Circuit	
Circuit Fault	Kinked or occluded breathing circuit
EEPROM Fault	EEPROM fails to accept a new value
Vent Inop	Internal ventilator fault has been detected
Output Alarms	
High Pressure	5–120 cmH_2O
Low Pressure	2–60 cmH_2O
Low Minute Volume	0.1–99.9 L/min
High Breath Rate	3–150 breaths per minute
Apnea	10–60 seconds

TABLE 9-36 Viasys Healthcare Vela Ventilator Capabilities

Modes	AC, SIMV, CPAP/PSV, Non-invasive with breath types of APRV, Volume, Pressure, TCPL, PRVC
Volume	2.0–2,500 L/min
Pressure	5–90 cmH_2O
Pressure Support	1–90 cmH_2O
Rate	1–150 BPM (neonatal); 1–120 BPM (adult)
Inspiratory Time	0.15–5.0 seconds
Peak Flow	0.4–150 L/min
Sigh Volume	150% of tidal volume
Inspiratory Pause	0.0–3.0 seconds
F_IO_2	0.21–1.00

TABLE 9-37 Flow and Pressure Controllers Classified

Ventilator	Input Power	Circuit	Drive Mechanism	Control Variable	Trigger Variable	Limit Variable	Cycling Variable	Alarms
Bear 1, 2	Electric	Single	Pneumatic	F/P	P/T/M	P/V/F	P/T	I/CC/P/V/T
Bear 3	Electric	Single	Pneumatic	F/P	P/T/M	P/V/F	P/F/T	I/CC/P/V/T
Bear 1000	Electric	Single	Pneumatic	F/P	P/T/M	P/V/F	P/V/F/T	I/CC/P/F/T
Bird 8400ST®i	Electric	Single	Pneumatic	F/P	P/F/T/M	P/V/F	P/F/T	I/CC/P/F/T
Bird TBird® AVS	Electric	Single	Pneumatic	P	F/T/M	P/V/F	P/F/T	I/CC/P/F/T
Dräger Evita 4	Electric	Single	Pneumatic	F/P	F/T/M	P/F	P/F/T	I/CC/P/V/F/T/IG
Nellcor Puritan-Bennett 840	Electric	Single	Pneumatic	F/P	P/F/T/M	P/V/F	P/F/T	I/CC/P/V/F/T
Hamilton Galileo	Electric	Single	Pneumatic	P	F/T/M	P/V/F	P/F/T	I/CC/P/F/T
Hamilton Veolar	Electric	Single	Pneumatic	F/P	P/T/M	P/V/F	P/F/T	I/CC/P/F/T/IG
Infrasonics Adult Star	Electric	Single	Pneumatic	F/P	P/T/M	P/V/F	P/F/T	I/CC/P/V/F/T
Newport Wave	Electric	Single	Pneumatic	F/P	P/T/M	P/F	P/F/T	I/CC/P/F
P-B 7200ae	Electric	Single	Pneumatic	F/P	P/F/T/M	P/V/F	P/F/T	I/CC/P/V/F/T
Siemens Servo 900C	Electric	Single	Pneumatic	F/P	P/T/M	P/V/F	P/F/T	I/P/F/T/IG
Servo 300	Electric	Single	Pneumatic	F/P	P/F/T/M	P/V/F	P/F/T	I/CC/P/F/T/IG
Servoi	Electric	Single	Pneumatic	F/P	P/F/T/M	P/V/F	P/F/T	I/CC/P/F/T/IG
Vela	Electric	Single	Pneumatic	P	P/F/T/M	P/V/F	P/F/T	I/CC/P/F/T

Key: ™P–Pressure, T–Time, F–Flow, CC–Control Circuit, IG–Inspired Gas, V–Volume, M–Manual, I–Input Power

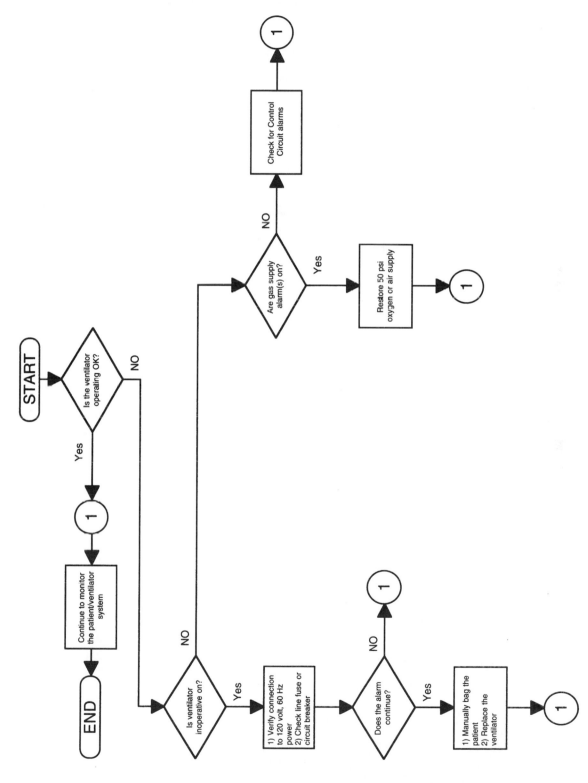

ALG 9-1 *An algorithm for troubleshooting input power alarms.*

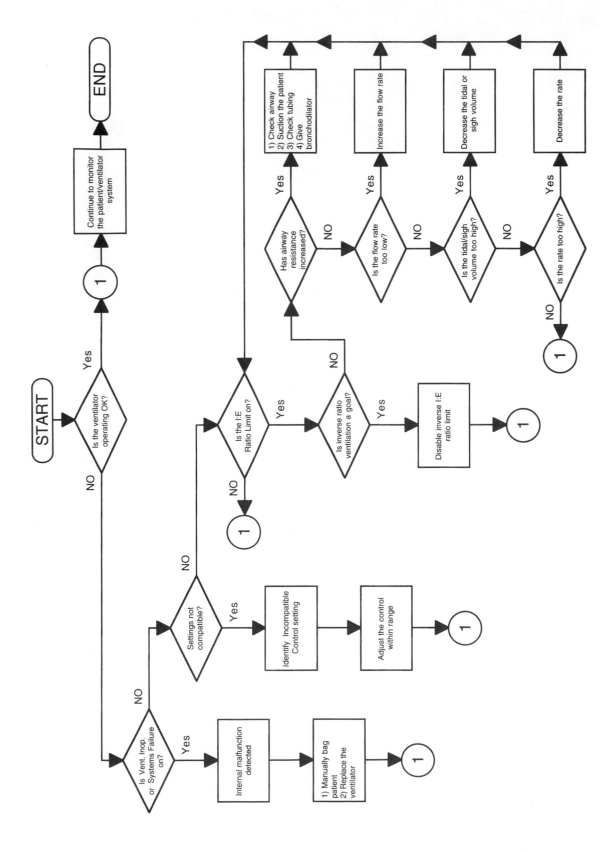

ALG 9-2 *An algorithm for troubleshooting control circuit alarms.*

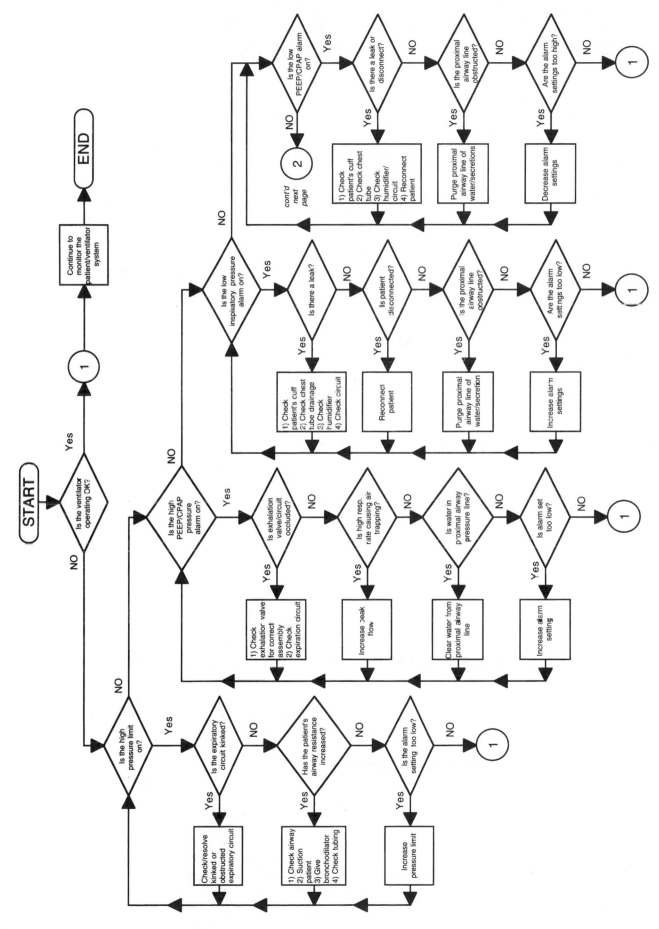

ALG 9-3 *An algorithm for troubleshooting output alarms.* **(continues)**

ALG 9-3 *(continues)*

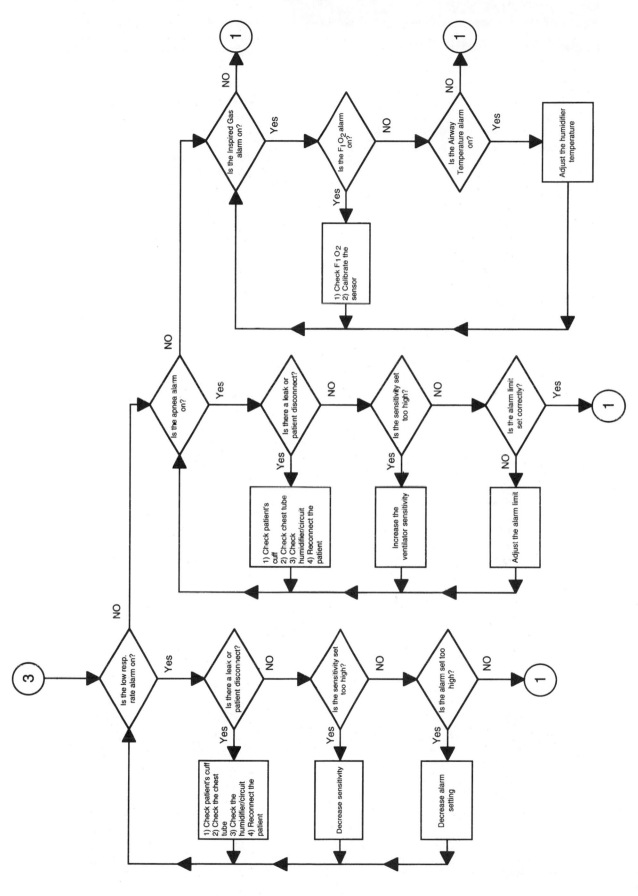

ALG 9-3 *(continued)*

CLINICAL CORNER

Bear 1000 Ventilator

1. You are adjusting the flow triggering for a patient who is on SIMV (volume controlled ventilation) with pressure support of 10 cmH$_2$O. Describe how you can assess whether your flow sensitivity adjustment is appropriate.
2. A physician wants you to correct for tubing compliance. In spite of your best efforts, you cannot locate the compliance factor for a clean circuit by looking at the package insert. How can you determine the tubing compliance for your patient's circuit?

Bird Products Corporation 8400ST®*i* Ventilator

1. You are asked to evaluate a patient who is being ventilated by a Bird 8400ST®*i*. The High Pressure alarm is sounding when you enter the room. Describe in sequence what you would do.

2. You are adjusting the alarms for a patient being ventilated by a Bird 8400ST®*i* ventilator. The patient is on pressure control (assist/control), with a rate of 10, pressure of 32 cmH$_2$O, and PEEP of 8 cmH$_2$O. Describe in detail how you would set your alarm limits.

Nellcor Puritan-Bennett 7200ae Ventilator

1. You are establishing flow triggering for a patient who is on a 7200ae ventilator and is being ventilated in pressure control mode. Describe in detail the key stroke sequence you would follow to change from pressure to flow triggering.
2. You place an in-line nebulizer with 2.5 mg Albuterol in 2.5 mL of normal saline on the circuit of a 7200ae ventilator. The patient is currently on volume control (tidal volume of 700 mL, rate of 12/min, PEEP of 5 cmH$_2$O, F$_I$O$_2$ of 0.40, and flow-by of 8/3 L/min). What must you remember to do when turning off the ventilator's nebulizer control?

Self-Assessment Quiz

1. Under which of the following conditions is pressure a control variable?
   I. mandatory volume breath delivery
   II. CPAP
   III. sigh breath delivery
   IV. pressure support
   a. I and II
   b. I and III
   c. II and III
   d. II and IV

2. Under which of the following situations is flow a control variable?
   I. mandatory volume breath delivery
   II. PEEP/CPAP
   III. sigh breath delivery
   IV. pressure support
   a. I and II
   b. I and III
   c. II and III
   d. II and IV

3. Which of the following ventilators have the capability of flow triggering?
   I. Bird 8400ST®*i*
   II. Siemens Servo 900C
   III. Puritan-Bennett 7200ae
   IV. Bear 1000

    a. I and II
    b. I and III
    c. II and III
    d. II and IV

4. Which of the following methods can be used to measure flow?
    a. differential pressure
    b. vortex sensing
    c. strain gauge technology
    d. all of the above

5. Which of the following are limit variables for the Bear 1000 ventilator?
    I. pressure
    II. volume
    III. flow
    IV. time
    a. I
    b. I and II
    c. I, II, and III
    d. I, II, III, and IV

6. If a ventilator is a flow controller, how is inspiratory volume delivery during mandatory breaths controlled?
    a. by measuring volume
    b. by integrating volume
    c. by measuring pressure
    d. by controlling inspiratory time

7. A ventilator becomes flow limited when:
    a. inspiratory flow reaches a maximum value.
    b. inspiratory flow no longer increases but remains constant.
    c. inspiratory flow reaches a maximum value then decreases.
    d. inspiratory flow starts at a maximum value then rapidly tapers.

8. A ventilator becomes volume limited when:
    a. inspiratory pause is used.
    b. sigh volume delivery is used.
    c. a preset volume has been reached and inspiration is terminated.
    d. inspiration terminates prior to the delivery of the complete volume.

9. Which of the following ventilators are not volume limited?
    a. Bear 1000
    b. Bird 8400ST®*i*
    c. Newport Wave
    d. Puritan-Bennett 7200ae

10. Which of the following ventilators can be volume cycled?
    a. Bear 1000
    b. Bird 8400ST®*i*
    c. Infrasonics Adult Star
    d. Puritan-Bennett 7200ae

11. Which of the following would be examples of a control circuit alarm?
    I. peak pressure
    II. I:E ratio
    III. low tidal volume
    IV. incompatible settings
    a. I and II
    b. II and III
    c. II and IV
    d. III and IV

12. Which of the following are examples of output alarms?
    I. peak pressure
    II. I:E ratio
    III. low tidal volume
    IV. incompatible settings
    a. I and II
    b. I and III
    c. II and III
    d. II and IV

13. Which of the following is an example of a flow output alarm?
    a. high respiratory rate
    b. low minute volume
    c. low tidal volume
    d. low PEEP/CPAP

14. The limit variables for the Infrasonics Adult Star ventilator are:
    I. pressure.
    II. volume.
    III. flow.
    IV. time.
    a. I
    b. I and II
    c. I, II, and III
    d. I, II, III, and IV

15. The Newport Wave is capable of delivering up to 45 cmH2O PEEP/CPAP; this variable is termed the:
    a. control variable.
    b. limit variable.
    c. cycling variable.
    d. baseline variable.

16. When the Hamilton Veolar is operating as a flow controller,
    a. flow is measured and used as a feedback signal.
    b. flow is a trigger variable.
    c. flow is regulated by a reducing valve.
    d. flow becomes independent of volume.

17. Which of the following ventilators require an external blender?
    I. Bear 1000
    II. Bird 8400ST®i
    III. Newport Wave
    IV. Siemens Servo 900C
    a. I and II
    b. I and III
    c. II and III
    d. I and IV

18. Which of the following ventilators have a sinusoidal flow output?
    I. Bear 1000
    II. Bird 8400ST®i
    III. Newport Wave
    IV. Siemens Servo 900C
    a. I and II
    b. I and III
    c. II and III
    d. II and IV

19. Which of the following ventilators have pressure control capability?
    I. Newport Wave
    II. Bird 8400ST®*i*
    III. Hamilton Veolar
    IV. Bear 3
    a. I and II
    b. I and III
    c. II and III
    d. II and IV

20. Which of the following ventilators have pressure support capability?
    I. Newport Wave
    II. Bird 8400ST®*i*
    III. Hamilton Veolar
    IV. Bear 3
    a. I
    b. I and II
    c. I, II, and III
    d. I, II, III, and IV

21. Which of the following ventilators rely on an independent exhalation valve on the patient circuit?
    I. Bear 1, 2
    II. BEAR 1000
    III. Newport Wave
    IV. Siemens Servo 300
    a. I
    b. I and II
    c. I, II, and III
    d. I, II, III, and IV

22. Which of the following ventilators utilizes an electromagnetic exhalation valve?
    a. Bear 1000
    b. Bird 8400ST®*i*
    c. Hamilton Veolar
    d. Newport Wave

23. "Inspiration ends and exhalation begins when a preset pressure has been reached" best describes:
    a. pressure control.
    b. pressure support.
    c. pressure limiting.
    d. pressure cycling.

24. "Inspiration begins when the expiratory flow drops to a preset value" best describes:
    a. flow triggering.
    b. flow limiting.
    c. flow cycling.
    d. flow controlling.

25. "Inspiration begins when the baseline pressure drops to a preset value" best describes:
    a. pressure limiting.
    b. pressure support.
    c. pressure triggering.
    d. pressure control.

26. An example of an inspired gas alarm is:
    a. peak pressure.
    b. low PEEP/CPAP pressure.
    c. F_1O_2.
    d. oxygen gas supply disconnect.

27. An example of an input power alarm would be:
    a. peak pressure.
    b. low PEEP/CPAP pressure.
    c. F_1O_2.
    d. oxygen gas supply disconnect.

28. "Delivery of a breath to a preset pressure for a specific inspiratory time" best describes:
    a. pressure support.
    b. pressure control.
    c. pressure limiting.
    d. pressure cycling.

29. "Termination of a breath when peak flow drops to 25% of the peak inspiratory flow level" best describes:
    a. pressure support.
    b. pressure control.
    c. pressure limiting.
    d. flow cycling.

30. Which of the following ventilators has an internal battery that can power it for a short time period following termination of the 115 volt, 60 Hz power supply?
    a. Bear 1000
    b. Bird 8400ST®i
    c. Siemens Servo 300
    d. Bear 5

Selected Bibliography

Barnes, T. A., et al. (1994). *Core textbook of respiratory care practice* (2nd ed.). Mosby-Yearbook.

Bear Medical Systems. (1977). *BEAR I ventilator instruction manual*. Riverside.

Bear Medical Systems. (1981). *BEAR II ventilator instruction manual*. Riverside.

Bear Medical Systems. (1987). *BEAR 5 ventilator instruction manual*. Riverside.

Bear Medical Systems. (1991). *BEAR 3 ventilator instruction manual*. Riverside.

Bear Medical Systems. (1992). *BEAR 1000 ventilator instruction manual*. Riverside.

Bird Productions Corporation. (1990). *8400ST®i volume ventilator instruction manual*. Palm Springs.

Bird Productions Corporation. (1997). *TBird® ventilator series service manual L1314*. Palm Springs.

Branson, R. D., & Chatburn, R. L. Technical description and classification of modes of ventilator operation. *Respiratory Care, 27*(9), 1026–1044.

Branson, R. D., et al. (2002). Closed-loop mechanical ventilation. *Respiratory Care, 47*(4), 437–453.

Campbell, R. S., et al. (2002). Pressure-controlled versus volume-controlled ventilation: Does it matter. *Respiratory Care, 47*(4), 415–426.

Chatburn, R. L. (1991). A new system for understanding mechanical ventilators. *Respiratory Care, 36*(10), 1123–1155.

Chatburn, R. L. (1992). Classification of mechanical ventilators. *Respiratory Care, 37*(9), 1009–1025.

Dräger, Inc. (1996). *Evita 4 intensive care ventilator operating instructions*. Telford.

Dupis, Y. (1992). *Ventilators: Theory and clinical application* (2nd ed.). Mosby-Yearbook.

Hamilton Medical. (1988). *Veolar operator's manual*. Reno.

Hamilton Medical. (2000). *Galileo intensive care ventilator operator's manual*. Reno.

Infrasonics, Inc. (1991). *Adult star ventilator operating instructions*. San Diego.

Newport Medical Instruments, Inc. (1991). *Newport wave ventilator operational instructions*. Newport Beach.

Puritan Bennett Corporation. (1990). *7200 series ventilator operator's manual*. Carlsbad.

Siemens-Elema AB. (2002). *Servo^i ventilator system user's manual*.

Siemens Medical Systems. (1984). *Servo ventilator 900C operating manual*. Danvers.

Siemens Medical Systems. (2003). *Servo ventilator 300 operating manual*. Danvers.

Viasys Healthcare. (2003). *Vela volume ventilator instruction manual*.

CHAPTER 10

PEDIATRIC AND NEONATAL VENTILATORS

INTRODUCTION

This chapter describes the many unique characteristics of pediatric and neonatal ventilators that merit the separation of this content into its own chapter. Chapters 8 and 9 described the adult acute care ventilators having volume, flow, and pressure as control variables. Like the ventilators described in Chapter 9, pediatric and neonatal ventilators utilize flow and pressure as control variables.

As discussed in Chapter 7, for a variable (pressure, volume, flow, or time) to be classified as a control variable, certain conditions must be met. Those conditions are that: (1) the variable must be measured, and (2) the variable must be used as a feedback signal to control the ventilator's output. Chatburn's ventilator classification system will be applied to classify the ventilators in this chapter.

OBJECTIVES

After completing this chapter, the student will accomplish the following objectives.
- Explain what is meant by the term *control variable* and how a specific ventilator may be classified as having flow or pressure as a control variable.
- For the ventilators described in this chapter, apply Chatburn's classification system and classify them according to:
  — Input power
  — Drive mechanism
  — Control scheme
  — Alarm systems

- Describe how to assemble and troubleshoot the following ventilators:
  — Bear Cub BP-2001
  — Bear Cub 750_{vs} and 750_{psv}
  — V.I.P. Bird
  — V.I.P. Bird Gold
  — Dräger Babylog 8000
  — Nellcor Puritan-Bennett Infant Star® 500/950
  — Newport Medical Instruments, Inc., Breeze
  — Sechrist Industries, Model IV-100B and IV-200

THE CONTROL VARIABLE

During a ventilator-supported breath, a mechanical ventilator can control one of the following variables: pressure, volume, flow, or time. In order for a ventilator to be classified as controlling one of these variables, two conditions must be met. First, that variable must

be measured, and second, it must be used as feedback to control the ventilator's output. Therefore, for a ventilator to be classified as a flow or pressure controller, flow or pressure must be measured and used as a signal to control the output from the ventilator. The ventilators discussed in this chapter meet these criteria and are classified as either flow or pressure controllers.

BEAR MEDICAL SYSTEMS, BEAR CUB BP-2001

The Bear Cub BP-2001 is a pressure or flow controller that can be time or manually triggered and time cycled (Figure 10-1). Gas flows continuously through the circuit, unless interrupted by the exhalation valve.

Input Power

The Bear Cub BP-2001 is pneumatically powered and electronically controlled. The drive mechanism is pneumatically powered, while the control circuit is electronically controlled. Both air and oxygen at 50 psi enter the ventilator through fittings on the rear panel. A power cord for 120 volts, 60 Hz electrical power is also connected to the rear of the ventilator.

Drive Mechanism

Air and oxygen, at 50 psi after entering the ventilator, flow past pressure switches, which will activate an alarm if pressure falls below

Figure 10-1 *The Bear Cub BP-2001 ventilator.*

22.5 psi. The gas supplies then pass through check valves (one-way valves), which prevent gas from leaving the ventilator and going back into the supply system (Figure 10-2).

Both the air and oxygen are then conducted to a single-stage reducing valve, which reduces the line pressure to 17 psi. From the regulators, the gases are mixed in a blender that operates using a proportioning valve. Figure 10-2 illustrates the pneumatic systems for the Bear Cub BP-2001 ventilator.

Control Circuit

The Bear Cub BP-2001 utilizes pneumatic and electronic components in its control circuit. The electronic components consist of electronic timers and popet valves.

The ventilatory rate and I:E ratios are controlled by an electronic timer. The rate control establishes the ventilatory rates of between 1 and 150 breaths per minute. The inspiratory time control sets the length of the inspiratory time to between 0.1 and 3.0 seconds. The inspiratory time control is also an electronic timer; however, it functions independently from the rate control.

For the Bear Cub BP-2001, the ventilator rate combined with the inspiratory time determines the I:E ratio. Once these controls are set, expiratory time is the duration left between end inspiration and the next breath. The I:E ratio is displayed on an LED display on the monitor panel.

The pneumatic components include a flow control valve, PEEP/CPAP and inspiratory pressure limit control, three-way solenoid, a metering valve, and the exhalation valve.

The flow control valve on the ventilator consists of an uncompensated Thorpe tube flowmeter (the needle valve is positioned upstream from the Thorpe tube). Low resistance humidifiers should be used to reduce the effects of back pressure on the flowmeter. Flows of between 3 and 30 L/min are available. The operation of Thorpe tube flowmeters was discussed in Chapter 1.

The PEEP/CPAP system provides elevated baseline pressures during CPAP and CMV/IMV modes. The levels of positive pressures are adjustable between 0.0 and 20 cmH$_2$O. Adjustment of the control varies flow sent to a venturi. The venturi provides the driving pressure of the PEEP/CPAP system. Adjustment of the control either restricts or opens the outlet of the venturi. In the Bear Cub BP-2001, gas pressure from the venturi is conducted to a

Figure 10-2 *A schematic of the Bear Medical Systems Bear Cub BP-2001 ventilator pneumatic system. (Courtesy Viasys Critical Care Inc., Riverside, CA)*

three-way solenoid that directs flow to the exhalation valve, partially closing it. The partially closed exhalation valve allows PEEP/CPAP pressure to build within the circuit.

The pressure limit control establishes the maximum pressure that can occur during inspiration. Pressure limits are available between 10 and 80 cmH$_2$O.

The Bear Cub BP-2001 pressure limit control uses a venturi system very similar to the PEEP/CPAP system. Adjustment of the control varies the pressure output from the venturi. Gas pressure from the venturi is applied through the three-way solenoid during inspiration to the exhalation valve. Once the pressure level in the circuit equals the value established by

the pressure limit control (applied to the exhalation valve), excess flow is vented past the exhalation valve to the atmosphere until the inspiratory time limit is reached.

The exhalation valve in the Bear Cub BP-2001 is pneumatically driven.

The sub-ambient pressure relief valve opens in the event that line pressure (gas source) fails when the circuit pressure drops approximately 2 cmH$_2$O below ambient pressure. This would allow the patient to obtain gas from the atmosphere in the event of line pressure failure.

The Bear Cub BP-2001 has a metering valve that shapes the inspiratory pressure waveform. At low flows, the inspiratory pressure waveform is nearly exponential. At high flows, the inspiratory waveform is more rectangular.

Control Variables

The Bear Cub BP-2001 ventilator is designed to control pressure. Pressure is limited by the adjustment made on the pressure limit control. The control is not calibrated; therefore, the pressure limit is set by observing the pressure manometer during inspiration. The pressure limit is adjustable between 0.0 and 72 cmH$_2$O.

Flow is a control variable in that inspiratory flow will not exceed the value established by the flow control. Flow is indicated by the Thorpe tube flowmeter and is adjusted with the flow control knob. Depending upon inspiratory time, a given flow may not be sufficient to achieve the set pressure limit, and the ventilator therefore becomes a flow controller.

Phase Variables

Trigger Variables

The trigger variables for the Bear Cub BP-2001 include time and manual triggering. Time is a trigger variable that is established by the rate control. The rate control is an electronic timer that divides 1 minute by the set ventilatory rate. The rate may be adjusted between 1 and 150 breaths per minute.

The ventilator may be manually triggered by depressing the manual breath button, delivering a ventilator supported breath.

Limit Variables

The limit variables for the Bear Cub BP-2001 include pressure and flow. Pressure limit is established using the pressure limit control. As already described, the control is not calibrated and the pressure manometer must be used when setting the control.

The ventilator may also be flow limited. Inspiratory flow will not exceed the value established using the flow control valve and is indicated on the Thorpe tube flowmeter. Tidal volume delivery may be estimated, during flow limited ventilation, by multiplying the inspiratory flow by the inspiratory time and correcting for the compressible volume in the patient circuit.

Cycle Variable

The cycle variable for the ventilator is time. The inspiratory time control determines the length of inspiration and, therefore, when expiration begins. Inspiratory time is adjustable between 0.1 and 3 seconds.

Baseline Variable

The baseline variable for the Bear Cub BP-2001 ventilator is pressure. PEEP/CPAP pressure may be adjusted between 0 and 20 cmH$_2$O.

Output Waveforms

The output waveform characteristics of the Bear Cub BP-2001 include pressure and flow waveforms. The pressure waveform may be almost square or exponential. The exponential waveform becomes a function of the pressure limit and flow settings. When the pressure limit is set for a maximum value, the pressure waveform rises exponentially. Simultaneously, the flow waveform is square.

When the ventilator is pressure limited and time cycled, with flow being the control variable, the pressure waveform assumes a nearly square-shaped morphology. The front portion of the square wave is rounded somewhat, so it is not truly a square wave pattern. Simultaneously, the flow waveform is nearly square, with a decelerating portion prior to exhalation.

Alarm Systems

Input Power Alarms

The input power alarms for the Bear Cub BP-2001 include loss of electrical power and loss of gas pressure. Should 120 v, 60 Hz power become lost or disconnected, an audible alarm will alert the practitioner to the event. The ventilator incorporates pressure switches that will activate if the gas pressure drops below 22.5 psi.

Control Circuit Alarms

Inspiratory Time/I:E Ratio. The ventilator incorporates a form of I:E ratio alarm. The Bear Cub BP-2001 will activate the I:E ratio alarm if the controls are set such that the I:E ratio is greater than 3:1. When the I:E ratio reaches this setting, both audible and visual alarms will be activated.

Rate/Time Incompatibility. The Bear Cub BP-2001 has an alarm that will alert the practitioner to rate and inspiratory time settings that result in an expiratory time less than 0.25 seconds. When this occurs, expiratory time will not be less than 0.25 seconds, and the displayed inspiratory time will be less than that set on the inspiratory time control. The Rate/Time incompatibility indicator will be illuminated, alerting the practitioner to the settings incompatibility.

Ventilator Inoperative. The Bear Cub BP-2001 incorporates a ventilator inoperative alarm that alerts the practitioner to the following conditions: failure to cycle, electric power failure, panel control malfunction, prolonged solenoid "on" time, high/low inspiratory time, and timing circuit failure.

Output Alarms

Pressure. The Bear Cub BP-2001 incorporates both low baseline and low inspiratory pressure alarms. The low baseline pressure is adjustable from 0.0 to 20 H_2O. The low inspiratory pressure is adjustable between 0.0 and 50 H_2O.

Tables 10-1 and 10-2 highlight the capabilities and alarm systems of the Bear Cub BP-2001.

VIASYS CRITICAL CARE BEAR CUB 750$_{vs}$ AND BEAR CUB 750$_{psv}$

The Viasys Critical Care Bear Cub 750$_{vs}$ and Bear Cub 750$_{psv}$ ventilators are manufactured by Viasys Critical Care, Palm Springs, California, a division of Viasys Healthcare (Figures 10-3A and 10-3B).

The ventilators are pressure or flow controllers that may be flow, time, or manually triggered, pressure or flow limited, and time or volume cycled. Since many similarities exist between the two ventilators, they will be considered together. When differences occur, they will be discussed on an individual basis.

Input Power

The Viasys Critical Care Bear Cub 750$_{vs}$ and Bear Cub 750$_{psv}$ ventilators are electrically powered using 112–120 v, 60 Hz AC power for the control circuitry. The drive mechanism utilizes compressed gases (50-psi air and oxygen). The rear of the ventilator contains DISS fittings for the high pressure gas connections as well as the electrical power cord.

Drive Mechanism

Air and oxygen at 50 psi, after entering the ventilators, flow past pressure switches, which will activate an alarm if the pressure falls below 24 psi. The gas supplies then pass through check valves (one-way valves), which prevent gas from leaving the ventilator and going back into the supply system (Figure 10-4).

Both air and oxygen are conducted to a single-stage reducing valve, which reduces the line pressure to 17 psi. From the regulators, the gases are mixed in a blender that operates using a proportioning valve.

Control Circuit

The control circuit of the Bear Cub 750$_{vs}$ and 750$_{psv}$ ventilators utilize both pneumatic and electronic components (Figure 10-4). Once the gas exits the blender, it passes through a filter and to the solenoid valve. The solenoid valve determines the ventilatory rate and

---

TABLE 10-1 Bear Cub BP-2001 Capabilities

Rate	1–150 BPM
Inspiratory Time	0.1–3.0 seconds
Press. Limit	0–72 cmH$_2$O
PEEP/CPAP	0–20 cmH$_2$O
Flow	3–30 L/min
F$_I$O$_2$	0.21–1.0

TABLE 10-2 Bear Cub BP-2001 Alarm Systems

Input Power	
Electric Power	X
Air Pressure	< 22.5 psi
Oxygen	< 22.5 psi
Control Circuit	
Insp. Time	X
I:E Ratio	X
Rate/Time Incompatible	X
Ventilator Inoperative	X
Output Alarms	
Low Inspiratory Pres.	X
Low Baseline Pres.	X

Figure 10-3A *A photograph of the Viasys Critical Care Bear Cub 750_{vs} ventilator.*

Figure 10-3B *A photograph of the Viasys Critical Care Bear Cub 750_{psv} ventilator.*

inspiratory time and is under electronic control. Feedback from the proximal airway flow transducer, a thermal anemometer, in conjunction with the ventilator settings provides feedback to the microprocessor that regulates the operation of the solenoid valve.

Gas exiting the solenoid valve is divided to two flow control valves, the base flow control valve and the inspiratory flow control valve. Both are needle valves that pneumatically determine the base flow and inspiratory flow, respectively.

Bear Cub 750psv Infant Ventilator Pneumatic Schematic

Figure 10-4 *A schematic diagram of the Viasys Critical Care Bear Cub 750_{psv} ventilator, (Courtesy Viasys Critical Care, Palm Springs, CA)*

Gas is then conducted to an adjustable over pressure relief valve and a dump solenoid. Both of these systems are designed to prevent excessive airway pressures from being applied to the patient circuit. The over pressure relief valve is adjustable between 15 to 75 cmH$_2$O.

The PEEP/CPAP system provides elevated baseline pressures during CPAP and CMV/IMV and PSV modes. The levels of positive pressure are adjustable between 0 to 30 cmH$_2$O. Adjustment of the PEEP/CPAP pressure control provides gas pressure to the diaphragm in the exhalation valve, partially closing it, which provides the PEEP/CPAP pressure in the patient circuit. The PEEP/CPAP and inspiratory pressure limit controls are regulated by a differential pressure transducer, which provides feedback signals to the microprocessor.

The exhalation valve on the ventilators is a diaphragm-type valve that operates as a pneumatic, servo-controlled regulator. The exhalation valve incorporates a venturi that reduces the pressure in the patient circuit during application of bias flow. This allows the ventilator to deliver a PEEP/CPAP pressure of zero even when bias flows are adjusted to 10 L/min.

Control Variables

The Bear Cub 750$_{vs}$ and 750$_{psv}$ ventilators are designed to control pressure. Pressure is limited by the adjustment made on the high pressure limit control. The control is adjustable to a maximum of 72 cmH$_2$O.

Flow is a control variable in that inspiratory flow will not exceed the value established by the flow control. Flow is indicated on the LED display and is adjusted with the flow control knob. Depending upon inspiratory time, a given flow may not be sufficient to achieve the set pressure limit, and the ventilator therefore becomes a flow controller. Flow is adjustable between 1 to 30 L/min.

Phase Variables

Trigger Variables

The trigger variables for the Bear Cub 750$_{vs}$ and 750$_{psv}$ include time, flow, and manual triggering. Time is a trigger variable that is established by the rate control. The rate control is an electronic timer that divides 1 minute by the set ventilatory rate. The rate may be adjusted between 1 and 150 breaths per minute.

The ventilators may also be flow triggered.

The ventilator's thermal anemometer flow sensor that is attached to the airway senses the patient's inspiratory flow. Trigger sensitivity is set using a graphic scale. Flow sensitivity is adjustable between 0.2 to 5.0 L/min.

The ventilators may be manually triggered by depressing the manual breath button, delivering a ventilator supported breath.

Limit Variables

The limit variables for the Bear Cub 750$_{vs}$ and 750$_{psv}$ ventilators include pressure and flow. Pressure limit is established using the high pressure limit control. As already described, the control is not calibrated, and the pressure manometer must be used when setting the control. Both ventilators also have an over pressure relief control (pop-off) that is adjustable between 15 to 75 cmH$_2$O.

The ventilators may also be flow limited. Inspiratory flow will not exceed the value established using the flow rate control. Tidal volume delivery may be estimated, during flow limited ventilation by multiplying the inspiratory flow by the inspiratory time and correcting for the compressible volume in the patient circuit.

The Bear Cub 750$_{psv}$ can also be pressure limited when operated using pressure support. During pressure support, an inspiratory pressure is set for the spontaneous breaths (CPAP portion) in which inspiratory pressure rises to assist the patient during spontaneous breaths.

Cycle Variables

The cycle variables for both ventilators are time and volume. The inspiratory time control determines the length of inspiration and, therefore, when expiration begins. Inspiratory time is adjustable between 0.1 and 3.1 seconds.

The ventilators may also be volume cycled when the volume limit control is used. The thermal anemometer flow sensor attached to the patient's airway measures flow when a breath is delivered, and the flow is electronically integrated into a volume. When the volume limit is reached, the breath is terminated and exhalation begins. The volume limit is adjustable between 5 to 300 mL. The control is technically a cycle control even though it is labeled as a limit control. If volume were limited, it would rise to the preset value and remain unchanged throughout the remainder of the breath.

Baseline Variable

The baseline variable for the Bear Cub 750_{vs} and 750_{psv} ventilators is pressure. PEEP/CPAP pressure may be adjusted between 0 and 30 cmH_2O.

Output Waveforms

The output waveform characteristics of the Bear Cub 750_{vs} and 750_{psv} include pressure and flow waveforms. The pressure waveform may be almost square or exponential. The exponential waveform becomes a function of the pressure limit and flow settings. When the pressure limit is set for a maximum value, the pressure waveform rises exponentially. Simultaneously, the flow waveform is square.

When the ventilator is pressure limited and time cycled, with flow being the control variable, the pressure waveform assumes a nearly square-shaped morphology. The resulting shape is a modified square wave. Simultaneously, the flow waveform is nearly square, with a decelerating portion prior to exhalation.

Alarm Systems

Input Power Alarms

The input power alarms for the Bear Cub 750_{vs} and 750_{psv} include loss of electrical power and loss of gas pressure. Should 120 v, 60 Hz power become lost or disconnected, an audible alarm will alert the practitioner to the event. The ventilator incorporates pressure switches that will activate if the gas pressure drops below 24 psi.

Control Circuit Alarms

A "Failed to Cycle" LED will illuminate if the ventilator detects either an internal or external malfunction.

A pressure setting incompatible LED will illuminate if the set inspiratory pressure is less than the PEEP/CPAP pressure setting.

A prolonged inspiratory pressure LED will illuminate if the airway pressure remains 10 cmH_2O above the PEEP/CPAP level for more than 3.5 seconds.

A flow sensor LED and alarm will be activated if the thermal anemometer flow sensor malfunctions or is disconnected.

Output Alarms

Pressure.   The Bear Cub 750_{vs} and 750_{psv} incorporate both low baseline and low inspiratory pressure alarms. The low baseline pressure is adjustable from −5.0 to 30 H_2O. The low inspiratory pressure is set using the following calculation:

$$\text{Low Insp. Pres.} = 0.25(\text{High Pres. Limit} - \text{Low PEEP/CPAP}) + \text{Low PEEP/CPAP}$$

Time.   Both ventilators have an Apnea alarm if the ventilator fails to detect the patient's inspiratory effort (flow trigger) for a set time interval. This is adjustable for 5, 10, 20, and 30 seconds. This alarm is not functional if the thermal anemometer flow sensor is removed from the patient's airway.

Tables 10-3 and 10-4 highlight the capabilities and alarm systems for the Bear Cub 750_{vs} and 750_{psv} ventilators.

TABLE 10-3 Bear Cub 750_{vs} and 750_{psv} Capabilities

	Bear Cub 750$_{vs}$	**Bear Cub 750$_{psv}$**
Rate	1–150 BPM	1–150 BPM
Inspiratory Time	0.1–3.0 seconds	0.1–3.0 seconds
Inspiratory Flow	1 to 30 L/min	1 to 30 L/min
Base Flow	1 to 30 L/min	1 to 30 L/min
Volume Limit	5 to 300 mL	5 to 300 mL
PEEP	0 to 30 cmH_2O	0 to 30 cmH_2O
Inspiratory Pressure	0 to 72 cmH_2O	0 to 72 cmH_2O
Manual Breath	x1	x1
Assist Sensitivity	0.20 to 5.0 L/min	0.20 to 5.0 L/min
Over Press. Relief	15 to 75 cmH_2O	15 to 75 cmH_2O
F_IO_2	0.21–1.00	0.21–1.00

TABLE 10-4 Bear Cub 750$_{vs}$ and 750$_{psv}$ Alarm Systems

	Bear Cub 750$_{vs}$	Bear Cub 750$_{psv}$
Input Power		
Electric Power	X	X
Gas Pressure	< 24 psi	< 24 psi
Control Circuit		
Failed to Cycle	X	X
Apnea	X	X
Patient Circuit	X	X
Prolonged Insp. Press.	X	X
PEEP/CPAP	X	X
Settings Incompatible	X	X
Press. Settings Incomp.	X	X
Flow Sensor	X	X
Output Alarms		
High Rate	3–255 BPM	3–255 BPM
Low PEEP/CPAP	–3 to 30 cmH$_2$O	–3 to 30 cmH$_2$O
Low Insp. Press.	1 to 65 cmH$_2$O	1 to 65 cmH$_2$O
High Press. Limit	10 to 75 cmH$_2$O	10 to 75 cmH$_2$O

ASSEMBLY AND TROUBLESHOOTING

Assembly—Bear CubBP-2001 and 750$_{vs}$ and 750$_{psv}$

To assemble the Bear Cub ventilators, follow the suggested assembly guide below.

1. Connect the high-pressure hoses to 50-psi sources of air and oxygen.

2. Connect the electrical power cord to a suitable 120 v, 60 Hz source.

3. Assemble the humidifier and attach it to the ventilator. Since many different humidifiers may be used, specific instructions are not included here.

4. Connect the inspiratory limb of the circuit to the humidifier. Attach the expiratory limb to the exhalation valve (fitting labeled "from patient").

5. Connect the proximal airway pressure line between the patient wye and the pressure monitor fitting.

6. Attach a short piece of tubing between the humidifier inlet and the ventilator outlet.

Troubleshooting

Refer to the troubleshooting algorithms found at the end of this chapter.

V.I.P. BIRD® AND V.I.P. BIRD® GOLD VENTILATORS

Viasys Critical Care, Palm Springs, CA, a division of Viasys Healthcare, manufactures and markets the V.I.P. Bird® and the V.I.P. Bird® Gold ventilators. The ventilators are microprocessor controlled, pneumatically actuated ventilators designed for neonatal, infant, and pediatric use (Figures 10-5, 10-6, 10-7, and 10-8). They are pressure and flow controllers that can be pressure, time, flow, or manually

Figure 10-5 *The Bird Products Corporation V.I.P. Bird® Ventilator. (Courtesy Viasys Critical Care, Palm Springs, CA)*

Figure 10-6 *The Bird Products Corporation V.I.P. Bird® Ventilator control panel. (Courtesy Viasys Critical Care, Palm Springs, CA)*

Figure 10-7 *The Viasys Critical Care, V.I.P. Bird®
Gold Ventilator. (Courtesy Viasys Critical Care, Palm
Springs, CA)*

triggered. They are capable of operating in a
time cycled continuous flow mode
(IMV/CPAP), Assist/Control, IMV, SIMV,
CPAP, volume cycled mode, or pressure support. Since many similarities exist between the
two ventilators, they will be considered

Figure 10-8 *The Viasys Critical Care, V.I.P. Bird®
Gold Ventilator's control panel. (Courtesy Viasys
Critical Care, Palm Springs, CA)*

together. When differences occur, they will be
discussed on an individual basis.

Input Power

Electric power at 120 v, 60 Hz provides
power to run the microprocessor for each ventilator, control systems, and alarm systems.

Two gas supply lines (oxygen and air) at
50 psi enter the rear of the ventilators and
pass through check valves and an inlet filter
(Figures 10-9 and 10-10). The two gas lines

Figure 10-9 *A schematic diagram of the Viasys Critical Care V.I.P. Bird® Ventilator's pneumatic system.
(Courtesy Viasys Critical Care, Palm Springs, CA)*

Figure 10-10 *A schematic diagram of the Viasys Critical Care V.I.P. Bird® Gold Ventilator's pneumatic system. (Courtesy Viasys Critical Care, Palm Springs, CA)*

continue to an oxygen proportioning valve (blender), where they are mixed to the desired F_IO_2. From the blender, the gas is conducted to a 1.1-liter accumulator.

Drive Mechanism

The accumulator provides additional flow during peak demands to augment the output from the blender. The 1.1-liter volume is sufficient to handle most patient care situations. The accumulator is a rigid structure; therefore, when it empties, large fluctuations in pressure could occur. However, the 200-mL pulsation dampener prevents this from affecting gas delivery.

From the accumulator, gas enters a reduc-

ing valve where the line pressure is reduced to 25 psi. The reducing valve is a single-stage reducing valve similar to those discussed in Chapter 1.

Gas flow from the reducing valve outlet goes to the blender bleed system, the pulsation dampener, and the flow control valve. The blender bleed system provides a continuous bleed rate of approximately 6 liters per minute during low flow demands. This assures a continuous flow of gas through the accumulator, which facilitates a more rapid change in F_IO_2, when required. The pulsation dampener is another rigid reservoir of approximately 200-mL volume. The pulsation dampener minimizes pressure changes caused by the rapid movement of the flow control valve and from the accumulator.

Control Circuit

The flow control valve is a linear, electro-mechanical valve controlled by a stepper motor (Figure 10-11). This valve has a rapid response through a relatively short travel. The rapid opening and closing of the valve would place excessive demands on the reducing valve if the pulsation dampener were not incorporated into the design. Gas flow through the valve is sonic up to a system back-pressure of 5 psi (350 cmH$_2$O). Flow rate range through the valve is between 0.0 and 120 liters per minute. From the flow control valve, the gas exits the ventilator to the patient circuit.

The exhalation valve is an electromechanical, linear actuator. Signals to the valve from the microprocessor control the opening and closing of the valve. PEEP/CPAP pressures are regulated by pressure feedback signals to the microprocessor, causing the microprocessor to partially close the exhalation valve.

Control Variables

The control variables for the V.I.P. Bird® and V.I.P.® Gold are pressure and flow. Pressure is limited by the adjustment made on the high pressure limit control. The control is adjustable between 3.0 and 80 cmH$_2$O during time-cycled, pressure-limited ventilation.

Flow is a control variable during time-cycled, pressure-limited ventilation, in that inspiratory flow will not exceed the value established by the flow control. Flow is adjustable between 3.0 and 40 liters per minute, using the flow control. Depending upon inspiratory time, a given flow may not be sufficient to achieve the set pressure limit, and the ventilator therefore becomes a flow controller.

During volume ventilation, the V.I.P. Bird® ventilators also operate as flow controllers. Flow from the flow control valve is based upon valve position. An optical sensor detects the valve's position. Gas flow exiting the valve is sonic up to a back-pressure of 350 cmH$_2$O. Mass flow from the flow control valve is unchanged up to the 350 cmH$_2$O maximum back-pressure. Therefore, flow from the valve is directly proportional to how far the valve has opened. The microprocessor uses an algorithm to determine flow based upon the feedback from the optical sensor, which senses valve position. Although flow is not directly measured, valve position is directly proportional to flow. Tidal volume delivery then becomes a function of flow and inspiratory time.

Figure 10-11 *The V.I.P. Bird® flow control valve. (Courtesy Viasys Critical Care, Palm Springs, CA)*

Phase Variables

Trigger Variables

The trigger variables for the V.I.P. Bird® ventilators include flow, pressure, time, and manual triggering. With the addition of the Partner Volume Monitor, mechanical breaths can also be flow triggered in the pressure-limited, time-cycled mode. The patient must exceed the flow sensitivity setting to trigger a breath. Flow sensitivity is adjustable between 0.2 and 5 L/min (V.I.P. Bird®), 0.2 to 3 L/min (infant sensor), and 1.0 to 5 L/min (V.I.P. Bird® Gold).

In the volume-controlled mode, mechanical breaths can be pressure triggered. The patient must exceed the pressure trigger threshold to obtain a mechanical breath. Sensitivity may be set between 1 and 20 cmH_2O below baseline pressure.

Time is a trigger variable, which is established by the breath rate control. The rate is adjustable from 0.0 to 150 breaths per minute (BPM V.I.P. Bird®) and 1 to 150 BPM V.I.P. Bird® Gold). The rate control sets a reference for the microprocessor, which controls the opening and closing of the exhalation valve. The exhalation valve servos to the high-pressure limit setting in the time-cycled mode.

Manual triggering occurs when the practitioner depresses the manual breath button. When pressed, the ventilator delivers a mandatory breath. The breath is given at the tidal volume, peak flow, and F_IO_2 set on the control panel.

Limit Variables

The limit variables for the V.I.P. Bird® ventilators include pressure and flow. The pressure limit is established during time-cycled ventilation using the high-pressure limit control. Pressure limits are adjustable between 3 and 80 cmH_2O.

The ventilator may also be flow limited. Inspiratory flow will not exceed the value established on the flow rate control. During time-cycled, pressure-limited ventilation, flows are adjustable between 3 and 40 liters per minute. In the volume-controlled mode, peak flow can be set from 3 to 100 L/min (V.I.P. Bird®) and 3 to 120 L/min (V.I.P. Bird® Gold), with 120 L/min available for spontaneous breaths.

Cycle Variables

The cycle variables for the V.I.P. Bird® ventilators are pressure, volume, flow, and time.

Pressure becomes a cycle variable when the ventilators are operated as volume ventilators. The high-pressure limit control establishes the pressure at which a volume-cycled breath will be terminated. This control is adjustable between 3.0 and 120 cmH_2O (V.I.P. Bird®) and 3 and 80 cmH_2O (V.I.P. Bird® Gold). Once the pressure limit is reached, inspiration is terminated and both audible and visual alarms will be activated.

The ventilators are volume cycled during volume-controlled ventilation. In this mode, the flow control valve's position and inspiratory time are used to determine delivered volume. Technically, flow and time are measured, and volume is derived from the two measurements.

Flow becomes a cycle variable during pressure support (V.I.P. Bird®). Inspiration is terminated when the inspiratory flow rate falls to a range of 5 to 25% of the peak inspiratory flow rate for that breath. Once flow decays to this point, inspiration is terminated and the ventilator cycles into exhalation. Pressure support may be adjusted between 1.0 and 50 cmH_2O.

The V.I.P. Bird® Gold ventilator also has the capability of delivering pressure support with a volume guarantee, termed volume assured pressure support (VAPS). In this mode, pressure support and volume control breaths are combined. If the patient fails to meet the targeted volume during a pressure supported breath, the ventilator reverts to volume support until the desired volume has been met or the inspiratory time for the breath has been exceeded. If the patient meets the targeted volume with a pressure supported breath, the breath is terminated when flow reaches 5 to 25% of the peak inspiratory flow rate for that breath.

Time is a cycle variable during pressure-limited, time-cycled ventilation. Inspiratory time is determined by the inspiratory time control. Inspiratory time may be adjusted to between 0.1 and 3.0 seconds for both ventilators.

Baseline Variable

The baseline variable for the V.I.P. Bird® ventilators is pressure. PEEP/CPAP pressure may be adjusted between 0 and 24 cmH_2O.

Output Waveforms

Pressure

The output pressure waveform characteristic of the V.I.P. Bird® ventilators is rectangular. The rectangular waveform is characteristic during time-cycled, pressure-limited ventilation, and in volume-cycled SIMV/CPAP mode with the addition of pressure support.

Flow

The flow output waveform is rectangular. This waveform occurs when the ventilators are operated in the volume control modes, and it functions as a flow controller.

Alarm Systems

Input Power Alarms

The input power alarms for the V.I.P. Bird® ventilators include loss of gas pressure and loss of electrical power. The low gas pressure alarm will be activated if the system pressure (distal to the reducing valve) falls below 22.5 psi or increases to greater than 27.5 psi (V.I.P. Bird®) and 22.5 and 27.4 psi (V.I.P. Bird® Gold). Both audible and visual alarms will result if these conditions are met.

In the event of a loss of electrical power, the ventilator inoperative alarm will be activated (audible and visual), and the safety and exhalation valves will be automatically opened.

Control Circuit Alarms

The control circuit alarms for the ventilators include ventilator inoperative and circuit fault. The ventilator inoperative alarm will be activated if the gas system pressure is less than 20 or greater than 30 psi for more than 1 second. It will also sound if an internal malfunction has been detected. The circuit fault alarm will be activated if a problem is detected in the patient circuit or with the pressure transducer.

Output Alarms

Pressure. Pressure alarms are available for high pressure limit, low peak pressure, low PEEP/CPAP and high/prolonged pressure. The pressure limit alarm is adjustable between 3 and 120 cmH_2O on both ventilators. The alarm is active in assist/control and SIMV/CPAP modes.

The low peak pressure alarm is adjustable between 3 and 120 cmH_2O. This alarm is available in all modes of operation.

The low PEEP/CPAP alarm is adjustable between –9 and 24 cmH_2O (V.I.P. Bird®). The V.I.P. Bird® Gold ventilator's low PEEP/CPAP is automatically set at 3 cmH_2O less than the setting on the PEEP/CPAP control (baseline pressure). This alarm is available in all modes of ventilation.

The high/prolonged pressure alarm works during pressure-controlled, time-cycled ventilation. This alarm is activated if the proximal pressure exceeds the high peak pressure limit setting by 10 cmH_2O (V.I.P. Bird®) and 6 cmH_2O (V.I.P. Bird® Gold). Once the alarm is activated, the flow control valve closes and the exhalation valve and safety valve are both opened, venting excess pressure in the circuit.

Time. The ventilators have an apnea alarm.

ASSEMBLY AND TROUBLESHOOTING

Assembly—V.I.P. Bird® and V.I.P. Bird® Gold Ventilators

To assemble the ventilator for use, complete the suggested assembly guide. Since this ventilator is designed for neonatal, infant, and pediatric patients, different circuits are required depending upon the ventilator's application. The circuits are similar as far as connections, but differ in size. Therefore, one set of circuit assembly instructions is provided.

1. Connect the ventilator to a 120 v, 60 Hz grounded power source. If used in the emergency or transport setting where AC current is not available, use a 12 v, 5 amp power supply.

2. Connect both air and oxygen supplies providing 50 psi to the fittings on the rear of the ventilator.

3. Assemble the patient circuit:
   a. Attach a bacteria filter to the ventilator outlet.
   b. Connect a sufficient length of 22-mm diameter tubing between the bacteria filter and a heated, high-efficiency humidifier.
   c. Install water traps onto the inspiratory and expiratory limbs of the circuit.
   d. Attach the expiratory limb of the circuit to the exhalation valve assembly.
   e. Pressure test the circuit.

Troubleshooting

Refer to the troubleshooting algorithms found at the end of this chapter.

This alarm is activated if the ventilator does not detect any inspiratory effort over a set time period. The range for the alarm is 20, 40, or 60 seconds (V.I.P. Bird®) and 10 to 60 seconds (V.I.P. Bird® Gold). Once activated, both audible and visual alarms result.

Tables 10-5 and 10-6 summarize the ventilators capabilities and alarm systems.

TABLE 10-5 V.I.P. Bird® and V.I.P. Bird® Gold Ventilator Capabilities

	V.I.P. Bird®	**V.I.P. Bird® Gold**
Modes		
Press. Controlled	SIMV, AC	AC, SIMV (PSV), CPAP
Flow-Controlled	AC	
Time Cycled	SIMV/CPAP, AC	
Volume Controlled		AC, SIMV (PSV)
Tidal Volume	20–995 mL	10–1200 mL
Rate	0.0–150 BPM	1–150 BPM
Inspiratory Time	0.10–3.0 seconds	0.10–3.0 seconds
Peak Flow		
Time Cycled	3–40 L/min	3–40 L/min
Volume Cycled	3–100 L/min	3–120 L/min
Press. Limit	3–80 cmH_2O	3–80 cmH_2O
PEEP/CPAP	0.0–24 cmH_2O	0.0–24 cmH_2O
Sensitivity	1–20 cmH_2O 0.2 to 5 L/min	1–20 cmH_2O 0.2 to 3 L/min
Pressure Support	1–50 cmH_2O	1–50 cmH_2O
Pressure Relief	0.0–130 cmH_2O	0.0–130 cmH_2O
F_IO_2	0.21–1.0	0.21–1.0

TABLE 10-6 V.I.P. Bird® and V.I.P. Bird® Gold Ventilator Alarm Systems

	V.I.P. Bird®	**V.I.P. Bird® Gold**
Input Power		
Low Gas Pressure		
System Pressure	< 22.5 psi	< 22.5 psi
System Pressure	> 27.5 psi	> 27.4 psi
Electrical Power	X	X
Control Circuit		
Ventilator Inoperative	X	X
Circuit Fault	X	X
Output Alarms		
High Pressure Limit	3–120 cmH_2O	3–120 cmH_2O
Low Peak Pressure	3–120 cmH_2O	3–120 cmH_2O
Low PEEP/CPAP	−9 to 24 cmH_2O	3 cmH_2O below baseline
High Pressure	+10 cmH_2O above pressure limit	
Apnea	20, 40, or 60 seconds	20, 40, or 60 seconds

DRÄGER BABYLOG 8000

The Dräger Babylog 8000 ventilator is designed for infant and pediatric use (Figure 10-12, A and B). The ventilator is a pneumatically powered, microprocessor-controlled flow controller, which is pressure, time, or manually triggered; pressure limited; and time cycled. It is capable of operating in assist/control, SIMV, and CPAP modes.

Figure 10-12A *Dräger, Inc. Babylog 8000 ventilator.*

Figure 10-12B *Dräger, Inc. Babylog 8000 control panel.*

Input Power

Gas supplies are connected using DISS fittings on the rear of the ventilator. Medical-grade air and oxygen are required at between 45 and 90 psi. Gases pass through a filter and check valves before pressure is reduced by means of two regulators (one for air and the other for oxygen). From the regulators, air and oxygen are taken through a solenoid valve blender system, which mixes them together to the desired F_IO_2.

Standard AC current provides the electrical power required to run the microprocessor control system and monitoring systems of the ventilator, 120/240 VAC, 50/60 Hz power is required.

Control Circuit

Blended gas flows through a pneumatic control valve and a flow rate control before entering the patient circuit (Figure 10-13). During inspiration, the exhalation valve closes and gas flows to the patient's lungs. Airway pressure is monitored by two pressure transducers, and pressure during inspiration is controlled by the exhalation valve.

PEEP/CPAP pressure is generated by the PEEP control valve applying partial pressure to the exhalation valve, partially closing it. PEEP/CPAP pressure may be adjusted between 0 and 15 cmH$_2$O.

Control Variable

The control variable of the Dräger Babylog 8000 is flow, which is controlled by the flow control valve and adjustable between 1 and 30 L/min. Flow is a control variable during pressure-limited, time-cycled ventilation.

Phase Variables

Trigger Variables

The trigger variables for the ventilator include flow, time, and manual triggering. Flow triggering is established by first calibrating the flow sensor, which is attached to the patient's airway. Once calibrated, flow triggering may be adjusted from a range of 1 to 10, which corresponds to flows of between 0 and 3 L/min. Once the patient exceeds the trigger threshold, a mandatory breath is delivered.

Time triggering occurs in the absence of the patient's spontaneous effort and is a function of the inspiratory and expiratory time settings. Frequencies of between 0 and 150 breaths per minute may be set. The frequency

Figure 10-13 *A schematic of the Babylog 8000 ventilator's pneumatic system.*

may be determined by dividing 60 by the sum of the inspiratory and expiratory times.

Manual triggering occurs when the practitioner depresses the manual inspiration button. When depressed, a manual breath is delivered up to the set inspiratory pressure limit. Inspiration is terminated when the button is released or 5 seconds have elapsed.

Limit Variables

The limit variables for the Dräger Babylog 8000 ventilator include pressure and flow. Pressure is a limit variable during pressure-limited, time-cycled ventilation. The pressure limit is set using the inspiratory pressure control and is adjustable between 10 and 80 cmH₂O. Once the pressure limit is reached, inspiration continues until the inspiratory time has lapsed.

Flow becomes a limit if, during inspiration, inspiratory flow reaches the setting established on the flow rate control. Inspiratory flows may be adjusted between 1 and 30 L/min.

Cycle Variables

The cycle variables of the ventilator include pressure and time. Pressure becomes a cycle variable when the airway pressure exceeds that of the automatically set upper pressure

limit value. The high airway pressure limit is automatically set to the peak pressure plus 10 cmH₂O or the PEEP/CPAP pressure plus 4 cmH₂O for spontaneous ventilation. When this threshold is exceeded, inspiration is terminated and audible and visual alarms result.

Time is a cycle variable during pressure-limited, time-cycled ventilation. Inspiratory time is adjusted by using the inspiratory time control and is adjustable between 0.1 and 2.0 seconds. Once the inspiratory time value has been met, inspiration ends and exhalation begins.

Baseline Variable

The baseline variable for the ventilator is pressure. PEEP/CPAP pressures may be adjusted from 0 to 15 cmH₂O. The PEEP control valve adjusts pressure against the exhalation valve, partially closing it and creating the PEEP/CPAP pressure.

Output Waveforms

Pressure

The output pressure waveform of the Dräger Babylog 8000 is rectangular. This is characteristic of most pressure-limited, time-cycled ventilators during mandatory breaths.

Pressure rises to the pressure limit value and is held until inspiration ends.

Flow

The flow waveform is also rectangular. Flow rate is limited by the setting on the inspiratory flow control. Flow rises to the value established (0 to 30 L/min) and is held at that value until inspiration is terminated.

Alarm Systems

Input Power Alarms

Input power alarms include loss of gas pressure and loss of electrical power. In the event either air or oxygen pressure falls below 43 psi, audible and visual alarms will alert the practitioner to the event. If electrical power is lost, a battery-powered alarm will sound.

Control Circuit Alarms

The control circuit alarms include flow measurement inoperative, pressure measurement inoperative, loss of stored data, ventilator malfunction, and I:E ratio. In the event signals from the flow sensor cannot be interpreted by the ventilator, an alarm will alert the clinician to this event. It is possible to continue using the ventilator; however, the clinician must maintain adequate minute ventilation and other parameters within safe levels without the information provided by the flow-sensing system. A qualified service technician should be contacted and the problem corrected as soon as possible.

If a fault in the pressure-monitoring system is detected, an alarm will alert the practitioner to the event. Some conditions that may cause this may be corrected by the practitioner, such as condensation in the circuit, liquid in the measuring system, or a circuit that is too small or offers too high a resistance. If a circuit fault is detected by the microprocessor, the ventilator should be removed from service and alternate ventilation provided for the patient.

The loss of stored data alarm will occur if the ventilator experiences a power failure. The clinician may enter the previous values and continue to use the ventilator. If the ventilator will not accept the new values after the initial power-up time, a qualified service technician should be contacted and the ventilator removed from service.

If the microprocessor detects a malfunction in the control or logic circuitry, an error code of xxx will be displayed. The ventilator should be removed from service and an alternate means of ventilation should be provided for the patient.

The I:E ratio alarm limits the I:E ratio to a maximum of 3:1. If the clinician attempts to exceed this ratio, an alarm will sound and ventilation will be limited to a ratio of 3:1. Settings should then be changed to maintain an acceptable I:E ratio.

Output Alarms

Pressure. Automatically set high-pressure and PEEP/CPAP pressure alarms alert the practitioner to these events. The high pressure limit is automatically set to the peak pressure plus 10 cmH_2O or CPAP pressure plus 4 cmH_2O. The PEEP/CPAP alarm is automatically set to the PEEP/CPAP pressure level minus 4 cmH_2O.

Flow. The Dräger Babylog 8000 ventilator incorporates both high and low minute ventilation alarms. The high minute ventilation alarm may be set between 0.13 and 15 L/min (upper limit), while the low minute ventilation alarm may be set between 0.03 and 14 L/min (lower limit).

Inspired Gas Alarms. The inspired gas alarm available on the ventilator is oxygen concentration. The alarm is automatically adjusted to ±4% of the set value on the oxygen percentage control.

Tables 10-7 and 10-8 summarize the Dräger Babylog 8000 ventilator capabilities and alarm systems.

TABLE 10-7 Dräger Babylog 8000 Ventilator Capabilities

Modes	Assist/control, time cycled SIMV/CPAP, CPAP
Tidal Volumes	0–999 mL
Inspiratory Time	0.1–2.0 seconds
Expiratory Time	0.2–30 seconds
Frequency	0–150 breaths/minute
Inspiratory Flow	1–30 L/min
Pressure Limit	10–80 cmH_2O
PEEP/CPAP	0–15 cmH_2O
Flow Sensitivity	0–3 L/min
F_IO_2	0.21–1.0

ASSEMBLY AND TROUBLESHOOTING

Assembly—Dräger Babylog 8000 Ventilator

To assemble the ventilator for use, complete the suggested assembly guide. Since this ventilator is designed for neonatal, infant, and pediatric patients, different circuits are required depending upon what application is desired. All circuits are similar as far as connections and components, but they differ in size.

1. Connect the ventilator to a suitable 120/240 VAC, 50/60 Hz power source.

2. Connect air and oxygen supplies at 50 psi to the rear of the ventilator using the DISS fittings.

3. Assemble the patient circuit:
   a. From the ventilator outlet, attach a short length of tubing between the outlet and a heated humidifier.
   b. Connect the inspiratory limb of the circuit to the outlet of the humidifier, making sure the temperature probe is placed close to the proximal airway. The use of condensation traps is recommended in both the inspiratory and expiratory limbs of the circuit.
   c. Connect the flow sensor to the patient airway connection and connect the sensing cable to the ventilator.
   d. Connect the expiratory limb of the circuit to the exhalation port on the ventilator.

Troubleshooting

Refer to the troubleshooting algorithms found at the end of this chapter.

TABLE 10-8 Dräger Babylog 8000 Ventilator Alarm Systems

Input Power

Loss of air pressure

Loss of oxygen pressure

Loss of electrical power

Control Circuit

Flow measurement inoperative

Pressure measurement inoperative

Loss of stored data

Ventilator malfunction

I:E ratio

Output

High airway pressure

Low PEEP/CPAP pressure

High and low minute volume

Inspired Gas

High and low oxygen concentrations

NELLCOR PURITAN-BENNETT, INFANT STAR 500 AND 950 VENTILATORS

Nellcor Puritan-Bennett, San Diego, CA manufactures and distributes the Infant Star ventilators. The ventilators are pneumatically powered, microprocessor-controlled infant ventilators (Figure 10-14). Since many similarities exist between the ventilators, they will be considered together. When differences occur, they will be discussed on an individual basis.

Both ventilators are pressure or flow controllers that are time triggered, pressure limited, and time cycled. They are capable of operating in continuous flow CPAP, continuous flow IMV, demand flow CPAP, and demand flow IMV. With the addition of the Star Sync patient-triggered interface, the Infant Star can provide patient-triggered breaths in Assist/Control, SIMV, and CPAP. The triggering mechanism used by the Star Sync is based on abdominal movement, which is detected by a change in pressure within an abdominal sensor (capsule). The Infant Star 500 is capable of operating in CPAP and IMV modes.

The Infant Star 950 has an option that may be added, which is a high-frequency module.

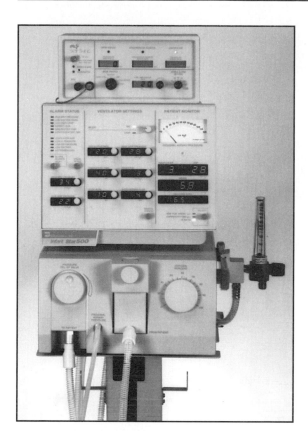

Figure 10-14 *The Nellcor Puritan-Bennett Infant Star 750$_{vs}$ Ventilator. (Courtesy Nellcor Puritan-Bennett, San Diego, CA)*

This allows the ventilator to be used as a high-frequency ventilator. When operated in this mode, the ventilator is a time controller.

Input Power

A 120 v, 60 Hz electrical power connection is provided on the rear of the upper electronic modules of the ventilators. Direct current from a 12-volt gell cell battery (120 v, 60 Hz power charges the battery) is used to operate the 8085 and 80C31 microprocessors and other components of the control and alarm systems in the ventilators. The battery power system offers both an uninterruptible power supply and protection from power surges.

Air and oxygen at 50 psi enter the rear of the lower pneumatics module through individual water traps and filters prior to entering the ventilators. Gases (air and oxygen) are conducted past pressure switches and to reducing valves, where line pressure is reduced to 38 psi, after which the gases enter the internal blender. The mixed gas exiting the blender

passes through a snap-acting regulator and into a 30-cubic-inch accumulator. (The snap-acting regulator closes when pressure rises to 36 psi and opens when pressure falls to 26 psi.) The gases are then conducted to another reducing valve, which reduces the pressure to 18 psi, whereupon the gases enter the proportional solenoid valve manifold.

Control Circuit

The proportional solenoid manifold consists of six proportional solenoid valves, 2 L/min, 4 L/min, 8 L/min, 16 L/min, 16 L/min, and 16 L/min. These valves open in combinations to provide flow rates for 4 to 40 L/min. When the desired flow rate is set on the electronic module, a control signal is sent to the microprocessor, activating one or more solenoid valves to produce the desired flow rate.

During mandatory breaths, a solenoid valve (SV10, Figure 10-15) sends pressurized gas to the exhalation valve diaphragm, closing it. Once the exhalation valve has closed, gas flow is directed into the patient circuit.

PEEP/CPAP pressure is also controlled through the exhalation valve diaphragm. When the practitioner adjusts the PEEP/CPAP control on the electronic module, a signal is sent to the microprocessor. The microprocessor opens a solenoid valve, which regulates output from the PEEP regulator. Pressure from the PEEP regulator is applied to the exhalation valve diaphragm, creating resistance to gas flow through the exhalation valve and PEEP/CPAP pressure in the circuit. PEEP/CPAP pressures are adjustable between 0.0 and 24 cmH$_2$O.

The ventilators have a heated exhalation block assembly. The heated exhalation block reduces water buildup in the exhalation block, which helps to minimize baseline pressure fluctuations.

Control Variables

The control variables for the ventilators include pressure and flow. Pressure becomes a control variable during pressure-controlled, time-cycled ventilation. The pressure limit is set using the peak inspiratory pressure control. The pressure limit is adjustable at 5 to 90 cmH$_2$O. During the first 75% of inspiration, gas flow matches the level set on the flow rate control. When 75% of the inspiratory phase

Figure 10-15 A schematic diagram of the Nellcor Puritan-Bennett Infant Star 500 pneumatic system. (Courtesy Nellcor Puritan-Bennett, San Diego, CA)

has passed, the Infant Star's microprocessor predicts when peak inspiratory pressure will be reached and gradually reduces flow from the solenoid manifold to prevent overshoot of the desired pressure limit. If the pressure limit is met prior to the end of inspiration, the 2 L/min solenoid valve may cycle on and off to compensate for leaks around the uncuffed endotracheal tube and to maintain the desired pressure limit. As with other infant ventilators, unless sufficient inspiratory time has been allowed, the pressure limit may not always be reached. Proximal (actual) pressure may be less than set if there is a significant leak.

Flow becomes a control variable for these ventilators in that inspiratory flow is set by the operator using the flow rate control. Flow is adjustable between 4 and 40 L/min. If the inspiratory time is not sufficient for the pressure limit to be reached, the ventilator becomes a flow controller.

The ventilators have an adjustable background (base flow), which can be set between 2 and 32 L/min. However, the background flow may not be set to a level greater than the flow rate setting. If the inspiratory pressure drops by 1 cmH_2O, the microprocessor progressively opens solenoid valves on the manifold to provide the flow needed to maintain the baseline pressure. Using this system, one flow can be set to meet the needs of mandatory ventilation, while the ventilator allows the patient to establish his or her inspiratory flow needs during spontaneous ventilation.

As was stated earlier, when the Infant Star 950 is equipped with the optional high-frequency module and operated as a high-frequency ventilator, time is the control variable.

Phase Variables

Trigger Variables

Trigger variables for the ventilators include pressure (Star Sync), time, and manual triggering.

When the Star Sync Patient Triggered Interface is used with either of the ventilators, pressure triggering can be used. The Star Sync senses inspiration using a pressure sensor that detects abdominal movement. Abdominal movement causes pressure changes to occur in the abdominal sensor, triggering a ventilator breath. Using the Star Sync, additional modes of Assist/Control, SIMV, and CPAP/Backup can be provided. The CPAP/Backup mode allows the patient to breathe spontaneously. However, if an apneic period occurs, the ventilator will revert to backup ventilation and deliver mechanical breaths, thus attempting to maintain an adequate minute ventilation.

Time is established using the ventilator's rate control on the electronic module. Respiratory rates may be set between 1 and 150 breaths per minute. The rate control setting establishes a reference for the microprocessor to control the output from the proportional solenoid manifold and the exhalation valve servo (SV10).

The ventilators become manually triggered when the practitioner depresses the manual breath button on the electronic control panel. Once depressed, a breath is delivered based upon the settings on the peak inspiratory pressure and inspiratory time controls.

Limit Variables

The limit variables for the ventilators include pressure and flow. The pressure limit is set using the peak inspiratory pressure control. Pressure limits may be adjusted between 5 and 90 cmH_2O. Pressures may also be limited by adjustment of the mechanical pop-off valve located on the front of the pneumatics module. If the pressure is limited by using the mechanical pop-off valve, many of the alarm and monitoring systems, which are based on proximal and internal pressure, may not be activated due to the limiting effect of the pop off valve. The mechanical pop-off valve is adjustable between 5 and 90 cmH_2O and 5 and 105 cmH_2O for both ventilators.

Flow becomes a limit variable when the pressure limit is not reached during inspiration. Under these conditions, flow is limited by the setting on the flow rate control. Flow rates may be adjusted between 4 and 40 L/min.

Cycle Variables

The cycle variables for the ventilators include pressure and time. If inspiratory pressure on the Infant Star reaches a level 5 cmH_2O greater than the peak inspiratory pressure setting, the exhalation valve opens, or both the exhalation valve and the safety valve may be opened to relieve circuit pressure. In either case, both an audible and visual alarm will result. The Infant Star ventilators incorporate a high inspiratory pressure alarm. This alarm is adjustable between 5 and 105 cmH_2O. If the alarm threshold is exceeded, the ventilator will open the exhalation valve and stop all inspiratory flow delivery. This alarm system allows the clinician to adjust pressures up to 15 cmH$_2$O above the peak inspiratory pressure setting.

The ventilators are normally time cycled. Inspiratory time is adjusted using the inspiratory time control. Inspiratory times may be adjusted between 0.1 to 3.0 seconds. Once the set inspiratory time has been reached, flow through the proportional solenoid manifold ceases and the exhalation valve opens.

Baseline Variables

The baseline variable for the Nellcor Puritan-Bennett Infant Star 750$_{vs}$ and Infant Star 750$_{psv}$ ventilators is pressure. PEEP/CPAP pressures may be adjusted between 0 and 24 cmH$_2$O.

Output Waveforms

Pressure

The output pressure waveform characteristic of the Infant Star ventilators is a rectangular waveform, which is characteristic during time-cycled, pressure-limited ventilation. This waveform may be modified by using lower flow rates, whereupon it will assume a more sinusoidal shape.

Flow

The flow output waveform is rectangular. This waveform occurs when the peak inspiratory pressure control is set high enough that it is not reached during inspiration. Under these circumstances, the ventilator is operating as a flow controller.

Alarm Systems

Input Power Alarms

The input power alarms include loss of electrical power and gas pressure. In the event that 120 v, 60 Hz electrical power is lost, a lamp will illuminate, indicating the loss of power. The internal battery can provide up to 30 minutes of power minimum, and usually 45 to 50 minutes when fully charged. When 5 to 10 minutes of battery time remain, both an audible and a visual alarm will be activated to alert the practitioner. Once the internal battery is fully discharged, reconnection to 120 v,

60 Hz power will fully charge the battery in about 1 hour.

If either air or oxygen inlet pressures fall below 45 psi, both audible and visual alarms will be activated. The Infant Star ventilators are capable of operating on either air or oxygen if one gas source is lost. If pressure in both gases is lost, both the internal safety valve and the exhalation valve are opened, permitting ambient gas flow to the patient circuit.

Control Circuit Alarms

The control circuit alarms for the ventilators include ventilator inoperative and insufficient expiratory time alarms. If the microprocessor detects a fault in the electronics or the exhalation valve operation, the ventilator stops cycling. All gas flow from the proportional solenoid manifold ceases and the safety valve and the exhalation valve are both opened, allowing gas to flow through the patient circuit. The ventilator inoperative alarm is both audible and visual, and codes will be displayed on the multiple display window on the electronics module to assist the practitioner in troubleshooting it.

The insufficient expiratory time alarm is activated when the rate and inspiratory time controls are incompatible. This occurs when the expiratory time is shorter than the minimum allowed for a given breath rate. For respiratory rates of up to 100 breaths per minute, the minimum expiratory time is 0.3 seconds. For respiratory rates greater than 100 breaths per minute, the minimum expiratory time is 0.2 seconds. When this alarm is activated, the respiratory rate is automatically decreased to ensure the minimum expiratory time. Simultaneously, a flashing rate indicator alerts the practitioner to the incompatibility of the settings.

Output Alarms

Pressure. Pressure alarms are available for peak and baseline pressures. A low peak pressure alarm is adjustable between the baseline pressure (PEEP/CPAP setting) and 60 cmH$_2$O. The low baseline pressure alarm setting varies depending upon the PEEP/CPAP level set.

Table 10-9 lists the pressures required to activate this alarm.

The alarm parameters are automatically established by the microprocessor. These variances in alarm threshold pressures allow for

TABLE 10-9 PEEP/CPAP Alarm Pressures

PEEP/CPAP Difference	Pressure Difference (Setting vs. Proximal Airway)
0–5 cmH$_2$O	2 cmH$_2$O
6–8 cmH$_2$O	3 cmH$_2$O
9–12 cmH$_2$O	4 cmH$_2$O
13–24 cmH$_2$O	5 cmH$_2$O

the normal fluctuations in baseline pressure that occur during PEEP/CPAP. The pressure difference (setting vs. proximal pressure) must be maintained below the threshold for 25 seconds to trigger an alarm.

The ventilators also include an obstructed tube alarm. This alarm will be activated under several circumstances.

If proximal pressure exceeds the peak inspiratory pressure setting by 10 cmH$_2$O, all gas flow will cease, the safety valve and exhalation valve will be opened, and the alarm code HI-PIP A05 will be displayed in the mul-

tiple display window. If proximal pressures exceed the peak inspiratory pressure setting by 5 cmH$_2$O, the Infant Star 500 is adjustable based upon the High Inspiratory Pressure alarm, all gas flow will cease, the safety valve and exhalation valve will be opened, and the alarm code HI-PIP-A02 will be displayed in the multiple display window.

If the expiratory limb of the circuit becomes partially blocked, the obstructed tube alarm will also be activated. This condition is detected by the pressure failing to drop by 50% of the difference between the peak inspiratory and the baseline pressure within 0.2 seconds after the end of inspiration. The alarm code HI-PIP-A03 will be displayed in the multiple display window. If the baseline pressure exceeds the PEEP/CPAP pressure setting by 6 cmH$_2$O for more than 5 seconds, the occluded airway alarm is activated and the error code HI-CPP-A04 will be displayed in the multiple display window.

If the machine (internal pressure) exceeds the proximal airway pressure by 15 cmH$_2$O, the obstructed tube alarm will also be activated and the alarm code HI-PIP-A05 will be displayed in the multiple display window.

Tables 10-10 and 10-11 summarize the Infant Star ventilator's capabilities and alarm systems.

ASSEMBLY AND TROUBLESHOOTING

Assembly—Infant Star Ventilators

To assemble the ventilator for use, complete the suggested assembly guide. Since this ventilator may be used with several different humidifiers, assembly instructions for these are not included.

1. Select an appropriate low compressible volume humidifier and mount it to the pedestal directly below the ventilator.

2. Connect the high pressure air and oxygen supply lines to an appropriate 50-psi gas source for each.

3. Connect the electrical power cord to a 120 v, 60 Hz electrical outlet.

4. Connect the inspiratory limb of the patient circuit to the ventilator outlet on the front of the pneumatics module. The use of water traps in the patient circuit is recommended.

5. Connect the expiratory limb of the patient circuit to the exhalation valve block on the front of the pneumatics module.

Troubleshooting

Refer to the troubleshooting algorithms found at the end of this chapter.

TABLE 10-10 Nellcor Puritan-Bennett Infant Star 500 and 950 Ventilator Capabilities

	500	950
Modes (Infant Star)	Continuous Flow (IMV, CPAP) Demand Flow (IMV, CPAP)	Continuous Flow (IMV, CPAP) Demand Flow (IMV, CPAP) HFV, HFV + IMV
Rate	1–150 BPM	1–150 BPM
Inspiratory Time	0.10–3.0 seconds	0.10–3.0 seconds
Flow Rate	4–40 L/min	4–40 L/min
Press. Limit	5–90 cmH$_2$O	5–90 cmH$_2$O
PEEP/CPAP	0.0–24 cmH$_2$O	0.0–24 cmH$_2$O
Sensitivity	1 cmH$_2$O below baseline	1 cmH$_2$O below baseline
Mech. Pressure Pop-Off	5–105 cmH$_2$O	5–105 cmH$_2$O
F$_I$O$_2$	0.21–1.0	0.21–1.0

TABLE 10-11 Nellcor Puritan-Bennett Infant Star Alarm Systems

	Infant Star 500	Infant Star 950
Input Power		
Low Gas Pressure		
Air Pressure	< 45 psi	< 45 psi
Oxygen Pressure	< 45 psi	< 45 psi
Electrical Power	X	X
Control Circuit		
Ventilator Inoperative	X	X
Internal Electronics Fault	X	X
Exhalation Valve Malfunction	X	X
Incompatible Settings	X	X
Expiratory Time Too Short	X	X
Output Alarms		
Pressure Limit	5–105 cmH$_2$O	5–105 cmH$_2$O
Low Insp. Pressure	3–60 cmH$_2$O	3–60 cmH$_2$O
Obstructed Tube		
Obstructed Tube		

Adjustable High Inspiratory Pressure range of 5–105 cmH$_2$O, limited to a maximum of 15 cmH$_2$O above the set peak inspiratory pressure

NEWPORT MEDICAL INSTRUMENTS, INC., BREEZE (E150) VENTILATOR

The Newport Medical Instruments, Inc., Breeze is a microprocessor-controlled, pneumatically powered ventilator designed for neonatal, infant, pediatric, and adult use (Figures 10-16 and 10-17). It is a pressure and flow controller that can be pressure, time, or manually triggered. It is capable of operating in time-cycled, pressure-controlled modes (Assist/Control, SIMV, or Spontaneous) and volume-controlled modes (Assist/Control + Sigh, Assist/Control, SIMV, or spontaneous).

Input Power

Electric power at 120-V AC, 60 Hz (220–240-V AC, 50–60 Hz switchable), provides power to run the microprocessor, control systems, and alarm systems. An internal battery provides a minimum of 1 hour of power in case of AC power failure.

Two gas supply lines (oxygen and air) at 50 psi enter the blender from the rear of the ventilator.

Control Circuit

The blender mixes the incoming air and oxygen to the desired oxygen concentration. Gas exiting the blender passes through a check valve assembly (CVA300, Figure 10-18) prior to entering the pneumatic interface valve. The Humphry interface (SOL200P) is an air-piloted valve. When opened, gas flows through the main flow control valve, which establishes the flow of gas into the patient circuit during mandatory breaths. A pilot control solenoid valve (PLV150P, Figure 10-18) prevents gas flow from the spontaneous flow pneumatic interface valve from entering the circuit during a mandatory breath. During expiration, the pilot control solenoid allows the spontaneous pneumatic interface valve to open so that gas can flow to the reservoir bag and through the patient circuit. Two independent flow rates may be established, one for mandatory breaths and the other for spontaneous breathing.

The expiratory drive line outlet delivers pressure to the diaphragm on the permanent exhalation valve. The PEEP and plateau actuators (VLV150A, Figure 10-18) provide pressure to the exhalation valve diaphragm to maintain PEEP/CPAP pressures and to control pressure delivery during time-cycled ventilation. During volume-controlled ventilation, the exhalation valve diaphragm is controlled by the PEEP actuator during exhalation; it is controlled by main flow outlet pressure during mandatory breath inspiration.

Control Variables

The control variables for the Breeze are pressure and flow. During pressure-controlled

Figure 10-16 *The Newport Breeze Ventilator (Model E150). (Courtesy Newport Medical Instruments, Inc., Newport Beach, CA)*

Figure 10-17 *The Newport Breeze Ventilator control panel. (Courtesy Newport Medical Instruments, Inc., Newport Beach, CA)*

ventilation, the peak inspiratory pressure control (PIP) is activated and controls the peak pressure during mandatory breaths. The peak inspiratory pressure level may be adjusted between 0.0 and 60 cmH$_2$O. A pressure relief level should be set using the pressure relief valve located on the upper left corner on the rear panel of the ventilator. The control is adjustable between 0.0 and 120 cmH$_2$O; the relief valve is functional during all modes of ventilation. The relief valve should always be set to a value greater than the high pressure alarm setting to act as a safety pop-off.

Flow is a control variable during volume-controlled ventilation in that inspiratory flow will not exceed the value established by the flow control. Flow is adjustable between 1 and 120 liters per minute using the flow control (mandatory breaths). Flow output is controlled by the combination of the main flow pneumatic interface valve and precision needle valve. Tidal volume delivery then becomes a function of flow rate and inspiratory time. The Breeze is unique in that two flow rates may be set, one for spontaneous ventilation

and the other for mandatory breaths. Spontaneous flow is adjusted using the spontaneous flow control, while mandatory flow is adjusted using the flow control knob found at the bottom center of the control panel.

Phase Variables

Trigger Variables

The trigger variables for the Newport Breeze include pressure, time, and manual triggering. Pressure triggering may be established by adjusting the trigger level control. Each time the proximal airway pressure drops below the set trigger level on the face of the manometer, a patient effort is recognized. Since the sensitivity trigger setting on the Breeze is an actual rather than a delta pressure setting, it is important to carefully adjust the trigger level so that each patient effort can be detected. If PEEP/CPAP is changed, the trigger level must be readjusted to be relative to the new baseline pressure.

If patient efforts do not exceed the trigger level setting during volume- or pressure-controlled, assist/control, or SIMV ventilation, time becomes the trigger variable. The rate control, which is adjustable between 1 and 150 breaths per minute, determines the ventilatory rate.

The ventilator may be manually triggered by depressing the manual inflation button located behind the fold-down door at the bottom face of the control panel. When the manual inflation button is depressed, gas is delivered to the patient at the mandatory flow setting until the manual inflation button is released, 2 seconds elapse, or the high pressure alarm is activated, whichever comes first.

Limit Variables

The limit variables for the Breeze include pressure and flow. As already described, during pressure-controlled ventilation, pressure is limited to the setting on the peak inspiratory pressure control (PIP). Pressure limits are adjustable from 0.0 to 60 cmH$_2$O.

Flow is a limit variable, both during pressure-controlled, time-cycled ventilation and during volume-controlled ventilation. Flow is adjusted using the spontaneous flow control valve (spontaneous breathing) and the flow control (mandatory breaths). During volume-controlled ventilation, mandatory inspiratory flow, which is adjustable between 1 and 120 L/min, will be delivered at the value set on the flow control. Spontaneous flow may be adjusted with the Spontaneous flow control between 0 and 50 L/min. During pressure-controlled ventilation, mandatory inspiratory flow, which is adjustable between 1 and 120 L/min, will be delivered at the value set on the flow control; but when airway pressure equals exhalation valve diaphragm pressure (PIP control), gas exits the exhalation valve rather than entering the patient airway. As in volume control, spontaneous flow may be adjusted with the Spontaneous flow control between 0 and 50 L/min.

Cycle Variables

The cycle variables for the Breeze ventilator include pressure and time. Pressure becomes a cycle variable if the value set on the high-pressure alarm is reached during mandatory breaths. If the pressure is reached, the Breeze cycles to exhalation, mandatory and nebulizer flows stop and, the spontaneous flow turns on.

Inspiratory time is set using the inspiratory time control. Inspiratory times are adjustable between 0.1 and 3.0 seconds. When the inspiratory time has been reached, the inspiratory phase will end and exhalation will begin.

Baseline Variable

The baseline variable for the Newport Medical Instruments Breeze (E150) is pressure. PEEP/CPAP pressures may be adjusted between 0 and 60 cmH$_2$O.

Output Waveforms

Pressure

The output pressure waveform characteristic of the Breeze during pressure-controlled ventilation is rectangular.

Flow

The flow output waveform is rectangular. This waveform occurs when the peak inspiratory pressure control is set high enough that it is not reached during inspiration. Under these circumstances, the ventilator is operating as a flow controller.

Alarm Systems

Input Power Alarms

Input power alarms include loss of pneumatic pressure and loss of electrical power. If pressure falls below 35 psi, an audible alarm will alert the practitioner to the event.

If electrical power is lost, the ventilator will automatically operate on an internal battery, which, when fully charged, can operate the ventilator for a minimum of 1 hour. A periodic audible alert reminds the practitioner that the battery is in use. An audible and visual low-battery alarm will alert the practitioner to a low-battery condition. When this alarm has been activated, less than 15 minutes of battery operation time remain.

Control Circuit Alarms

The control circuit has a system failure alarm. If all the LEDs on the front panel remain on for longer than 2 seconds during the power-on self-test, an internal problem has been detected on the microprocessor board. In the event this alarm has occurred, contact an authorized service representative and use a different ventilator.

Figure 10-18 *A schematic of the Newport Breeze pneumatic system. (Courtesy Newport Medical Instruments, Inc., Newport Beach, CA)* *(continues)*

Output Alarms

Pressure. The Newport Breeze includes both high and low inspiratory pressure alarms and a low CPAP alarm. The high pressure alarm is set using the HI PRESS alarm control. It is adjustable between 10 and 120 cmH$_2$O. The low pressure alarm is set using the LO PRESS alarm control. It is adjustable between 3 and 99 cmH$_2$O. Both pressures are sensed using

the proximal airway line and a transducer located inside the ventilator. Both alarms function in all modes except the spontaneous modes. In spontaneous modes, the low inspiratory pressure alarm setting display goes dark (unless the low CPAP alarm is in use).

The low CPAP alarm is available only in the spontaneous modes of ventilation. In these modes, the apnea alarm control may be set to

Figure 10-18 *(continued)*

the first, left-most position, thus deactivating the apnea alarm and activating the low CPAP alarm. When you choose to use the low CPAP alarm in place of the apnea alarm, the total rate display on the panel will display "OFF" and the LO PRESS display will display the low CPAP alarm pressure setting. The low CPAP alarm is adjusted using the LO PRESS alarm control. The low CPAP pressure alarm is adjustable between 0 and 99 cmH$_2$O. The alarm is activated if the baseline pressure falls below the alarm limit for longer than 4 seconds.

Time. An apnea alarm alerts the practitioner to periods of apnea. The interval is adjustable between 5 and 60 seconds in 5-second increments. Once the detection delay has been set, if no breaths (spontaneous or mandatory) have been sensed by the sensitivity trigger control in that time interval, the apnea alarm will be activated and both audible and visual alarms will be triggered.

The I:E ratio alarm is activated if the inspiratory time and rate controls are set such that an inverse I:E ratio of greater than 4:1 has been set. If this occurs, the inspiratory time and I:E ratio display flashes and alerts the practitioner to the excessive inverse ratio. The flashing inspiratory time will indicate the actual inspiratory time for the set ventilatory rate. The ventilator will not allow an I:E ratio of greater than 4:1. Once this ratio is reached, the inspiratory time will automatically decrease.

Tables 10-12 and 10-13 summarize the Newport Breeze ventilator's capabilities and alarm systems.

TABLE 10-12 Newport Medical Instruments, Inc., Breeze Ventilator Capabilities

Modes	
Pressure Controlled	Spontaneous, SIMV, Assist/Control
Volume Controlled	Spontaneous, SIMV, Assist/Control, Assist/Control + Sigh
Rate	1–150 BPM
Inspiratory Time	0.10–3.0 seconds
Flow Rate	3–120 L/min (mechanical); 0.0–50 L/min (spontaneous)
Press. Limit	0–60 cmH$_2$O
Maximum Inverse I:E	4:1
Tidal Volume	10–2500 mL
PEEP/CPAP	0.0–60 cmH$_2$O
Sensitivity	0.0–60 cmH$_2$O (actual pressure, not delta pressure)
Mech. Pressure Pop-Off	0–120 cmH$_2$O
F$_I$O$_2$	0.21–1.0

TABLE 10-13 Newport Medical Instruments, Inc., Breeze Ventilator Alarm Systems

Input Power	
Inlet Gas Pressure	< 35 psi
Electrical Power	Loss of 115 v, 60 Hz (Battery power for 60 minutes is available if fully charged.) Also, if operated on 220–240 v, 50–60 Hz, similar loss of electrical power alarms function.
Low Battery	Less than 15 minutes of battery time remaining.
Control Circuit	
Systems Failure	Fault detected on the microprocessor board
Output Alarms	
Pressure Limit	10–120 cmH$_2$O
Low Insp. Pressure	3–99 cmH$_2$O
Low PEEP/CPAP	0–99 cmH$_2$O
Time	
I:E Ratio	Inspiratory time and rate exceed an inverse ratio of 4:1
Apnea	No breaths detected for 5, 10, 15, 20, or 25 seconds

ASSEMBLY AND TROUBLESHOOTING

Assembly—Newport Medical Instruments, Breeze Ventilator

To assemble the ventilator for use, complete the suggested assembly guide. Since this ventilator may be used with several different humidifiers, assembly instructions for these are not included.

1. Select an appropriate low compressible volume humidifier and mount it to the pedestal or cart directly below the ventilator.

2. Connect the high pressure air and oxygen supply lines to an appropriate 50-psi gas source for each.

3. Connect the electrical power cord to a 115 v, 60 Hz electrical outlet (220–230 v, 50–60 Hz, international).

4. Connect the inspiratory limb of the patient circuit to the ventilator outlet beneath the right-hand side of the face panel. The use of water traps or a heated wire system in the patient circuit is recommended.

5. Connect the expiratory limb of the patient circuit to the permanent exhalation valve and secure it to the exhalation valve mounting block beneath the ventilator on the lower left.

6. Connect the proximal airway line to the proximal airway nipple beneath the ventilator on the lower right.

7. Connect a reservoir bag to the large-bore outlet beneath the ventilator at the right rear of the ventilator or use the reservoir bag cap if ventilating neonates.

Troubleshooting

Refer to the troubleshooting algorithms found at the end of this chapter.

SECHRIST INDUSTRIES, MODEL IV-100B AND IV-200

Sechrist Industries, Inc., markets two infant ventilators, the IV-100B and the IV-200. Both ventilators are pneumatically-powered, micro-processor- and fluidically-controlled ventilators (Figures 10-19 and 10-20). They are capable of operating as pressure or flow controllers; pressure, time, or manually triggered, pressure or

Figure 10-19 *The Sechrist Industries IV-100B ventilator. (Courtesy Sechrist Industries, Inc., Anaheim, CA)*

Figure 10-20 *The Sechrist Industries IV-200 ventilator. (Courtesy Sechrist Industries, Inc., Anaheim, CA)*

flow limited; and pressure or time cycled ventilators. Both ventilators may be patient triggered with the addition of the SAVI (for Synchronized Assisted Ventilation of Infants) module. Being continuous flow ventilators, mechanical breaths are delivered when the exhalation valve has closed. Since many similarities exist between the ventilators, they will be considered together. When differences occur, they will be discussed on an individual basis.

Input Power

The electronic control circuitry is configured to operate on either AC input (120 volt or 220 volt) or 12-volt DC input. Both the alarm system and electronic manometer have a battery backup. Electrical power enters the rear of the ventilator via a standard AC electric cord and plug or via the supplied DC input cord and plug.

Both ventilators rely on 50-psi air and oxygen for their respective drive mechanisms. The IV-100B uses an external blender to mix the supply gases to the desired output concentration. On the IV-100B, the blender is mounted as an integral part of the ventilator on the left side. A gas flowmeter is used to adjust the continuous flow through the patient circuit.

The IV-200's blender and flowmeter are internal and have been integrated into the design of the front panel (Figure 10-20). For both ventilators, blended gas passes through a 7-micron filter and then to a regulator, which then reduces the 50-psi line pressure to 20 psi to power the internal fluidic system.

Control Circuit

The control circuit of both ventilators consists of both electronic and fluidic elements (Figure 10-21). To initiate inspiration, the microprocessor sends signals to a solenoid valve which, when closed, sends a reference signal to a back-pressure switch and an OR/NOR gate. The back-pressure switch serves as an on-off control, determining whether the ventilator is in the inspiratory phase (mandatory breath) or expiratory phase.

In the output 02 state (stable state), the ventilator is in the expiratory phase. Gas flows from 02 on the back-pressure sense gate, and then to a negative pressure jet and the proxi-

mal airway pressure line. The negative pressure jet is a venturi that supplies sub-ambient pressure at the exhalation valve. This reduces resistance to flow in the expiratory limb of the circuit from the continuous flow (refer to the exhalation valve in Figure 10-21). Gas supplied to the proximal airway pressure line helps to keep it clear from condensate. A restriction in the line minimizes flow through it.

Either a control signal from the microprocessor, depression of the manual breath control, or a signal from the SAVI patient synchronizer module closes the solenoid valve and causes the S control port to be blocked on the back-pressure switch. This causes beam deflection, and the output changes to 01. Output from 01 results in the removal of pressure from the negative pressure jet and proximal airway line. Additionally, a control signal is sent from the back-pressure switch to the OR/NOR gate.

The OR/NOR gate controls pressure when inspiratory or expiratory pressure is applied to the exhalation valve diaphragm. The control signal from the back-pressure switch (or absence of one) determines whether the ventilator is in the inspiratory or expiratory phase.

In the expiratory phase, output from the OR/NOR gate is directed to the expiratory pressure control, through a check valve to the waveform adjust control, and on to the exhalation valve.

When a control signal from the back-pressure switch is applied to the control port, C3, the OR/NOR gate switches from the stable state, 02, to 01. Output from 01 flows through the inspiratory pressure control, through a check valve, to the waveform adjust control and the exhalation valve.

PEEP/CPAP pressure is controlled by the expiratory pressure control. PEEP/CPAP levels may be adjusted between −2 and 20 cmH$_2$O. The expiratory pressure control is a needle valve that reduces gas pressure from the 20-psi regulator and applies it to the exhalation valve. The needle valve creates a back pressure (expiratory pressure); the excess flow is vented to the atmosphere. Pressure from this control is applied through a check valve to the waveform adjust control and then to the exhalation valve diaphragm, partially closing it. The partially closed diaphragm acts as a threshold resistor, creating the PEEP/CPAP pressure.

Figure 10-21 *A schematic diagram of the pneumatic system of the Sechrist Industries IV-100B ventilator. (A) Inspiration, (B) Exhalation. (Courtesy Sechrist Industries, Inc., Anaheim, CA)*

Control Variables

The control variables for both ventilators are pressure and flow. During pressure-limited ventilation, the peak inspiratory pressure is controlled by the inspiratory pressure control. This control determines the pressure applied to the exhalation valve diaphragm during the inspiratory phase. Inspiratory pressure may be adjusted between –5 and 70 cmH_2O.

A pressure relief level should be set, using the pressure relief valve located on the rear panel of the ventilator above the DISS air and oxygen inlets (IV-100B) or at the lower left on the front (IV-200). The mechanical relief valve is adjustable between 5 and 80 cmH_2O, with the relief valve being functional during all modes of ventilation. The relief valve should always be set to a value greater than the expiratory pressure setting in order to act as a safety pop-off.

Flow is a control variable during time cycled, pressure-limited ventilation, in that inspiratory flow will not exceed the value established using the flowmeter. Flow is adjustable between 0.0 and 32 liters per minute using the flowmeter. Depending on inspiratory time, a given flow may not be sufficient to achieve the set pressure limit, and the ventilator therefore becomes a flow controller.

Phase Variables

Trigger Variables

The trigger variables for the ventilators include time, manual, and electronic triggering. Time triggering is established by the inspiratory and expiratory time control. Inspiratory time is adjustable between 0.1 and 2.9 seconds. An oscillating quartz timer is used to accurately establish inspiratory time. The inspiratory time is displayed using LEDs in the "Insp. Time" display window. Setting the control determines how long the microprocessor will hold the exhalation valve closed through the fluidic control circuit. The expiratory time control sets the time limit for expiration. The same quartz oscillator is used to accurately establish expiratory time. The expiratory time is displayed by LEDs in the "Exp. Time" display window. Expiratory times may be set between 0.3 and 60 seconds. The ventilatory rate is 60 divided by the sum of the inspiratory and expiratory time in seconds. The rate and I:E ratio are calculated and displayed above the "Insp." and "Exp." time displays.

Manual triggering occurs when the practitioner depresses the manual breath button. When depressed, the S control port of the back-pressure switch becomes occluded. This causes the control signal to be sent to the OR/NOR gate, changing its output and closing the exhalation valve. Inspiration will occur as long as the button is depressed and will not be synchronized with the electronic timing circuit.

With the addition of the SAVI monitor, the IV-100B and IV-200 are capable of electronic, patient-triggered ventilation. The ventilator may be servoed to an external impedance, plethysmographic cardiorespiratory monitor. The analog output signal from the cardiorespiratory monitor provides a triggering signal to the SAVI system. By adjusting the sensitivity control, the trigger point may be moved to early or late in the inspiratory phase. Furthermore, the ventilator is able to analyze the impedance of the signal and detect the onset of exhalation. Once exhalation has been detected, the inspiratory phase is terminated and the patient is allowed to exhale. Signals from the respiratory monitor override the normal electronic control and timing mechanism. However, in the absence of any inspiratory effort, the normal timing mechanism acts as a backup system.

Limit Variables

The limit variables for the ventilators include pressure and flow. As already described, pressure is limited to the setting on the inspiratory pressure control. Pressure limits are adjustable from 0 to 70 cmH_2O. The inspiratory pressure control is a needle valve that obtains gas from the main, 20-psi regulator. The needle valve creates a back pressure (inspiratory pressure), and excess flow is vented to the atmosphere. Pressure from this control is applied through a check valve to the waveform adjust control and then to the exhalation valve diaphragm, partially closing it.

Flow is a limit variable if the inspiratory pressure is not met during the inspiratory phase. Under these conditions, the ventilator becomes flow limited. Flow is adjusted using the flowmeter, and is adjustable from 0.0 to 32 L/min.

Cycle Variable

The cycle variable for the IV-100B and IV-200 is time. Once the time established on the inspiratory time control has elapsed, exhalation begins.

Besides time cycling, the IV-100B and IV-200 may be electronically cycled with the addition of the SAVI module. Using the analog output from an external plethysmographic cardiorespiratory monitor, spontaneous patient ventilatory effort can be traced, and the ventilator can be synchronized to the patient's breathing efforts. Once the microprocessor has detected the onset of exhalation by analyzing the electronic impedance signal, inspiration is terminated and exhalation begins.

Baseline Variable

The baseline variable for the Sechrist Industries IV-100B and IV-200 is pressure. PEEP/CPAP pressure may be adjusted between –2 and 20 cmH$_2$O.

Output Waveforms

Pressure

The output pressure waveform characteristic of the Sechrist IV-100B and IV-200 is rectangular. The rectangular waveform is characteristic during time-cycled, pressure-limited ventilation.

The waveform control can be adjusted such that the output approaches a sinusoidal waveform. The waveform adjust control determines the proximal airway pressure waveform by controlling the rate of the exhalation valve closure and opening. If flow is unimpeded, the valve operation rate is rapid and is essentially a square wave. If the valve impedes flow (sending it through a fixed resistance), the valve operation rate is slowed. This mimics a sine wave flow pattern.

Flow

The flow output waveform for the ventilators is rectangular. This waveform occurs when the peak inspiratory pressure control is set high enough that it is not reached during inspiration. Under these circumstances, the ventilator is operating as a flow controller.

ASSEMBLY AND TROUBLESHOOTING

Assembly—IV-100B, IV-200 Ventilators

To prepare the IV-100B and the IV-200 for use, complete the suggested assembly guide. Since the ventilators are very similar, one set of instructions will suffice for both.

1. Assemble and fill a low compressible volume humidifier and attach it to the mounting pole of the ventilator (Figure 10-22). Since a variety of humidifiers may be used, assembly instructions are not included here.

2. Connect the large-bore circuit tubing between the flowmeter outlet and the humidifier inlet.

3. Connect the patient circuit's inspiratory limb to the humidifier outlet and the expiratory limb to the exhalation valve.

4. Connect the proximal airway pressure line to the proximal airway nipple on the exhalation valve block.

5. Connect the temperature probe to the patient wye for the humidifier servo controller.

6. Connect the air and oxygen supply lines to 50-psi gas sources.

7. Connect the power cord to an appropriate AC outlet.

8. If electronic triggering is desired, interface an external impedance, plethysmographic cardiorespiratory monitor to the SAVI Synchronizing Module, using the supplied cable.

Troubleshooting

Refer to the troubleshooting algorithms found at the end of this chapter.

Alarm Systems

Input Power Alarms

Both ventilators have alarms for low gas pressure and loss of electrical power. If either the air or oxygen inlet pressure falls below 25 psi, an audible alarm results. If both source gases fail simultaneously, the ventilator low inspiratory pressure alarm will sound.

If electrical power is lost, audible and visual alarms will result; these are powered by a backup battery supply.

Control Circuit Alarms

The IV-100B and IV-200 incorporate a self-test circuit, which checks the microprocessor function. In the event a malfunction has been detected, an audible and visual alarm will alert the practitioner to the failure.

Output Alarms

Pressure. The IV-100B, when supplied with an analog manometer, incorporates a low

TABLE 10-14 Ventilator Capabilities

IV-100B

Modes	VENT (CMV or IMV)
Rate	1–150 BPM
Inspiratory Time	0.10–2.9 seconds
Expiratory Time	0.30–60 seconds
Expiratory Pressure	–2–20 cmH$_2$O
Flow Rate	0.0–32 L/min
Press. Limit	–5–70 cmH$_2$O
Mechanical Pop-Off	5–85 cmH$_2$O
F$_I$O$_2$	0.21–1.0

IV-200 and IV-100B (with an Electronic Manometer)

Modes	VENT (CMV or IMV)
Rate	1–150 BPM
Inspiratory Time	0.10–2.9 seconds
Expiratory Time	0.30–60 seconds
Expiratory Pressure	–2–20 cmH$_2$O
Flow Rate	0.0–32 L/min
Press. Limit	–5–70 cmH$_2$O
Mechanical Pop-Off	5–85 cmH$_2$O
F$_I$O$_2$	.21–1.0

TABLE 10-15 Sechrist Ventilators Alarm Systems

	IV-100B	IV-200
Input Power		
Low Gas Pressure	X	X
Electrical Power	X	X
Control Circuit		
Systems Failure	X	X
Output Alarms		
Pressure:		
High Pressure Limit		X
Low Insp. Pressure	X	X

inspiratory pressure alarm. This alarm consists of a movable needle, which is set at a pressure 1 to 2 cmH2O below the peak inspiratory pressure. The alarm incorporates an infrared sensor into the manometer. The manometer needle must pass the set point within the detection delay time or it will cause the alarm to sound. Primarily, it serves to alert the practitioner to leaks in IMV and disconnects in the CPAP mode.

The detection delay sets the time delay before the alarm is activated. This delay is adjustable between 3 and 60 seconds.

The IV-100B, when used with an electronic manometer, and the IV-200 incorporate a high-pressure alarm in addition to the low-pressure alarm system.

Tables 10-14 and 10-15 summarize the Sechrist Industries IV-100B and IV-200 ventilator capabilities and alarm systems.

CHAPTER SUMMARY

Several ventilators have been presented in this chapter that are designed for the pediatric and neonatal patient. These ventilators all have a common characteristic in that flow or pressure is measured and used as a control variable. Table 10-16 may help you to learn the similarities and differences between the ventilators presented in this chapter.

To assist you in troubleshooting, refer to the algorithms found in ALG 10-1 and ALG 10-2.

Figure 10-22 *The Sechrist IV-100B and IV-200 circuit.*

CLINICAL CORNER

Bear Cub BP-2001

1. You have set an inspiratory time of 0.25 seconds and a flow of 9 L/min. What is your approximate tidal volume delivery at these settings?
2. The infant you are assigned to is on a Bear Cub ventilator. The pressure alarm has been going off about every 5 minutes. What should you check and do to correct the situation?

V.I.P. Bird® Ventilator

1. You have a pediatric patient being ventilated with a V.I.P. Bird® ventilator. Her settings are as follows: rate, 20/min; tidal volume, 125 mL; flow, 60 L/min; pressure, 22 cmH$_2$O; F$_I$O$_2$, 0.45. How would you set your alarm limits?
2. The low inlet gas alarm is sounding— what does this mean?

Sechrist IV-100B and IV-200 Ventilators

1. You have set an inspiratory time of 0.20 seconds and an expiratory time of 1.8 seconds. What are the rate and I:E ratio?
2. In order to use the SAVI triggering capability of the IV-200, what equipment must you have on hand?

TABLE 10-16 Pediatric/Neonatal Ventilator Classifications

Ventilator	Input Power	Circuit	Control Mechanism	Trigger Variable	Limit Variable	Cycling Variable	Alarms
Bear Cub 750$_{vs}$ and 750$_{psv}$	Electric	Single	Pneumatic	T/M	P/F	T	I/CC/P
Bird® V.I.P.	Electric	Single	Pneumatic	P/T/F/M	P/F	P/V/F/T	I/CC/P/T
Bird® V.I.P. Gold	Electric	Single	Pneumatic	P/T/F/M	P/F	P/V/F/T	I/CC/P/T
Dräger Babylog 8000	Electric	Single	Pneumatic	F/T/M	P/F	P/T	I/CC/P/F/IG
Nellcor Puritan-Bennett Infant Star 500 and 950	Electric	Single	Pneumatic	T/M	P/F	P/T	I/CC/P
Newport Breeze	Electric	Single	Pneumatic	P/T/M	P/F	P/T	I/P/T
Sechrist IV-100B	Electric	Single	Fluidic	T/M	P/F	T	I/P
Sechrist IV-200	Electric	Single	Fluidic	T/M/E	P/F	T/E	I/CC/P

Key: P—Pressure, T—Time, F—Flow, CC—Control Circuit, V—Volume, M—Manual, I—Input Power, E—Electronic, IG—Inspired Gas.

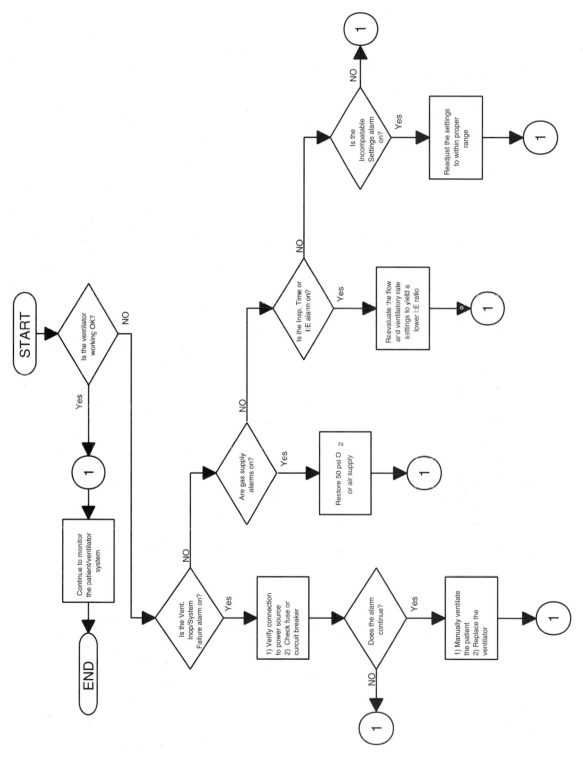

ALG 10-1 A troubleshooting algorithm for input power and control circuit alarms.

ALG 10-2 *A troubleshooting algorithm for output alarms.*

Self-Assessment Quiz

1. An infant ventilator is operating in pressure-limited, time-cycled ventilation. The inspiratory time is insufficient to allow for the pressure to reach the pressure limit. Under these conditions, which of the following is the control variable?
   a. pressure
   b. volume
   c. flow
   d. time

2. An infant ventilator is operating in pressure-limited, time-cycled ventilation. The pressure limit is reached early in the inspiratory phase and is held for the duration of inspiration. Which of the following is the control variable?
   a. pressure
   b. volume
   c. flow
   d. time

3. Which of the following infant/pediatric ventilators is (are) capable of pressure support ventilation?
   I. V.I.P. Bird®
   II. Newport Breeze
   III. Nellcor Puritan-Bennett Infant Star 500
   IV. Sechrist IV-200
   a. I
   b. I and II
   c. II and III
   d. I, II, III, and IV

4. Which of the following infant/pediatric ventilators must be used with an external monitoring/alarm system?
   a. Nellcor Puritan-Bennett Infant Star 500
   b. Bear Cub BP-2001
   c. Sechrist IV-100B
   d. Newport Breeze

5. What fluidic element do the Sechrist ventilators use to initiate inspiration?
   a. a back-pressure switch
   b. a flip-flop
   c. an OR/NOR gate
   d. an AND/NAND gate

6. Which of the following infant/pediatric ventilators are pressure triggered?
   I. V.I.P. Bird®
   II. Newport Breeze
   III. Nellcor Puritan-Bennett Infant Star 500
   IV. Sechrist IV-200
   a. I and II
   b. I and III
   c. II and III
   d. III and IV

7. Which of the following ventilators are time cycled only?
   I. Bear Cub BP-2001
   II. Nellcor Puritan-Bennett Infant Star 500
   III. Newport Breeze
   IV. Sechrist IV-100B
   a. I and II
   b. I and IV
   c. II and III
   d. II and IV

8. What is the purpose of the mechanical pressure pop-off valve on an infant/pediatric ventilator?
   a. It acts as the pressure limit control.
   b. It determines when inspiration ends.
   c. It is a safety pop-off.
   d. It controls the PEEP/CPAP.

9. Which of the following infant/pediatric ventilators utilizes a manifold of solenoid valves providing flow rates between 4 and 40 L/min?
   a. V.I.P. Bird®
   b. Newport Breeze
   c. Nellcor Puritan-Bennett Infant Star 500
   d. Sechrist IV-200

10. Which of the following infant/pediatric ventilators allows the operator to set one flow rate for spontaneous breaths and another for mechanical breaths?
    a. V.I.P. Bird®
    b. Newport Breeze
    c. Nellcor Puritan-Bennett Infant Star 500
    d. Sechrist IV-200

11. Which of the following infant/pediatric ventilators can be interfaced with an external respiratory monitor for triggering?
    a. V.I.P. Bird®
    b. Newport Breeze
    c. Nellcor Puritan-Bennett Infant Star 500
    d. Sechrist IV-200

12. Which of the following are limit variables for infant/pediatric ventilators?
    I. pressure
    II. volume
    III. flow
    IV. time
    a. I and II
    b. I and III
    c. I, II, and III
    d. I, II, III, and IV

13. Which of the following infant/pediatric ventilators utilize flow as a cycle variable?
    a. V.I.P. Bird®
    b. Newport Breeze
    c. Nellcor Puritan-Bennett Infant Star 500
    d. Sechrist IV-200

14. Which of the following would be examples of a control circuit alarm?
    I. peak pressure
    II. I:E ratio
    III. low inspiratory pressure
    IV. incompatible settings
    a. I and II
    b. II and III
    c. II and IV
    d. III and IV

15. Which of the following are examples of output alarms?
    I. peak pressure
    II. I:E ratio
    III. low inspiratory pressure
    IV. incompatible settings
    a. I and II
    b. I and III
    c. II and III
    d. II and IV

16. The Newport Breeze is capable of delivering up to 60 cmH$_2$O PEEP/CPAP. This variable is termed the:
    a. control variable.
    b. limit variable.
    c. cycling variable.
    d. baseline variable.

17. Which of the following ventilators can deliver a sinusoidal-like waveform?
    a. Bear Cub
    b. Nellcor Puritan-Bennett Infant Star 500
    c. Newport Breeze
    d. Sechrist IV-100B

18. Which of the following ventilators require an exhalation valve as a part of the patient circuit?
    a. Bear Cub
    b. Nellcor Puritan-Bennett Infant Star 500
    c. Newport Breeze
    d. Sechrist IV-100B

19. An infant/pediatric ventilator is pressure cycled when:
    a. pressure reaches a preset level and is held for the duration of inspiration.
    b. pressure reaches a preset level and inspiration is terminated.
    c. inspiration begins when a preset pressure level is reached.
    d. when the inspiratory pressure falls to baseline.

20. Which of the following is an example of an input power alarm?
    a. peak pressure
    b. low PEEP/CPAP pressure
    c. F$_1$O$_2$
    d. oxygen gas supply disconnect

21. "Exhalation begins when the inspiratory flow drops to a preset value" best describes:
    a. flow triggering.
    b. flow limiting.
    c. flow cycling.
    d. flow controlling.

22. "Inspiration begins when the baseline pressure drops to a preset value" best describes:
    a. pressure limiting.
    b. pressure support.
    c. pressure triggering.
    d. pressure controlling.

23. "Delivery of a breath to a preset pressure for a specific inspiratory time" best describes:
    a. pressure support.
    b. pressure control.
    c. pressure limiting.
    d. pressure cycling.

24. Which of the following ventilators have an internal battery that can power them if the main electrical power fails?
    I. V.I.P. Bird®
    II. Newport Breeze
    III. Nellcor Puritan-Bennett Infant Star 500
    IV. Sechrist IV-200
    a. I and II
    b. II and III
    c. I and IV
    d. II and IV

25. Which of the following ventilators have a control circuit alarm?
    I. Bear Cub BP-2001
    II. V.I.P. Bird®
    III. Nellcor Puritan-Bennett Infant Star 500
    IV. Sechrist IV-200
    a. I
    b. I and II
    c. I, II, and III
    d. I, II, III, and IV

26. When calculating tidal volume delivery when using an infant/pediatric ventilator operating in pressure-limited, time-cycled ventilation, which of the following must be known?
    I. inspiratory time
    II. pressure limit
    III. flow
    IV. expiratory time
    a. I and II
    b. I and III
    c. II and III
    d. I and IV

27. You are using a Sechrist IV-100B ventilator. The inspiratory time is 0.2 seconds and the expiratory time is 0.8 seconds. What is the ventilatory rate?
    a. 120 BPM
    b. 90 BPM
    c. 60 BPM
    d. 30 BPM

28. What is the most common output waveform when the inspiratory pressure limit is set such that flow becomes a control variable?
    a. rectangular
    b. ascending ramp
    c. descending ramp
    d. sinusoidal

29. You are using a Bear Cub with the following settings:
    Inspiratory Time   0.6 seconds
    Pressure Limit   20 cmH$_2$O
    Ventilator Rate   60 BPM
    Flow Rate   20 L/min

    What is the delivered tidal volume (neglecting loss in the ventilator circuit)?
    a. 20 mL
    b. 60 mL
    c. 120 mL
    d. 200 mL

30. Given an inspiratory time of 0.2 seconds and a flow rate of 20 L/min, what is the estimated tidal volume?
    a. 140 mL
    b. 96 mL
    c. 66 mL
    d. 46 mL

Selected Bibliography

Barnes, T. A., et al. (1994). *Core textbook of respiratory care practice* (2nd ed.). Mosby-Yearbook.

Chatburn, R. L. (1991). A new system for understanding mechanical ventilators. *Respiratory Care, 36*(10), 1123–1152.

Chatburn, R. L. (1992). Classification of mechanical ventilators. *Respiratory Care, 27*(9), 1009–1025.

Dupuis, Y. (1992). *Ventilators: Theory and clinical application* (2nd ed.). Mosby-Yearbook.

Mallinckrodt, Inc. (1989). *Infant Star neonatal ventilator operating instructions, form 9910005*. San Diego.

Mallinckrodt, Inc. (1992). *InfantStar ventilator service and repair instructions, form 9910103*. San Diego.

Newport Medical Instruments, Inc. (1991). *Newport Breeze ventilator operating manual*. Newport Beach.

Sechrist Industries, Inc. *Operational instructions and routine maintenance infant ventilator model IV-100B, part number 1000006*. Anaheim.

Viasys Critical Care. (1982). *BEAR CUB infant ventilator model BP 2001, part number 2937*. Palm Springs.

Viasys Critical Care. (1991). *Bird® VIP infant-pediatric ventilator instruction manual, part number L1194*. Palm Springs.

CHAPTER 11

NON-INVASIVE, HOMECARE, AND TRANSPORT VENTILATORS

INTRODUCTION

Non-invasive mechanical ventilation by definition is the application of positive pressure via the upper respiratory tract for the purpose of augmenting alveolar ventilation. For the purposes of this chapter, non-invasive ventilation will be defined as positive-pressure ventilation applied to the airway via a full face or nasal mask without intubation. By this definition, any critical care ventilator could be applied in this manner. However, certain specialized bi-level positive airway pressure ventilators have been adapted and meet this particular role and application very well; they will be the focus of discussion for this chapter.

Homecare and extended care are two of the most rapidly growing segments of the health care environment. Maintenance of mechanically ventilated patients in the home and in extended care and skilled nursing facilities is very common. It is important to understand the unique characteristics of these ventilators and how their capabilities differ from one another.

Transport ventilators are commonly used for ground, airborne, and intrahospital patient transports. The use of these ventilators for such special applications is becoming more common. As a practitioner, you should understand how these ventilators operate, how the controls function, and how the ventilators differ in their capabilities and operation.

OBJECTIVES

After completing this chapter, the student will accomplish the following objectives:

- Define non-invasive positive-pressure ventilation.
- Describe the indications and hazards of non-invasive positive-pressure ventilation.
- Discuss the patient interface used for non-invasive positive-pressure ventilation.
- For the non-invasive positive-pressure ventilators in this chapter, apply Chatburn's classification system according to:
  — Input power
  — Drive mechanism
  — Control scheme
  — Alarm systems

- For the homecare ventilators described in this chapter, apply Chatburn's classification system and classify them according to:
  — Input power
  — Drive mechanism
  — Control scheme
  — Alarm systems
- For the transport ventilators described in this chapter, apply Chatburn's classification system and classify them according to:
  — Input power
  — Drive mechanism
  — Control scheme
  — Alarm systems

KEY TERM

Non-invasive Positive-Pressure Ventilation

DEFINITION OF NON-INVASIVE POSITIVE-PRESSURE VENTILATION

Non-invasive positive-pressure ventilation (NPPV) is the application of positive pressure to the airway without the use of an endotracheal tube, or tracheostomy tube (artificial airway). Rather, positive pressure is applied to the airway via a full face or nasal mask. The advantages of this form of ventilation include improved ability of the patient to communicate and the ability of the patient to take fluids and food orally.

INDICATIONS FOR NON-INVASIVE POSITIVE-PRESSURE VENTILATION (NPPV)

Indications for positive-pressure ventilation include acute exacerbation of chronic obstructive pulmonary disease (COPD), acute hypoxemic respiratory failure, acute cardiogenic pulmonary edema, weaning from ventilatory support, community-acquired pneumonia, postoperative respiratory failure, severe acute asthma, and do not resuscitate/do not intubate orders.

By far, the greatest application of NPPV in the literature is for exacerbation of COPD. In many instances, the patient can be provided time to overcome the period of acute respiratory failure without intubation. NPPV allows the patient to normalize their $PaCO_2$ and PaO_2 without the additional risks associated with intubation.

Hypoxic respiratory failure responds well to positive-pressure ventilation. NPPV augments alveolar ventilation, improving PaO_2. In some cases, the patient's family requests that the patient not be intubated or resuscitated. Sometimes NPPV can provide a time window to overcome the initial cause of hypoxic failure and to allow time for the patient to recover.

In cardiogenic pulmonary edema, NPPV has been effective in augmenting alveolar ventilation. When used concomitantly with diuretic therapy and cardiac drugs, NPPV can provide time and support for the patient's recovery. The augmentation NPPV provides helps the patient to overcome their work of breathing, while recruiting FRC and improving PaO_2.

NPPV has been used for patients who have been supported with conventional positive-pressure ventilation via an endotracheal tube and have failed weaning attempts following the removal of the artificial airway. NPPV can provide a means to augment the patient's alveolar ventilation, supporting them while reducing the patient's work of breathing. NPPV can again provide a time window, allowing for recovery without re-intubation.

Community-acquired pneumonia can lead to respiratory failure. NPPV can provide the necessary alveolar ventilatory support until antibiotics and other medications can take effect. NPPV can reduce the patient's dyspnea and help to normalize $PaCO_2$ and PaO_2. Complications associated with an artificial airway can be avoided as well.

Postoperatively, some patients have difficulty resuming full ventilatory self-support. Typically, patients are hypoxemic and hypercarbic due to hypoventilation induced by the anesthesia. NPPV can augment their alveolar ventilation, supporting them until the anesthetic has been excreted or reversed effectively.

NPPV has been applied effectively in the management of patients in acute asthma crisis and ventilatory failure. In acute asthmatic crisis, patients present with hypercarbia and hypoxemia. NPPV can help improve the patient's ventilation to overcome their work of breathing and improve their gas exchange.

Some patients with terminal chronic disease have made the decision to not be intubated or placed on "life support." NPPV can provide temporary ventilatory support without intubation, and can sometimes allow sufficient time to overcome the cause of ventilatory failure.

HAZARDS OF NON-INVASIVE POSITIVE-PRESSURE VENTILATION

Hazards include leaks, nasal, sinus, or patient discomfort, gastric insufflation, eye irritation, barotrauma, aspiration pneumonia, mucous plugging, and hypoxemia.

Leaks in the circuit or around the patient interface (mask) are common in NPPV. Mask and head gear fit is critical to the success of this mode of ventilation. There are numerous mask sizes, styles, cushions, and head gear types. If the leak(s) is excessive, poor tidal volume and alveolar ventilation may result. Most ventilators have the ability to compensate some for leaks, however they should be kept to a minimum. Proper sizing and type of cushion are important in mask fitting. Several types and styles may need to be tried before one with a minimal leak is finally fit.

Nasal, sinus, or patient discomfort is sometimes experienced by patients who are ventilated with NPPV. Sometimes the mask can cause pressure sores if it does not fit properly. Some practitioners attempt to compensate for a poor fit by tightening the straps on the head gear, increasing the pressure of the mask against the patient's face. This only exacerbates the pain and discomfort. Correct mask fit is the way to prevent pressure sores. Some patients also find that the flow through the NPPV ventilator dries their respiratory mucosa and increases their discomfort. Use of humidification can reduce this discomfort.

Gastric insufflation can occur with NPPV. Since an artificial airway is not placed, some positive pressure can be directed into the stomach via the esophagus. There is an increased risk of aspiration, especially with the use of a full face mask. Placement of a nasal gastric tube can help prevent insufflation and aspiration by decompressing the stomach and removing gastric contents.

Barotrauma can be caused by NPPV. It is possible to over-distend the lungs by applying too much pressure. There have been reported instances of pneumothorax and other barotraumas when using NPPV. It is important to titrate the pressures until sufficient alveolar ventilation has been achieved, without use of excessive pressures to accomplish the ventilatory goals.

Mucous plugging and bronchial casts have been reported with the application of NPPV without humidification. If the patient is likely to remain on NPPV for an extended period of time, humidification should be used in conjunction with NPPV. Appropriate hydration is also important with oral and or parenteral fluid administration while the patient is being ventilated using NPPV. Both humidification and adequate hydration can help to prevent this complication.

Hypoxemia can occur with NPPV if adequate alveolar ventilation cannot be maintained via this technique. Sometimes, NPPV should be abandoned in favor of intubation and conventional positive-pressure ventilation if adequate blood gases and ventilatory goals can't be met.

PATIENT INTERFACE

Several styles and types of mask/interfaces are available for the application of NPPV. These include nasal mask, full face mask, and the Total® face mask.

Nasal masks often work for patients who are claustrophobic. The nasal mask fits over the patient's nose, resting on the upper lip and bridge of the nose (Figure 11-1). Nasal masks are available with air, foam, and gel cushions to improve the fit and maximize patient comfort. Many sizes and styles are available. It is important that the fit be correct, resulting in minimal force being exerted by the head gear to hold it in place. Advantages of the nasal mask include decreased risk of aspiration, ability to eat and drink, and improved verbal communication.

The full face mask covers both the mouth and the nose (Figure 11-2). This type of mask helps to assure better ventilation (fewer leaks), but comes with an increased risk of aspiration. Therefore, a nasal gastric tube is often placed with this type of mask to decompress the stomach and remove gastric contents. With

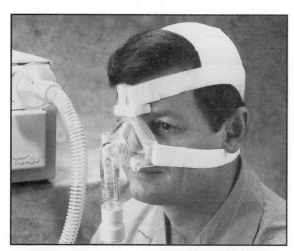

Figure 11-1 *A photograph of a nasal mask correctly fitted and secured to a patient's face. (Courtesy Respironics, Inc., Murrysville, PA)*

Figure 11-2 *A photograph of a full face mask correctly fitted to the patient's face. (Courtesy Respironics, Inc., Murrysville, PA)*

Figure 11-3 *A photograph of the Total® face mask.*

this type of mask, the patient is not able to take fluids or eat orally and their communication is limited.

The Total® face mask, manufactured and distributed by Respironics, Inc., Murrysville, PA, is similar to the full face mask in that the mouth and nose are both covered. However, the Total® face mask is made of a hard acrylic plastic that has an inflatable seal around the perimeter (Figure 11-3). As positive pressure is applied, the seal inflates against the skin, providing a tight seal. Since the cushion is very large (greater surface area), less pressure is applied and some patients find it more comfortable compared with conventional nasal or full face masks. Like the full face mask, the Total® face mask has similar hazards and complications.

NON-INVASIVE POSITIVE-PRESSURE VENTILATORS

RESPIRONICS, INC., BIPAP® VISION™ VENTILATOR

Respironics, Inc., Murrysville, PA manufactures and distributes the BiPAP® Vision™ Ventilator (Figure 11-4). The Vision™ is an electrically powered, blower-driven microprocessor-controlled ventilator. It is a flow controller that is time or flow triggered and time or flow cycled. It is specifically designed for non-invasive ventilatory support of the critically ill patient, in that the graphical monitoring capability and alarm systems improve its safety and efficacy.

Figure 11-4 *A photograph of the BiPAP® Vision™ ventilatory support system.*

Input Power

The BiPAP® Vision™ is electrically powered. A power cord on the rear of the unit may be connected to 100/120 v, 60 Hz or 220/240 v, 60 Hz AC power (switchable). The electricity powers both the blower drive mechanism and the microprocessor control system of the ventilator.

A 50-psi oxygen inlet on the rear of the ventilator is provided when supplemental oxygen is required. The ventilator mixes the oxygen with room air from the blower and adjusts the F_IO_2 to the desired level, and any F_IO_2 is available from 0.21 to 1.00. At low concentrations (<0.30) the F_IO_2 can vary by +0.3. At F_IO_2 levels above 0.30, the oxygen can vary by 0.10 (as concentration increases, percentage varies proportionally). It is also important to note, as the oxygen concentration increases, flow from the blower must decrease to maintain the higher concentration. Therefore, flow can decrease by up to 110 L/min between F_IO_2 levels of 0.64 to 1.00 (Figure 11-5).

Drive Mechanism

The drive mechanism of the BiPAP® Vision™ ventilator is a rotary compressor or blower. It is electrically powered and micro-

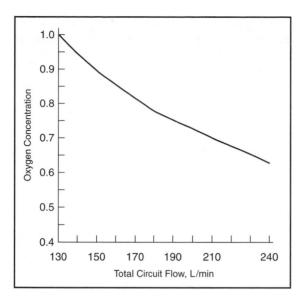

Figure 11-5 *A graph showing oxygen concentration versus flow rate. (Courtesy Respironics, Inc., Murrysville, PA)*

processor controlled (Figure 11-6). Air is drawn in through a filter that removes the gross particles from ambient air. It then is compressed by the rotary compressor. Gas exits the compressor through two pressure valve assemblies arranged in tandem.

The pressure valve assemblies (PVAs) regulate the pressure from the blower, working in tandem with one another. The PVAs regulate both inspiratory and expiratory pressures in the patient circuit.

Once gas passes through the PVAs, it passes through a pneumotachometer (air flow module) and pressure transducer before exiting the ventilator to the patient circuit connection. The pneumotachometer measures inspiratory flow and transmits this data along with the inspiratory/expiratory pressure to the microprocessor, closing the feedback loop to the blower.

Baseline pressure is maintained by partially exhausting gas to the ambient air through the PVAs, maintaining the desired pressure in the patient circuit. Excess gas flow above the set expiratory positive airway pressure (EPAP) is exhausted to the ambient air, and the remaining flow maintains pressure in the circuit during exhalation.

Control Variable

The control variable for the BiPAP® Vision™ ventilator is flow. Flow is measured by the pneumotachometer and used as a feedback signal to regulate the output of the blower drive mechanism.

Figure 11-6 *A schematic of the BiPAP® Vision™ ventilator's pneumatic system. (Courtesy Respironics, Inc., Murrysville, PA)*

Phase Variables

Trigger Variables

The trigger variables for the BiPAP® Vision™ ventilator are volume and flow. Volume triggering is automatically adjusted to 6 mL of volume above the baseline leak in the circuit. When inspired volume exceeds this trigger threshold, inspiration begins.

Inspiratory and expiratory flows are continuously monitored. The patient's flow pattern is off-set or delayed by 15 L/min and 300 msec from the actual flow pattern. When the patient's actual flow varies from the delayed flow (shadow or signal shape), the flows "cross over" and inspiration begins (Figure 11-7). The shape signal provides an alternative to pressure or volume sensing to trigger inspiration.

Figure 11-7 *A graph of inspiratory pressure and flow with illustrating the shape signal and the crossover point. (Courtesy Respironics, Inc., Murrysville, PA)*

Limit Variable

The limit variable for BiPAP® Vision™ ventilator is pressure. Pressure is adjusted by means of the inspiratory positive airway pressure (IPAP) and expiratory positive airway pressure (EPAP) controls. Adjustment of the controls varies both inspiratory and expiratory pressures, which may be set independent of one another.

Inspiratory pressures are adjustable between 4 to 40 cmH$_2$O in 1-cmH$_2$O increments. The pressure set is monitored by the proximal airway pressure transducer and is maintained in the circuit during inspiration.

Expiratory pressures are adjustable between 2 and 20 cmH$_2$O in 1-cmH$_2$O increments. Pressure in the patient circuit is monitored during exhalation, and excess flow is exhausted into the ambient air, maintaining the desired expiratory pressure in the circuit.

Cycle Variables

The cycle variables for the ventilator are flow and time. As described previously in the trigger variable section, inspiratory flow is continuously monitored. The actual measured flow is "shadowed" by 15 L/min and 300 msec behind the actual flow. When the flow between measured and the shadow or shape changes, the ventilator cycles into exhalation (Figure 11-7).

A second method of flow monitoring is used during the spontaneous/timed mode to end inspiration. An electronic flow signal is generated that is proportional to the inspiratory flow signal. When the inspiratory flow level reaches the electronic signal (spontaneous expiratory threshold), exhalation begins (Figure 11-8).

Time is a cycle variable during timed inspiration. When the timed inspiration soft key is depressed, it may be adjusted between 0.5 to 3.0 seconds. Once that time interval has passed, exhalation begins.

Baseline Variable

The baseline variable for the BiPAP® Vision™ ventilator is pressure. Pressure is set using the EPAP control and is adjustable from 2 to 20 cmH$_2$O in 1-cmH$_2$O increments. Adjustment of the control causes excess flow to be vented past the PVA valves, reducing pressure in the circuit to the set EPAP level.

Output Waveforms

In general, the pressure waveform output is roughly square, while the flow waveform output is a decelerating ramp. However, being a pressure ventilator, the actual waveform varies depending upon pulmonary compliance.

Alarm Systems

Input Alarms

Loss of Electrical Power. In the event of loss of electrical power, the Vent Inop alarm will be activated (audible and visual). The ventilator does not have a backup battery for power, therefore, loss of power will render it inoperative. The backup battery only powers the alarm system and not the ventilator blower or the control mechanism.

O$_2$ Flow. This alarm is activated if oxygen supply pressure is lost. The ventilator will continue to operate; however, only room air oxygen concentration will be delivered.

System Alarms

Check Ventilator Alarm. The Check Vent alarm is activated if the microprocessor detects a system error. Check the codes. The ventilator may require service from a qualified biomedical engineer.

Pressure Regulation Alarm. The pressure regulation alarm is a non-adjustable system alarm that activates both audible and visual

Figure 11-8 *A graph illustrating inspiratory pressure and flow and the electronically generated Spontaneous Expiratory Threshold (SET) used to terminate inspiration. (Courtesy Respironics, Inc., Murrysville, PA)*

alarms if the measured proximal pressure differs more than +5 cmH$_2$O from the set pressure for greater than 5.0 seconds.

Proximal Pressure Line Disconnect. This alarm is activated if the proximal pressure measures less than 1 cmH$_2$O for more than 1 second. Both audible and visual alarms are activated if this condition is met.

Disconnect. This alarm monitors flow output from the ventilator. If continuous excessive flow is measured (patient disconnect), both audible and visual alarms are activated. Should spontaneous breathing resume, the alarm will reset itself.

Exhalation Port. This alarm monitors circuit baseline flow. If baseline flow falls to less than 5 L/min or 50%, whichever is greater, both audible and visual alarms will be activated. If spontaneous ventilation resumes and the above conditions are exceeded, the alarm will self-cancel.

Output Alarms

Pressure. The pressure alarms for the BiPAP® Vision™ ventilator include high pressure and low pressure. The high pressure alarm is adjustable between 5 and 50 cmH$_2$O in increments of 1 cmH$_2$O. Pressure is monitored in the patient circuit during inspiration

(IPAP), and if the pressure exceeds the set value for more than 0.5 seconds, inspiration is terminated and audible and visual alarms are activated.

The low-pressure alarm is adjustable between 0 and 40 cmH$_2$O in 1-cmH$_2$O increments. EPAP pressure is monitored, and if the pressure falls below the baseline pressure for the time interval set (0 to 60 seconds), both audible and visual alarms are activated.

Flow Alarms

The BiPAP® Vision™ ventilator has a low minute ventilation alarm. This alarm is adjustable between 0 to 99 L/min in 1-L/min increments. If the minute ventilation falls below the set threshold, both audible and visual alarms will be activated.

Time. The BiPAP® Vision™ ventilator has high and low respiratory rate alarms. The alarms are adjustable between 4 to 120 BPM in 1-BPM increments for both high and low respiratory rates, respectively.

The BiPAP® Vision™ ventilator also has an adjustable apnea alarm. This alarm has three settings: disabled, 20, and 40 seconds. If a spontaneous breath is not detected within the set window, both audible and visual alarms will be activated. The alarm will self-cancel if two consecutive breaths are detected.

ASSEMBLY AND TROUBLESHOOTING

Assembly—BiPAP® Vision

To assemble the Respironics BiPAP® Vision™ ventilator for use, complete the following suggested assembly guide.

1. Connect the ventilator to a suitable AC power source. Either 120 v, 60 Hz or 220–230 v, 50–60 Hz electrical power may be used.

2. Connect a 50-psi oxygen source to the DISS fitting on the rear of the ventilator using a high-pressure hose.

3. Assemble the patient circuit:
   a. Connect the 22-mm diameter smooth-bore tubing to the ventilator's outlet.
   b. Connect the small diameter pressure line to the proximal pressure port above it.

4. Move the Start/Stop switch on the rear of the ventilator to the Start position.

5. Occlude the 22-mm diameter tubing's distal end tightly, and press the "Test Exh Port" soft key at the upper right of the screen to test the circuit/ventilator integrity.

6. Press the "monitoring" key on the lower left corner of the control panel.

7. Select an appropriate interface for the patient (nasal or full face mask).

8. Make the desired settings (mode, IPAP, EPAP, F_IO_2, etc.).

Assembly—BiPAP® S/T

To assemble the BiPAP® S/T system for use, follow the suggested assembly guide.

1. Connect the ventilator to a suitable AC power source. Either 120 v, 60 Hz or 220–230 v, 50–60 Hz electrical power may be used:
   a. Rotate the voltage selector switch to the correct current setting.

2. Assemble the patient circuit:
   a. Connect the patient tubing to the outlet of the ventilator.

(1) If supplemental oxygen is desired, attach the oxygen enrichment fitting between the ventilator outlet and the patient circuit.
   b. Connect the whisper swivel to the distal end of the patient circuit.
   c. Connect either nasal pillows or a nasal mask to the outlet of the whisper swivel.
   d. Connect a spacer to the top of the mask and adjust the spacer/mask assembly to fit the patient using the headgear.

3. Adjust the pressure levels:
   a. Adjust the IPAP pressure using the IPAP control on the rear of the ventilator.
   b. Adjust the EPAP pressure using the EPAP control on the rear of the ventilator.

4. Select the mode of operation:
   a. *CPAP:* Select either the IPAP or EPAP position. Whichever position is selected, the ventilator will operate in CPAP mode delivering either IPAP or EPAP pressure to the circuit.
   b. *Spontaneous:* The ventilator will cycle between the IPAP and EPAP pressure based upon its flow sensing logic.
   c. *Spontaneous/Timed:* This setting allows spontaneous ventilation with a backup ventilatory rate in the absence of spontaneous efforts.
   d. *Timed:* This mode delivers augmented ventilation at the set ventilatory rate and percent IPAP time.

5. Turn the unit on by pressing the on/off switch on the right front of the control panel.

Troubleshooting

Use the troubleshooting algorithm at the end of this chapter to assist you with troubleshooting problems associated with intermittent bi-level positive airway pressure systems.

RESPIRONICS, INC., BIPAP® S/T-D VENTILATOR

Respironics, Inc., Murrysville, PA manufactures and distributes the BiPAP® S/T-D Ventilatory Support System (Figure 11-9). The BiPAP® S/T-D is an electrically powered, noncontinuous, ventilatory augmentation system designed to support a patient's ventilatory efforts with inspiratory (IPAP) and expiratory (EPAP) pressures. The BiPAP® S/T-D system is a pressure controller that is flow or time triggered, pressure limited, and flow or time cycled. The BiPAP® S/T may operate in spontaneous, spontaneous/time cycled, time cycled, and CPAP modes. The BiPAP® S/T-D differs from the BiPAP® S/T in that it is equipped with an output interface that can be connected to digital or oscilloscope recorders to monitor estimated tidal volume, estimated flow rate, total flow rate, and inspiratory pressures.

Input Power

The input power for the BiPAP® S/T-D ventilatory support system is AC electrical power. Either 120 v, 60 Hz (domestic) or 220–230 v, 50–60 Hz (international) AC current may be used. Either may be selected by rotating the voltage selector switch on the rear of the ventilator to the right of the power cord receptacle.

Control Circuit

The control circuit consists of an electrically powered fan (flow generator) and an electrodynamic pressure control valve. Adjustment of the IPAP and EPAP pressure controls on the rear of the unit causes electrical current to the coils in the valve to vary, increasing or decreasing magnetic attraction between the valve core and the permanent magnet housing (Figure 11-10). The magnetic attraction

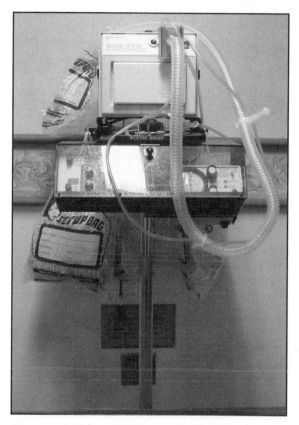

Figure 11-9 *A photograph of the Respironics, Inc. BiPAP® S/T-D ventilator.*

Figure 11-10 *A schematic diagram of the Respironics, Inc. flow control system. (Courtesy Respironics, Inc., Pittsburgh, PA)*

between the valve core and the valve disc causes pressure to build within the pressure chamber. As magnetic attraction increases, so does the pressure. Once pressure exceeds the magnetic attraction, excess pressure is vented through the exhaust valve.

Inspiration and expiration is determined by flow-sensing logic in the ventilator. Flow is detected by a flow transducer. When the total flow increases above the leak threshold by 40 cc/second for 0.03 seconds, inspiration is triggered and pressure rises to the IPAP level. When flow tapers below the estimated leak threshold, inspiration is terminated and pressure falls to the EPAP level.

If supplemental oxygen is desired, it may be bled in by placing the oxygen enrichment attachment between the ventilator outlet and the patient circuit (Figure 11-11). Oxygen is bled in until the desired oxygen concentration is reached and verified with an oxygen analyzer.

Control Variable

The control variable for the BiPAP® S/T-D is pressure. IPAP and EPAP levels are adjustable between −4 and 20 cmH$_2$O. As already described, the pressure control valve (Figure 11-10), determines the delivered pressure.

Phase Variables

Trigger Variables

The trigger variables for the BiPAP® S/T-D system include flow and time. When operated in the spontaneous mode, flow is the trigger variable. As already described, the flow-sensing logic determines when inspiration begins and ends, cycling the ventilator into and out of IPAP.

Figure 11-11 *A photograph illustrating supplemental oxygen being bled into the circuit at the ventilator outlet.*

When the ventilator is operated in the spontaneous/timed mode, the ventilator may be flow or time triggered. If the patient has spontaneous efforts that are detected by the flow-sensing logic at a rate equal to or greater than the breath per minute control setting (respiratory rate), the BiPAP® S/T-D system functions using flow as a cycle variable. If the patient's spontaneous rate falls below the set respiratory rate, the ventilator becomes time triggered, delivering pressure augmented breaths at the set rate (breaths per minute).

If the ventilator is operated in the timed mode, the BiPAP® S/T-D system delivers pressure augmented breaths at the set ventilator rate (breaths per minute) and percent IPAP time. Rates may be adjusted between 4 and 30 breaths per minute. Percent IPAP times may be adjusted between 10 and 90%.

Limit Variable

The limit variable is pressure. Pressure increases during inspiration to the IPAP pressure setting. IPAP is adjustable between −4 and 20 cmH$_2$O. Once inspiration begins, pressure increases to the IPAP level and plateaus until exhalation begins.

Cycle Variables

The cycle variables include flow and time. Flow cycling occurs when inspiratory flow falls to a level less than the estimated leak flow. When this flow threshold is reached, inspiratory assistance is terminated and pressure falls to the EPAP level.

Time cycling occurs when the BiPAP® S/T-D system is operated in the timed mode. Inspiration is terminated when the percent IPAP time has been reached. The percent IPAP time may be adjusted between 10 and 90%.

Baseline Variable

The baseline variable is pressure. EPAP pressures may be adjusted between −4 and 20 cmH$_2$O. It is important to adjust the EPAP pressure to a lower value than the IPAP pressure.

Output Waveforms

Pressure

The pressure waveform output is generally rectangular. However, with changes in pulmonary compliance, the pressure waveform becomes more exponential.

Flow

The flow waveform is generally decelerating. However, with changes in pulmonary compliance, the characteristic of the flow waveform will change.

Alarm Systems

There are no built-in alarm systems on the BiPAP® S/T-D ventilator. It may be used with an external pressure monitor (Figure 11-9) that contains a pressure manometer to visually measure IPAP and EPAP as well as low and high pressure alarm thresholds and a detection delay adjustable between 0.5 to 60 seconds.

HOMECARE VENTILATORS

BEAR MEDICAL SYSTEMS, INC., BEAR 33

The Bear 33 volume ventilator is a microprocessor-controlled, rotary-driven piston ventilator capable of control, assist/control, and SIMV modes (Figure 11-12). It is a volume controller, which may be flow limited and may be pressure, volume, or time cycled.

Input Power

The Bear 33 ventilator may be powered by AC power (120 v, 60 Hz or 220–230 v, 50–60 Hz), an internal 12-V DC battery, or an external, deep-cycle 12-V DC battery.

If supplemental oxygen is required, an oxygen source may be connected to the oxygen accumulator nipple on the front of the ventilator. A 9-inch-long section of 22-mm, large-bore tubing is then connected between the accumulator outlet and the gas inlet port directly above it. The percentage of oxygen delivered to the patient varies depending upon the tidal volume and respiratory rate.

Drive Mechanism

On the reverse stroke of the piston, gas is drawn into the cylinder from the oxygen accumulator through a filter and a check valve (Figure 11-13). As already described, if oxygen-enriched gas is desired, the oxygen accumulator may be connected to an oxygen source.

During the inspiratory phase (forward piston stroke), gas flows through a check valve into the patient circuit (Figure 11-13). Two other gas lines originate near the output of the cylinder. These include a line that powers the

Figure 11-12 *A photograph of the Bear Medical Systems, Inc., Bear 33 Volume Ventilator. (Courtesy Bear Medical Systems, Inc., Riverside, CA)*

Figure 11-13 *The Bear Medical Systems, Inc., Bear 33 Volume Ventilator's pneumatic system. (Courtesy Bear Medical Systems, Inc., Riverside, CA)*

exhalation valve and a line that purges the proximal airway line.

The line powering the exhalation valve is attached to the overpressure relief valve, the pressure limit valve, and the sigh solenoid. Should excessive pressure build within the circuit, two relief valves ensure that excessive pressure is not delivered to the patient. The sigh solenoid delivers 1.5 times the tidal volume (up to 80 cmH₂O) when the sigh system is on.

The proximal airway purge line reduces the condensate in the proximal airway line by purging it with a small volume of gas during inspiration. The inspiratory pressure transducer and other electronic components inside the ventilator could be harmed if excessive moisture were to enter the ventilator.

PEEP may be accomplished by adding an external threshold resistor valve to the patient circuit. This valve should be added proximal to the exhalation valve to minimize any potential volume losses through the exhalation valve. If the PEEP valve is located distal to the exhalation valve, a pressure gradient may develop between the PEEP valve and the

exhalation valve diaphragm, preventing it from completely sealing and, under some circumstances, resulting in a loss of delivered volume. This effect may be more prominent when using disposable circuits.

Control Variable

The control variable for the Bear 33 ventilator is volume. The tidal volume control allows adjustment of the tidal volumes between 100 mL and 2,200 mL, with incremental adjustments of 10 mL. The tidal volume control determines the stroke of the piston, and therefore, the volume of gas contained within the cylinder.

Phase Variables

Trigger Variables

The trigger variables for the Bear 33 ventilator are pressure and time. The trigger variable is adjusted using the assist/sensitivity control. Sensitivity is adjustable between −9 and 19 cmH₂O in increments of 1 cmH₂O.

Adjustment of the control establishes a reference value that the microprocessor uses to compare with what the proximal pressure transducer measures. When the values equal one another, a ventilator-assisted breath is delivered. When operated in Control mode, the sensitivity control is inactive and inspiratory efforts will not be recognized by the microprocessor.

The ventilator is time triggered in the absence of any spontaneous ventilatory efforts. The rate control establishes the length of time for the ventilatory cycle (inspiration and expiration). Ventilatory rates are adjustable between 2 and 40 breaths per minute. Between the rates of 2 and 20 breaths per minute, the rate may be adjusted in increments of 0.5 breaths per minute. Between the rates of 10 and 40 breaths per minute, the rate may be adjusted in increments of 1 breath per minute.

Limit Variable

Flow is the limit variable for the Bear 33 ventilator. Flow becomes a limit variable if the peak flow control is set such that the flow rate value is met early during inspiration and is held for the remainder of the inspiratory time. Peak flow rates are adjustable between 20 and 120 L/min in 1-L/min increments. The peak flow control changes the speed of the electric drive motor during the forward stroke of the piston, adjusting the flow rate.

Cycle Variables

The cycle variables for the Bear 33 ventilator include pressure, volume, and time. Pressure becomes a cycle variable when the inspiratory pressure exceeds the value set on the high pressure alarm. The high pressure alarm is adjustable between 10 and 80 cmH$_2$O. Once the alarm limit is reached, the piston stops its forward travel (terminating the breath), the alarm indicator illuminates, the pressure limit solenoid valve opens, and the exhalation valve on the circuit depressurizes. If two consecutive breaths exceed the pressure limit, an audible alarm will sound as well.

Volume becomes a cycle variable if the ventilator-assisted breath is not terminated before either the pressure limit or inspiratory time has been met. Under these circumstances, inspiration ends following delivery of the volume contained within the piston.

Volume is also a cycle variable when sighs have been selected. Under these circumstances,

a volume of 1.5 times the set tidal volume or 3,300 mL (whichever is less) will be delivered 6 times per hour. Both the high-pressure alarm and the expiratory time are automatically lengthened by 50% whenever sigh mode is selected. This precludes the delivery of stacked breaths.

Time may be a cycle variable if the inspiratory time control is adjusted so that inspiration is terminated prior to the delivery of the volume contained within the piston. Inspiratory time is adjustable between 0.25 and 4.99 seconds. Under these circumstances, the inspiratory time LCD will flash 0.25 and another parameter (tidal volume or peak flow) will also flash, indicating that the limiting factor is insufficient inspiratory time.

Output Waveforms

Pressure, Volume, and Flow

The flow waveform output for the ventilator is sinusoidal. This results from the fact that the piston accelerates at different rates, depending upon the wheel and connecting rod positions (refer to Chapter 7). Although the flow waveform is sinusoidal, the pressure waveform assumes a sigmoidal shape, with the peak values occurring at different times.

Alarm Systems

Input Alarms

Input Power. The Bear 33 ventilator low-battery alarm will be triggered if the internal battery falls below 25% of its operating capacity. This represents approximately 15 minutes of operation. The alarm is a continuous, audible alarm accompanied by a flashing alarm indication. This alarm may not be reset. If the ventilator is being powered by the internal battery and the alarm sounds, an alternative power source must be provided (wall AC or an external battery).

The power change alarm will activate when the ventilator switches power sources. For example, if an external, deep-cycle battery becomes discharged or the AC power cord becomes disconnected, the ventilator will automatically switch to internal battery power. Under these circumstances, the visual and audible power change alarm will alert the practitioner to the event. This alarm may be reset using the visual reset control.

Control Circuit Alarms

In the event that a microprocessor error or problem has been detected, the Bear 33 ventilator will default to the parameters listed in Table 11-1.

Under these circumstances, make sure the patient is receiving alternative ventilation and turn the power switch off and then back on. If the ventilator enters the default condition again, remove it from service and contact a qualified biomedical repair facility.

Output Alarms

Pressure. As already described ("cycle variables" section), the Bear 33 ventilator has a high-pressure alarm, which is adjustable between 10 and 80 cmH$_2$O. The Bear's low-pressure alarm is adjustable between 3 and 70 cmH$_2$O. During inspiration, if the inspiratory pressure fails to reach the alarm threshold, the low-pressure alarm will flash. If on a second breath the same event occurs, an audible alarm will sound and the flashing display will change to a steady illumination. If, on the second breath, inspiratory pressure exceeds the threshold value, the visual indicator will automatically reset to the off condition.

Time. An apnea alarm will be triggered if a breath has not occurred for 20 seconds during mechanical or spontaneous breathing. Both audible and visual alarms will trigger after

TABLE 11-1 Default Parameters

Rate	16 BPM
Volume	500 mL
Flow	35 L/min
Hi Press.	40 cmH$_2$O
Lo Press.	10 cmH$_2$O
Mode	Assist/Control
Sensitivity	−1.0 cmH$_2$O

TABLE 11-2 Bear 33 Ventilator Capabilities

Modes	Control, Assist/Control, SIMV, Sigh
Volume	100 to 2,200 mL
Breath Rate	2 to 10 BPM (0.5-breaths-per-minute increments)
	10 to 40 BPM (1-breath-per-minute increments)
Insp. Time	0.25 to 3.99 seconds
Peak Flow	20 to 120 L/min
Sigh Volume	150% of tidal volume at 6 sighs per hour
Sensitivity	−9 to 19 cmH$_2$O
F$_I$O$_2$	0.21 to 1.0

ASSEMBLY AND TROUBLESHOOTING

Assembly—Bear 33

To assemble the Bear Medical Systems, Inc., Bear 33 volume ventilator, follow the suggested assembly guide.

1. Connect the ventilator to an appropriate power source:
   a. External, deep-cycle 12-V DC battery.
   b. AC wall electrical supply (120 v, 60 Hz or 220–230 v, 50–60 Hz).
   c. Internal battery, if fully charged.

2. Assemble the patient circuit:
   a. Attach one end of the 18-inch, 22-mm diameter tubing to the ventilator outlet and the other end to a heated humidifier. Suitable humidifiers would include the Bear VH-820, Bird Wick, Fisher Paykel, or any other high-efficiency humidifier.

   b. Connect one end of the 60-inch, 22-mm diameter tubing to the humidifier outlet and the other end to the patient manifold.
   c. Attach the proximal pressure tee to the patient manifold and a 4- or 6-inch tracheostomy flextube to its outlet.
   d. Connect the exhalation valve to the balloon fitting on the ventilator.
   e. Connect the proximal pressure line to the Prox. Tee fitting on the ventilator.

Troubleshooting

To assist you in troubleshooting the ventilators, refer to the algorithms at the end of this chapter.

TABLE 11-3   Bear 33 Ventilator Alarm Systems

Input Power

Low Battery

Power Switch-over

Control Circuit

Ventilator Inoperative

Output Alarms

Pressure	
High Pressure	10 to 80 cmH$_2$O
Low Pressure	3 to 70 cmH$_2$O
Time	
Apnea	

this time interval. If a breath occurs after the alarm condition has been met, the audible alarm will cancel and the visual display will continue to be illuminated until it is reset.

Tables 11-2 and 11-3 summarize the BEAR 33 volume ventilator's capabilities and alarm systems.

NELLCOR PURITAN-BENNETT LP20 VENTILATOR

The Nellcor Puritan-Bennett LP20 volume ventilator is designed to meet the needs of the homecare and sub-acute care patient (Figure 11-14). The ventilator is electrically powered and microprocessor controlled. It is a volume controller and is either time or pressure triggered. It may be pressure limited and pressure, volume, or time cycled. The ventilator may be powered by AC current (120 or 220 volts) or by an external 12-V DC battery. The ventilator may be operated in assist/control, SIMV, or pressure cycled modes.

Input Power

The LP20 ventilator is electrically powered. The practitioner may choose between 120 v, 60 Hz or 220–230 v, 50–60 Hz AC power; external, 12-V DC battery; or if charged, an internal battery. If fully charged and in good condition, the internal battery can power the ventilator for 30 to 60 minutes.

If supplemental oxygen is desired, an oxygen elbow may be attached to the ventilator

outlet. When so configured, approximately 40% oxygen may be delivered. Alternatively, an oxygen source may be connected to the rear of the ventilator, and when using an external reservoir (3-L anesthesia bag), up to 100% oxygen delivery may be achieved.

Drive Mechanism

The ventilator's drive mechanism consists of an electrically powered, rotary-driven piston. Gas enters the piston during its backstroke through a one-way valve and an inlet filter. During the forward stroke, gas is compressed and delivered to the ventilator outlet through another one-way valve. A secondary port adjacent to the ventilator outlet powers the exhalation valve on the patient circuit.

If desired, PEEP can be accommodated by adding an external threshold resistor to the patient circuit. The PEEP valve should be placed proximally to the exhalation valve to minimize volume loss through the latter. Volume loss may be more of a concern when using disposable circuits.

Control Variables

The control variables of the LP20 ventilator are volume and pressure. Volume is a control variable during mandatory breath delivery. Adjustment of the tidal volume control varies the stroke of the piston drive mechanism. Tidal volumes are adjustable between 100 and 2,200 mL.

Pressure becomes a control variable when the pressure limit control is set to a level lower than the high alarm limit control that would normally be reached during a mandatory

Figure 11-14   *A photograph of the Puritan-Bennett LP20 Volume Ventilator. (Courtesy Puritan-Bennett, Pleasanton, CA)*

breath. When the pressure limit is adjusted in this way, excess pressure is vented to the atmosphere and the set pressure limit is maintained. The pressure limit is adjustable between 15 and 50 cmH$_2$O.

Phase Variables

Trigger Variables

The trigger variables of the LP20 ventilator include pressure and time. Pressure triggering is accomplished by adjusting the breathing effort (sensitivity) control, which may be adjusted between 15 and 50 cmH$_2$O below baseline pressure. When the trigger pressure has been reached, the ventilator will deliver a mandatory breath (assist/control mode), or if in the SIMV mode, the breathing effort lamp will be illuminated.

Time is a trigger variable in the absence of spontaneous breathing efforts. The rate control establishes the length of time for the ventilatory cycle (inspiration and expiration). Ventilatory rates are adjustable between 22 and 38 breaths per minute in increments of 2 breaths per minute.

Limit Variable

The limit variable for the LP20 is pressure. As already described, if the pressure limit is set lower than the normal peak pressure for a given tidal volume, the pressure will rise to that level and be held constant. Excess pressure during inspiration will be vented to the atmosphere.

Cycle Variables

The cycle variables for the LP20 include pressure, volume, and time. Pressure becomes a cycle variable when the peak inspiratory pressure exceeds the value set on the high-pressure alarm. When this condition is met, inspiration is terminated and both audible and visual alarms are activated. High-pressure alarm limits may be set between 15 and 90 cmH$_2$O in increments of 5 cmH$_2$O.

Volume is a cycle variable during mandatory breath delivery if neither the high-pressure limit nor the pressure limit setting is met. Under these circumstances, gas delivery ceases when the piston reaches the end of its stroke. Tidal volumes are adjustable between 100 and 2,200 mL.

Time becomes a cycle variable if the pressure limit has been reached before the end of inspiration. Under these circumstances, the breath will be time cycled (determined by the inspiratory time). Inspiratory times are adjustable between 0.5 and 1.0 second in increments of 0.1 and 1.2 seconds. Inspiratory times may also be adjusted between 1.5 and 5.5 seconds in increments of 0.5 seconds.

Output Waveforms

The flow output of the ventilator is a sinusoidal waveform. This results from the ventilator having a rotary-driven, piston drive mechanism (refer to Chapter 7). Although the flow waveform is sinusoidal, the pressure assumes a sigmoidal shape, with peak pressures occurring at differing times from the peak flow values.

Alarm Systems

Input Power

When operating on an external battery, the ventilator will indicate this condition by the illumination of the amber-colored, external battery LED.

When the ventilator is operating on the internal battery, a flashing amber LED and an audible tone, which sounds every 5 minutes, will alert the clinician that the ventilator is operating on the internal battery. If fully charged and in good condition, the internal battery can power the ventilator for up to 10 hours.

If the ventilator switches from a higher power source to a lower one (i.e., from an AC to a DC power source), a pulsating tone will signify the event. However, no alarm sounds will occur when switching from a lower power source to a higher one.

Control Circuit Alarm

Microprocessor Failure. In the event that a microprocessor malfunction is detected, a steady-tone (audible) alarm will result. In this event, the clinician should provide an alternate means of ventilation for the patient and remove the ventilator from service.

Settings Error. If the clinician establishes settings beyond the capabilities of the ventilator, an audible alarm will sound and a flashing setting error/pre-silence LED will be illuminated. Control settings must be within range for the alarm to silence.

Output Alarms

Pressure. The LP20 ventilator has both high and low airway pressure alarms. Both alarms

TABLE 11-4 Nellcor Puritan-Bennett LP20 Ventilator Capabilities

Modes	Assist/Control, SIMV, Pressure Cycle
Volume	100 to 2,200 mL
Breath Rate	1 to 20 BPM (1-breath-per-minute increments); 22 to 38 BPM (2-breaths-per-minute increments)
Pressure Limit	15 to 50 cmH$_2$O
Inspiratory Time	0.5 to 1.0 seconds (0.1- and 1.2-second increments); 1.5 to 5.5 seconds (0.5-second increments)
Sensitivity	−10 to +10 cmH$_2$O
F$_I$O$_2$	0.40 to 1.0

TABLE 11-5 Nellcor Puritan-Bennett LP20 Alarm Systems

Input Power

Low Battery

Power Switch-Over

Control Circuit

Microprocessor Failure

Settings Error

Output Alarms

High Pressure	15 to 90 cmH$_2$O
Low Pressure	2 to 32 cmH$_2$O

incorporate LEDs and an audible, pulsating tone. The low-pressure alarm is adjustable between 2 and 32 cmH$_2$O in 2-cmH$_2$O increments. The high-pressure alarm is adjustable between 15 and 90 cmH$_2$O in 5-cmH$_2$O incre-

ments. (The high-pressure alarm was already described in the "cycling variables" section.) The low-pressure alarm helps alert the clinician to patient disconnects and leaks and is activated following two ventilator breaths.

Tables 11-4 and 11-5 summarize the LP20 ventilator's capabilities and alarm systems.

ASSEMBLY AND TROUBLESHOOTING

Assembly—Nellcor Puritan-Bennett LP20 Ventilator

To assemble the Nellcor Puritan-Bennett LP20 ventilator for use, follow the suggested assembly guide.

1. Select a power source:
   a. Connect the ventilator to an appropriate AC power source.
   b. Connect the ventilator to an external 12-V DC, deep-cycle battery using the supplied cables and observing the correct polarity (red = positive and black = negative).
   c. If the internal battery is charged, the ventilator may be operated for 30 to 60 minutes.

2. Assemble the patient circuit:
   a. Attach one end of the 16-inch, 22-mm diameter tubing to the ventilator outlet and the other end to a heated humidifier.
   b. Connect one end of the 60-inch, 22-mm diameter tubing to the humidifier outlet and the other end to the exhalation manifold.
   c. Attach the proximal line and the exhalation valve drive line to the exhalation manifold.
   d. Attach a 4- or 6-inch tracheostomy flextube to the exhalation manifold and the appropriate patient interface to the other end.
   e. Connect the exhalation valve to the exhalation valve port fitting on the ventilator, using ⅛-inch, small-diameter tubing.
   f. Connect the proximal pressure line to the patient pressure fitting on the ventilator using ¼-inch tubing.

Troubleshooting

To assist you in troubleshooting the ventilator, refer to the algorithms at the end of this chapter.

NELLCOR PURITAN-BENNETT LP6 PLUS AND LP10

The Nellcor Puritan-Bennett LP6 PLUS volume ventilator is designed to meet the needs of homecare patients (Figure 11-15).

The LP10 volume ventilator differs from the LP6 PLUS in that a pressure limit control is provided for pressure-limited ventilation (Figure 11-16).

The LP10 ventilator is intended to meet the needs of those patients requiring volume and/or pressure ventilation modalities. Both ventilators are microprocessor-controlled volume controllers which can be time or pressure triggered. The ventilators may be pressure limited and pressure, volume, or time cycled. The ventilators may be operated from 120- or 220-volt electrical power or operated by an internal or external 12-volt DC battery. Since so many features are common between the two ventilators, they will be presented together. When differences occur, they will be presented and compared.

Input Power

The ventilators are electrically powered, and the practitioner has several choices regarding the power source. Standard electrical

Figure 11-15 *A photograph of the Puritan-Bennett LP6 PLUS Volume Ventilator. (Courtesy Puritan-Bennett, Pleasanton, CA)*

power of 120 v, 60 Hz (United States) or 220–230 v, 50–60 Hz (international) may be selected. Additionally, the ventilators may be powered for up to 1 hour using the internal 12-volt DC battery, if fully charged. Alterna-

Figure 11-16 *A photograph of the Nellcor Puritan-Bennett, LP10 Volume Ventilator. (Courtesy Puritan-Bennett, Pleasanton, CA)*

tively, an external, deep-cycle, 12-volt DC battery may be used to power the ventilators.

If supplemental oxygen is required, an oxygen elbow may be added to the outlet of the ventilators, which can provide an F_IO_2 of up to 0.4. Oxygen concentration is increased by bleeding in oxygen at the elbow to achieve the desired F_IO_2. If a higher oxygen concentration is required, an oxygen enrichment kit may be added to the filter port on the rear of the ventilator to increase the oxygen concentration delivered to the patient. Through the use of this kit, the F_IO_2 may be increased to 1.0.

Drive Mechanism

Both ventilators utilize an electrically powered, rotary-driven 2.2-liter piston. Gas enters the piston during its backstroke through a one-way valve and an inlet filter (Figures 11-17A and 11-17B). During the

Figure 11-17A *A schematic diagram of the Nellcor Puritan-Bennett, LP6 PLUS Volume Ventilator pneumatic system. (Courtesy Puritan Bennett, Pleasanton, CA)*

Figure 11-17B *A schematic diagram of the Nellcor Puritan-Bennett, LP10 Volume Ventilator pneumatic system. (Courtesy Puritan-Bennett, Pleasanton, CA)*

forward stroke, gas is compressed and delivered to the patient air port through another one-way valve. A port adjacent to the patient air port powers the exhalation valve, closing it.

If desired, an optional PEEP valve may be added to the patient circuit's exhalation valve. This valve should be added proximally to the exhalation valve to minimize any potential volume losses through the latter. If the PEEP valve is located distal to the exhalation valve, a pressure gradient may develop between the PEEP valve and the exhalation valve diaphragm, preventing it from completely sealing under some circumstances and resulting in a loss of delivered volume. This effect may be more prominent when using disposable circuits.

Control Variables

The control variable for the LP6 PLUS ventilator is volume, while the control variables for the LP10 ventilator are both pressure and volume.

Pressure is a control variable for the LP10 when the pressure limit control is set to a level that is lower than the high alarm limit control and the peak pressure that would normally be reached during a mechanical breath. When the pressure limit is adjusted in this way and the pressure limit has been reached, excess pressure is vented to the atmosphere and the set pressure limit is maintained. When operated in this way, the ventilator becomes a pressure controller. The pressure limit is adjustable between 15 and 50 cmH$_2$O.

The volume control determines the tidal volume delivered with each breath. Adjustment of this control varies the stroke of the piston, and therefore the tidal volume. Tidal volumes may be adjusted between 100 and 2,200 mL. Volume is adjusted at a rate of 100 mL per machine cycle (piston stroke) until the desired volume has been reached.

Phase Variables
Trigger Variables

The trigger variables for the ventilators include pressure and time. The ventilators may be pressure triggered by adjusting the breathing effort control. This control sets the trigger sensitivity level and is adjustable from −10 to +10 cmH$_2$O. When the pressure in the patient circuit (measured at the proximal airway) falls to the adjusted level, a ventilator-assisted breath is triggered (Assist/Control), or if in the spontaneous portion of SIMV, the breathing effort lamp will be illuminated.

The ventilators are time triggered in the absence of any spontaneous ventilatory efforts. The breath rate control establishes the length of time for the ventilatory cycle (inspiration and expiration). Ventilatory rates are adjustable between 1 and 20 breaths per minute (in 1-breath-per-minute increments), and 22 to 38 breaths per minute (in 2-breath-per-minute increments).

Limit Variables

As already described, if the mechanical pressure limit valve (LP10) is adjusted to less than the high alarm limit control and less than the peak inspiratory pressure, airway pressure will not exceed that level of adjustment. Under these circumstances, the ventilator is a pressure controller. Excess pressure is vented through the pressure limit valve to the atmosphere, maintaining the set pressure limit for the remaining tidal volume delivery.

Cycle Variables

The cycle variables for the ventilators include pressure, volume, and time. The ventilators are pressure cycled when the peak inspiratory pressure exceeds the pressure level set on the high alarm limit control. When this condition is met, inspiration is terminated and both audible and visual alarms are activated. High alarm limits are adjustable between 15 and 90 cmH$_2$O in 5-cmH$_2$O increments.

The ventilators are volume cycled during mechanical breath delivery if both the high alarm limit and pressure limit settings are not reached. Under these circumstances gas delivery ceases when the piston reaches the end of its travel. Tidal volumes are adjustable between 100 and 2,200 mL.

If the pressure limit has been reached prior to the end of inspiration, the breath will be time cycled and will be terminated after the set inspiratory time has elapsed. Inspiratory times are adjustable between 0.5 and 1.0 seconds in 0.1-second increments, between 1.0 and 1.2 seconds in 0.2-second increments, and between 1.5 and 5.5 seconds in 0.5-second increments. The inspiratory time control adjusts the motor speed and determines the time required to deliver the selected tidal volume. The inspiratory time control, in conjunction with the tidal volume control, determines the inspiratory flow. Inspiratory flow is equal to the tidal volume divided by the inspiratory time.

Output Waveforms

The flow waveform output for the ventilators is sinusoidal. This results from the fact that the piston accelerates at different rates depending upon the wheel and connecting rod positions (refer to Chapter 7). Although the flow waveform is sinusoidal, the pressure waveform assumes a sigmoidal shape, with the peak values occurring at differing times.

Alarm Systems

Input Alarms

When operating on an external battery, the ventilators will indicate this condition by the illumination of the amber-colored external battery LED.

When the ventilators are operating on the internal battery, an amber LED will flash and an audible tone will sound every 5 minutes, alerting the practitioner that the ventilator is operating on the internal battery. If the internal battery fails to charge or if its charge is low, both audible and visual (Low Power LED) alarms will alert the practitioner to the event.

If the ventilators switch from a higher power source to a lower one, a pulsating tone will signify the event (i.e., from an AC to a DC power source). No alarm sounds will occur when switching from a lower power source to a higher one (i.e., a DC power source to an AC source; internal battery to external battery).

Control Circuit Alarms

General Systems Failure. In the event that a microprocessor malfunction is detected, a steady-tone audible alarm will result. In the event this occurs, ensure that the patient is being ventilated by other means and remove the ventilator from service.

Settings Error. The setting error alarm is activated when the practitioner sets control settings that are out of the range the ventilators can achieve. Control settings must be within range for the alarm to silence. The alarm consists of a pulsating audible tone.

Output Alarms

Pressure. The ventilators incorporate high- and low-pressure alarms. Both alarms incorporate LEDs and an audible, pulsating tone. The low-pressure alarm is adjustable between 2 and 32 cmH$_2$O in 2-cmH$_2$O increments. The high alarm limit is adjustable between 15 and 90 cmH$_2$O in 5-cmH$_2$O increments. (The func-

tion of the high-pressure alarm was described in the "cycling variables" section.) The low-pressure alarm is helpful in alerting the practitioner to patient disconnects and leaks and is activated following two ventilator breaths.

Tables 11-6 and 11-7 summarize the Nellcor Puritan-Bennett LP6 PLUS and LP10 ventilators' capabilities and alarm systems.

TABLE 11-6 Nellcor Puritan-Bennett LP6 PLUS and LP10 Volume Ventilator Capabilities

Modes	Assist/Control, SIMV, Pressure Control
Volume	100 to 2,200 mL
Breath Rate	1 to 20 (1-breath-per-minute increments)
	22 to 38 (2-breaths-per-minute increments)
Press. Limit	15 to 50 cmH$_2$O (LP10 only)
Insp. Time	0.5 to 1.0 second (0.1-second increments)
	1.0 to 1.2 seconds (0.2-second increments)
	1.5 to 5.5 seconds (0.5-second increments)
Sensitivity	−10 to 10 cmH$_2$O
F$_I$O$_2$	0.21 to .40 (oxygen elbow attachment)
	0.40 to 1.0 (oxygen enrichment kit attachment)

TABLE 11-7 Nellcor Puritan-Bennett LP6 PLUS and LP10 Volume Ventilator Alarm Systems

Input Power	
Low Battery	
Power Switch-Over	
Control Circuit	
Microprocessor Failure	
Settings Error	
Output Alarms	
High Pressure	15 to 90 cmH$_2$O
Low Pressure	2 to 32 cmH$_2$O

ASSEMBLY AND TROUBLESHOOTING

Assembly—Puritan-Bennett LP6 PLUS and LP10 Volume Ventilators

To assemble the Aequitron Medical, Inc., volume ventilators for use, follow the suggested assembly guide.

1. Select a power source:
   a. Connect the ventilator to an external power source (120 v, 60 Hz, or 220–230 v, 50–60 Hz) outlet and select the appropriate power source on the rear of the ventilator.
   b. Connect the ventilator to an external, 12-V DC deep-cycle battery using the supplied cables and observing the correct polarity (red is "+" and black is "−").
   c. If the internal battery is charged, the ventilator may be operated for 45 to 60 minutes on the internal battery.

2. Assemble the patient circuit:
   a. Attach one end of the 16-inch, 22-mm diameter tubing to the ventilator outlet and the other to a heated humidifier. Suitable humidifiers include the Bird Wick, Fisher Paykel MR 410 or MR 480, Puritan-Bennett Cascade, or any other high-efficiency, heated humidifier.
   b. Connect one end of the 60-inch, 22-mm diameter tubing to the humidifier outlet and the other end to the exhalation manifold.
   c. Attach the proximal line and the exhalation valve drive line to the exhalation manifold.
   d. Attach a 4- or 6-inch tracheostomy flextube to the exhalation manifold and an appropriate patient interface to the other end.
   e. Connect the exhalation valve to the exhalation valve port fitting on the ventilator.
   f. Connect the proximal pressure line to the patient pressure fitting on the ventilator.

Troubleshooting

To assist you in troubleshooting the ventilators, refer to the algorithms at the end of this chapter.

RESPIRONICS, INC., PLV-100 AND PLV-102

The Respironics, Inc. PLV-100 and PLV-102 volume ventilators are electrically powered, linearly-driven piston ventilators. The PLV-100 (Figure 11-18) is capable of operating in control, assist/control, and SIMV modes. The PLV-102 (Figure 11-19) is capable of operating in control, assist/control, and SIMV modes and providing sighs in control and assist/control modes. Both ventilators are volume controllers that are pressure or time triggered and volume or pressure cycled.

Figure 11-18 *A photograph of the Respironics PLV-100 Volume Ventilator. (Courtesy Respironics, Inc., Murrysville, PA)*

Figure 11-19 *A photograph of the Respironics PLV-102 Volume Ventilator. (Courtesy Respironics, Inc., Murrysville, PA)*

Input Power

The ventilators may be powered from three power sources: AC electrical current, 12-V DC, deep-cycle, external batteries, and a 12-V DC internal battery. When powered by AC current, either 120 v, 60 Hz (U.S. model) or 220 v, 60 Hz (international model) may be used.

If supplemental oxygen is required, a 50-psi medical oxygen source must be connected to the DISS fitting on the rear of the ventilator (PLV-102). To provide supplemental oxygen for the PLV-100, an oxygen inlet adapter must be added between the ventilator outlet and the humidifier (Figure 11-20), and oxygen must be bled in to provide the desired F_IO_2.

Drive Mechanism

Both ventilators utilize a linearly-driven piston. During the backstroke of the piston, gas is drawn through a check valve and an intake filter to the piston (Figure 11-20, PLV-100; Figure 11-21, PLV-102). The piston compresses the gas during the forward stroke (inspiration), causing gas to flow to the patient

circuit exhalation valve, safety pop-off (mechanical), solenoid dump valve, and a pressure transducer.

PEEP may be accomplished by adding an external threshold resistor valve to the patient circuit. This valve should be added proximal to the exhalation valve to minimize any potential volume losses through the exhalation valve. If the PEEP valve is located distal to the exhalation valve, a pressure gradient may develop between the PEEP valve and the exhalation valve diaphragm, preventing it from completely sealing under some circumstances, and resulting in a loss of delivered volume. This effect may be more prominent when using disposable circuits.

Control Variable

The control variable for both ventilators is volume. The tidal volume control determines the length of the piston's backward stroke and, therefore, the volume within the cylinder. During the forward stroke (inspiration), the volume in the cylinder (tidal volume) is delivered to the patient. Tidal volumes are adjustable between 50 mL and 3,000 mL.

Figure 11-20 *A schematic diagram of the Respironics PLV-100 pneumatic system. (Courtesy Respironics, Inc., Murrysville, PA)*

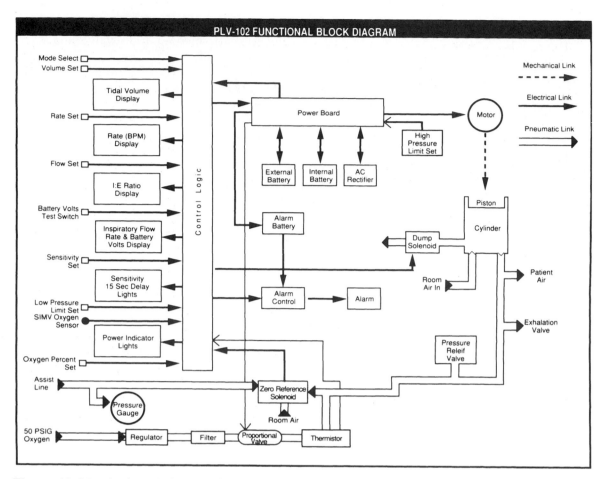

Figure 11-21 *A schematic diagram of the Respironics PLV-102 pneumatic system. (Courtesy Respironics, Inc., Murrysville, PA)*

Phase Variables

Trigger Variables

The trigger variables for the ventilators include pressure and time. Pressure is a trigger variable during assist/control ventilation. Pressure triggering is adjusted using the sensitivity control. The sensitivity may be adjusted between −6 and 3 cmH₂O (PLV-100) and −5 and 18 cmH₂O (PLV-102). This control determines the patient effort required to trigger a breath.

Time becomes a trigger variable for both ventilators in the absence of any spontaneous patient effort. This trigger variable is adjusted using the rate control. Respiratory rates may be adjusted between 2 and 40 breaths per minute.

Limit Variable

The limit variable for the ventilators is pressure. The pressure limit is adjustable between 5 and 89 cmH₂O (PLV-100) and 10

and 100 cmH₂O (PLV-102). When the pressure limit is reached, excess pressure is vented to the atmosphere and the piston continues its forward stroke. Thus inspiration does not end when the pressure limit is met.

Cycle Variable

The cycle variable for the PLV-100 and PLV-102 is volume. Volume is a cycle variable during mechanical breath delivery. Under these circumstances, the delivery of the full tidal volume determines the end of inspiration. Volume is also a cycle variable during sigh delivery (PLV-102). When sigh delivery is selected, a volume equal to 150% of the set tidal volume is delivered every 100 breaths.

Output Waveforms

Pressure, Volume, and Flow

The flow waveform output for the ventilators is sinusoidal. This results from the fact that the piston accelerates at different rates.

Even though the piston is linearly driven, the microprocessor alters its acceleration to mimic a rotary-driven piston's flow pattern. Thus, although the flow waveform is sinusoidal, the pressure waveform is sigmoid in shape. The peak values of the flow and pressure waveforms occur at different times.

Alarm Systems

Input Alarms

Loss of Electrical Power.   In the event that the ventilators are turned on and no power is connected (no AC or external 12-V DC battery or a deeply discharged, internal battery), an alarm will sound.

An audible alarm will be activated if the practitioner attempts to attach a battery with the leads reversed (positive lead connected to the negative battery terminal and vice versa). This alarm will activate even when the ventilators are in the "off" position. The circuitry of the ventilators has been designed such that improper connection will not cause any internal damage. The ventilators should be turned off, the battery terminal connections reversed, and normal operation then resumed.

If the ventilators automatically switch power sources (AC to internal battery or external battery to internal battery), an alarm will be activated. When operated on the internal battery, a maximum of 60 minutes' operation time is provided.

Oxygen System (PLV-102).   If the oxygen flow is inadequate or if the medical source gas pressure falls below 35 psi, the oxygen system alarm will be activated. The alarm code "A-4" will appear in the flow LCD window, alerting the practitioner to this event.

Control Circuit Alarms

Ventilator Malfunction (PLV-100), Internal Failure (PLV-102).   This alarm condition will be activated if a fault is found in the pressure transducer, if the piston has stalled, if an internal battery circuit has failed, or if a microprocessor failure has been detected. A fast-beeping (audible) alarm will result and the code "A-5" (PLV-102) will be displayed in the flow LCD window.

Incompatible Settings.   If the practitioner has set an insufficient inspiratory flow rate for the tidal volume and rate settings, the increase inspiratory flow LED will flash and the ventilator will automatically increase the inspiratory flow up to the maximum flow of 120 L/min. The ventilators will also alert the practitioner to inverse I:E ratio conditions by flashing the I:E ratio LCD display off and on.

Output Alarms

Pressure.   Both ventilators incorporate high- and low-pressure alarms. The high-pressure alarm was discussed earlier in the "cycling variables" section, and it is the pressure limit control. The low-pressure alarm is adjustable between 2 and 50 cmH$_2$O. This alarm is helpful in detecting leaks and patient disconnect conditions.

Time.   Both ventilators incorporate a 15-second delay alarm. If a breath (mechanical or spontaneous) has not been detected for 15 seconds, the low-pressure alarm will be activated. If a spontaneous effort or mechanical breath occurs, a green LED illuminates, alerting the practitioner to the patient's ventilatory condition.

Tables 11-8 and 11-9 summarize the Respironics PLV-100 and PLV-102 capabilities and alarm systems.

TABLE 11-8   Respironics, Inc., PLV-100 and PLV-102 Ventilator Capabilities

	PLV-100	**PLV-102**
Modes	Cont., Asst./Cont., SIMV	Cont., Asst./Cont., SIMV Sigh (Cont., Asst./Cont.)
Volume	50 to 3,000 mL	50 to 3,000 mL
Breath Rate	2 to 50 BPM	2 to 40 BPM
Peak Flow	20 to 120 L/min	20 to 120 L/min
Sigh Volume		150% of tidal volume every 100th breath
Sensitivity	−6 to 3 cmH$_2$O	−5 to 18 cmH$_2$O
F$_I$O$_2$	0.21 to 1.00	0.21 to 1.0

TABLE 11-9 Respironics, Inc., PLV-100 and PLV-102 Alarm Systems

	PLV-100	**PLV-102**
Input Power		
Loss of Electrical Power	X	X
Low Battery	X	X
Power Switch-Over	X	X
Control Circuit		
General Systems Failure	X	X
Incompatible Settings	X	X
Inverse I:E Ratio	X	X
Output		
High Pressure	5 to 95 cmH$_2$O	10 to 100 cmH$_2$O
Low Pressure	2 to 50 cmH$_2$O	2 to 50 cmH$_2$O
Time		
Apnea	15-second delay	15-second delay

ASSEMBLY AND TROUBLESHOOTING

Assembly—Respironics, Inc., PLV-100 and PLV-102 Ventilators

To assemble the Respironics, Inc., PLV-100 and PLV-102, follow the suggested assembly guide.

1. Connect the ventilator to a power source:
   a. AC current 120 v, 60 Hz (U.S. model) or 220–230 v, 50–60 Hz (international model).
   b. External, deep-cycle 12-V DC battery.
   c. Fully-charged internal battery (good for approximately 1 hour).
2. Assemble the patient circuit:
   a. Attach one end of the 18-inch, 22-mm diameter tubing to the ventilator outlet and the other end to a heated humidifier. Suitable humidifiers would include all those that are capable of body humidity at high flow rates.
   b. Connect one end of the 60-inch, 22-mm diameter tubing to the humidifier outlet and the other end to the exhalation valve assembly.
   c. Attach the proximal pressure adapter to the patient manifold and a 4- or 6-inch tracheostomy flextube to its outlet.
   d. Attach an appropriate patient interface to the tracheostomy flextube to mate to the patient's airway.
   e. Connect the exhalation valve drive line to the exhalation valve and the exhalation valve fitting on the ventilator.
   f. Connect the proximal pressure line to the proximal airway adapter and to the PAP fitting on the ventilator.
   g. If supplemental oxygen is desired:
      (1) Attach the oxygen adapter between the ventilator outlet and the humidifier inlet and bleed in oxygen to the desired F$_I$O$_2$ (PLV-100).
      (2) Attach a 50-psi oxygen source to the DISS fitting on the rear of the ventilator and adjust the oxygen percent control to the desired level, verifying it with an oxygen analyzer.

Troubleshooting

To assist you in troubleshooting the ventilators, refer to the algorithms at the end of this chapter.

NONCONTINUOUS VENTILATORY AUGMENTATION

Two of the primary treatments for obstructive and mixed sleep apnea syndromes include CPAP and bi-level positive airway pressure systems. These non-invasive ventilatory support systems may also be used to augment the ventilation of patients unable to adequately maintain normal blood gases spontaneously but not acutely ill enough to require continuous mechanical ventilatory support. There are several advantages to augmenting a patient's ventilation using these devices. These include lack of complications from an artificial airway, a patient who may communicate effectively, and patients who have control of their ventilatory rate and tidal volumes.

Both CPAP and bi-level positive airway pressure systems are effective in the management of obstructive sleep apnea syndromes by acting as a pneumatic splint and preventing the upper airway from closing. The positive pressure created in the nasopharynx forces the tongue anteriorly, maintaining an open airway and preventing the airway from collapsing during inspiration. (The airway collapses during obstructive sleep apnea due to the loss of muscle tone in the upper airway and the pressure gradient between the airway and atmospheric pressure.)

PURITAN-BENNETT GOODKNIGHT® 420S NASAL CPAP SYSTEM

The Puritan-Bennett Goodknight 420S CPAP system is a continuous flow pressure controller that is designed to provide intermittent CPAP ventilatory support for patients with obstructive sleep apnea (Figure 11-22). The Puritan-Bennett Goodknight 420S has the ability to detect and record apnea, hypopnea, and snoring events. The unit will not titrate pressure based upon the events detected, rather the events are counted and stored in memory that can later be downloaded for analysis. The CPAP system may operate in the normal (on) or ramp setting. Some patients experience difficulty adjusting to their prescribed pressures when initially falling asleep. The ramp feature allows up to 30 minutes to elapse prior to delivery of the full prescribed

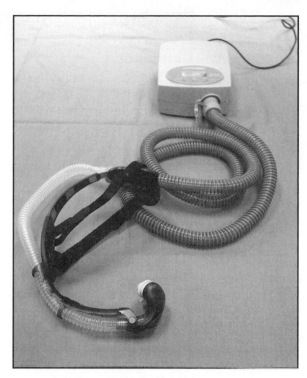

Figure 11-22 *A photograph of the Companion 420S CPAP system.*

CPAP pressure. (explained in more detail under "control variables").

Input Power

The Goodknight 420S CPAP system is electrically powered. It is powered by standard AC current. A selector switch on the bottom of the unit allows usage of 120 v, 60 Hz (domestic) or 220–230 v, 50–60 Hz (international) electric power.

Control Circuit

The control circuit of the Goodknight 420S consists of an electronically controlled fan, a pressure regulator, and a flow transducer. Signals from the pressure regulator and flow transducer are monitored by the microprocessor, and the fan's output is adjusted to maintain the desired pressure. CPAP pressure is adjusted using a control on the bottom of the unit and is adjustable between 4 and 20 cmH$_2$O.

If supplemental oxygen is desired, oxygen may be bled into the desired concentration by using an oxygen adapter between the CPAP system outlet and the patient tubing. Oxygen flow from the oxygen source is then adjusted until the desired concentration is verified using an oxygen analyzer.

ASSEMBLY AND TROUBLESHOOTING

Assembly—Companion 418G CPAP

To prepare the Companion 318 CPAP system for use, complete the suggested assembly guide.

1. Connect the CPAP system to a suitable AC power source. Either 120 v, 60 Hz or 220–230 v, 50–60 Hz electrical power may be used.

2. Connect the patient tubing to the outlet of the CPAP system.

3. Attach either nasal pillows or a nasal mask to the outlet of the patient tubing.

4. Adjust the CPAP pressure to the prescribed level using the CPAP adjustment control on the bottom of the unit.

CPAP pressures should be titrated for each individual patient based upon the results of a polysomnographic sleep study.

5. Turn on the unit:
   a. Depress the "on" button on the control panel.
   b. If a ramp pressure delay is desired, depress the ramp button on the control panel.

Troubleshooting

Use the troubleshooting algorithm at the end of this chapter to assist you with troubleshooting problems associated with intermittent CPAP systems.

Control Variable

The control variable for the Goodknight 420S CPAP system is pressure. Pressure is controlled using CPAP control on the base of the unit. Adjustment of the control results in a change in gas flow through the control valve, causing a higher or lower pressure to be delivered.

The ramp feature allows the inspiratory pressure to be ramped over a period of time. Many patients find it difficult to go to sleep with the CPAP system set at the prescribed pressure. The ramp control may be set between 0 and 30 minutes, in 5-minute increments. Once the ramp time has passed (presumably the patient has reached stage II sleep), the unit will automatically increase the pressure to the set pressure level at a rate of 2 cmH$_2$O per minute. Many patients are more comfortable as the pressure gradually ramps to the set level. The ramp feature is activated by setting the ramp time (four-position switch on the bottom of the unit) and then depressing the ramp button on the front control panel.

Phase Variable
Baseline Variable

The baseline variable for the Goodknight 420S is pressure. As already described, pressure is adjusted using the inspiratory pressure control valve. CPAP pressures may be adjusted between 4 and 20 cmH$_2$O.

RESPIRONICS, INC., REMSTAR® PLUS CPAP SYSTEM

The Respironics, Inc., REMstar® Plus CPAP system is an electrically powered intermittent CPAP system designed to be used for patients with obstructive sleep apnea (Figure 11-23). It is a pressure controller that is capable of delivering CPAP pressures between 4 and 20 cmH$_2$O. The pressure may be ramped or delayed for up to 45 minutes before the REMstar® Plus CPAP system reaches the prescribed pressure setting. The REMstar® Plus CPAP system includes a battery-powered, infrared remote control to activate the unit and initiate the ramp feature.

Input Power

The input power for the REMstar® Plus CPAP system is either 120 v, 60 Hz (domestic) or 220–230 v, 50–60 Hz (international) AC electrical power. A selector switch on the rear of the unit allows the selection of either power source.

Control Circuit

The control circuit consists of an electrically powered fan (flow generator) and an electronic controlling circuit. Adjustment of the CPAP pressure control on the rear of the unit causes the speed of the fan to change, changing the delivered pressure. A pressure manometer is

Figure 11-23 *A photograph of the REMstar® Plus CPAP system.*

used to verify the desired pressure. Once the desired pressure is reached, the electric motor speed powering the fan remains constant.

Control Variable

The control variable for the REMstar® Plus CPAP system is pressure. As already described, pressure is varied using the CPAP control and results in changes in the motor speed. CPAP pressures may be adjusted between 4 and 20 cmH$_2$O in 1-cmH$_2$O increments by depressing the pressure on/off button until the desired pressure is displayed in the LED window.

The ramp feature allows the inspiratory pressure to be delayed over a period of time. Many patients find it difficult to go to sleep with the CPAP system set at the prescribed pressure. The ramp control may be set between 0 and 45 minutes, in 5-minute increments. By setting the delay period, the REMstar® Plus CPAP system calculates a linear pressure slope to achieve the desired pressure setting. The pressure increases gradually until the set pressure is reached at the end of the delay period. Many patients are more comfortable as the pressure gradually ramps to the set level. The ramp feature is activated by depressing the ramp switch and then depressing the pressure on/off switch until the desired setting is displayed in the LED window.

Phase Variable

Baseline Variable

The baseline variable for the REMstar® Plus CPAP system is pressure.

ASSEMBLY AND TROUBLESHOOTING

Assembly—REMstar® Plus

1. Connect the CPAP system to a suitable AC power source. Either 120 v, 60 Hz or 220–230 v, 50–60 Hz electrical power may be used.

2. Assemble the patient circuit:
   a. Connect a Sanders® CPAP valve to the patient circuit. Alternatively, the Whisper swivel may be used.
   b. Connect the opposite end of the patient tubing to the outlet of the REMstar® Plus.
   c. Connect either nasal pillows or a nasal mask to the distal end of the tubing.
   d. Connect a spacer to the top of the mask and adjust the spacer/mask

   assembly to fit the patient using the headgear.

3. Adjust the CPAP pressure to the prescribed level using the CPAP adjustment control on the unit. CPAP pressures should be titrated for each individual patient based upon the results of a polysomnographic sleep study.

4. Turn on the unit by pressing the on/off switch on the right front of the control panel.

Troubleshooting

Use the troubleshooting algorithm at the end of this chapter to assist you with troubleshooting problems associated with intermittent CPAP systems.

BI-LEVEL POSITIVE AIRWAY PRESSURE SYSTEMS

Bi-level positive airway pressure systems are similar to CPAP systems except that two pressure levels are delivered. One pressure is delivered during inspiration (inspiratory positive airway pressure, or IPAP), which is greater; and the other during exhalation (expiratory positive airway pressure, or EPAP), which is less. By applying a lower pressure during exhalation (EPAP), the patient exhales against a lower resistance, which many find more comfortable. Bi-level positive airway pressure ventilators sense inspiration and expiration by monitoring flow, and therefore are flow triggered and flow cycled.

PURITAN-BENNETT KNIGHTSTAR® 330 BI-LEVEL VENTILATOR

The Puritan-Bennett KnightStar® 330 Bi-Level® Ventilator is a bi-level positive airway pressure ventilator system (Figure 11-24). As described earlier, a practitioner may adjust two independent pressures IPAP (inspiratory) and EPAP (expiratory). The bi-level positive airway pressure ventilator is an electrically powered pressure controller, which is flow triggered and flow cycled. The KnightStar® 330 Bi-Level® Ventilator also incorporates a delay feature similar to the KnightStar® 330 Nasal CPAP System, allowing a gradual ramping of pressure to the preset level for patient comfort.

Input Power

The input power for the KnightStar® 330 Bi-Level® Ventilator is AC electrical power. The unit may be operated from 120 v, 60 Hz (domestic) or 220–230 v, 50–60 Hz (international) AC power by adjusting a selector switch on the rear of the ventilator.

Control Circuit

The control circuit of the KnightStar® 330 Bi-Level® Ventilator consists of an electrically powered fan and an adjustable pressure controlling valve. As IPAP and EPAP pressures are adjusted using controls on the bottom of the ventilator, the pressure controlling valve opens or closes, creating the threshold resistance required against the fan to create the desired pressure levels. A flow transducer senses changes in flow to the patient.

When inspiration begins, flow is high, signaling the beginning of a breath. When flow tapers to a level lower than the leak threshold, IPAP delivery ceases and inspiration ends.

If supplemental oxygen is desired, it may be bled into the desired concentration by using an oxygen adapter between the CPAP system outlet and the patient tubing. Oxygen flow from the oxygen source is then adjusted until the desired concentration is verified using an oxygen analyzer.

Control Variable

The control variable for the KnightStar® 330 Bi-Level® Ventilator is pressure. Pressures are adjusted using the IPAP and exhale EPAP pressure controls on the bottom of the ventilator. Both pressures are adjustable between 3 and 30 cmH_2O. The EPAP control must always be set to a lower pressure than the IPAP control. Adjustment of the pressure control causes the pressure control valve to open or close changing the threshold resistance.

The delay/ramp feature allows the inspiratory pressure to be ramped over a period of

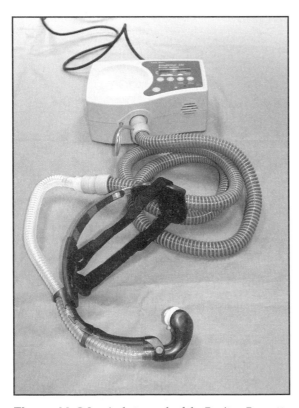

Figure 11-24 *A photograph of the Puritan-Bennett KnightStar® 330 Bi-Level Respiratory System.*

time. Many patients find it difficult to go to sleep with the bi-level positive airway pressure system set with IPAP at the prescribed pressure. The delay/ramp control may be set between 5 and 30 minutes, in 5-minute increments. Once the delay time has passed (presumably the patient has reached stage II sleep), the unit will automatically increase the pressure to the set pressure level at a rate of 1, 2, or 3 cmH$_2$O per minute. Many patients are more comfortable as the pressure gradually ramps to the set level. The delay/ramp feature is activated by using the settings button and depressing the delay/ramp button to decrease pressure and the alarm silence button to increase pressures to the desired settings for the delay/ramp period.

Phase Variables

Trigger Variable

As already described, the trigger variable is flow. Changes in flow sensed by the flow transducer signal the start and end of inspiration. The trigger sensitivity may be adjusted using two controls located on the back of the unit. Both inspiratory and expiratory sensitivity may be adjusted to better match the patient's spontaneous ventilatory efforts. These controls are labeled inhale and exhale.

Limit Variable

The limit variable is pressure. Once inspiration begins, pressure rises to a preset level and is maintained at that level until the end of inspiration. The pressure level reached is established using the IPAP control on the rear of the ventilator.

Cycle Variable

The cycle variable is flow. Once inspiratory flow decays to a level less than the leak threshold, pressure falls from the IPAP level to the EPAP level.

Baseline Variable

The baseline variable is pressure and it is set using the EPAP control on the rear of the ventilator. Once inspiration ends, the delivered pressure falls to the EPAP level and is maintained at that level until the next breath is sensed.

ASSEMBLY AND TROUBLESHOOTING

Assembly— KnightStar® 330 Bi-Level® Ventilator Respiratory System

1. Connect the CPAP system to a suitable AC power source. Either 120 v, 60 Hz or 220–230 v, 50–60 Hz electrical power may be used.

2. Connect the patient tubing to the outlet of the CPAP system.

3. Attach either nasal pillows or a nasal mask to the outlet of the patient tubing.

4. Adjust the pressure levels:
   a. IPAP pressure is adjustable between 3 and 30 cmH$_2$O using the IPAP control on the rear of the ventilator.
   b. Set the EPAP pressure (3 to 30 cmH$_2$O) using the EPAP control on the rear of the ventilator.

5. Turn on the unit:
   a. Depress the on button on the control panel.
   b. If a ramp pressure delay is desired:
      (1) Set the delay time using the delay control on the rear of the ventilator (5 to 30 minutes).
      (2) Set the ramp rate (1, 2, or 3 cmH$_2$O/minute).
      (3) Activate the delay feature by depressing the delay control on the front control panel.

Troubleshooting

Use the troubleshooting algorithm at the end of this chapter to assist you with troubleshooting problems associated with intermittent bi-level positive airway pressure systems.

RESPIRONICS, INC., BIPAP® SYNCHRONY™ VENTILATORY SUPPORT SYSTEM

The BiPAP® Synchrony™ ventilatory support system is designed to augment a patient's breathing by providing positive pressure through the breathing circuit. It is an electrically powered ventilator support system with electronic pressure control (Figure 11-25). The BiPAP® Synchrony™ ventilatory support system is a flow pressure controller that is flow or pressure triggered and flow or time cycled. The ventilator can operate in Spontaneous (S), CPAP, Spontaneous/Timed (S/T), Timed (T), or Pressure Control (PC) modes.

Input Power

The BiPAP® Synchrony™ ventilatory support system is electrically powered using either 100–110 v or 220–240 v 50–60 Hz AC power. The electrical power drives the blower drive mechanism and powers the electronic control circuit.

Control Circuit

The control circuit of the BiPAP® Synchrony™ ventilatory support system consists of an electrically powered fan, an adjustable pressure controlling valve, and flow and pressure transducers. IPAP and EPAP pressures are adjusted using the up/down arrow keys and the LED screen display. The pressure control valve opens or closes, creating the threshold resistance against the fan to create the desired pressure levels. Feedback from the flow and pressure transducers are used by the microprocessor to control the pressure control valve.

Control Variable

The control variable of the BiPAP® Synchrony™ ventilatory support system is pressure. Pressures are adjustable between 4 to 30 cmH$_2$O (IPAP), 4 to 15 cmH$_2$O (EPAP), and 4 to 20 cmH$_2$O (CPAP). Adjustment of the pressure control valve adjusts the closure of the pressure control valve, which regulates the pressure in the patient circuit.

The BiPAP® Synchrony™ ventilatory support system has a ramp feature that gradually increases the inspiratory pressures over time. The ramp settings can be adjusted between 0.5, 1.0, 2.0, and 3.0 cmH$_2$O per breath. Pressure is slowly increased at the set pressure increase per breath until the desired IPAP pressure is obtained.

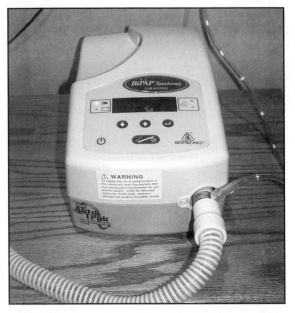

Figure 11-25 *A photograph of the BiPAP® Synchrony™ ventilatory support system.*

Phase Variables
Trigger Variables

The trigger variables for the BiPAP® Synchrony™ ventilatory support system are volume and flow. Volume triggering is automatically adjusted to 6 mL of volume above the baseline leak in the circuit. When inspired volume exceeds this trigger threshold, inspiration begins.

Inspiratory and expiratory flows are continuously monitored. The patient's flow pattern is offset or delayed by 15 L/min and 300 msec from the actual flow pattern. When the patient's actual flow varies from the delayed flow (shadow or signal shape), the flows "cross over" and inspiration begins (Figure 11-7). The shape signal provides an alternative to pressure or volume sensing to trigger inspiration.

Limit Variable

The limit variable for the BiPAP® Synchrony™ ventilatory support system is pressure. Pressure is adjusted by means of the inspiratory positive airway pressure (IPAP) and expiratory positive airway pressure (EPAP) controls. Adjustment of the controls varies both inspiratory and expiratory pressures, which may be set independently of one another.

Inspiratory pressures are adjustable between 4 to 30 cmH$_2$O in 1-cmH$_2$O increments. The pressure set is monitored by the proximal airway pressure transducer and is maintained in the circuit during inspiration.

Expiratory pressures are adjustable between 4 and 15 cmH$_2$O in 1-cmH$_2$O increments (EPAP) and 4 and 20 cmH$_2$O in 1-cmH$_2$O increments (CPAP). Pressure in the patient circuit is monitored during exhalation, and excess flow is exhausted into the ambient air, maintaining the desired expiratory pressure in the circuit.

Cycle Variables

The cycle variables for the ventilator are flow and time. As described previously in the "trigger variables" section, inspiratory flow is continuously monitored. The actual measured flow is "shadowed" by 15 L/min and 300 msec behind the actual flow. When the flow between measured and the shadow or shape changes, the ventilator cycles into exhalation (Figure 11-7).

A second method of flow monitoring is used during the spontaneous/timed mode to end inspiration. An electronic flow signal is generated that is proportional to the inspiratory flow signal. When the inspiratory flow level reaches the electronic signal (spontaneous expiratory threshold), exhalation begins (Figure 11-8).

Time is a cycle variable during timed inspiration. When the timed inspiration soft key is depressed, it may be adjusted between 0.5 to 3.0 seconds. Once that time interval has passed, exhalation begins.

Baseline Variable

The baseline variable for the BiPAP® Synchrony™ ventilatory support system is pressure. Baseline pressures CPAP and EPAP are adjustable between 4 and 20 cmH$_2$O and 4 and 15 cmH$_2$O, respectively.

Alarm Systems

Input Power

In the event of loss of electrical power, the BiPAP® Synchrony™ ventilatory support system will activate a continuous audible alarm for two minutes.

Control Circuit

In the event of an internal failure, an alarm will sound in single beeps until power is removed from the unit. The only way to silence the alarm is to disconnect the power cord from the AC power supply.

Output Alarms

Pressure. The BiPAP® Synchrony™ ventilatory support system has a high-pressure, low-pressure, and low-pressure support alarms. The high pressure alarm is activated when the circuit pressure exceeds the set pressure by 5 cmH$_2$O for 0.5 seconds. The alarm is terminated when the pressure is within the 5-cmH$_2$O setting window for more than 0.5 seconds.

The low-pressure alarm is caused by the circuit pressure falling by more than 5 cmH$_2$O for 0.5 seconds. Like the high-pressure alarm, the low-pressure alarm will correct itself if the pressure increases above the 5-cmH$_2$O threshold for more than 0.5 seconds.

ASSEMBLY AND TROUBLESHOOTING

Assembly—Respironics, Inc., BiPAP® Synchrony™ Ventilatory Support System

1. Install the inlet air filter on the rear of the ventilator.

2. Assemble and attach the patient circuit.

3. Connect the power cord to the rear of the ventilator and connect it to an appropriate AC power source. Either 120 v, 60 Hz or 220–230 v, 50–60 Hz electrical power may be used.

4. Connect the patient interface to the circuit using a mask or nasal pillows.

5. Set the pressure levels:
   a. IPAP may be set between 4 to 30 cmH$_2$O in 2-cmH$_2$O increments.

   b. EPAP may be set between 4 and 15 cmH$_2$O in 2-cmH$_2$O increments.

6. Turn on the unit:
   a. Depress the Standby key on the control panel.
   b. If a ramp pressure delay is desired:
      (1) Activate the delay feature by depressing the delay control on the front control panel.

Troubleshooting

Use the troubleshooting algorithm at the end of this chapter to assist you with troubleshooting problems associated with intermittent bi-level positive airway pressure systems.

The low-pressure support alarm is activated using the following formula:

Press. Support Setting − Measured Press. Support > 2 cmH₂O for 60 seconds continuously

The alarm will be terminated once the measured pressure support falls below the 2-cmH₂O window for 5 seconds or more.

Flow. A low minute volume alarm will be activated if the minute volume falls below the setting established by the practitioner for this alarm.

Time. The BiPAP® Synchrony™ ventilatory support system has an apnea alarm that will be activated if the time between spontaneous breaths exceeds the setting on the apnea alarm. The alarm will reset itself after two consecutive spontaneous breaths.

TRANSPORT VENTILATORS

Transport ventilators are commonly used for ground, airborne, and intrahospital patient transports. Examples of intrahospital transports include moving the patient from the emergency room to ICU or transporting the patient from ICU to CT scan, MRI scan, or fluoroscopy for special procedures. As a practitioner, you should understand how these ventilators operate, how controls function, and how these ventilators differ in their capabilities and operation from conventional critical care adult and pediatric ventilators.

AMBU, INC., TRANSCARE 2

Ambu, Inc., markets the TransCARE 2 portable, pneumatically-powered, transport ventilator, which incorporates an electronic monitoring system (Figure 11-26). The Trans-CARE 2 ventilator has many similarities to the Omni-Vent ventilator (described later in this chapter). The ventilator is pneumatically powered and controlled. It is a flow controller that is pressure or time triggered, pressure or flow limited, and time cycled. It may be operated in volume control, pressure control, IMV (volume or pressure controlled modes), and CPAP modes.

Figure 11-26 *A photograph of the Ambu, Inc., TransCARE 2 Ventilator. (Courtesy Ambu, Inc.)*

Input Power

The TransCARE 2 is pneumatically powered and controlled. A medical gas source of between 25 and 140 psi may be used to power the ventilator. A 50-psi source is the recommended pressure. However, if desired, the ventilator may be calibrated to run at lower pressures (25 psi) to utilize liquid systems, which may be desirable in some situations, or higher pressure sources (140 psi), which may be used for the TransCARE 1-HB for hyperbaric clinical applications.

The electronic monitoring system may be powered by an internal "AAA" battery pack (350 hours), or an external 12- to 24-V DC power source. Additionally, an optional AC power adapter may be purchased to utilize commercial AC power.

Control Circuit

Gas to power the ventilator enters through a filter in the gas inlet assembly (Figure 11-27). It then passes through an on/off valve in the same assembly and on to the inspiratory-and-expiratory valve block. From the inspiratory/expiratory valve block, the gas is conducted to a flow accelerator and then to a flow control valve. From the flow control valve, the gas flow is split, with one path flowing to a pressure relief valve and patient circuit and the other path flowing to the exhalation valve diaphragm.

PEEP/CPAP may be added using an external threshold resistor valve attached to the patient circuit. PEEP/CPAP pressures of between 0 and 20 cmH₂O may be added using the external valve.

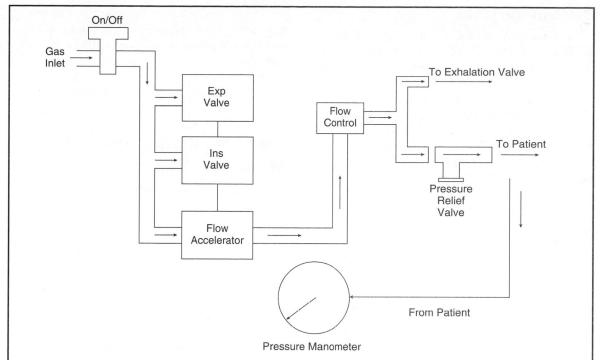

INSPIRATORY PHASE

Source gas is introduced through a filter in the gas inlet assembly; then gas flows to the pneumatic valve supply inlet. The gas flows to the flow control, then to the tee assembly which directs gas simultaneously to the exhalation valve and pressure relief valve to the patient.

As gas pressure increases in the lung, it is transmitted to the manometer through a tubing independent from the tubing wye connector.

EXPIRATORY PHASE

Source gas follows the identical path of the inspiratory phase to the pneumatic valves and is then held until the inspiratory phase begins.

Figure 11-27 *A schematic diagram of the Ambu, Inc., TransCARE 2 Ventilator during inspiration and expiration. (Courtesy Ambu, Inc.)*

Control Variable

The control variable for the TransCARE 2 ventilator is flow, which is determined by the flow control valve. Flow rates may be adjusted between 0 and 85 L/min. The flow control valve is a variable orifice needle valve. Opening or closing the valve regulates the flow of gas through it. Since flow is constant, volume delivery becomes a function of inspiratory flow and inspiratory time (volume is equal to flow multiplied by time).

Phase Variables

Trigger Variables

The trigger variables include pressure and time. Pressure is a trigger variable during IMV ventilation. When inspiratory effort is sufficient to open a one-way valve in the IMV reservoir, gas is delivered to the patient. An IMV flow rate may be adjusted from 0 to 60 L/min by using the IMV flow knob (needle valve) on the left front of the control panel. IMV gas flows out of the ventilator via the nipple on the left side of the ventilator.

Time is the control variable for volume- and pressure-controlled ventilation, as well as the mandatory portion of IMV. The expiratory time control acts as a rate control. The expiratory valve is a needle valve, which controls the rate of gas leakage through a timing cartridge. If gas flow leaking from the cartridge is high, expiratory time is less. Conversely, if gas leakage is slow, expiratory time is longer. Respiratory rates are adjustable between 0 and 150 breaths per minute.

Limit Variables

The limit variables for the TransCARE 2 include pressure and flow. Pressure becomes a limit variable if the pressure relief valve is set lower than the peak inspiratory pressure for a given inspiratory time and flow rate. Under these circumstances, pressure will rise to the pressure limit setting and plateau until the inspiratory time has elapsed with the ventilator operating in pressure control mode. The pressure limit may be adjusted between 0 and 120 cmH$_2$O.

The ventilator may also be flow limited. If the flow rate is set at a lower setting and inspiratory time is set such that flow increases and plateaus, the ventilator is then flow limited.

Cycle Variable

The cycle variable for the ventilator is time. Inspiratory time is determined by the inspira-

tory time needle valve. The control, like the expiratory time control, is a pneumatic timing cartridge. Adjustment of the needle valve controls the rate of gas leakage from the cartridge, which either lengthens or shortens inspiratory time. Inspiratory times may be adjusted between 0.2 and 2.0 seconds.

Alarm/Monitoring Systems

Monitoring System

The TransCARE 2 incorporates a compact electronic monitoring and alarm package into its design. The monitoring/alarm system measures pressure in the patient circuit and can integrate that electronic pressure signal over time. All data is displayed on a back-lit LCD displaying both a circular bar graph and alphanumeric data. The monitoring capability is summarized in Table 11-10.

Control Circuit Alarms

The TransCARE 2 incorporates a failure-to-cycle alarm into its alarm system. If the ventilator fails to cycle, the alarm will be activated.

Output Alarms

Pressure. Both high- and low-pressure alarms are incorporated in the alarm system. The high-pressure alarm alerts the practitioner to pressures that exceed the alarm setting. The alarm may be set between −10 and 120 cmH$_2$O. The low-pressure alarm may be set between (−0 and 120 cmH$_2$O.) The low-pressure alarm is helpful in detecting leaks and patient disconnect situations.

A leak detection alarm may also be used in addition to the low-pressure alarm. The leak detection alarm is an adjustable pressure alarm that may be set between 0 and 10 cmH$_2$O below the high-pressure alarm, independent of the low-pressure alarm.

Tables 11-11 and 11-12 summarize the TransCARE 2 ventilator's capabilities and alarm systems.

TABLE 11-10 TransCARE 2 Monitoring Systems

Pressure	−10 to 120 cmH$_2$O
Respiratory Rate	4 to 400 BPM
Inspiratory Time	0.01 to 10 seconds
Expiratory Time	0.01 to 60 seconds
I:E Ratio	2:1 to 1:99

TABLE 11-11 TransCARE 2 Ventilator Capabilities

Modes	Volume and Pressure Control, IMV, CPAP
Tidal Volume	0 to 2,000 mL
Respiratory Rate	0 to 150 BPM
Inspiratory Time	0.2 to 2 seconds
Expiratory Time	0.2 to 60 seconds
Flow Rate	0 to 85 L/min
IMV Flow Rate	0 to 60 L/min
Pressure Relief	0 to 120 cmH_2O
PEEP/CPAP	0 to 20 cmH_2O (external threshold resistor)

TABLE 11-12 TransCARE 2 Alarm Systems

Control Circuit

Failure to Cycle

Output

High Pressure	-10 to 120 cmH_2O
Low Pressure	-10 to 120 cmH_2O
Leak Detection	0 to 10 cmH_2O below high pressure

ASSEMBLY AND TROUBLESHOOTING

Assembly—TransCARE 2

To prepare the Ambu, Inc., TransCARE 2 for use, follow the suggested assembly guide.

1. Select a power source for the monitoring/alarm system:
   a. Internal "AAA" battery pack.
   b. External 12- to 24-V DC source.
   c. AC power adapter.
2. Connect the ventilator to a medical gas source (25 to 140 psi). If an F_IO_2 of less than 1.0 is desired, the ventilator may be powered from a blender operating from independent sources of medical air and oxygen.
3. Assemble the patient circuit:
   a. Connect one end of the 22-mm diameter patient circuit to the ventilator outlet.
   b. Connect the patient manifold assembly to the distal end of the 22-mm diameter patient circuit.
   c. Connect one end of the 1/8-inch diameter line to the exhalation valve nipple on the side of the ventilator and the other end to the exhalation valve on the patient manifold assembly.
   d. Connect the other 1/8-inch diameter line between the airway pressure nipple on the ventilator and the proximal airway tap on the patient manifold.
   e. Connect a 6-inch flextube to the patient manifold assembly and attach a mask adapter or tracheostomy adapter to the distal end to interface with the patient airway.
4. Turn on the gas supply and calibrate the ventilator by depressing the blue "*" switch on the side of the ventilator. Next press and hold the two gray up/down keys on the monitor simultaneously to calibrate the ventilator and set the zero. Once the word "calibrate" and "0000.00" appear on the display, the ventilator has been calibrated.
5. Confirm the ventilator's operation:
   a. Connect the patient circuit to a test lung and rotate the on/off switch to the on position.
   b. Adjust flow, inspiratory, and expiratory time to the desired settings.
   c. Confirm rate and volume delivery using a Wright respirometer or other volume-measuring device and a watch.
   d. Occlude the patient circuit and adjust the pressure relief valve to the desired pressure.

Troubleshooting

To assist you in troubleshooting the TransCARE 2 ventilator, refer to the troubleshooting algorithm at the end of this chapter.

BIO-MED DEVICES CROSSVENT 4

The Bio-Med Devices Crossvent 4 is an electronically controlled, electrically powered (battery or AC) ventilator (Figure 11-28). It may be operated in control, assist/control, SIMV, CPAP, pressure support, and pressure-limited, time-cycled ventilation modes. The ventilator is a flow controller that is pressure, time, or manually triggered; pressure or flow limited; and pressure, volume, or time cycled.

Input Power

The electronic control circuit is powered by either an internal battery (up to 11 hours' operation when the LCD back-light is used for approximately 1 of the 11 hours), external battery, or AC power source (120 or 220 volts). When using external power sources, the electrical power should be connected to the left side of the ventilator, utilizing the factory supplied plug.

The pneumatic systems of the ventilator require a compressed gas source of between 44 and 66 psi (55 psi average). An external blender may be used to mix air and oxygen to the desired F_IO_2.

Control Circuit

Gas enters the ventilator through a DISS inlet fitting via a 40-micron inlet filter and on to an internal pressure regulator. The pressure regulator drops the inlet pressure to approximately 20 psi (Figure 11-29). From the regulator, the gas flows to a solenoid-controlled, two-way pilot valve. From the pilot valve, gas flows to an electronically-controlled solenoid valve. The solenoid valve position is controlled by a needle valve. Since inlet pressure is constant (20 psi) and outlet pressure is negli-

Figure 11-28 *A photograph of the Bio-Med Devices, Inc., Crossvent 4 Ventilator.*

gible (patient pressure), the flow rate through the valve is solely a function of the size of the valve's orifice. Maximum flow from the ventilator is dependent upon the gas supply pressure (from 120 L/min at 55 psi to 100 L/min at 45 psi). Gas is delivered from the flow control valve to the patient circuit.

During gas delivery to the patient through the flow control valve, gas flows through another solenoid valve to pressurize the diaphragm of the exhalation valve. During exhalation, gas pressure may be partially removed from the exhalation valve, creating PEEP/CPAP pressure.

Control Variable

The control variable of the Crossvent 4 is flow, which is controlled by the orifice size of the flow control valve. The position of the flow control valve (orifice size) is relayed to the electronic control circuit by a precision potentiometer connected to the flow rate's needle valve. Volume delivery is a function of flow (L/sec) multiplied by inspiratory time.

Phase Variables

Trigger Variables

The trigger variables of the Crossvent 4 include pressure, time, and manual triggering. Pressure triggering is adjusted using the inspiratory effort control. Pressure triggering may be adjusted from 0 to 10 cmH_2O below baseline pressure (PEEP or atmospheric). Pressure triggering will not function during time-cycled, pressure-limited ventilation or at respiratory rates greater than 60 breaths per minute.

Time triggering is a variable used during assist/control, the mandatory portion of SIMV, and time-cycled, pressure-limited ventilation. Time triggering is established by using the rate control. Respiratory rates of between 5 and 150 breaths per minute may be set.

Manual triggering is accomplished by depressing the manual screen button. Doing so delivers a manual breath at the set rate, tidal volume, and inspiratory time. This control is only operational in the CPAP mode.

Limit Variables

The Crossvent 4 may be pressure or flow limited. The ventilator is pressure limited in the infant mode (pressure-limited, time-cycled ventilation). The pressure limit is set using the maximum pressure control. Pressure is adjustable between 0 and 120 cmH_2O.

Figure 11-29 *A schematic diagram of the Bio-Med Devices, Inc., Crossvent-4 pneumatic system. (Courtesy Bio-Med Devices, Inc., Guilford, CT)*

Flow becomes a limit variable when the inspiratory flow rate is adjusted low enough that the ventilator reaches that flow and plateaus during inspiration while in volume control ventilation. Flow is also a limit variable during pressure-limited, time-cycled ventilation.

Cycle Variables

Cycle variables of the Crossvent 4 include pressure, volume, and time. Pressure becomes a cycle variable when the pressure exceeds that set by the high-peak pressure alarm limit (adjustable between 1 and 120 cmH$_2$O). When this pressure value is reached, inspiration is terminated and the alarm sounds. This feature is not operative during time-cycled, pressure-limited ventilation.

Volume is a cycle variable during sigh breath delivery (CMV mode). When depressed, a sigh breath of 1.5 times the tidal volume is delivered (up to 2,500 mL) for every 100 mandatory breaths.

Time is a cycle variable during infant ventilation (time-cycled, pressure-limited ventilation). Inspiratory time is adjustable between 0.1 and 1.5 seconds.

Alarm Systems

Input Power Alarms

While operating on the ventilator's internal battery, an alarm will sound and the indication "BATT LOW" will be displayed when approximately 20 minutes of battery power remain. Additionally, a bar graph continuously displays battery power remaining, decreasing in 20% increments.

Control Circuit Alarms

I:E Ratio Alarm. The Crossvent 4 incorporates an I:E ratio alarm, which will flash and audibly sound when the I:E ratio is greater than 3:1, inspiratory time is greater than 3 seconds or less than 0.1 seconds, or expiratory time is less than 0.2 seconds. The alarm can be permanently silenced only by changing the ventilation parameters or by correcting the I:E ratio or the inspiratory or expiratory time.

ASSEMBLY AND TROUBLESHOOTING

Assembly—Bio-Med Devices, Inc., Crossvent 4

1. Connect a 50-psi gas source to the ventilator using the DISS fitting on the ventilator's right-hand side.

2. If using an external power source or AC power, connect the external power connector to its receptacle on the left side of the ventilator.

3. Assemble the patient circuit for use:
   a. Attach the exhalation valve manifold to the 22-mm, large-diameter tubing.
   b. Attach a 6-inch piece of 22-mm, large-diameter tubing to the patient outlet side of the exhalation valve manifold, securing a mask adapter or elbow fitting to interface with the patient's airway.
   c. Attach the exhalation valve drive line to the exhalation valve and the proximal pressure monitoring line to the circuit.
   d. If the optional pneumotachometer is used, use a standard patient wye fitting to interface with the patient's airway and connect the pneumotachometer to the expiratory side of the wye, between the wye and the exhalation valve assembly.
   e. Connect the exhalation valve drive line, proximal airway pressure line, and pneumotachometer lines to their respective fittings on the left side of the ventilator.

Troubleshooting

To assist you in troubleshooting the ventilator, follow the troubleshooting algorithm at the conclusion of this chapter.

Output Alarms

Pressure. The Crossvent 4 has a peak pressure alarm, which is adjustable between 0 and 125 cmH$_2$O. During sigh breath delivery, the peak pressure alarm is automatically increased by 1.5 times the display setting, to a maximum of 125 cmH$_2$O.

A mean airway pressure alarm may be used to alert the practitioner of changes in the mean airway pressure. Pressures may be adjusted between 0 and 125 cmH$_2$O. Both high- and low-pressure limits may be established.

The PEEP/CPAP pressure alarm has high and low limits, which may be adjusted between 0 and 99 cmH$_2$O. In the event of a loss of PEEP/CPAP pressure, the alarm will flash and an audible alarm will sound.

Volume. The Crossvent 4 may be equipped with an optional exhaled tidal volume alarm. The alarm is adjustable between 0 and 2,500 mL. The ventilator must be configured with an external pneumotachometer, which is accurate between 200 and 2,500 mL and at flows from 13 to 140 L/min. Both high and low parameters may be set when using this alarm.

Flow. The Crossvent 4 may be purchased with an optional minute ventilation alarm for use when using the external pneumotachometer. Alarm limits may be adjusted between 0 and 200 L/min. Both upper and lower minute volume limits may be set.

Time. The Crossvent 4 ventilator incorporates a high breath rate alarm, which is adjustable between 0 and 199 breaths per minute.

Inspired Gas. When equipped with the optional oxygen sensor, the Crossvent 4 can alert the practitioner to changes in oxygen delivery. Both high and low alarm limits may be set between 21 and 100%. Tables 11-13 and 11-14 summarize the Crossvent 4 ventilator's capabilities and alarm systems.

TABLE 11-13 Crossvent 4 Transport Ventilator Capabilities

Modes	Assist/Control, SIMV, CPAP, Pressure Support, and Time-Cycled, Pressure-Limited Ventilation
Rate	5 to 150 BPM
Flow	1 to 120 L/min
Pressure Limit	1 to 120 cmH$_2$O
Pressure Support	0 to 50 cmH$_2$O
PEEP/CPAP	0 to 35 cmH$_2$O
Inspiratory Time	0.1 to 1.5 seconds
Tidal Volume	5 to 2,500 mL
Sensitivity	−1 to −10 cmH$_2$O
Sigh	1.5 times the tidal volume every 100th breath

TABLE 11-14 Crossvent 4 Transport Ventilator Alarm Systems

Input Power

Low Battery

Control Circuit

I:E Ratio

Output Alarms

Pressure	
High Pressure	0 to 125 cmH$_2$O
Low Pressure	0 to 125 cmH$_2$O
Mean Airway Pressure	0 to 125 cmH$_2$O
PEEP/CPAP Pressure	0 to 99 cmH$_2$O
Volume	
Exhaled Tidal Volume	0 to 2,500 mL
Flow	
Exhaled Minute Volume	0 to 200 L/min
Time	
Breath Rate	0 to 199 BPM
Inspired Gas Alarm	
Oxygen Percent	21 to 100%

BIRD PRODUCTS CORPORATION, AVIAN™

The Avian™ Transport Ventilator is a microprocessor-controlled, battery-powered ventilator (Figure 11-30). It is capable of operating in control, assist/control, SIMV, and CPAP modes. The ventilator is a flow controller, which is pressure or time triggered, pressure or flow limited, and pressure, volume (in sigh mode), or time cycled.

Input Power

The microprocessor control system of the Avian™ Transport Ventilator is powered by an internal, rechargeable, 6-volt DC battery. The ventilator may also be powered by a 120/230-volt AC power source using an external power adapter supplied with the ventilator. Additionally, the ventilator may be powered from an external 11- to 30-volt DC power source. An automotive-style cigarette lighter power cord is also supplied with the ventilator.

Gas to the pneumatic system must be provided between 40 and 60 psi. A blender may be used to mix air and oxygen to the desired F_IO_2. The ventilator does not have a blender incorporated into its design.

Control Circuit

Gas enters the ventilator through a DISS gas inlet port. The gas then flows through a pressure regulator, where pressure is reduced to 30 psi (Figure 11-31). From the pressure regulator, gas is conducted to a main and a demand solenoid valve. Gas flow from the main solenoid valve passes through the flow control valve and a check valve to the patient circuit. Gas flow from the demand solenoid passes through a fixed orifice and then to the patient circuit.

A potentiometer is attached to the poppet of the flow control valve to sense the valve's position. Valve position is directly proportional to flow. The mass flow through the valve is unaffected by downstream pressures of up to 3 psig or 210 cmH$_2$O.

PEEP/CPAP pressure is generated by a user adjustable manual PEEP valve. PEEP pressures may be adjusted between 0 and 20 cmH$_2$O.

Control Variable

The control variable for the Avian™ Transport Ventilator is flow. Flow is directly proportional to valve position and is sensed by a potentiometer attached to the flow control valve's poppet. The feedback signal from the potentiometer (valve position) is used by the microprocessor to calculate tidal volume delivery (volume equals flow multiplied by time). Mass flow through the valve is not affected by back pressure in the patient circuit up to a pressure of 3 psig or 210 cmH$_2$O.

Figure 11-30 *A photograph of the Bird Avian™ transport ventilator. (Courtesy Bird Products Corporation)*

Figure 11-31 *A schematic diagram of the Bird Products Corporation Bird Avian's™ pneumatic system. (Courtesy Bird Products Corporation)*

Phase Variables

Trigger Variables

The trigger variables for the Avian™ include pressure, time, and manual triggering. Pressure is a trigger variable during assist/control, SIMV (spontaneous breaths), and CPAP modes. Inspiratory pressure is sensed in the patient circuit by a pressure transducer. The electronic signal is used as a feedback signal to the microprocessor to initiate a breath or open the demand valve. Trigger sensitivity may be adjusted between −2 and −8 cmH$_2$O.

Time is a trigger variable during control mode, assist/control mode (in the absence of spontaneous efforts), and during the mandatory portion of SIMV. The breath rate control is used to set the respiratory rate and time triggering. Respiratory rates may be adjusted between 0 and 150 breaths per minute.

The ventilator is manually triggered if the practitioner depresses the manual breath button. When depressed, the ventilator delivers a mandatory breath at the set volume and inspiratory flow rate or at the set inspiratory time and flow rate.

Limit Variables

The limit variables include pressure and flow. Pressure becomes a limit variable if the pressure relief valve is adjusted to a pressure lower than the peak inspiratory pressure for the set tidal volume. Under these conditions, the inspiratory pressure reaches a plateau (pressure relief limit) and is held until the inspiratory time ends. Pressure relief is adjustable between 10 and 100 cmH$_2$O.

Flow may become a limit variable if the inspiratory flow is adjusted such that the flow reaches the control's set value and plateaus, delivering a square waveflow pattern.

Cycle Variables

The cycle variables for the Avian™ Transport Ventilator include pressure, volume, and time. Pressure becomes a cycle variable if the peak inspiratory pressure exceeds the value set on the peak inspiratory pressure control. Peak inspiratory pressure is adjustable between 1 and 100 cmH$_2$O. If the pressure limit is reached, inspiratory flow is terminated, the exhalation valve opens, and an audible and visual alarm will result.

Volume becomes a cycle variable when sigh breath delivery is selected. When sighs are activated, a sigh breath equal to 1.5 times the current tidal volume setting (2,000 mL maximum volume) or 1.5 times the current inspiratory time setting (maximum of 3.0 seconds), will be delivered every 100th breath or every 7 minutes, whichever occurs first. The high-pressure limit and inspiratory time are automatically increased by 1.5 times when a sigh breath is delivered, up to a maximum value of 100 cmH$_2$O pressure limit and 3.0 seconds inspiratory time.

Time becomes a cycle variable when the ventilator is in time cycled mode. Under these circumstances, inspiration ends when the inspiratory time has elapsed. Inspiratory time is adjustable between 0.1 and 3.0 seconds or until an I:E ratio of 1:1 is reached.

Alarm Systems

Input Power Alarms

Battery Low/Fail. In the event that no external power is applied and the internal battery is less than 5.6 volts ±0.2 volts, the "Battery Low/Fail" LED will be illuminated on the front panel. The alarm may be silenced for 5-minute intervals.

External Power Low/Fail. In the event that an external power source is out of range, the ventilator automatically switches to the internal battery and activates the "External Power Low/Fail" LED on the front control panel. This alarm may be silenced until the internal battery voltage falls to 5.6 volts, activating the Battery Low/Fail alarm.

Control Circuit Alarms

Ventilator Inoperative. Ventilator inoperative alarms may be classified into recoverable and nonrecoverable conditions. A recoverable alarm will occur if external power is interrupted and the internal battery is low, the mode switch is momentarily set to the off position, or the power supply voltages are out of range. Once the condition has been corrected, the ventilator will return to normal operation.

Nonrecoverable conditions occur if the microprocessor or control system fails a self-check. Under these conditions, the ventilator ceases to operate; however, the antisuffocation valve and exhalation valve are designed to allow a patient to spontaneously breathe from the ambient air.

I:E Ratio. If the inspiratory time exceeds 50% of the total breath period (inspiratory plus expiratory time), the I:E alarm flashes and inspiration is limited to 50% of the total breath time. This alarm alerts the practitioner to inspiratory time and tidal volume, or flow and breath rate control settings, which result in this condition.

Disconnect. If the airway pressure fails to rise at least 2 cmH$_2$O above the initial inspiratory pressure (baseline) during a breath period (inspiratory plus expiratory time), both audible and visual alarms will result.

Output Alarms

Pressure. As already described, the Avian™ incorporates a high peak pressure alarm. This alarm is adjustable between 1 and 100 cmH$_2$O and results in the termination of inspiration and an audible and visual alarm condition.

The Avian™ also has a low peak pressure alarm. This alarm has an off position and is adjustable between 2 and 50 cmH$_2$O. When activated, both an audible and a visual alarm will result. This alarm is helpful in the detection of leaks or patient disconnects.

PEEP Not Set. In the event that the PEEP/CPAP pressure varies more than 5 cmH$_2$O from the selected reference value, a visual LED indicator will be illuminated. The practitioner may adjust the reference value between 0 and 20 cmH$_2$O. Once set, this electronic reference value is used to compare the circuit pressure to the desired setting established using the manual PEEP valve on the expiratory port.

Time: Apnea. If no breath (inspiratory start) is detected for a 20-second time window, both audible and visual alarms will result and a backup breath rate of 12 BPM will be initiated. All other ventilator parameters (tidal volume, inspiratory time, etc.) will be as previously set by the practitioner.

Tables 11-15 and 11-16 summarize the Avian™ Transport Ventilator capabilities and alarm systems.

TABLE 11-15 Avian™ Transport Ventilator Capabilities

Modes	Control, Assist/Control, SIMV, CPAP
Rate	0 to 150 BPM
Flow	5 to 100 L/min
Insp. Time	0.1 to 3.0 seconds
Tidal Volume	50 to 2,000 mL
Sensitivity	-2 to -8 cmH$_2$O
Pressure Limit	1 to 100 cmH$_2$O
PEEP/CPAP	0 to 20 cmH$_2$O
Sigh	1.5 times tidal volume every 100th breath or every 7 minutes

TABLE 11-16 Avian™ Transport Ventilator Alarm Systems

Input Power

Battery Low/Fail

External Power Low/Fail

Control Circuit

Ventilator Inoperative

I:E Ratio

Ventilator Disconnect

Output Alarms

Pressure	
High Pressure	1 to 100 cmH$_2$O
Low Pressure	Off, 2 to 50 cmH$_2$O
PEEP Not Set	

Time

Apnea	No trigger for 20 seconds

ASSEMBLY AND TROUBLESHOOTING

Assembly—Avian™ Transport Ventilator

To assemble the Avian™ Transport Ventilator for use, follow the suggested assembly guide.

1. Connect the ventilator to a 50-psi medical gas source. If an F$_I$O$_2$ less than 1.0 is desired, operate the ventilator by connecting it to an oxygen blender having separate air and oxygen gas sources at 50 psi.

2. Choose the desired power source:
   a. Internal 6-V DC battery
   b. External 11–30 V DC battery
   c. 120 v, 60 Hz or 220–230 v, 50–60 Hz AC power using the AC power adapter

3. Assemble the patient circuit:
   a. Connect one end of the 22-mm, large-bore patient tubing to the ventilator outlet.
   b. Connect the distal end of the 22-mm, large-bore tubing to the patient manifold assembly (exhalation valve assembly).
   c. Connect the exhalation valve drive tubing to the exhalation valve nipple and the opposite end to the exhalation valve drive port on the side of the ventilator.
   d. Connect the proximal airway pressure tubing between the proximal airway pressure nipple on the patient manifold and the airway pressure port on the side of the ventilator.
   e. Connect a 6-inch flextube to the outlet of the patient manifold and use a mask adapter or tracheostomy adapter to interface the patient circuit with the patient's airway.

Troubleshooting

To assist you in troubleshooting the Avian™ Transport Ventilator, refer to the troubleshooting algorithm at the end of this chapter.

HAMILTON MEDICAL, INC., MAX

Hamilton Medical, Inc., markets and distributes the MAX transport ventilator (Figure 11-32). The MAX is a pneumatically-powered, electronically-controlled transport ventilator. It is a flow controller, which is pressure, time, or manually triggered, pressure or flow limited, and time cycled. The ventilator may operate in control and spontaneous (IMV) modes of ventilation.

Input Power

The ventilator is pneumatically powered and requires a medical gas source of between 50 and 90 psi. Once gas enters the ventilator, it is reduced in pressure by a single-stage reducing valve to 50 psi.

The electronic control system may be powered by alkaline batteries, rechargeable NiCad batteries, or by an AC adapter. NiCad batteries can operate the ventilator for approximately 8 hours. If alkaline batteries are used, the ventilator may be operated for over 30 hours.

Control Circuit

Gas flows from the single-stage reducing valve to an electronically controlled solenoid valve (Figure 11-33). When opened, the sole-

Figure 11-33 *A schematic diagram of the Hamilton Medical, Inc., MAX ventilator's pneumatic system. (Courtesy Hamilton Medical, Inc.)*

Figure 11-32 *A photograph of the Hamilton MAX ventilator. (Courtesy Hamilton Medical, Inc.)*

noid valve allows gas to flow through the flow control valve (tidal volume) and into the patient circuit. Between mandatory breaths, the patient's spontaneous inspiratory effort opens a demand valve, admitting gas to the patient circuit. A manual breath button when depressed allows gas to bypass the solenoid valve and flow directly through the flow control valve to the patient circuit.

PEEP may be provided by adding an external threshold resistor valve to the patient circuit. PEEP pressures may typically range from 0 to 20 cmH$_2$O when using these devices.

Control Variable

The control variable for the MAX ventilator is flow. Flow is adjusted using the tidal volume control. The control is a variable orifice valve, which throttles flow from the elec-

tronic solenoid. Flow rate is adjustable between 0 and 90 L/min through the flow control valve. Since inspiratory time is fixed at 1 second, volume becomes a function of flow (valve position) and time.

Phase Variables

Trigger Variables

The trigger variables for the MAX ventilator include pressure, time, and manual triggering. During spontaneous ventilation, if the patient inspiratory effort (pressure) is sufficient to open the demand valve, gas will flow into the patient circuit. The trigger sensitivity is not adjustable, but is preset to -2 cmH$_2$O.

Time is the trigger variable during mandatory breaths. Time triggering is adjusted using the rate control. Respiratory rates of between

---

ASSEMBLY AND TROUBLESHOOTING

Assembly—MAX Ventilator

To assemble the Hamilton Medical, Inc., MAX ventilator for use, follow this suggested assembly guide.

1. Select an electrical power source:
   a. Internal rechargeable NiCad or alkaline batteries (4 "AA" batteries).
   b. Use 120 v, 60 Hz power and the AC adapter.

2. Connect the ventilator to a 50-psi medical gas supply using the DISS fitting on the left side of the ventilator.

3. Assemble the patient circuit:
   a. Connect one end of the 22-mm diameter patient circuit to the outlet of the ventilator located on the left side.
   b. Connect the distal end of the 22-mm diameter patient circuit to the patient manifold assembly.
   c. Connect the ⅛-inch diameter exhalation valve drive line between the exhalation valve nipple on the left side of the ventilator and the exhalation valve on the patient manifold assembly.
   d. If PEEP is desired, connect an exter-

nal PEEP threshold device to the outlet of the patient manifold.
   e. Connect a 6-inch flextube to the patient connection on the manifold assembly. Attach a mask adapter or a tracheostomy adapter to the flextube to interface the ventilator to the patient's airway.

4. Check the ventilator for proper operation:
   a. Connect the patient circuit to a test lung.
   b. Set the tidal volume control for 500 mL and the rate control for 10 breaths per minute.
   c. Use a watch to verify the rate and a Wright respirometer or other volume measuring device to verify volume delivery.
   d. Disconnect the test lung and obstruct the patient circuit. Observe the pressure limit setting and adjust as required.

Troubleshooting

To troubleshoot the MAX ventilator, follow the troubleshooting algorithm at the conclusion of this chapter.

0 and 30 breaths per minute may be set. The respiratory rate control is a timer, which determines the cycling rate of the electronic solenoid valve.

The ventilator is manually triggered when the practitioner depresses the manual breath button on the right of the control panel. When depressed, gas flow bypasses the electronic solenoid valve and flows through the flow control valve and on to the patient circuit. Inspiration is terminated once the manual breath button is released. When the manual breath button is depressed, there is no fixed inspiratory time.

Limit Variables

The limit variables for the ventilator are pressure and flow. Pressure in the patient circuit is limited by an internal adjustable pressure relief valve. The pressure relief limit may be adjusted between 10 and 100 cmH$_2$O. To adjust the pressure relief, the ventilator cover must be removed, the patient circuit must be occluded, and the internal pressure regulator adjusted to the desired pressure limit during inspiration. If the pressure limit is set to a level that is lower than the peak inspiratory pressure for a given tidal volume, pressure will rise and plateau at the set pressure limit. When operated in this way, the ventilator is pressure limited. Inspiratory pressure is displayed on a circular pressure manometer located at the left side of the control panel.

The pressure limit control operates by adjusting the pressure applied to the exhalation valve. Once pressure in the patient circuit exceeds the pressure in the exhalation valve, excess pressure is vented past the exhalation valve to ambient air. When this occurs, a loud noise results as gas flows through the partially closed exhalation valve.

Flow is a limit variable when tidal volume is set at a low setting, and flow rises and plateaus during the inspiratory phase. Since inspiratory time is fixed at 1 second, it is possible at low tidal volume settings to be flow limited. The tidal volume control, as discussed earlier, is really a flow rate control, which is calibrated in mL.

Cycle Variable

The cycle variable for the ventilator is time. Inspiratory time is not adjustable and is set at 1 second. With a constant inspiratory time, volume delivery is a function of the flow rate through the flow control valve (tidal volume control).

Alarm Systems

Input Power Alarms

When less than 30 minutes of operation remain (when using the internal battery pack), the battery light will illuminate on the front control panel and an audible alarm will sound. The battery pack consists of four "AA" batteries.

A low oxygen alarm will result if the pressure powering the ventilator falls to less than 27 psi. If this occurs, both audible and visual alarms will result.

Tables 11-17 and 11-18 summarize the Hamilton Medical, Inc., MAX ventilator's capabilities and alarm systems.

TABLE 11-17 The Hamilton Medical, Inc. MAX Ventilator Capabilities

Modes	Control, IMV
Respiratory Rate	2 to 30 BPM
Inspiratory Time	1 second
Tidal Volume	50 to 1,500 mL
Flow Rate	0 to 90 L/min (mandatory)
	0 to 145 L/min (spontaneous)
Pressure Limit	10 to 100 cmH$_2$O
Sensitivity	−2 cmH$_2$O

TABLE 11-18 The Hamilton Medical, Inc. MAX Ventilator's Alarm Systems

Input Power	
Low Battery	Less than 30 minutes' operation remaining
Low Gas Pressure	Gas supply pressure less than 27 psi

IMPACT MEDICAL CORPORATION UNI-VENT® MODEL 750

Impact Medical Corporation's Uni-Vent® Model 750 is a microprocessor-controlled portable ventilator (Figure 11-34). The ventilator is capable of operating in control, assist/control, and SIMV modes. It is a flow controller that may be pressure, time, or manually triggered, and pressure, volume, or time cycled.

Input Power

The ventilator may be powered by internal batteries for up to 9 hours when fully charged. The ventilator may also be operated using a multivoltage power supply (120/230 v, 50 to 400 Hz) or 11- to 30-volt DC external deep-cycle battery. When operated on the multivoltage power supply, the internal batteries are automatically charged.

A medical gas source at 50 to 90 psi is required to power the pneumatic system of the ventilator. If an F_IO_2 of less than 1.0 is desired, the ventilator may be operated from an external blender with independent gas sources for air and oxygen at 50 to 90 psi.

Control Circuit

The gas enters the ventilator through a DISS fitting on the top of the ventilator. Once gas enters the ventilator, it is reduced in pressure to 50 psi by a single-stage reducing valve (Figure 11-35). Gas flow from the reducing valve then flows to two inspiration solenoids and a demand solenoid valve. Duplication of the inspiration solenoid valves provides a safety feature in the event that a solenoid valve should fail. Gas flows from the second inspiration solenoid to a flow control valve and then to the patient circuit. Gas flow from the demand solenoid flows to the patient circuit. Pressure in the patient circuit is measured by a pressure transducer connected to the patient manifold.

PEEP pressure can be provided by using an external PEEP valve. Sensitivity can be PEEP compensated using the auto-PEEP compensation system. When activated, the pressure transducer measures the baseline pressure and uses it as the baseline pressure to reference the sensitivity setting.

Control Variable

The control variable for the ventilator is flow. Flow is controlled by the flow control valve. Flow is adjustable between 0 and 100 L/min. Volume delivery becomes a function of flow and inspiratory time (flow multiplied by inspiratory time).

Figure 11-34 *A photograph of the Impact Medical Corporation's Uni-Vent® Model 750 ventilator. (Courtesy Impact Medical Corporation)*

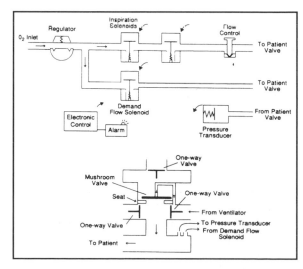

Figure 11-35 *A schematic diagram of the Uni-Vent® Model 750 pneumatic system. (Courtesy Daedalus Enterprises, Inc.)*

Phase Variables

Trigger Variables

The trigger variables for the ventilator include pressure, time, and manual triggering. Pressure is a trigger variable during assist/control and SIMV modes. When pressure sensed in the airway by the pressure transducer is less than the trigger threshold, the inspiration solenoid valves open, delivering gas flow to the circuit. During spontaneous ventilation, a drop in circuit pressure results in the demand solenoid opening, providing gas flow to the patient. Sensitivity is adjustable between -2 and -8 cmH_2O in 2-cmH_2O increments.

Time becomes a trigger variable in control and assist/control modes. Time triggering is adjusted using the ventilation rate control. Respiratory rates are adjustable between 1 and 150 breaths per minute.

The ventilator may be manually triggered by the practitioner depressing the manual trigger button. Once depressed, the ventilator delivers a breath at the set flow and inspiratory time. Manual breaths may be delivered during all modes of ventilation.

Limit Variable

The limit variable for the ventilator is flow. Flow is adjustable between 0 and 100 L/min.

Cycle Variables

The cycle variables include pressure, volume, and time. Pressure is a cycle variable when the peak inspiratory pressure exceeds the value set on the high-pressure alarm. The high-pressure alarm may be adjusted between 15 and 100 cmH_2O. Once the set pressure level has been reached, the alarm is activated.

Volume becomes a cycle variable when the sigh mode is activated. When activated, the ventilator delivers a sigh breath equal to 150% of the volume setting every 100th breath, or every 7 minutes, whichever occurs first.

Time is a cycle variable during mechanical breath delivery. Inspiratory time is set using the inspiration time control. Inspiratory times are adjustable between 0.1 and 3.0 seconds in 0.1-second increments. Once the inspiratory time has lapsed, inspiration ends.

Alarm Systems

Input Power Alarms

The ventilator alerts the practitioner to both loss of external power as well as a discharged internal battery pack. If the external multivoltage power supply becomes disconnected, the ventilator automatically switches to the internal batteries and activates the external power low/fail alarm.

ASSEMBLY AND TROUBLESHOOTING

Assembly—Uni-Vent® Model 750

To assemble the Impact Medical Corporation's Uni-Vent® Model 750 for use, follow the suggested assembly guide.

1. Select a power source:
   a. Multivoltage power supply (external battery or 120/230 v, 60 Hz AC power).
   b. Internal batteries if charged.

2. Connect the ventilator to a 50- to 90-psi medical gas source using the DISS fitting on the top of the ventilator.

3. Assemble the patient circuit:
   a. Connect the 22-mm diameter, large-bore tubing (patient circuit) to the outlet of the ventilator.
   b. Connect the patient manifold to the distal end of the 22-mm diameter patient circuit.
   c. Connect the 3/16-inch diameter tubing to the patient manifold and the proximal end to the outlet of the demand flow solenoid.
   d. Connect the 1/8-inch diameter tubing from the patient manifold to the pressure transducer nipple on the top of the ventilator.
   e. Connect a 6-inch flextube to the outlet of the patient manifold and attach a mask adapter or tracheostomy adapter to interface the circuit with the patient's airway.

Troubleshooting

To assist you in troubleshooting the ventilator, follow the troubleshooting algorithm at the conclusion of this chapter.

If the internal battery's voltage drops to less than 11 volts, the battery low/fail alarm will be activated. Once the internal batteries reach this voltage, approximately 1 hour of operation time remains.

Control Circuit Alarms

The control circuit alarm consists of an inverse I:E ratio alarm. When inspiration becomes greater than 50% of the breath cycle time, the alarm is activated. Once activated, inspiration is terminated and the ventilator cycles into exhalation.

Output Alarms

Pressure. As described earlier, the ventilator has a high-pressure alarm that is adjustable between 15 and 100 cmH$_2$O. In addition, the ventilator also has a low-pressure/disconnect alarm. It is adjustable between 0 and 50 cmH$_2$O. This alarm is helpful in detecting leaks and patient disconnects.

The PEEP not set alarm alerts the practitioner to baseline pressure changes from that set on the manual display setting. Changes in baseline pressure may be caused by leaks or patient disconnects.

Time. The ventilator also incorporates an apnea alarm. If the ventilator does not detect a breath trigger for 20 seconds, the alarm will be activated. This is helpful in detecting disconnects as well as apneic events.

Tables 11-19 and 11-20 summarize the Uni-Vent® capabilities and alarm systems.

TABLE 11-19 Uni-Vent® Ventilator Capabilities

Modes	Control, Assist/Control, SIMV, Sigh
Pressure	0 to 100 cmH$_2$O
Flow	0 to 100 L/min
Inspiratory Time	0.1 to 3.0 seconds
Expiratory Time	0.1 to 59.9 seconds
Rate	1 to 150 BPM
Sigh	150% of tidal volume
Sensitivity	−2 to −8 cmH$_2$O
PEEP	0 to 20 cmH$_2$O

TABLE 11-20 Uni-Vent® Alarm Systems

Input Power

External Power Low/Fail

Battery Low/Fail

Control Circuit

Inverse I:E Ratio

Output

High Pressure	15 to 100 cmH$_2$O
Low Pressure	0 to 50 cmH$_2$O
PEEP Not Set	

Time

Apnea	No breath detected for 20 seconds

LIFE SUPPORT PRODUCTS, INC., AUTOVENT 2000/3000

Life Support Products, Inc., produces two portable transport ventilators, the AutoVent 2000 and AutoVent 3000 (Figure 11-36). Both ventilators are pneumatically powered and controlled. They are flow controllers, which are time or pressure triggered, pressure or flow limited, and time cycled. Since many similarities exist between the ventilators, they will be considered together. When differences occur, they will be discussed on an individual basis.

Input Power

Power input for both the AutoVent 2000 and AutoVent 3000 is a medical gas supply between 40 and 90 psi. Since the ventilator is a single circuit ventilator, if an F$_I$O$_2$ different from the source gas is desired, the ventilator may be operated from a blender using a separate air and oxygen supply.

Control Circuit

Gas enters the ventilator through a DISS fitting on the left side of the ventilator. Once gas enters the ventilator, it is filtered and reduced in pressure by a single-stage reducing valve to 30 psi.

Figure 11-36 *A photograph of the Life Support Products, Inc., AutoVent 2000 and AutoVent 3000. (Courtesy Life Support Products, Inc.)*

During the inspiratory phase, gas flow is split (Figure 11-37A), with one path flowing through the timing cartridge and the other path flowing through the tidal volume control (flow control valve). The volume control is a variable orifice flow control valve, which regulates the continuous flow of gas through the patient circuit. Gas flow through the timing cartridge is also split, with one path going through a fixed orifice valve (adjustable in the AutoVent 3000), which is the inspiratory time control and to a volume accumulation chamber. The other gas pathway is to the exhalation valve diaphragm in the patient manifold. Once the volume accumulation chamber is filled, gas pressurizes the right portion of the timing cartridge, sliding it left and cycling the ventilator into exhalation.

During exhalation, pressurized gas in the volume accumulation chamber and inspiratory time control is exhausted to the atmosphere (Figure 11-37B). Gas flow from the reducing valve is conducted to the rate control. The rate control has an adjustable orifice, which regulates gas flow to its accumulation chamber. Once the accumulation chamber becomes pressurized, the timing cartridge

slides to the right, cycling the ventilator into inspiration.

Control Variable

The control variable for both ventilators is flow. Flow is controlled by the tidal volume control. Flow is adjustable between 16 and 48 L/min. Since gas flow through the patient circuit is continuous, volume delivery becomes a function of inspiratory time and flow.

Phase Variables

Trigger Variables

The trigger variables for both ventilators include pressure and time. Pressure is a trigger variable during spontaneous ventilation. If the patient's inspiratory effort is sufficient, gas can be drawn from the continuous flow through the patient manifold. Sensitivity is not adjustable, but is preset at −2 cmH$_2$O. Gas flow is available up to 48 L/min.

Time is the trigger variable during mandatory ventilation. Time triggering is adjusted using the respiratory rate control (labeled in BPM).

Figure 11-37A *A schematic diagram of the Life Support Products, Inc., AutoVent 2000/3000 pneumatic system during inspiration. (Courtesy Life Support Products, Inc.)*

Figure 11-37B *A schematic diagram of the Life Support Products, Inc., AutoVent 2000/3000 pneumatic system during expiration. (Courtesy Life Support Products, Inc.)*

The rate control, as described earlier, is a pneumatic timing cartridge that controls expiratory time. The AutoVent 2000 has ventilatory rates adjustable between 0 and 20 breaths per minute. The AutoVent 3000 may be adjusted between 0 and 28 breaths per minute.

Limit Variables

The limit variables for both ventilators are pressure and flow. The pressure limit is adjusted using the pressure limit alarm incorporated into the patient manifold assembly. The pressure limit is set at 50 cmH$_2$O, ±5 cmH$_2$O. Once the pressure limit is reached, excess pressure is vented to the atmosphere until the inspiratory time has lapsed.

The ventilators may also be flow limited. If the tidal volume is set at a lower setting and the inspiratory time is such that flow increases and plateaus, the ventilator is then flow limited. Since inspiratory time is fixed (1.5 or 0.75 seconds), this may occur under some circumstances.

Cycle Variable

The cycle variable for both ventilators is time. Inspiratory time for the AutoVent 2000 is fixed at 1.5 seconds. The inspiratory time for the AutoVent 3000 is selectable between 0.75 seconds (child) and 1.5 seconds (adult). As described earlier, the inspiratory time control is a pneumatic timer, controlling the length of inspiration.

Alarm Systems

Output Alarm

The output alarm for both ventilators is pressure. When the pressure limit is reached, an audible pneumatic reed alarm will also sound. As described earlier, the pressure limit is set at 50 cmH$_2$O, ±5 cmH$_2$O.

Tables 11-21 and 11-22 summarize the Life Support Products, Inc., AutoVent 2000 and 3000 ventilator capabilities and alarm systems.

ASSEMBLY AND TROUBLESHOOTING

Assembly—AutoVent 2000 and 3000

To assemble the AutoVent 2000 or AutoVent 3000 for use, follow the suggested assembly guide.

1. Connect the ventilator to a medical gas source between 40 and 90 psi. The ideal pressure input is 50 psi. If a different F$_I$O$_2$ from the source gas is desired, an oxygen blender may be used with separate oxygen and air gas sources.

2. Assemble the patient circuit:
   a. Connect the patient valve supply tubing to the ventilator outlets on the right side of the ventilator. The outlets are indexed with internal and external threads to prevent accidental mismatching.
   b. Connect the patient valve supply tubing to the patient manifold, observing the indexing of the tubing.
   c. Connect a 6-inch flextube to the outlet of the patient manifold and a mask adapter or tracheostomy adapter to its distal end to interface with the patient's airway.

3. Verify the ventilator's operation:
   a. Set the BPM control for 12 breaths per minute.
   b. Set the tidal volume control to 800 mL.
   c. Set the inspiratory time to the adult setting on the AutoVent 3000 (1.5 seconds).
   d. Connect the patient manifold to a test lung.
   e. Use a watch and a Wright respirometer or other volume-measuring device to verify the rate and tidal volume delivery.
   f. Occlude the patient outlet and verify that the pressure limit alarm is operational.

Troubleshooting

To troubleshoot the AutoVent 2000 and AutoVent 3000, refer to the troubleshooting algorithm at the conclusion of this chapter.

TABLE 11-21 AutoVent 2000 and AutoVent 3000 Capabilities

	AutoVent 2000	**AutoVent 3000**
Flow Rate	16–48 L/min	6–48 L/min
Tidal Volume	400–1,200 mL	200-1,200 mL
Rate	8–20 BPM	8–28 BPM
Inspiratory Time	1.5 seconds	0.75 or 1.5 seconds
Expiratory Time	1.5 to 6.0 seconds	1.5 to 6.0 seconds
Pressure Limit	50 cmH$_2$O, ±5 cmH$_2$O	50 cmH$_2$O, ±5 cmH$_2$O
Sensitivity	−2 cmH$_2$O	−2 cmH$_2$O

TABLE 11-22 AutoVent 2000 and AutoVent 3000 Alarm Systems

	AutoVent 2000	**AutoVent 3000**
Output Alarm		
Pressure	50 cmH$_2$O, ±5 cmH$_2$O	50 cmH$_2$O, ±5 cmH$_2$O

NEWPORT MEDICAL INSTRUMENTS, INC., NEWPORT E100M

Newport Medical Instruments, Inc., produces the E100M transport ventilator (Figure 11-38). The E100M is a microprocessor-controlled, pneumatically-powered ventilator. It is a flow controller that is time, pressure, or manually triggered, pressure or flow limited, and time cycled. The ventilator may operate in assist/control, SIMV, and spontaneous ventilation modes.

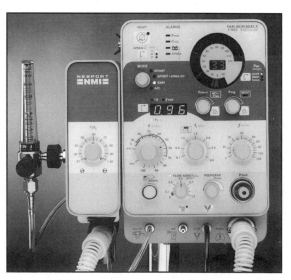

Figure 11-38 *Photographs of the Newport Medical Instruments, Inc., (A) E100M ventilator and (B) the E100M ventilator's control panel. (Courtesy Newport Medical Instruments, Inc., Newport Beach, CA)*

Input Power

The Newport E100M incorporates an integral blender into its design. Both air and oxygen are connected to the blender using the DISS fittings located on the rear of the blender. Medical gas sources between 35 and 70 psi may be used, with 50 psi being the recommended input pressure.

The ventilator may be operated from three different electrical power sources. Standard AC current (100–120 VAC or 220–240 VAC, 50–60 Hz), external battery, or internal battery. When fully charged, the internal battery can power the ventilator for approximately 6 to 8 hours.

Control Circuit

Gas from the blender is split into three paths (Figure 11-39). One path flows to the spontaneous toggle switch. This switch has two positions: off (no gas flow for spontaneous breathing) and 8 L/min. When toggled to the 8 L/min setting, approximately that amount is delivered to the reservoir bag and then enters the patient circuit during spontaneous ventilation. Gas flow from this toggle switch also provides pneumatic power to the pilot valve, which, in conjunction with the flow control valve, determines inspiration.

Another gas path directs blended gas to the transport toggle switch, which is designed to conserve gas during transport. This is accomplished by blocking the air/oxygen blender bleeds, thus limiting gas consumption to about 15 L/min. This feature may cause the F_IO_2 to vary by more than 0.03; therefore, when using this feature, careful monitoring of oxygen delivery is important.

The third gas path is to the main flow control valve. When the pilot valve is electronically actuated, gas from the pilot valve activates the main flow valve, delivering gas through the flow control valve and a muffler and then into the patient outlet. Bleed gas from the outlet of the main flow valve powers the nebulizer and the exhalation solenoid valve.

The exhalation valve is controlled by an exhalation solenoid, which inflates the exhalation valve during inspiration, thus delivering gas to the patient. PEEP/CPAP pressure is generated by bleed gas from the pilot valve. The bleed gas is directed through the PEEP regulator and provides pressure, partially closing the exhalation valve, which acts as a threshold resistor, thus creating PEEP/CPAP pressure in the circuit.

Control Variable

The control variable for the Newport E100M ventilator is flow. Flow is controlled by the flow control valve and is adjustable between 1 and 100 L/min. Volume delivery becomes a function of inspiratory flow and inspiratory time (volume equals flow multiplied by inspiratory time).

Phase Variables

Trigger Variables

The trigger variables of the ventilator include pressure, time, and manual triggering. Pressure triggering occurs when the patient's inspiratory effort exceeds the level set on the pressure trigger control. Pressure triggering may be adjusted between −10 and 25 cmH_2O. By depressing the automatic trigger control (ATC) button, a function is activated that maintains the pressure triggering as sensitively as possible within a specified range while preventing artifacts or autotriggering. When using this feature, the ventilator attempts to maintain a trigger threshold of −2 cmH_2O below baseline pressure.

Time triggering occurs during assist/control and the mandatory portion of SIMV. Time triggering is set using the respiratory rate control. Respiratory rates are adjustable between 1 and 120 breaths per minute. The rate control functions with the microprocessor control system and determines the opening and closing of the pilot valve.

Manual triggering occurs when the practitioner depresses the manual button. When depressed, gas flow is directed through the flow control valve and into the patient circuit. The breath ends when the button is released, the maximum pressure alarm threshold is met, or 4 seconds have elapsed.

Limit Variables

The limit variables of the Newport E100M include pressure and flow. The pressure limit is adjusted using the pressure limit control, which is a manually adjustable pop-off valve. The pressure limit may be adjusted between 0 and 120 cmH_2O. When the pressure limit is reached, pressure is held constant and excess pressure is vented through the relief valve to the atmosphere. Inspiration is terminated once the inspiratory time has passed.

Flow becomes a limit variable if the flow rate is set at a lower setting and inspiratory time is set such that flow increases and plateaus. Under these conditions, the

Figure 11-39 *A schematic of the Newport Medical Instruments, Inc., E100M ventilator's pneumatic system. (Courtesy Newport Medical Instruments, Inc., Newport Beach, CA)* **(continues)**

ventilator becomes flow limited. Inspiratory flow rates may be set between 1 and 100 L/min.

Cycle Variables

The cycle variables for the Newport E100M include pressure and time. Pressure becomes a cycle variable if the inspiratory pressure exceeds the setting on the high-pressure alarm. If the high-pressure alarm threshold is met,

inspiration is terminated and audible and visual alarms result. The high-pressure alarm is an adjustable pressure sensor. The alarm is set by pushing in the "P" alarm knob, and then rotating it clockwise, to increase, or counter-clockwise, to decrease, the setting. The high-pressure alarm settings may be set between 5 and 120 cmH$_2$O.

Time becomes a cycle variable when the microprocessor control system deactivates the

Figure 11-39 *(continued)*

pilot valve, thus closing it. Time cycling is adjusted using the inspiratory time control. Inspiratory times are adjustable between 0.1 and 3.0 seconds.

Baseline Variable

The baseline variable for the ventilator is pressure. PEEP/CPAP pressures are adjustable between 0 and 25 cmH$_2$O. The PEEP/CPAP control regulates pressure transmitted against the exhalation valve diaphragm, creating a

threshold resistor that generates PEEP/CPAP pressure.

Modes of Ventilation
Assist/Control

When operated in this mode, the ventilator delivers breaths at the set rate, flow, and inspiratory time. If the patient has spontaneous efforts sufficient enough to be detected by the sensitivity system, a ventilator-supported breath will be delivered.

SIMV

The E100M ventilator SIMV system allows the patient to breathe spontaneously between mandatory breaths. The first patient-triggered breath during a mandatory breath interval will be ventilator assisted. Following the initial assisted breath, any breaths taken during the rest of the time interval are spontaneous breaths. If no spontaneous breaths are taken, the ventilator will deliver mandatory breaths at the rate established by the setting on the frequency control.

Time-Cycled, Pressure-Limited Ventilation (Assist/Control or SIMV)

During this mode of ventilation, the practitioner sets a pressure plateau level using the mechanical pressure relief valve. The ventilator will deliver breaths at the set rate and inspiratory time, but all breaths will be pressure-limited at the set plateau level. All pressure in excess of the pressure limit setting will be vented to the atmosphere.

Spontaneous

In this mode of ventilation, the E100M ventilator will deliver gas to the patient exclusively through the reservoir system. The constant-flow toggle switch must be opened and/or flow from the auxiliary flowmeter must be added in order to provide gas flow to the reservoir system. All gas flowing through the system is blended gas from the integral blender.

Mandatory and spontaneous flows may be adjusted independently using the DuoFlow system incorporated into the E100M ventilator. The mandatory flow rate control will set the flow delivered during mandatory breaths, while the spontaneous toggle switch and the auxiliary flowmeter may be set to establish an independent flow for the spontaneous breaths.

Flow assist may be used to augment a patient's peak flow needs during spontaneous breathing. During the flow assist time interval, a high flow (the flow setting on the mandatory flow control) is delivered. After the flow assist time has lapsed, the flow rate becomes the combination of the spontaneous toggle switch and auxiliary flowmeter settings. The flow assist may be set between 0.0 and 1.0 seconds.

Alarm Systems

Input Power Alarms

The input power alarms include loss of electric power, low battery, and low gas inlet pressure. If electrical power has been lost, a continuous alarm will result to indicate the loss of electrical power. If the external battery pack has become discharged, the same alarm will result. In addition, in the event that either air or oxygen pressure is lost, a pneumatic reed alarm will sound continuously.

Control Circuit Alarms

The control circuit alarms of the E100M ventilator include I:E ratio and fault system alarms. The I:E ratio alarm is activated if the inspiratory time is longer than the expiratory time. When this occurs, a yellow LED will blink, indicating that the 1:1 ratio has been exceeded.

If the microprocessor detects a function problem with the ventilator or its control system, a continuous audible alarm results and an error code is displayed in the control monitor. In the event this occurs, provide an alternate source of ventilation for the patient and remove the ventilator from service.

Output Alarms

Pressure. The E100M ventilator incorporates both high- and low-pressure alarms and an automatic baseline pressure alarm. The high-pressure alarm is adjustable between 5 and 120 cmH$_2$O, and the low-pressure alarm is adjustable between 3 and 118 cmH$_2$O.

The automatic baseline pressure alarm provides for both high and low baseline pressure indications. The high baseline pressure alarm is activated if the airway pressure remains above the minimum pressure alarm setting at the end of exhalation. The minimum baseline pressure alarm is activated if the airway pressure remains below the low baseline alarm setting for more than 3 seconds.

Time. The ventilator incorporates an apnea alarm. If the ventilator is operated in the spontaneous mode, the apnea alarm will alert the practitioner to apneic events. The detection delay has three settings: 0, or off; 15 seconds; and 30 seconds. If the sensitivity system fails to detect any spontaneous breaths within the detection delay time period, both audible and visual alarms will result. This alarm is also helpful in detecting patient disconnects.

TABLE 11-23 Newport Medical Instruments, Inc., E100M Ventilator Capabilities

Modes	Assist/Control, SIMV, Time-Cycled, Pressure-Limited A/C or SIMV; Spontaneous
Rate	1 to 120 BPM
Pressure	0 to 120 cmH$_2$O
Pressure Limit	0 to 120 cmH$_2$O
Inspiratory Time	0.1 to 3.0 seconds
Tidal Volume	5 to 5,000 mL
Sensitivity	−10 to 25 cmH$_2$O
Flow Rate	1 to 100 L/min
PEEP/CPAP	0.0 to 25 cmH$_2$O
F$_I$O$_2$	0.21 to 1.0

Tables 11-23 and 11-24 summarize the Newport E100M ventilator capabilities and alarm systems.

TABLE 11-24 Newport Medical Instruments, Inc., E100M Ventilator Alarm Systems

Input Power

Loss of Electrical Power

Low Battery

Low Air/Oxygen Pressure

Control Circuit

Inverse I:E Ratio

Fault System

Output

Pressure

   High Pressure

   Low Pressure

   High Baseline Pressure

   Low Baseline Pressure

Time

Apnea

ASSEMBLY AND TROUBLESHOOTING

Assembly—Newport Medical Instruments, Inc., E100M Ventilator

To prepare the Newport Medical Instruments E100M ventilator for use, follow this suggested assembly guide.

1. Select a power source:
   a. 120/230 v, 60 Hz electrical power.
   b. External 12-V DC battery.
   c. Internal battery (if fully charged).

2. Connect the ventilator to 50-psi medical gas supplies (air and oxygen) using the DISS fittings on the rear of the blender.

3. Assemble the patient circuit:
   a. Connect a high-range flowmeter to the DISS fitting on the left of the integral blender.
   b. Connect oxygen supply tubing between the flowmeter and the reservoir bag inlet.
   c. Connect a 2-liter reservoir bag to the reservoir bag adapter fitting.
   d. Connect the inspiratory limb of the patient circuit to the main flow ventilator outlet, the expiratory limb of the patient circuit to the exhalation valve, and the proximal pressure sensing line to the proximal connection.
   e. Connect the ⅛-inch diameter exhalation valve drive line to the exhalation valve nipple on the front of the ventilator.
   f. Connect the distal end of the ⅛-inch exhalation valve drive line to the exhalation valve on the patient circuit manifold assembly.

Troubleshooting

To assist you in troubleshooting the Newport Medical Instruments E100M ventilator, refer to the troubleshooting algorithms at the end of this chapter.

OMNI-TECH MEDICAL, INC., OMNI-VENT

Omni-Tech Medical, Inc., produces the Omni-Vent portable pneumatically-powered transport ventilator (Figure 11-40). The ventilator is pneumatically powered and controlled. It is a flow controller, which is pressure or time triggered, pressure or flow limited, and time cycled. It may be operated in volume control, pressure control, IMV (volume- or pressure-controlled modes), and CPAP modes.

Input Power

The Omni-Vent is pneumatically powered and controlled. A medical gas source of between 25 and 140 psi may be used to power the ventilator. A 50-psi source is the recommended pressure to power the ventilator. However, if desired, the ventilator may be calibrated to run at lower pressures (25 psi) to utilize liquid systems which may be desirable in some situations.

Control Circuit

Gas powering the ventilator enters through a filter in the gas inlet assembly (Figure 11-41). It then passes through an on/off valve in the same assembly and on to the inspiratory and expiratory valve block. From the inspiratory/expiratory valve block, the gas is conducted to a flow accelerator and then to a flow control valve. From the flow control valve, the gas flow is split, with one path flowing to a pressure relief valve and patient circuit and the other path flowing to the exhalation valve diaphragm.

IMV may be provided by the addition of an external reservoir and one-way valve assembly. Gas is diverted to the reservoir through a needle valve located on the top of the ventilator.

PEEP/CPAP may be added using an external threshold resistor valve attached to the patient circuit. PEEP/CPAP pressures of between 0 and 20 cmH$_2$O may be added using the external valve.

Control Variable

The control variable for the Omni-Vent is flow. Flow is determined by the flow control valve. Flow rates may be adjusted between 0 and 98 L/min. The flow control valve is a variable orifice needle valve. Opening or closing the valve regulates the flow of gas through it. Since flow is constant, volume delivery

Figure 11-40 *A photograph of the Omni-Tech Medical, Inc., Omni-Vent portable ventilator. (Courtesy Omni-Tech Medical, Inc.)*

becomes a function of inspiratory flow and inspiratory time (volume is equal to flow multiplied by time).

Phase Variables

Trigger Variables

The trigger variables include pressure and time. Pressure is a trigger variable during IMV ventilation. When inspiratory effort is sufficient to open a one-way valve in the IMV reservoir, gas is delivered to the patient.

Time is the control variable for volume- and pressure-controlled ventilation, as well as the mandatory portion of IMV. The expiratory time control acts as a rate control. The expiratory valve is a needle valve, which controls the rate of gas leakage through a timing cartridge. If gas flow leaking from the cartridge is high, expiratory time is less. Conversely, if gas leakage is slow, expiratory time is longer. Respiratory rates are adjustable between 0 and 150 breaths per minute.

Limit Variables

The limit variables for the Omni-Vent include pressure and flow. Pressure becomes a limit variable if the pressure relief valve is set lower than the peak inspiratory pressure for a given inspiratory time and flow rate. Under these circumstances, pressure will rise to the pressure limit setting and plateau until the

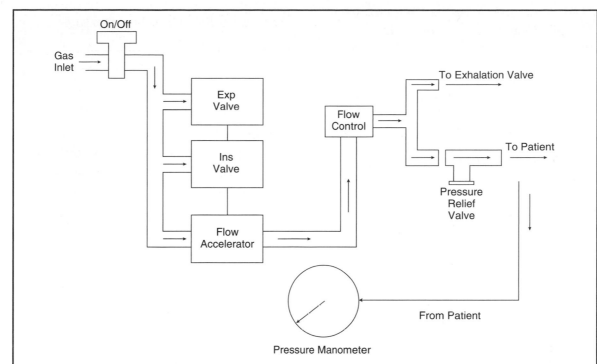

INSPIRATORY PHASE

Source gas is introduced through a filter in the gas inlet assembly; then gas flows to the pneumatic valve supply inlet. The gas flows to the flow control, then to the tee assembly which directs gas simultaneously to the exhalation valve and pressure relief valve to the patient.

As gas pressure increases in the lung, it is transmitted to the manometer through a tubing independent from the tubing wye connector.

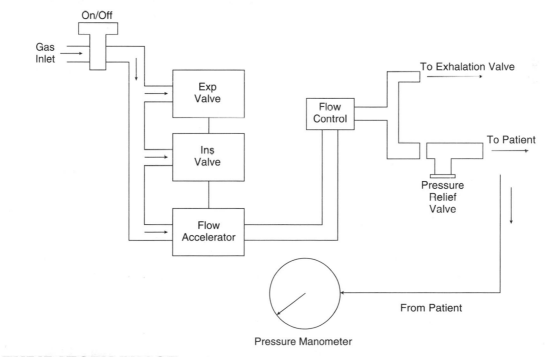

EXPIRATORY PHASE

Source gas follows the identical path of the inspiratory phase to the pneumatic valves and is then held until the inspiratory phase begins.

Figure 11-41 *A schematic diagram of the Omni-Tech Medical, Inc., Omni-Vent pneumatic system. (Courtesy Omni-Tech Medical, Inc.)*

inspiratory time has elapsed, with the ventilator operating in pressure control mode. The pressure limit may be adjusted between 0 and 120 cmH$_2$O.

The ventilator may also be flow limited. If the flow rate is set at a lower setting and inspiratory time is set such that flow increases and plateaus, the ventilator is then flow limited.

Cycle Variable

The cycle variable for the ventilator is time. Inspiratory time is determined by the inspiratory time needle valve. The inspiratory time like the expiratory time control is a pneumatic timing cartridge. Adjustment of the needle valve controls the rate of gas leakage from the cartridge, which either lengthens or shortens inspiratory time. Inspiratory times may be adjusted between 0.2 and 3.0 seconds.

Monitoring System

The Omni-Vent monitoring system consists of an analog pressure gauge located on the upper left of the control panel. The gauge is connected to the patient circuit via the proximal airway line and reflects pressures at the proximal airway.

TABLE 11-25 Omni-Vent Ventilator Capabilities

Modes	Volume and Pressure Control, IMV, CPAP
Tidal Volume	30 to 3,000 mL
Respiratory Rate	0 to 150 BPM
Inspiratory Time	0.2 to 3.0 seconds
Expiratory Time	0.2 to 60 seconds
Flow Rate	0 to 98 L/min
Pressure Relief	0 to 120 cmH$_2$O
PEEP/CPAP	0 to 20 cmH$_2$O (external threshold resistor)

Alarm Systems

The Omni-Vent has no built-in alarm systems. Table 11-25 summarizes the Omni-Vent's capabilities.

ASSEMBLY AND TROUBLESHOOTING

Assembly—Omni-Vent

To prepare the Omni-Tech Medical, Inc., Omni-Vent for use, follow the suggested assembly guide.

1. Connect the ventilator to a medical gas source (25 to 140 psi). If an F$_I$O$_2$ of less than 1.0 is desired, the ventilator may be powered from a blender operating from independent sources of medical air and oxygen.

2. Assemble the patient circuit:
   a. Connect one end of the 22-mm diameter patient circuit to the ventilator outlet.
   b. Connect the patient manifold assembly to the distal end of the 22-mm diameter patient circuit.
   c. Connect one end of the 1/8-inch diameter line to the exhalation valve nipple on the side of the ventilator and the other end to the exhalation valve on the patient manifold assembly.
   d. Connect the other 1/8-inch diameter line between the airway pressure nipple on the ventilator and the proximal airway tap on the patient manifold.
   e. Connect a 6-inch flextube to the patient manifold assembly and attach a mask adapter or tracheostomy adapter to the distal end to interface with the patient airway.

3. Confirm the ventilator's operation:
   a. Connect the patient circuit to a test lung and rotate the on/off switch to the on position.
   b. Adjust flow, inspiratory, and expiratory time to the desired settings.
   c. Confirm rate and volume delivery using a Wright respirometer or other volume-measuring device and a watch.
   d. Occlude the patient circuit and adjust the pressure relief valve to the desired pressure.

Troubleshooting

To assist you in troubleshooting the Omni-Vent ventilator, refer to the troubleshooting algorithm at the end of this chapter.

CHAPTER SUMMARY

This chapter has covered a diverse group of ventilators and noncontinuous ventilatory support devices. Tables 11-26 and 11-27 will assist you in learning the similarities and differences among the ventilators presented in this chapter.

TABLE 11-26 Homecare Ventilators and Noncontinuous Ventilatory Support Ventilators

Ventilator	Input Power	Circuit	Control Mechanism	Trigger Variable	Limit Variable	Cycling Variable	Alarms
Homecare Ventilators							
Puritan-Bennett LP6 PLUS	Electric	Single	Electronic	P, T		P, V, T	I, CC, P
Puritan-Bennett LP10	Electric	Single	Electronic	P, T	P	P, V, T	I, CC, P
Puritan-Bennett LP20	Electric	Single	Electronic	P, T	P	P, V, T	I, CC, P
Bear Medical Systems, Inc.							
Bear 33	Electric	Single	Electronic	P, T	F	P, V, T	I, CC, P, T
Respironics, Inc.							
PLV-100	Electric	Single	Electronic	P, T	P	V	I, CC, P, T
PLV-102	Electric	Single	Electronic	P, T	P	V	I, CC, P, T
Noncontinuous Ventilatory Augmentation Ventilators							
Nellcor Puritan-Bennett Corporation							
KnightStar 420S Nasal CPAP System	Electric	Single	Electronic	F	P	P	F
KnightStar 330 Bi-level Ventilator	Electric	Single	Electronic	F	P	P	F
Respironics, Inc.							
REMstar	Electric	Single	Electronic	F	P	P	F
BiPAP Synchrony	Electric	Single	Electronic	F	P	P	F

Key: *F—Flow, P—Pressure, V—Volume, T—Time, I—Input Power, CC—Control Circuit.*

TABLE 11-27 Transport Ventilators

Ventilator	Input Power	Circuit	Control Mechanism	Trigger Variable	Limit Variable	Cycling Variable	Alarms
AMBU, Inc.							
TransCARE 2	Pneumatic	Single	Pneumatic	P, T	P, F	T	CC, P
Bird Products Corporation							
Avian™	Pneumatic	Single	Electronic	P, T, M	P, F	P, V, T	I, CC, P, T
Hamilton Medical, Inc.							
MAX	Pneumatic	Single	Electronic	P, T, M	P, F	T	I
Impact Medical Corporation							
Uni-Vent®	Pneumatic	Single	Electronic	P, T, M	F	P, V, T	I, CC, P, T
Life Support Products, Inc.							
AutoVent 2000/3000	Pneumatic	Single	Pneumatic	P, T	P, F	T	P
Newport Medical Instruments, Inc.							
E100M	Pneumatic	Single	Electronic	P, T, M	P, F	P, T	I, CC, P, T
Omni-Tech Medical, Inc.							
Omni-Vent	Pneumatic	Single	Pneumatic	P, T	P, F	T	

Key: *F—Flow, M—Manual, P—Pressure, V—Volume, T—Time, I—Input Power, CC—Control Circuit.*

ALG 11-1 *A troubleshooting algorithm for homecare ventilator input power and control circuit alarm.*

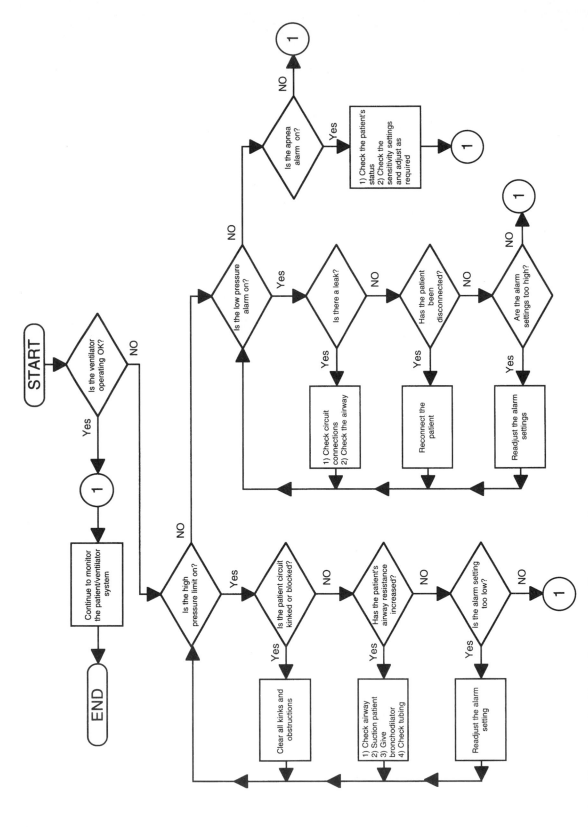

ALG 11-2 A troubleshooting algorithm for homecare ventilator output alarms.

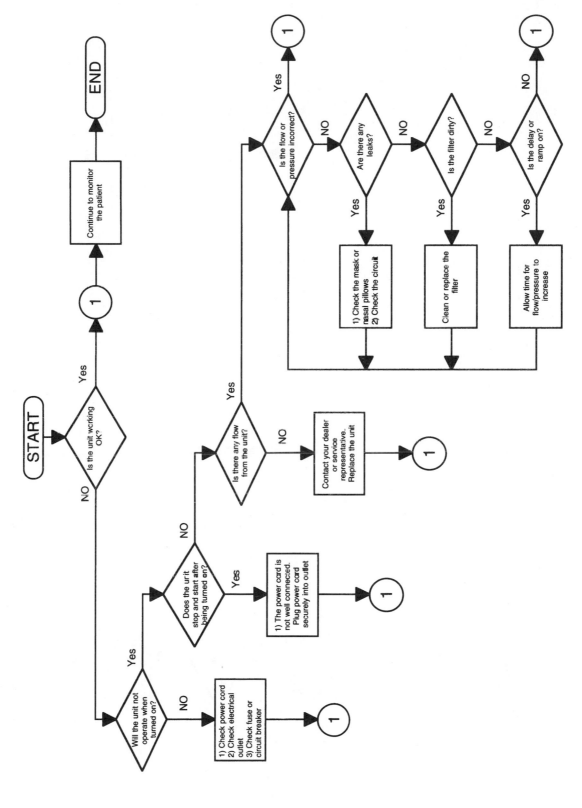

ALG 11-3 *A troubleshooting algorithm for noncontinuous ventilator augmentation devices.*

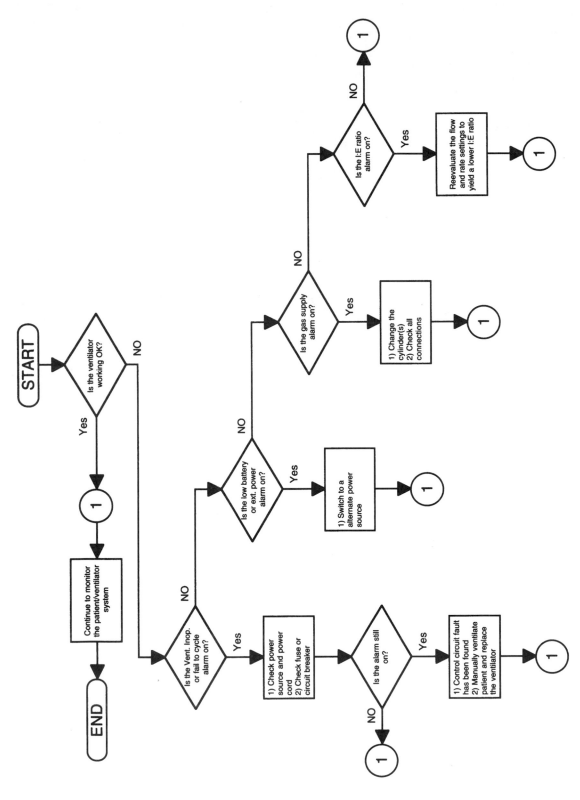

ALG 11-4   *A troubleshooting algorithm for transport ventilator input power and control circuit alarms.*

ALG 11-5 *A troubleshooting algorithm for transport ventilator output alarms.*

CLINICAL CORNER

Homecare Ventilators

1. You are making your biweekly visit to a homecare patient who is ventilator dependent. The patient's caregiver expresses concern that the pressure alarm frequently goes off. What should you assess and what might you do?
2. You are helping a caregiver prepare to take a ventilator-dependent patient on a day trip to an art gallery. List the equipment that the caregiver should take along.

Noncontinuous Ventilatory Augmentation Equipment

1. A doctor asks you to explain the difference between a home CPAP and home bi-level positive airway pressure system. What would you say?
2. A patient on a Puritan-Bennett Goodknight has an order to increase the nocturnal pressure by 10 cmH$_2$O. How can you assist the patient in adjusting to this new pressure level?

Transport Ventilators

1. When maintaining a patient on a transport ventilator during transport, what other equipment should you always have with you (besides the ventilator)?
2. During a helicopter flight, a transport ventilator's low-pressure alarm (visual alarm) goes off. What should you check?

Self-Assessment Quiz

1. Which of the following is the common control variable among the homecare ventilators discussed in this chapter?
   a. pressure
   b. flow
   c. volume
   d. time

2. Which of the following is a common power source between the homecare ventilators discussed in this chapter?
   a. electric
   b. pneumatic
   c. both electric and pneumatic
   d. none of the above

3. Which of the following homecare ventilators may be pressure limited?
   I. Puritan-Bennett LP10
   II. Bear 33
   III. Respironics, Inc. PLV-102
   IV. Puritan-Bennett LP6 PLUS
   a. I
   b. I and II
   c. I, II, and III
   d. I, III, and IV

4. "Pressure rises to a preset value and remains at that level until inspiration is terminated" best describes:
   a. pressure cycling.
   b. pressure controlling.
   c. pressure limiting.
   d. baseline pressure.

5. Which of the following homecare ventilators have an apnea alarm?
   I. Puritan-Bennett LP10
   II. Bear 33
   III. Respironics, Inc. PLV-100
   IV. Puritan-Bennett LP6 PLUS
   a. I
   b. I and II
   c. I, II, and III
   d. II, III, and IV

6. Which of the following ventilators utilize a rotary-driven piston as the drive mechanism?
   I. Puritan-Bennett LP10
   II. Bear 33
   III. Respironics, Inc. PLV-100
   IV. Puritan-Bennett LP6 PLUS
   a. I
   b. I and II
   c. I, II, and III
   d. I, II, and IV

7. When adding an external PEEP threshold resistor to the circuit, the device should be located:
   a. proximal to the exhalation valve in the circuit.
   b. distal to the exhalation valve in the circuit.
   c. at the end of the 6-inch flextube near the patient's airway.
   d. none of the above.

8. Proper location of an external PEEP threshold resistor is important because it may cause:
   a. interference with pressure triggering.
   b. loss of volume.
   c. interference with pressure limiting.
   d. interference with flow limiting.

9. The trigger variables common to the homecare ventilators include:
   I. pressure.
   II. flow.
   III. volume.
   IV. time.
   a. I and II
   b. I and III
   c. I and IV
   d. III and IV

10. Which of the following homecare ventilators may be flow limited?
    a. Nellcor Puritan-Bennett Medical LP10
    b. Bear 33
    c. Lifecare PLV-100
    d. Lifecare PLV-102

11. When a homecare ventilator is operated as a pressure-limited ventilator, the cycle variable is:
    a. pressure.
    b. flow.
    c. volume.
    d. time.

12. Which of the following are examples of control circuit alarms?
    I. ventilator inoperative
    II. I:E ratio
    III. microprocessor error
    IV. control circuit fault
    a. I
    b. I and II
    c. I, II, and III
    d. I, II, III, and IV

13. CPAP is an effective treatment for sleep apnea because:
    a. the positive pressure inflates the lungs.
    b. the artificial airway keeps the patient's airway patent.
    c. the CPAP pressure splints the airway open.
    d. gas exchange is improved.

14. The control variable for CPAP systems is:
    a. pressure.
    b. flow.
    c. volume.
    d. time.

15. The trigger variable for the bi-level positive airway pressure systems discussed in this chapter is:
    a. pressure.
    b. flow.
    c. volume.
    d. time.

16. The limit variable for the bi-level positive airway pressure systems discussed in this chapter is:
    a. pressure.
    b. flow.
    c. volume.
    d. time.

17. Common patient interfaces for both CPAP and bi-level positive airway pressure systems include:
    I. a nasal mask.
    II. an endotracheal tube.
    III. nasal pillows.
    IV. a tracheostomy tube.
    a. I and II
    b. I and III
    c. II and III
    d. II and IV

18. Which of the following transport ventilators are not pneumatically controlled?
    a. Ambu, TransCARE 2
    b. Impact Medical, Uni-Vent®
    c. Omni-Tech Medical, Omni-Vent
    d. Life Support Products, AutoVent 3000

19. Which of the following transport ventilators may be manually triggered?
    I. Ambu, TransCARE 2
    II. Viasys Critical Care, Avian™
    III. Impact Medical, Uni-Vent®
    IV. Hamilton Medical, MAX
    a. I and II
    b. I and III
    c. II and III
    d. II, III, and IV

20. You are using a transport ventilator, which is a flow controller. You set the inspiratory time for 0.3 seconds and the flow rate at 50 L/min. What is the delivered tidal volume?
    a. 150 mL
    b. 500 mL
    c. 900 mL
    d. 1,500 mL

21. Which of the following transport ventilators may be pressure limited?
    I. Ambu, TransCARE 2
    II. Viasys Critical Care, Avian™
    III. Hamilton Medical, MAX
    IV. Newport Medical Instruments, E100M
    a. I
    b. I and II
    c. I, II, and III
    d. I, II, III, and IV

22. Which of the following transport ventilators incorporates an integral blender?
    a. Ambu, TransCARE 2
    b. Viasys Critical Care, Avian™
    c. Hamilton Medical, MAX
    d. Newport Medical Instruments, E100M

23. When a transport ventilator delivers a volume of gas based upon inspiratory time and flow rate, what is the cycle variable?
    a. pressure
    b. flow
    c. volume
    d. time

24. If a transport ventilator has inspiratory and expiratory time and flow controls, which control determines time triggering once tidal volume delivery has been determined?
    a. inspiratory time
    b. expiratory time
    c. flow rate
    d. none of the above

25. "Inspiratory pressure rises to a preset level and remains constant until the inspiratory time has lapsed" best describes:
    a. pressure controlling.
    b. pressure limiting.
    c. pressure cycling.
    d. none of the above.

26. Which of the following transport ventilators may be operated in IMV or SIMV mode without the addition of an external IMV manifold assembly?
    I. Viasys Critical Care, Avian™
    II. Ambu, TransCARE 2
    III. Newport Medical Instruments, E100M
    IV. Life Support Products, AutoVent 3000
    a. I and II
    b. I and III
    c. II and III
    d. II and IV

27. Which of the following transport ventilators have PEEP/CPAP incorporated into their design?
    I. Viasys Critical Care, Avian™
    II. Ambu, TransCARE 2
    III. Newport Medical Instruments, E100M
    IV. Life Support Products, AutoVent 3000
    a. I and II
    b. I and III
    c. II and III
    d. II and IV

28. Which of the following transport ventilators may be flow limited?
    I. Ambu, TransCARE 2
    II. Viasys Critical Care, Avian™
    III. Omni-Tech Medical, Omni-Vent
    IV. Life Support Products, AutoVent 3000
    a. I
    b. I and II
    c. I, II, and III
    d. I, II, III, and IV

29. Which of the following ventilators can be volume cycled?
    I. Viasys Critical Care, Avian™
    II. Impact Medical, Uni-Vent®
    III. Omni-Tech Medical, Omni-Vent
    IV. Newport Medical Instruments, E100M
    a. I and II
    b. I and III
    c. II and III
    d. III and IV

30. "Inspiration is terminated when a preset pressure is reached" best describes:
    a. pressure controlling.
    b. pressure limiting.
    c. pressure cycling.
    d. none of the above.

Selected Bibliography

Aequitron Medical, Inc. (1994). *LP6 PLUS volume ventilator and LP10 volume ventilator with pressure limit user's manual.* Minneapolis.

Ambu, Inc. (1994). *Ambu TransCARE series ventilators (TransCARE 1, TransCARE 1-HB, TransCARE 2) operator's manual.* Linthicum.

Bear Medical Systems. (1987). *Bear 33 volume ventilator clinical instruction manual.* Riverside.

Bio-Med Devices, Inc. (1996). *Crossvent 4 intensive care/transport ventilator operation and service manual.* Guilford.

Bird Products Corporation. (1994). *Bird Avian™ operators/service manual.* Palm Springs.

Branson, R. D. (1992). Intrahospital transport of critically ill, mechanically ventilated patients. *Respiratory Care, 37*(7), 775–795.

Campbell, R. S., et al. (1992). Laboratory and clinical evaluation of the impact Uni-Vent 750 portable ventilator. *Respiratory Care, 27*(1), 29–36.

Chatburn, R. L. (1991). A new system for understanding mechanical ventilators. *Respiratory Care, 36*(10), 1123–1152.

Chatburn, R. L. (1992). Classification of mechanical ventilators. *Respiratory Care, 37*(9), 1009–1025.

Gietzen, J. W., et al. (1991). Effect of PEEP-value placement on function of a homecare ventilator. *Respiratory Care, 26*(10), 1093–1098.

Hamilton Medical. (1989). *Operator's manual MAX.* Reno.

Hill, N. (1997). Complications of noninvasive positive pressure ventilation. *Respiratory Care, 42*(4), 432–442.

Life Support Products, Inc. (1991). *AutoVent 2000/3000 operating manual.* Irvine.

Lifecare, Inc. (1991). *PLV-100 operating manual.* Westminster.

Lifecare, Inc. (1991). *PLV-102 operating manual.* Westminster.

McPherson. S. P. (1990). *Respiratory th. rapy equipment* (4th ed.). Mosby-Yearbook.

Newport Medical Instruments, Inc. (1998). *The Newport E100M ventilator operating manual.* Newport Beach.

Newport Medical Instruments, Inc. (1998). *The Newport E100M ventilator service manual.* Newport Beach.

Omni-Tech Medical, Inc. (1994). *Omni-Vent operators/service manual.* Topeka.

Puritan-Bennett Corporation. (1990). *Companion 2801 volume ventilator operating instruction manual.* Lenexa.

Puritan-Bennett Corporation. (1993). *Companion 318 nasal CPAP system patient guide.* Lenexa.

Puritan-Bennett Corporation. (1993). *Companion 320I/E bi-level respiratory system patient guide.* Lenexa.

Respironics, Inc. (1992). *BiPAP® S/T ventilatory support system operator's manual.* Murrysville.

Respironics, Inc. (1992). *BiPAP® systems guidebook: A discussion of the systems and their applications.* Murrysville.

Respironics, Inc. (1993). *BiPAP® service manual.* Murrysville.

Respironics, Inc. (2000). *BiPAP® Synchrony ventilatory support system provider manual.* Murrysville.

Respironics, Inc. (1994). *REMstar Choice nasal CPAP system patient pamphlet.* Murrysville.

Respironics, Inc. (1994). *REMstar Choice service manual.* Murrysville.

Respironics, Inc. (2001). *REMstar Plus CPAP system home care provider setup instructions.* Murrysville.

Turner, R. (1997). NPPV: Face versus interface. *Respiratory Care, 42*(4), 389–393.

HIGH-FREQUENCY MECHANICAL VENTILATION

INTRODUCTION

By definition, high-frequency ventilators administer smaller tidal volumes (equal to or less than anatomical dead space) at high frequencies. The U.S. Food and Drug Administration defines a high-frequency ventilator as any ventilator that delivers breaths at a rate greater than 150 breaths per minute or any jet ventilator regardless of its frequency or rate. Today, there are four primary types of high-frequency ventilators: high-frequency positive-pressure ventilators, high-frequency flow interrupters, high-frequency jet ventilators, and high-frequency oscillatory ventilators.

High-frequency ventilators are employed in patient care in situations in which the patient has intractable hypoxemia and hypercarbia that is not responsive to conventional positive-pressure ventilation. In other circumstances, high-frequency ventilation is used when there is pulmonary insult or damage that results in large air leaks (bronchopulmonary fistulae). Some surgical cases (laser bronchoscopy, laryngoscopy, and tracheal surgery) also support the use of high-frequency ventilation, in which it is desirable to maximize the airway caliber while supporting the patient adequately without an airtight seal.

High-frequency ventilation accomplishes the goal of adequately supporting gas exchange without using large tidal breaths at low frequencies. The mechanism of gas exchange with the alveoli is different when compared with bulk convection (as understood with conventional mechanical ventilation). There are several theories of how gas is exchanged during high-frequency ventilation, including asymmetric velocity profiles, pendelluft, Taylor dispersion, cardiogenic mixing, and molecular diffusion.

In this chapter you will learn about the different types of high-frequency ventilators, the circumstances when high-frequency ventilation is employed clinically, the different theories of gas exchange, and the specifics of some of the high-frequency ventilators currently being marketed.

OBJECTIVES

After completing this chapter, the student will accomplish the following objectives:

- Describe the following types of high-frequency ventilators.
  - High-frequency positive-pressure ventilator
  - High-frequency jet ventilator
  - High-frequency flow interrupter
  - High-frequency oscillatory ventilator
- Discuss the different mechanisms of gas exchange in the lungs.
  - Bulk convective ventilation
  - Asymmetric velocity profiles
  - Pendelluft
  - Taylor dispersion
  - Cardiogenic mixing
  - Molecular diffusion
- Describe the different clinical situations in which high-frequency ventilators are employed.
  - Failure of conventional ventilation
  - Pulmonary insult resulting in air leaks
  - Surgical ventilatory support
  - Refractory hypoxemia and hypercarbia
- For the ventilators in this chapter, describe the following:
  - Input power
  - Drive mechanism

— Control scheme
— Alarm systems
• Describe how to assemble and trouble-
shoot the following ventilators:

— Percussionaire® VDR 4
— Viasys Critical Care 3100A and 3100B
Oscillator

KEY TERMS

Asymmetric velocity profiles
Cardiogenic mixing
Convective ventilation
High-Frequency Flow
Interrupter (HFFI)

High-Frequency Jet
Ventilator (HFJV)
High-Frequency Oscillatory
Ventilator (HFOV)

High-Frequency Positive-
Pressure Ventilator (HFPPV)
Molecular diffusion
Pendelluft

TYPES OF HIGH-FREQUENCY VENTILATORS

There are several different types of high-frequency ventilators. These include high-frequency positive-pressure ventilators, high-frequency flow interrupters, high-frequency jet ventilators, and high-frequency oscillatory ventilators. Each of these ventilator types has the commonality of delivering small tidal breaths at high frequencies; however, some rely on passive exhalation (recoil of the lung tissue and chest wall) while others are active during exhalation (active movement of the gas during exhalation).

HIGH-FREQUENCY POSITIVE-PRESSURE VENTILATOR (HFPPV)

The **high-frequency positive-pressure ventilator (HFPPV)** was first described and developed by Swedish investigators Sjöstrand and associates. A high-frequency positive-pressure ventilator (HFPPV) consists of a conventional mechanical ventilator with a modified circuit employing a low compliance and compressible volume. These modifications allow tidal breath delivery at higher frequencies, which is not possible with the conventional circuit. Fresh gas is introduced into the circuit through a side arm, which functions as a fluidic valve using the Coanda effect (refer to Chapter 7). The exhalation valve on the circuit

permits control of baseline pressures for the application of PEEP/CPAP. Gas delivery is achieved at flows of 175 to 250 L/min and tidal volumes of 3 to 4 mL/kg. Exhalation with this ventilator is passive, relying on the recoil of the lungs and chest wall.

Advantages of this type of ventilator when compared to conventional positive-pressure mechanical ventilation include diminished cardiac side effects, including blood pressure fluctuations, and the ability to ventilate through small catheters or cannulas. This type of ventilator is frequently used during laryngoscopy, bronchoscopy, and upper airway surgery. The application of the ventilator through a small cannula or catheter allows an improved operative field for the surgeon.

HIGH-FREQUENCY JET VENTILATOR (HFJV)

The **high-frequency jet ventilator (HFJV)** employs high-pressure, short puffs or bursts of gas at high frequencies to accomplish gas exchange. These high-frequency bursts of gas are introduced into the airway through a small catheter at the endotracheal tube port via a special adapter or through a specialized endotracheal tube (High-Lo Jet Tracheal Tube). Through viscous shearing, additional gas flow is entrained around the cannula with each jet pulse, making the tidal volume the sum of the entrained gas and the volume delivered with the pulse, or burst, of gas. Ventilatory rates of 100 to 200 breaths per minute, with I:E ratios of 1:2 to 1:8, are possible. Since tidal volume delivery is a function of the jet pulse and gas entrainment, precise tidal volume measurement is difficult. Exhalation is passive with these ventilators; instead, the elastic recoil of the lungs and chest wall provide the force for exhalation.

HIGH-FREQUENCY FLOW INTERRUPTER (HFFI)

The **high-frequency flow interrupter (HFFI)** ventilator is similar to the HFJV in that small bursts of gas are delivered to the airway by interrupting a high-pressure or high-flow gas source. However, no injector cannula is used. The most common types of HFFI ventilators use a rotating ball with a single orifice or gas pathway (Figure 12-1) to interrupt the gas flow into short bursts. Frequency is determined by the rate at which the ball is rotating,

and volume delivery is controlled by varying the pressure proximal to the rotating ball and through bias flow entrainment (Figure 12-1). Exhalation is passive, relying on the recoil of the lungs and chest wall.

HIGH-FREQUENCY OSCILLATORY VENTILATOR (HFOV)

The **high-frequency oscillatory ventilator (HFOV)** is active both during inspiration and exhalation. Most HFOV ventilators employ a diaphragm, piston, or modified acoustic speaker to oscillate the gas into and out of the airway (Figure 12-2). Typically, a bias flow

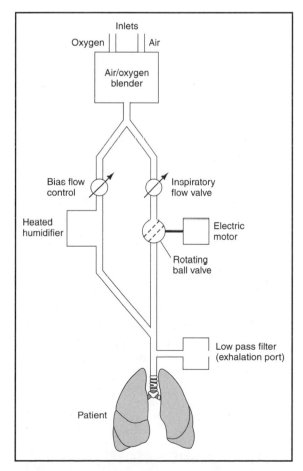

Figure 12-1 *A high-frequency flow interrupter that uses a rotating ball assembly.*

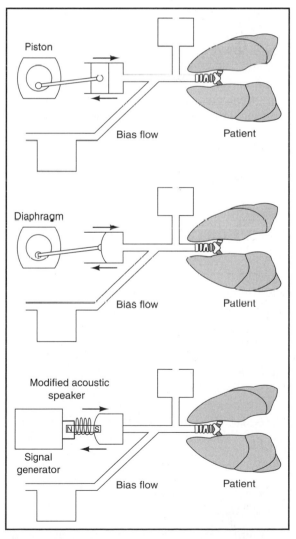

Figure 12-2 *Three types of high-frequency oscillatory ventilators: with piston drive, with diaphragm drive, and with an acoustic speaker drive.*

past the airway provides the fresh gas source, while the HFOV provides forward (inspiration) and backward (exhalation) movement of gas into and out of the artificial airway. The forward and backward motion of the oscillatory device causes a typical sinusoidal flow waveform. HFOV ventilators typically deliver volumes of between 0.8 and 2.0 mL/kg at frequencies of 180 to 1,000 breaths per minute. Tidal breath delivery is dependent on the stroke volume of the oscillator, bias flow, size of the artificial airway, and impedance of the low-pass filter.

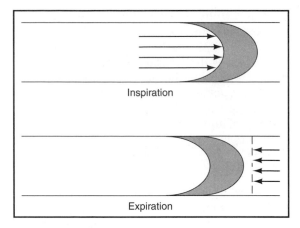

Figure 12-3 *A schematic drawing of asymmetric velocity profiles. Notice how flow is greatest in the central portion of the airway.*

GAS EXCHANGE IN THE LUNGS DURING HIGH-FREQUENCY VENTILATION

High-frequency ventilation relies on small tidal volumes (often equal to or less than dead space) moving at high rates to accomplish gas exchange. Since large volumes of gas are not moving into and out of the lungs by convection, other mechanisms of gas exchange must be at work in order to normalize oxygen and carbon dioxide tensions in the blood. Several mechanisms have been hypothesized besides convective ventilation, including asymmetric velocity profiles, pendelluft, Taylor dispersion, cardiogenic mixing, and molecular diffusion.

CONVECTIVE VENTILATION

Convective ventilation, or the bulk flow of gas into and out of the lungs, is how gas exchange is most readily understood. Large tidal volumes (greater than the anatomic dead space) enter the pulmonary conduction system, with velocity slowing as the airways narrow and the cross-sectional area increasing as the gas moves distally toward the parenchyma. Eventually, the alveoli (comprising the respiratory zone) come into contact with gas that has passed through the conduction zone and oxygen and carbon dioxide are exchanged with the blood.

ASYMMETRIC VELOCITY PROFILES

Asymmetric velocity profiles comprise an attempt to account for differences in the relative shape of the inspiratory and expiratory velocity gradient, or profile. During inspiration, the velocity at the center of the airway is greatest whereas the velocity near the periphery of the airway is less (Figure 12-3). This can be accounted for by the difference in resistance to flow, whereby resistance is greater near the bronchial wall (frictional loss) compared with the central lumen of the airway.

During exhalation, the velocity profile of the exhaled gas is relatively flat when compared with the parabolic inspiratory profile. During oscillatory ventilation, it is hypothesized that the inspiratory gases tend not to decelerate (due to momentum). Therefore, there is a net gas movement during inspiration down the center of the airway, while expiratory gases tend to move out the peripheral portions of the airway. It has been theorized that inspiratory and expiratory flow can occur simultaneously (due to the net inspiratory and expiratory flow gradients).

PENDELLUFT

Pendelluft, a compound word of German origin, means air swinging back and forth freely, or in an oscillatory fashion. Pendelluft occurs due to the fact that different areas of the lung have different time constants, resulting in their filling and emptying at different rates. This results in a net gas flow from one lung region to another, which improves the overall uniformity of gas distribution.

TAYLOR DISPERSION

Taylor described a model in which turbulent gas flow in the airways enhances diffusion by augmenting the mixing process caused by the eddies formed in the turbulent flow. Fredberg expanded the work of Taylor and described the flow of gas during high-frequency ventilation as being dependent upon turbulence and dispersion. Fredberg hypothesized that to increase turbulence, flow must be increased, and that at low tidal volumes, the most efficient way to increase flow is to increase frequency. Frequency is optimal in his model when minute ventilation is the greatest at a given pressure, which is dependent on the mechanics of the respiratory system.

CARDIOGENIC MIXING

Cardiogenic mixing is a theory proposed by Slutsky in which the motion of the heart during the cardiac cycle is hypothesized to help with the distribution of gas during high-frequency ventilation. The continuous cardiac motion should help to vibrate the airways, thus further enhancing gas distribution and mixing.

MOLECULAR DIFFUSION

Molecular diffusion theory supports the concept that with the increased frequencies associated with high-frequency ventilation, the kinetic activity of the molecules at the alveolar level should increase. This greater kinetic activity should enhance the transport of gases across the alveolar capillary membrane.

CLINICAL APPLICATION OF HIGH-FREQUENCY VENTILATION

Unlike conventional positive-pressure ventilation, high-frequency ventilation can provide adequate gas exchange by using lower tidal volumes at high respiratory rates and lower mean airway pressures. When ventilating patients, there are several potential advantages in the unique aspects of high-frequency ventilation. These advantages, when compared with conventional ventilation, include lower mean airway and intrathoracic pressures; minimum cardiac side effects caused by positive intrathoracic pressure; a stable, motionless operative field; and improvement in gas exchange in some patients.

REDUCED MEAN AIRWAY AND INTRATHORACIC PRESSURE

High-frequency mechanical ventilation accomplishes gas exchange by using small tidal volumes at high respiratory rates. Several investigators have demonstrated that it is possible to maintain adequate gas exchange using high-frequency ventilation at lower mean airway pressures when compared with the pressures required using conventional ventilation. The decrease in mean and peak airway pressures helps to prevent ventilator-induced lung injury and undesirable cardiac side effects associated with elevated intrathoracic pressures. While a reduction in mean and intrathoracic pressures is often a goal of high-frequency ventilation, it has been shown that it is also important to initially recruit lung volumes while providing adequate pressures to sustain those volumes once those regions have been initially recruited.

HFJV has been used for patients who have a bronchopulmonary fistula, resulting in large air leaks when conventional mechanical ventilation had been employed. The reduced mean airway pressures and minimal chest wall excursion associated with HFJV help with the resolution of such air leaks.

STABLE, MOTIONLESS OPERATIVE FIELD

HFJV has been successfully used for bronchoscopies, tracheal surgery, and laryngoscopy to ventilate patients and provide a stable, motionless operative field. Since HFJV can be accomplished through a small cannula (even percutaneously), it offers a large operative field. Furthermore, since ventilation is accomplished using small tidal volumes at lower pressures, it causes minimal chest wall and airway motion.

REFRACTORY HYPOXEMIA AND HYPERCARBIA

Because high-frequency ventilation achieves gas exchange by other mechanisms besides convection, it is often helpful in patients who have refractory hypoxemia and hypercarbia while being supported by conventional ventilatory methods. Often, when these patients are switched to high-frequency ventilation, gas exchange improves, resulting in increases in oxygenation and an improvement in ventilation.

The success of high-frequency ventilation has been found in infants with respiratory failure and patients with adult respiratory distress syndrome (ARDS), using HFPPV, HFJV, and HFOV.

REPRESENTATIVE HIGH-FREQUENCY VENTILATORS

Three high-frequency ventilators currently account for the majority of sales: the Percussionaire Corporation VDR 4 and the Viasys Critical Care Corporation 3100A and 3100B Oscillators. In this section the functional characteristics of these ventilators will be explained and you will learn how to assemble and troubleshoot them in preparation for their clinical application.

PERCUSSIONIARE® VDR 4

The Percussionaire® VDR 4 ventilator is a pneumatically powered and controlled, high-frequency ventilator (Figures 12-4A and 12-4B). Some authors have described the VDR 4 as an HFFI, an HFOV, or an HFJV. In reality, the VDR 4 is classified as a pneumatically powered and controlled, time-triggered, time-cycled, pressure-limited ventilator. It is unique in that it has the ability to provide both convective and percussive (high-frequency) ventilation simultaneously.

Input Power

The Percussionaire® VDR 4 is pneumatically powered and requires a 50-psi source of both air and oxygen. DISS fittings are located on the right rear side of the ventilator. The gases enter the ventilator, pass through check valves, and are then conducted to a Bird® air/oxygen blender, where F_IO_2 levels may be adjusted between 0.21 and 1.00.

Drive Mechanism and Control Circuit

Gas from the air/oxygen blender is reduced from 50 psi to, typically, between 35 and 40 psi before being conducted to the master switch, the drive mechanism, and the control circuits (Figure 12-5). The master switch is an on/off rotary switch, which allows the clinician to select either phasic (percussive,

Figure 12-4A *Photo of the Percussionaire® VDR 4 ventilator. (Courtesy Percussionaire Corporation, Sandpoint, ID)*

Figure 12-4B *Control panel of the VDR 4 (Courtesy Percussionaire Corporation, Sandpoint, ID)*

high-frequency) ventilation or demand CPAP and manual ventilation (spontaneous CPAP breathing or manual breath delivery).

The drive mechanism of the VDR 4 is a high-frequency pulse generator (HFPG). The clinician can program the pulse frequency, pulsatile flow rate, and inspiratory and expiratory times. Together, these controls determine the number of subtidal breaths delivered during each oscillatory interval. The pulse frequency control is a needle valve, which controls the breath rate or frequency. It is adjustable from 40 to over 900 breaths per minute. The pulsatile flow rate control determines the inspiratory flow rate of the subtidal volume delivery. Pulsatile flow rates may be adjusted up to 125 liters per minute at an operating

Figure 12-5 *A schematic drawing of the VDR 4 pneumatic system.*

Figure 12-6 *Phasitron® during inspiration.*

pressure of 40 psi. Peak pressure is controlled by the convective pressure rise control, which is found on the upper right portion of the control panel. The inspiratory and expiratory times determine the duration of the inspiratory and expiratory time intervals, and each may be adjusted independently of the other.

An important component in the overall drive mechanism of the VDR 4 ventilator is the Phasitron®. The Phasitron® is a spring-loaded, sliding venturi, which allows the HFPG to be interfaced with the patient's airway (Figures 12-6 and 12-7). During inspiration, the diaphragm inflates, and simultaneously, gas is injected into the venturi. Forward displacement of the diaphragm slides the venturi body forward, closing the exhalation port. Simultaneously, humidified gas is entrained through the venturi, augmenting flow to the patient. When gas pressure is removed from the diaphragm (expiratory phase), spring

Figure 12-7 *Phasitron® during expiration.*

tension opens the exhalation port by sliding the venturi backward and the patient exhales passively.

The output of the nebulizer is adjustable via a needle valve labeled "nebulization." The nebulizer is powered by source gas pressure. Rotation of the control in the counterclockwise direction increases the nebulizer's output.

Control Variable

The control variable for the VDR 4 ventilator is time. The pulse frequency control determines the ventilatory rate, which may be adjusted from 40 to over 900 breaths per minute. Time is a control variable since both pressure and flow vary with changes in resistance and compliance of the pulmonary system.

Phase Variables
Trigger Variables

The trigger variables for the VDR 4 include time and manual triggering. Time triggering is established by setting the pulse frequency control. Manual triggering is accomplished by depressing the manual inspiration button, which delivers a single convective breath up to the pressure set on the operational pressure control.

Cycle Variable

The cycle variable for the VDR 4 is time. The inspiratory time control determines the length of the inspiratory phase before the ventilator cycles into exhalation. The control is adjustable between 0.5 seconds and infinity (breath hold).

Baseline Variable

The baseline variable for the VDR 4 ventilator is pressure. The oscillatory CPAP/PEEP control regulates baseline pressure for the percussive portions of the scheduled breath pattern, and demand CPAP/PEEP regulates the baseline pressure during the static portion of the scheduled breath pattern.

Conditional Variable

The conditional variable of the VDR 4 is time. Control of convective or diffusive (high-frequency) ventilation is governed by the "pulse i/e ratio" control. In its fully counterclockwise position, an I:E ratio of 1:1 is delivered. At this ratio, the baseline profile of the waveform remains constant at the set oscillatory CPAP/PEEP level. When the I:E ratio approaches 1:1, the net effect is to improve pulmonary distribution and improve the PaO_2. When the pulse I:E ratio control is rotated clockwise until the I:E ratio becomes 1:3, the baseline profile will be sinusoidal with the percussive, high-frequency, subtidal breaths superimposed on it (Figures 12-8A and 12-8B). As the breath delivery becomes more convective, CO_2 elimination is enhanced.

Output Waveforms

The pressure waveform output of the VDR 4 ventilator may be varied from an oscillatory waveform without variation in base pressure to a sinusoidal waveform with oscillatory ventilation superimposed on it (Figure 12-8). As already discussed, the "pulse i/e ratio" control determines the waveform output of the ventilator.

Alarm and Monitoring Systems

The Percussionaire® VDR 4 has several alarm and monitoring features. These include pneumatic pressure, a fail-safe sensitivity, pressure-sensing alert/alarm system, and an external oscilloscope/waveform analyzer, which provides real-time graphical analysis of the VDR 4's performance.

Figure 12-8A   *A graphic tracing of diffusive ventilation.*

Figure 12-8B   *A graphic tracing illustrating diffusive and convective ventilation.*

ASSEMBLY AND TROUBLESHOOTING

Assembly—Percussionaire® VDR 4

1. Assemble the Phasitron® (Figure 12-9):

   a. Connect the green (inspiratory) fail-safe tee to the port closest to the patient outlet of the Phasitron®.

   b. Connect the red (expiratory) fail-safe tee to the port closest to the patient outlet of the Phasitron®.

   c. Install a snap-lock plug onto the small port at the end of the Phasitron®.

   d. Install the rubber-nosed plug into one end of the swivel tee and install the tee onto the outlet of the Phasitron®.

2. Assemble the patient circuit (Figure 12-10):

   a. Assemble the aerosol generator and volume regulator by attaching the volume-regulator cross tee to the nebulizer (Figure 12-10). Before installing it, inspect the three one-way valves for integrity and proper operation (inspiratory valve opens outward, purge valve opens outward, expiratory valve opens inward).

   b. Connect a length of green 22-mm diameter aerosol tubing to the outlet of the nebulizer.

   c. Install a water trap to the open end of the green aerosol tubing.

   d. Connect another length of green aerosol tubing to the open port of the water trap and connect the remaining end to the inlet of the green (inspiratory) fail-safe tee.

   e. Connect one end of the long red (expiratory) 22-mm diameter tubing to the outlet of the red (expiratory) fail-safe tee and the other end to the expiratory valve of the volume-regulator cross tee.

   f. Attach a 3-liter anesthesia bag to the reservoir bag fitting of the volume-regulator cross tee.

3. Assemble the small-diameter drive and monitoring lines:

   a. Connect the small-diameter red monitoring line to the small port on the swivel tee. Be certain that the check valve points toward the tee. Connect the opposite end to the red gauge fitting on the VDR 4 control panel.

   b. Connect the white small-diameter Phasitron® drive line to the small fitting on the white end cap of the Phasitron®. Attach the opposite end to the white fitting on the VDR 4 ventilator labeled Phasitron®.

   c. Attach the yellow small-diameter nebulizer drive line to the bottom fitting on the nebulizer, and attach the opposite end to the yellow fitting labeled aerosol on the VDR 4 ventilator.

   d. Connect the green small-diameter tubing to the remaining port on top of the aerosol generator and its opposite end to the green fitting on the VDR 4 labeled accessory.

Troubleshooting

Refer to the troubleshooting algorithms found at the end of this chapter.

Input Power Alarms

A pneumatic reed alarm is incorporated into the Bird® blender. In the event that either air or oxygen pressure is lost, the alarm will sound, alerting the practitioner.

Control Circuit Alarms

The fail-safe sensitivity monitors the VDR 4 gas delivery through the patient circuit. If the patient circuit were to accidentally become obstructed, the fail-safe sensitivity system opens, allowing the excess pressure in the circuit to be vented. Simultaneously, an audible alarm sounds, alerting the practitioner. The fail-safe sensitivity system may be reset by manually depressing the reset alert thumb-button for several seconds after the obstruction has been cleared or resolved.

It is important to properly adjust the fail-safe sensitivity system to match the pressure delivery required for each patient. If the pulmonary

Figure 12-9 *An assembly drawing of the VDR 4 manifold assembly.*

THE FORREST M. BIRD CONCEIVED VDR FAILSAFE DIFFUSIVE/CONVECTIVE BREATHING CIRCUIT.
UNIVERSAL STANDARD FOR NEONATAL, PEDIATRIC AND ADULT APPLICATION.

U.S. and FOREIGN PATENTS ISSUED AND PENDING

© 1988 COPYRIGHT PERCUSSIONAIRE®CORPORATION

Figure 12-10 *An assembly drawing of the Percussionaire® VDR 4 ventilator's circuit. (Courtesy Percussionaire Corporation, Sandpoint, ID)*

system is very compliant (requiring low driving pressures), rotate the fail-safe sensitivity system control counterclockwise. Conversely, if compliance is low and drive pressures are high, rotate the control clockwise.

Output Alarms

The battery-powered, pressure-sensing alert/alarm system is located on the right side of the ventilator. The alert/alarm system provides for clinician alert/alarms for high-

Figure 12-11 *The Oscilloscope Waveform analyzer or monitor.*

pressure (pressure rise) and low-pressure (pressure drop) conditions. The pressure drop delay control allows for the time interval between the time when the pressure drops below the set value on the pressure drop control and the time when the audible alarm is activated. This system provides for the sensing of patient disconnects as well as high-pressure alert conditions.

Oscilloscope Waveform Analyzer

The Oscilloscope/Waveform analyzer (Figure 12-11) provides real-time analysis of the VDR 4 ventilator's performance through a CRT oscilloscope display. The clinician may adjust the pressure scale and sweep speed of the display. A frequency counter is also incorporated into the monitor to assist the clinician with setup and monitoring of the ventilator. The monitor also has high- and low-pressure alarms, which may be clinician adjusted to provide disconnect and high-pressure alerts.

VIASYS CRITICAL CARE 3100A AND 3100B HIGH-FREQUENCY OSCILLATORY VENTILATOR

The Viasys Critical Care 3100A and 3100B high-frequency oscillatory ventilator is an HFOV approved for the ventilatory support of neonates ranging in weight between 0.54 and 4.6 kg and pediatric patients for whom conventional ventilation has failed (Figures 12-12A and 12-12B). The Viasys Critical Care 3100B high-frequency oscillatory ventilator is designed for adults and large children weighing more

Figure 12-12A *The Viasys Critical Care 3100A High-Frequency Oscillatory Ventilator. (Courtesy SensorMedics Corporation)*

Figure 12-12B *The control panel of the Viasys Critical Care 3100A High-Frequency Oscillatory Ventilator. (Courtesy SensorMedics Corporation)*

than 35 kg (Figures 12-13A and 12-13B). The ventilators are pneumatically powered and electronically-controlled, time-triggered, time-cycled, pressure-limited HFOV. Since many

Figure 12-13A *A photograph of the Viasys Critical Care 3100B HFOV ventilator. (Copyright SensorMedics Corporation)*

Figure 12-13B *The control panel of the Viasys Critical Care 3100A High-Frequency Oscillatory Ventilator. (Courtesy SensorMedics Corporation)*

similarities exist between the two ventilators, they will be considered together. When differences occur, they will be discussed on an individual basis.

Input Power

Input power for the 3100A and 3100B ventilators requires two pneumatic gas sources and one electrical source. The DISS connection located at the upper left of the rear control panel must be connected to the outlet of an air/oxygen blender, which must be capable of providing between 30 and 50 psi nominal pressure output. Adjustment of the blender determines the F_IO_2 delivered to the patient. The second pneumatic connection is for cooling air for the oscillator; it is located at the

lower right of the rear control panel. This pneumatic connection is an air DISS fitting and must be powered by a 50-psi source capable of providing a minimum 15 L/min flow. Electrical power is provided by a standard three-prong electrical cord and plug and is adjustable between 120 v, 60 Hz and 220 v, 50 Hz power supply systems.

Drive Mechanism

The drive mechanism for the 3100A and 3100B ventilators consists of a square-wave driver, which powers an electric linear motor and a piston (Figure 12-14). The electric drive motor consists of a permanent magnet suspended in an electric coil. When alternating square-wave current passes through the coil, positively charged current displaces the piston/diaphragm toward the patient circuit, while negatively charged current displaces the piston/diaphragm away from the patient circuit. The stroke of the piston is determined by the amplitude of the applied current. The piston/diaphragm assembly has a maximum displacement of around 365 mL. The 3100B ventilator is capable of delivering higher mean airway pressures and amplitudes due to a larger magnet in the drive mechanism.

The electric linear motor, when operating at the frequencies required to support a

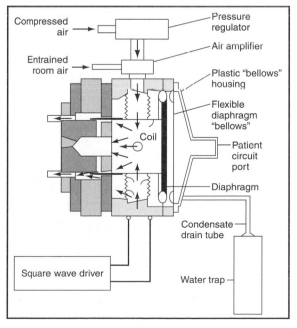

Figure 12-14 *A schematic drawing of the Viasys Critical Care 3100A High-Frequency Oscillatory Ventilator's drive mechanism. (Courtesy SensorMedics Corporation, Yorba Linda, CA)*

patient's ventilation, requires cooling. There-fore, a 50-psi air source (at 15 L/min) entrains additional air through a venturi, which augments the flow to 60 L/min. Should the temperature of the coil exceed 190°C, the oscillator will shut down to protect itself. Prior to oscillator shutdown, a yellow caution light will illuminate (at 175°C) to alert the clinician of a potential overtemperature condition.

Amplitude of the square-wave drive signal is controlled by the power/DP control. This control is adjustable on a percentage scale of 0 to 100%. Setting the control to a higher per-centage results in a greater amplitude of the drive signal, which increases piston displace-ment. As the piston displacement varies (increases or decreases), the DP (inspiration to expiration) also changes.

When operating the ventilator, it is impor-tant to center the piston. This is done by using the piston centering control located on the lower-left part of the support column, just opposite the power switch. Rotating this con-trol varies the center position of the piston and is graphically displayed on the centering bar graph on the control panel. Piston centering determines the Paw (limits or increases dis-placement) and also prevents the piston from striking mechanical stops, which may result in damage to the drive system.

Control Circuit

The control circuit of the 3100A and 3100B ventilators consists of electronic and micro-processor systems that control the oscillator drive system and the pneumatic logic and control subsystems (Figure 12-15). The oscilla-tor subsystem develops square-wave pulses, resulting in subtidal volume delivery into the patient circuit. Bias flow from the external blender and humidifier into the circuit augments the volume delivered to the patient. Bias flow is adjustable between 0 and 40 L/min (3100A) and 0 to 60 L/min (3100B) and is controlled by a flowmeter located on the upper right of the control panel.

Control Variable

The control variable of the 3100A and 3100B ventilators is time. The frequency con-trol determines the oscillator frequency, which is calibrated in hertz (cycles per second). Fre-quencies may be adjusted between 3 and 15 hertz (180 to 900 breaths per minute) for both ventilators. A digital LED displays the frequency at which the HFOV is operating.

Figure 12-15 *An assembly drawing of the Viasys Critical Care 3100A High-Frequency Oscillatory Ventilator's circuit. (Courtesy SensorMedics Corporation, Yorba Linda, CA)*

Phase Variables

Trigger Variable

The trigger variable for the ventilators is time. The frequency control determines the rate at which the oscillator cycles and, therefore, when inspiration occurs.

Limit Variables

The limit variables for the 3100A and 3100B ventilators are pressure and time. The pressure limit is adjusted using the mean pressure limit control. The mean pressure may be limited between 10 and 45 cmH$_2$O (3100A) and 10 to 55 cmH$_2$O (3100B). The control consists of a needle valve that adjusts a pneumatic valve, limiting mean pressures. The pressure limit may be adjusted below the operating pressure (Paw); however, it is intended as a safety to prevent barotrauma in the event of an over-pressure condition and is usually set above the Paw.

Time may be a limit variable and is adjusted using the percent inspiratory time control. This control determines for what percentage of the inspiratory time the piston is displaced at its maximum forward position (closest to the patient circuit). This control is adjustable between 30 and 50%. The inspiratory time percentage is displayed on a digital LED. Changing the percent inspiratory time will have an effect on the Paw and the change in pressure (inspiration to expiration) since it alters the symmetry of the oscillatory waveform.

Cycle Variable

The cycle variable of the 3100A and 3100B ventilators is time. The cycle variable is not directly set but is a function of the frequency and inspiratory time percentage. Once the allotted inspiratory time has passed, the piston travels away from the patient circuit, initiating exhalation. Exhalation on the 3100A HFOV is active, and gas is withdrawn from the patient circuit and airway by the backward displacement of the piston.

Output Waveforms

The pressure waveform output of the 3100A and 3100B ventilators is square. The oscillator and electronic driver produce a true square wave with each breath or oscillation.

Alarm Systems

Input Power Alarms

Input power alarms are included for electrical and source gas power interruptions. In the event of an electrical power failure, a 3-kilohertz, modulated, audible alarm will sound. Once activated, the alarm can only be silenced by depressing the reset button. The power failure alarm is powered by a battery that is independent of the main power supply for the ventilator.

If the line pressure from the external blender falls below 30 psi, a yellow lamp will illuminate to alert the clinician to this condition. This type of alarm is considered a caution alarm and, therefore, no audible condition will result.

Control Circuit Alarms

The control circuit alarm is an overheated oscillator alarm (already discussed). When the oscillator temperature reaches 175 degrees Celsius, a yellow LED will illuminate to alert the clinician to the condition.

Output Alarms

Output alarms include minimum mean airway pressure, maximum mean airway pressure, mean airway pressure greater than 50 cmH$_2$O (3100A) and 60 cmH$_2$O (3100B), mean airway pressure less than 20% of set maximum mean airway pressure (3100A), and peak airway pressure less than 5 cmH$_2$O (3100B). The minimum and maximum mean airway pressure alarms are adjustable between 0 and 49 cmH$_2$O (3100A) and 0 and 59 cmH$_2$O (3100B). Both are thumbwheel switches located on the lower left portion of the control panel. Adjustment of the alarms can make them serve as high- and low-pressure alarm indicators; they will automatically reset if the condition corrects itself or if the operator depresses the 45-second-silence button.

The mean airway pressure greater than 50 cmH$_2$O (3100A) and greater than 60 cmH$_2$O (3100B) alarm will activate if the mean airway pressure exceeds this value. Once the alarm condition is met, a red LED will illuminate; a 3-kilohertz, modulating, audible tone will sound; the oscillator will automatically shut down; a dump valve will open to the atmosphere; and bias flow will continue. The purpose of this alarm is to protect the patient from barotrauma, which may result from the increased pressures. The alarm can be reset

ASSEMBLY AND TROUBLESHOOTING

Assembly—Viasys Critical Care 3100A and 3100B Ventilators

1. Assemble the patient circuit (Figure 12-14):

   a. Attach the patient circuit body to the bellows/water trap assembly (Figure 12-14).

   b. Place the three diaphragms onto their respective seats in the circuit and snap the diaphragm valve caps over them, completing the valve assembly. These components are identical and, therefore, interchangeable.

   c. Attach the bellows/water trap assembly to the front of the ventilator by positioning it correctly and rotating the four T-handles to lock it into place.

   d. Connect the small-diameter control and monitoring tubes to the correct valve caps and connectors:

      (1) Connect the blue tube to the limit valve and limit valve fitting on the ventilator.

      (2) Connect the green tube to the control valve cap and the stop/start fitting on the ventilator.

      (3) Connect the red tube to the dump valve and to the dump valve fitting on the ventilator.

      (4) Connect the clear, ⅛-inch tubing to the pressure port on the patient wye and to the airway pressure fitting on the ventilator.

2. Connect the gas supply lines:

   a. Connect a 50-psi air and oxygen source to an external blender and connect the 50-psi outlet of the blender to the inlet on the ventilator.

   b. Connect a 50-psi air source to the DISS air fitting on the ventilator.

3. Connect an appropriate electrical supply to the ventilator and ensure that the switch is set for the correct voltage.

Troubleshooting

Refer to the troubleshooting algorithms in ALG 12-1 and 12-2.

---

only by the clinician correcting the situation and depressing the reset button manually. The oscillator must be started following the startup procedure.

The alarm signaling that mean airway pressure is less than 20% of the set maximum mean airway pressure is another safety alarm. This alarm is indicated by a red LED, a 3-kilohertz modulating tone, shutdown of the oscillator, opening of the dump valve, and continuation of the bias flow through the circuit. This alarm occurs when the mean airway pressure drops to this value. The alarm will reset itself if the condition corrects itself. If the clinician must correct the problem, the reset

button must be depressed and the oscillator must be started by following the startup procedure.

If peak airway pressure falls to less than 5 cmH$_2$O on the 3100B ventilator, a red LED will illuminate, a 3-kilohertz modulating tone will sound, the oscillator will shut down, a dump valve opens, and bias flow continuously flows through the circuit. This alarm occurs when the peak airway pressure drops below this value. The alarm will reset itself if the condition corrects itself. If the clinician must correct the problem, the reset button must be depressed and the oscillator must be started by following the startup procedure.

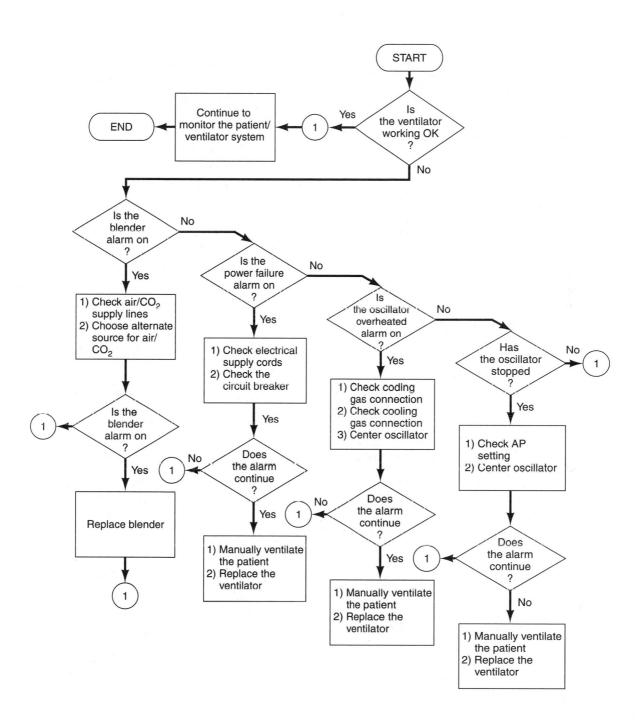

ALG 12-1 *An algorithm for troubleshooting input power and control circuit alarms.*

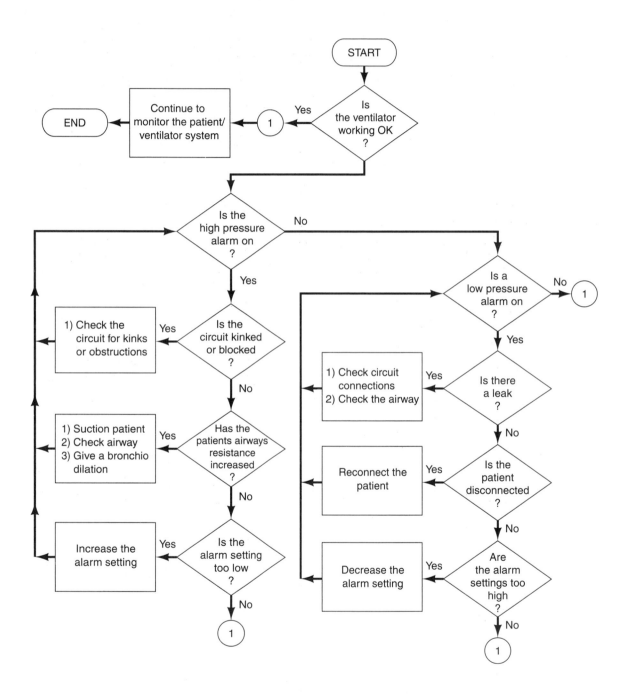

ALG 12-2 *An algorithm for troubleshooting output alarms.*

CLINICAL CORNER

High-Frequency Ventilators

1. Describe two circumstances in which high-frequency ventilators would be used instead of conventional ventilators.
2. Explain why it is important to center the piston of the Viasys Critical Care 3100A and 3100B ventilators.
3. What control on the Percussionaire® VDR 4 ventilator causes ventilation to become more convective rather than diffusive?
4. Describe what occurs when you depress the manual inspiration button on the Percussionaire® VDR 4 ventilator.

Self-Assessment Quiz

1. Which of the following ventilators depend upon the elastic recoil of the lungs and chest wall for exhalation?
   I. HFPPV
   II. HFFI
   III. HFJV
   IV. HFOV
   a. I
   b. I and II
   c. I, II, and III
   d. II, III, and IV

2. Which of the following ventilators has an active expiratory phase?
   a. HFPPV
   b. HFFI
   c. HFJV
   d. HFOV

3. Which of the following is a primary application of HFPPV?
   a. support of neonates in respiratory distress
   b. support of adults in respiratory distress
   c. ventilation of patients with lung injury
   d. surgical cases involving the upper airway

4. Which of the following ventilators employs a small catheter or a specialized endotracheal tube to interface with the patient's airway?
   a. HFPPV
   b. HFFI
   c. HFJV
   d. HFOV

5. Which of the following types of high-frequency ventilators employs a rotating-ball valve to determine the respiratory frequency?
   a. HFPPV
   b. HFFI
   c. HFJV
   d. HFOV

6. Which of the following theories suggests that areas of the lung with a given time constant contribute to gas exchange by emptying into adjacent areas with different time constants?
   a. Taylor dispersion theory
   b. pendelluft theory
   c. molecular diffusion theory
   d. cardiogenic mixing theory

7. Which of the following theories suggests that gas exchange during high-frequency ventilation is enhanced by turbulent flow within the airways?
   a. Taylor dispersion theory
   b. pendelluft theory
   c. molecular diffusion theory
   d. cardiogenic mixing theory

8. Which of the following theories suggests that the increased velocities and respiratory rates associated with high-frequency ventilation contribute to a greater molecular kinetic activity, which achieves adequate ventilation at low tidal volumes?
   a. Taylor dispersion theory
   b. pendelluft theory
   c. molecular diffusion theory
   d. cardiogenic mixing theory

9. Which of the following best describes the asymmetric velocity profile theory of ventilation during high-frequency ventilation?
   a. increased turbulence resulting in the diffusion and mixing of gases
   b. cardiac oscillations, resulting in the agitation of the airways and thus enhancing molecular mixing
   c. a difference in velocity profiles between inspiration and expiration, causing a greater net flow of gases during inspiration
   d. increased kinetic activity of gases caused by the increased frequencies

10. Which of the following are advantages of high-frequency ventilation?
    I. low mean airway and intrathoracic pressures
    II. minimal cardiac side effects
    III. minimal motion of the airways and chest wall
    IV. stability of the upper airway structures during ventilation
    a. I
    b. I and II
    c. I, II, and III
    d. I, II, III, and IV

11. Which of the following accounts for the reports of success with high-frequency ventilation being used to ventilate patients with large air leaks?
    I. low mean airway and intrathoracic pressures
    II. minimal cardiac side effects
    III. minimal motion of the airways and chest wall
    IV. stability of the upper airway structures during ventilation
    a. I and II
    b. I and III
    c. II and III
    d. III and IV

12. The improvement in cardiovascular side effects of high-frequency ventilation when compared with conventional ventilation is best accounted for by:
    a. decreased mean airway and intrathoracic pressures.
    b. decreased expansion of the chest wall.
    c. decreased motion of the upper airways.
    d. cardiogenic mixing.

13. Which of the following procedures may benefit from the use of high-frequency ventilation?
    I. laryngoscopy
    II. laser bronchoscopy
    III. laryngeal surgery
    IV. tracheal surgery
    a. I
    b. I and II
    c. I, II, and III
    d. I, II, III, and IV

14. Which of the following types of high-frequency ventilation may be achieved percutaneously via a small cannula or catheter?
    a. HFPPV
    b. HFJV
    c. HFOV
    d. HFFI

15. High-frequency ventilation has been used successfully in patients who had refractory hypoxemia and hypercarbia while being maintained on conventional ventilation. What best accounts for the success of high-frequency ventilation in these circumstances?
    a. the reliance of high-frequency ventilation on convective ventilation
    b. the lower mean airway pressures associated with high-frequency ventilation
    c. the decreased cardiac side effects of high-frequency ventilation
    d. the difference in the way high-frequency ventilation accomplishes gas exchange

16. What is the drive mechanism of the Percussionaire® VDR 4 ventilator?
    a. an electrodynamic motor
    b. a rotating-ball valve
    c. a high-frequency pulse generator
    d. a reducing valve

17. What is the input power of the Percussionaire® VDR 4 ventilator?
    I. 50-psi air
    II. 50-psi oxygen
    III. 120 v, 60 Hz electrical power
    a. I
    b. I and II
    c. I, II, and III
    d. II and III

18. Which of the following are functions of the Percussionaire® VDR 4 ventilator's Phasitron®?
    I. provides an interface to the patient's airway
    II. acts to entrain additional gas augmenting flow and tidal volumes
    III. acts as a pneumatic clutch
    a. I
    b. I and II
    c. II and III
    d. I, II, and III

19. How is the control circuit of the Percussionaire® VDR 4 ventilator classified?
    a. electronic
    b. electric
    c. pneumatic
    d. mechanical

20. Which of the following is the control variable for the Percussionaire® VDR 4 ventilator?
    a. pressure
    b. volume
    c. flow
    d. time

21. Which of the following is the cycle variable for the Percussionaire® VDR 4 ventilator?
    a. pressure
    b. volume
    c. flow
    d. time

22. Which of the following is the baseline variable for the Percussionaire® VDR 4 ventilator?
    a. pressure
    b. volume
    c. flow
    d. time

23. Which of the following is classified as the input power alarm of the Percussionaire® VDR 4 ventilator?
    a. the fail-safe sensitivity
    b. the pressure drop alarm
    c. the blender alarm
    d. the ventilator inoperative alarm

24. What is the input power of the Viasys Critical Care 3100A ventilator?
    I. 50-psi air
    II. 50-psi oxygen
    III. 120 v, 60 Hz electrical power
    a. I
    b. I and II
    c. I, II, and III
    d. II and III

25. What is the drive mechanism for the Viasys Critical Care 3100A and 3100B ventilators?
    a. an electrodynamic motor
    b. a rotating-ball valve
    c. a high-frequency pulse generator
    d. a reducing valve

26. What is the control variable for the Viasys Critical Care 3100A and 3100B ventilators?
    a. pressure
    b. volume
    c. flow
    d. time

27. What is the cycle variable for the Viasys Critical Care 3100A ventilator?
    a. pressure
    b. volume
    c. flow
    d. time

28. What determines the tidal volume delivery of the Viasys Critical Care 3100A and 3100B ventilators?
    a. the frequency
    b. the amplitude of the alternating signal
    c. percentage inspiratory time
    d. the oxygen percentage

29. What control manipulates time as a phase variable for the Viasys 3100A ventilator?
    a. frequency
    b. bias flow
    c. percentage inspiratory time
    d. mean pressure limit

30. Which of the following alarms on the Viasys 3100A ventilator is powered by an independent battery?
    a. max. mean airway pressure
    b. min. mean airway pressure
    c. mean airway pressure greater than 50 cmH$_2$O
    d. power failure

Selected Bibliography

Allen, J., et al. (1985). Alveolar pressure magnitude and asynchrony during high-frequency oscillations of excised rabbit lungs. *American Review of Respiratory Diseases, 132,* 343–349.

Bird, F. M. (1987). *Percussionaire® state of the art, universal mechanical cardiopulmonary support for the nineteen nineties.* Percussionaire Corporation: Sandpoint.

Bird, F. M. (1987). *The evolutionary concept and functional logic of the VDR-4 servolator percussionator (ventilator) conceived and developed by Forrest M. Bird.* Percussionaire Corporation: Sandpoint.

Bird, F. M. (1987). VDR servitor VDR-4 Percussionaire®. Percussionaire Corporation: Sandpoint.

Boynton, B. R. (1986). High frequency ventilation in newborn infants. *Respiratory Care, 31,* 480–490.

Cioffi, W. G., et al. (1989). High-frequency percussive ventilation in patients with inhalation injury. *Journal of Trauma, 29,* 350–364.

Coghill, C. H., et al. (1991). Neonatal and pediatric high-frequency ventilation: Principles and practice. *Respiratory Care, 36,* 596–612.

Cordero, L., et al. (1992). High frequency ventilation: Comparison of fan electronic flow interrupter and a new pneumatic oscillator. *Respiratory Care, 37,* 1241–1249.

Cordero, L., et al. (1992). The high-frequency pneumatic flow interrupter: Effects of different ventilatory strategies. *Respiratory Care, 37,* 348–356.

Davis, K., Jr., et al. (1989). High frequency percussive ventilation. *Problems in Respiratory Care, 2,* 39–47.

Franz, I. D., III, et al. (1983). High-frequency ventilation in premature infants with lung disease: Adequate gas exchange at low tracheal pressure. *Pediatrics, 71,* 483–488.

Fredberg, J. J. (1980). Augmented diffusion in the airways can support pulmonary gas exchange. *Journal of Applied Physiology, 49,* 232–238.

Gallagher, J. T. (1989). High-frequency percussive ventilation compared with conventional mechanical ventilation. *Critical Care in Medicine, 17,* 364–366.

Herridge, M. S., et al. (1996). High-frequency ventilation: A ventilatory technique that merits revisiting. *Respiratory Care, 41,* 385–396.

Hurst, J. M., et al. (1987). The role of high-frequency ventilation in post-traumatic respiratory insufficiency. *Journal of Trauma, 27,* 236–241.

Lehr, J. L., et al. (1985). Photographic measurement of pleural surface motion during lung oscillation. *Journal of Applied Physiology, 59,* 623–633.

Rodeberg, D. A. (1992). Decreased pulmonary barotraumas with the use of volumetric diffusive respiration in pediatric patients with burns. *Journal of Burn Care and Rehabilitation, 13,* 506–511.

Sjöstrand, U. H., et al. (1980). High rates and low volumes in mechanical ventilation—not just a matter of ventilatory frequency. *Anesthesia and Analgesia, 59,* 567–576.

Slutsky, A. S. (1981). Gas mixing by cardiogenic oscillations: A theoretical quantitative analysis. *Journal of Applied Physiology, 51,* 1287–1293.

Slutsky, A. S. (1984). Mechanisms affecting gas transport during high frequency oscillation. *Critical Care in Medicine, 12,* 713–717.

Viasys Critical Care. (1995). *3100A high frequency oscillatory ventilator operator's manual.* Yorba Linda.

Viasys Critical Care. (2001). *3100B high frequency oscillatory ventilator operator's manual.* Yorba Linda.

Weber, K., et al. (1994). Lung-volume-dependent effects of varying inspiratory time during high-frequency oscillation of surfactant-deficient rabbits. *Respiratory Care, 37,* 973–978.

APPENDIX

ANSWER KEYS TO SELF-ASSESSMENT QUESTIONS

Chapter 1 • Medical Gas Supply Equipment

1. b	6. a	11. a	16. c	21. c	26. b
2. c	7. a	12. a	17. e	22. c	27. c
3. c	8. c	13. a	18. d	23. b	28. b
4. d	9. a	14. c	19. c	24. c	29. a
5. c	10. d	15. e	20. c	25. b	30. a

Chapter 2 • Medical Gas Therapy Equipment

1. d	6. d	11. d	16. b	21. d	26. c
2. a	7. b	12. d	17. b	22. b	27. a
3. d	8. b	13. a	18. c	23. d	28. d
4. c	9. b	14. d	19. c	24. b	29. a
5. c	10. c	15. b	20. d	25. a	30. d

Chapter 3 • Humidity and Aerosol Therapy Equipment

1. c	6. c	11. c	16. a	21. a	26. c
2. a	7. b	12. a	17. a	22. c	27. d
3. c	8. c	13. c	18. a	23. a	28. c
4. a	9. d	14. c	19. b	24. a	29. c
5. c	10. c	15. d	20. b	25. a	30. c

Chapter 4 • Hyperinflation Therapy Equipment

1. b	6. c	11. c	16. c	21. a	26. b
2. a	7. b	12. a	17. d	22. c	27. b
3. c	8. c	13. c	18. a	23. a	28. c
4. a	9. d	14. d	19. e	24. a	29. c
5. c	10. a	15. d	20. c	25. c	30. d

Chapter 5 • Emergency Resuscitation Equipment

1. c	6. d	11. c	16. b	21. a	26. b
2. b	7. d	12. d	17. d	22. b	27. c
3. a	8. d	13. c	18. d	23. d	28. b
4. b	9. c	14. d	19. d	24. b	29. b
5. b	10. d	15. b	20. c	25. d	30. c

Chapter 6 • Physiological Measurement and Monitoring Devices

1. b	6. c	11. a	16. c	21. d	26. b
2. a	7. d	12. b	17. b	22. c	27. a
3. a	8. b	13. b	18. d	23. a	28. a
4. c	9. d	14. a	19. b	24. d	29. c
5. d	10. a	15. c	20. a	25. b	30. d

Chapter 7 • Mechanical Ventilator Theory and Classification

1. d	6. a	11. d	16. c	21. d	26. c
2. d	7. b	12. b	17. a	22. d	27. b
3. d	8. b	13. b	18. d	23. d	28. c
4. d	9. a	14. d	19. b	24. c	29. d
5. b	10. d	15. c	20. c	25. a	30. a

Chapter 8 • Adult Acute Care Ventilators: Ventilators Having Volume as a Control Variable

1. b	3. d	5. c	7. b	9. c
2. a	4. b	6. b	8. c	10. d

Chapter 9 • Adult Acute Care Ventilators: Ventilators Having Flow and Pressure Control Variables

1. d	6. d	11. c	16. a	21. a	26. c
2. b	7. b	12. b	17. d	22. b	27. d
3. b	8. b	13. b	18. d	23. b	28. b
4. d	9. c	14. c	19. c	24. a	29. d
5. c	10. a	15. d	20. d	25. c	30. c

Chapter 10 • Pediatric and Neonatal Ventilators

1. c	6. d	11. d	16. d	21. c	26. b
2. a	7. b	12. b	17. d	22. c	27. c
3. a	8. c	13. b	18. c	23. c	28. a
4. a	9. c	14. c	19. b	24. b	29. c
5. a	10. b	15. b	20. d	25. d	30. c

Chapter 11 • Non-Invasive, Homecare, and Transport Ventilators

1. c	6. d	11. d	16. a	21. d	26. b
2. a	7. a	12. d	17. b	22. d	27. b
3. d	8. b	13. c	18. b	23. d	28. d
4. c	9. c	14. a	19. d	24. b	29. a
5. d	10. b	15. b	20. c	25. b	30. c

Chapter 12 • High-Frequency Mechanical Ventilation

1. c	6. b	11. b	16. c	21. d	26. d
2. d	7. a	12. a	17. b	22. a	27. d
3. d	8. c	13. d	18. d	23. c	28. b
4. c	9. c	14. b	19. c	24. c	29. c
5. b	10. d	15. d	20. d	25. a	30. d

GLOSSARY

Absolute Humidity   The amount of water vapor contained in a gas at a given temperature. Absolute humidity is expressed in mg/L.

Absolute Temperature   The temperature expressed in the absolute scale, which is referenced to absolute zero. In the Systems Internationale (SI) units, the absolute scale is Kelvin while in the United States Customary scale it is Rankine.

Accumulator   A rigid reservoir of 1 to 2 liters, used by ventilator manufacturers to help to meet instantaneous flow demands.

A/D Card   An electronic card in a computer that converts analog data to digital data, which can be interpreted by the computer program.

Adsorption   The physical adhesion of a thin layer of molecules to the surface of a porous substance.

Aerosol   Particulate matter suspended in a gas. Aerosols can be solids as well as liquids.

Airway Pressure Release Ventilation (APRV)   A combination of two separate levels of CPAP pressures. The patient may breathe spontaneously from both CPAP levels.

American Standard Safety System (ASSS)   A safety system designed by the Compressed Gas Association for large medical gas cylinder valve connections. The system incorporates varying diameters, thread pitches, and internal and external threading to prevent the mismatching of regulators or connections with the incorrect cylinder.

Amplitude   The extent of a periodic vibratory motion that reflects the height of the waveform. For ultrasonic nebulizers, amplitude represents the energy transmitted and therefore governs aerosol output or density.

Anatomic Reservoir   The anatomic reservoir consists of the nasopharynx and oropharynx and in the adult is approximately 50 mL in volume. Most low-flow oxygen delivery devices depend upon filling this anatomic space with relatively pure oxygen, enriching the inspired oxygen concentration.

And/Nand Gate   A monostable fluidic element used to control specific functions when interrupted by a control signal. The Monaghan 225/SIMV ventilator uses this element to control the operation of the exhalation valve mushroom.

Aneroid Barometer   A mechanical barometer that employs an evacuated chamber to measure changes in air pressure.

Anhydrous   Free from water or water vapor.

Anterior Mandibular Displacement   A manual positional maneuver used to open the airway. The ramus of the mandible is grasped bilaterally, and the mandible is advanced anteriorly. As this maneuver is performed, the tongue is also displaced anteriorly, opening the airway.

Apnea Monitors   Apnea monitors are devices that monitor a patient's breathing and sound an alarm if the patient stops breathing (apnea). These devices operate using inductive plethysmography or impedance plethysmography.

Assist Control   In this mode of ventilation the ventilator has a sensitivity or assist system that will respond to the patient's inspiratory effort by opening the main solenoid valve, delivering a breath. If the patient fails to initiate a breath, the ventilator functions automatically, as in CMV, and ventilates the patient.

Assisted Mechanical Ventilation   A mode of mechanical ventilation where there is no set respiratory rate. All breaths are patient triggered.

Asymmetric Velocity Profiles   The theory that describes a net flow of gas through the central lumen of the airway during inspiration and expiratory gas simultaneously flowing out the peripheral portion of the airway lumen.

Asynchronous Ventilation   Asynchronous ventilation can be observed when the patient is "fighting the ventilator." An example is if the patient is exhaling while the ventilator is attempting to give a breath. Most often, the sensitivity is improperly adjusted, or the patient is receiving controlled breaths when breathing spontaneously.

Atelectasis   Atelectasis is the collapsing of lung tissue. Atelectasis can include microatelectasis, the collapsing of alveoli and small structures of the lung, or it can involve entire lobes.

Atomizer   A jet-type aerosol generator that produces a wide range of particle sizes. An atomizer lacks a baffle, which helps to stabilize particle size in a nebulizer.

Augmented Mandatory Ventilation (AMV)
A mode of ventilation in which the respiratory care practitioner sets a minimum minute volume, tidal volume, respiratory, peak flow, assist sensitivity, and oxygen percent. If the patient's spontaneous ventilation falls below the minimum minute volume, the ventilator delivers mandatory breaths until that volume is reached.

Babbington Principle The production of an aerosol using a pressurized glass sphere and a baffle. Water forms a sheet over the sphere and is aerosolized when it encounters a high velocity gas stream exiting the pressurized sphere through a small hole.

Back Pressure Compensated A device that is designed such that back pressure (pressure distal to the device) will not affect its accuracy. Back pressure compensation is common in Thorpe tube flowmeters.

Bacteria Filter A low-resistance, high-efficiency filter capable of removing particles as small as .3 microns in diameter.

Baffle An object placed in the path of an aerosol flow to remove the larger particles of greater size (mass) by means of inertial impaction.

Beam Deflection The disruption of the coanda effect by a control pressure from one or more control ports on a fluidic element. Once the coanda effect has been disrupted, the beam may be directed to another output port, changing the logic of the output.

Bellows Drive Mechanism A ventilator that uses a bellows to convert its power source to ventilatory work. Examples of these ventilators include the Puritan-Bennett MA-1 and MA-2+2 and the Monaghan 225/SIMV.

Bellows Spirometer A spirometer that measures volume displacement using a flexible bellows. The bellows expands and contracts with inspiration and expiration.

Bernoulli's Principle A reduction in pressure that occurs near the walls of a tube as gas flow is increased through the tube. This effect only occurs as long as the gas is contained within a tube and if the flow is laminar.

Bi-Level Positive Airway Pressure A mode of ventilation which combines pressure support with airway pressure release ventilation.

Independent airway pressures for inspiration and expiration may be set.

Biofeedback Biofeedback is the application of a monitoring or indicating device to give patient feedback regarding their effort, performance, or physiological function. Incentive spirometry is one application of this technique to improve a patient's effort during inspiration.

Blender A blender is a device that mixes air and oxygen to precise concentrations. Air and oxygen at 50 psi are mixed internally by means of proportioning valve. Blended gas exits the blender via check-valved DISS fittings.

Body Humidity The humidity conditions at body temperature and pressure saturated (BTPS). Body humidity is defined as 37 degrees Celsius, 100% saturation, 43.9 mg/L water vapor content, and a partial pressure of 47 mmHg.

Body Plethysmograph A body plethysmograph is a device that relies on Boyle's law to measure thoracic volume changes. A body plethysmograph completely encloses the patient in an airtight sealed chamber.

Body Plethysmography The technique of measuring the residual volume and expiratory reserve volume, indirectly using Boyle's law. A device known as a body plethysmograph is used in the determination of these volumes.

Boeringer Valve A type of PEEP/CPAP valve that depends upon gravity and a weighted ball to generate the expiratory resistance.

Bourdon Gauge A mechanical pressure gauge that employs a coiled tube to measure gas pressure. As pressure increases the tube straightens, causing a needle to indicate the increased pressure.

Bourdon Gauge Flowmeter A type of flowmeter that regulates the flow of a gas using a Bourdon tube and a single-stage reducing valve. The Bourdon gauge is recalibrated to read flow although it measures a change in pressure.

Boyle's Law A gas law that relates a change in volume to a change in pressure at a constant temperature. The law states that if pressure increases, volume will decrease provided the temperature remains constant.

Brownian Motion The random motion of small particles, such as smoke observed under a microscope, caused by the kinetic activity of gas molecules.

Calibration   The comparison of an instrument to a known physical standard to assess its accuracy and reproducibility.

Capacity   Capacity is the maximum amount of water vapor (humidity) that a gas can contain at a given temperature when fully saturated.

Cardiogenic Mixing   The motion of the heart during its cycle acting to further agitate the airways, enhancing gas distribution during high-frequency ventilation.

Carlens Tube   The Carlens tube is designed to intubate the left mainstem bronchus. It has two cuffs, the distal cuff seals the left mainstem bronchus, while the proximal one seals the trachea.

Capnography   The graphic display of CO_2 concentration versus time. The shape of the waveform is more important clinically than the actual concentration displayed numerically.

Capnometry   The measurement of end tidal CO_2 concentration. This data is a numeric display that changes with time and the ventilatory cycle.

Carrier Gas   Carrier gas is the primary gas flow from a device that contains the aerosol generated from the device.

Centrifugal Compressor   A centrifugal compressor is an electrically powered compressor that uses an impeller mounted eccentrically within the compressor housing. The compressor works by the application of centrifugal force.

Charles' Law   Charles' law relates the volume and the temperature of a gas when the pressure remains constant. The law states that as the temperature of a gas increases, its volume will increase as well.

Chest Physiotherapy   A therapeutic technique which involves clapping on a patient's chest wall to promote vibration for secretion removal. Chest physiotherapy may be done manually, using one's hands, or mechanically, using a mechanical percussor.

Choked Flow   The phenomenon of choked flow occurs when an increase in the head pressure to a nozzle will no longer increase the gas velocity exiting the nozzle. This velocity is usually close to sonic velocities. Once this maximum velocity is reached, the flow is choked.

Clark Electrode   The PO_2 measuring electrode in a blood gas system, oxygen analyzer, or transcutaneous electrode.

Closed Loop Control Circuit   A closed loop control circuit is one where the desired output is selected and then the ventilator measures a specific parameter or variable (flow, pressure, or volume) continuously. The input is constantly adjusted to match the desired output.

Coanda Effect   The attachment of a high-velocity flow of gas to an adjacent wall by the formation of a separation bubble.

Combined Gas Law   A law that relates temperature, pressure and volume of a gas under ideal conditions. This is often referred to as the ideal gas law. The law states that $P_1V_1/T_1 = P_2V_2/T_2$.

Combitube Airway   The Combitube airway is a double lumen airway with the features of an esophageal gastric airway and an endotracheal tube. It is designed to be inserted blindly without the use of a laryngoscope.

Communi-Trach (Pitt speaking tube)   The Communi-Trach (Pitt speaking tube) is a tracheostomy tube that facilitates speech when the cuff is inflated. A second line and tube are attached to the tracheostomy tube, which directs oxygen flow above the cuff through small holes. The additional flow of gas allows the patient to use the vocal cords to communicate even when the cuff is inflated.

Compliance   A change in volume divided by a change in pressure. This measurement is reflective of elastic properties.

Compressible Volume   The volume of gas that is not delivered to a patient but is lost in the ventilator circuit due to compression. Compressible volume may be found by multiplying the peak inspiratory pressure times the tubing compliance.

Compressor   A device that is designed to compress a gas (usually air). Compressors operate using a diaphragm, piston or a centrifugal impeller, to compress the gas entering the device.

Constant Flow Generator   A classification of ventilators that delivers a constant flow during the inspiratory phase. These are often referred to as square wave generators.

Constant Pressure Generator   A classification of ventilators that delivers a constant pressure during the inspiratory phase. The driving pressure may be high (greater than 4,000 cmH$_2$O) or low (less than 45 cmH$_2$O).

Continuous Mandatory Ventilation A mode of mechanical ventilation where the respiratory care practitioner sets the ventilator to deliver a respiratory rate and tidal volume for the patient. Any spontaneous efforts generated by the patient will be ignored by the ventilator.

Continuous Positive Airway Pressure (CPAP) A spontaneous mode of ventilation where positive pressure is applied during inspiration and expiration.

Control Circuit The system that governs or controls the ventilator's drive mechanism. This system may be mechanical, electrical, electronic, fluidic, pneumatic, or microprocessor-controlled. Both open and closed loop control systems are utilized.

Control Variable A variable (volume, pressure, flow, or time), which is measured and utilized as a feedback signal to control the ventilator's output.

Convective Ventilation The process of gas exchange whereby gas transport occurs via bulk flow at low respiratory rates. The net result is alveoli coming into contact with the gases, which are directly conducted through the airways.

Conventional Laryngoscopes Laryngoscopes that are similar in design and function to a typical battery-powered flashlight. Lifting the handle and locking it at a right angle activates light at the distal tip of the blade, illuminating the airway.

Corrected Tidal Volume The actual volume delivered to the patient's lungs by a mechanical ventilator. Corrected tidal volume is calculated by subtracting the compressible volume from the measured volume.

Cuff A cuff is an inflatable balloon located at the distal tip of some artificial airways (endotracheal tubes, tracheostomy tubes, and esophageal obturator airways). The purpose of the cuff is to seal the airway so that positive pressure may be applied to the lungs and to protect the natural airway from aspiration.

Cycle Variable A variable (pressure, volume, flow, or time), which is measured and used to terminate inspiration.

Cylinder Manifold Two or more gas cylinders connected together, in series, to provide a larger supply of gas.

Dalton's Law Dalton's law of partial pressures states that the total pressure of a gas mixture is equal to the sum of the partial pressures of the gases that comprise the gas mixture. For example, if a gas mixture is composed of gases A, B, and C, the total pressure is equal to the partial pressures of A + B + C.

Demand Flow Pulsed Oxygen Delivery Device An oxygen delivery device that is designed to deliver a pulsed dose of oxygen during inspiration only. The device senses inspiration and only delivers gas during the inspiratory phase, conserving oxygen.

Demand Valve A type of mechanical valve that provides gas to a spontaneously breathing patient in response to the pressure gradient developed by the patient's inspiratory effort.

Diameter Index Safety System (DISS) A safety system designed by the compressed gas association for low pressure (less than 200 psi) applications. The system incorporates varying diameters, thread pitches, and internal and external threading to prevent the mismatching of delivery devices with the incorrect gas source.

Diaphragm Compressors A type of compressor utilize a flexible diaphragm driven by an electric motor to compress the air. These are commonly used to power small-volume nebulizers for home use.

Differential Pressure Transducer A type of pressure transducer with two pressure ports separated by a diaphragm. Since two pressures are exerted on the diaphragm, the displacement of it is equal to the pressure difference. These transducers may be strain gauge or variable reluctance transducers.

Direct Acting Cylinder Valve A cylinder valve that operates by a valve stem opening and closing the valve seat. The stem itself acts directly upon the seat to open or close it.

Disposable, Self-Inflating Manual Resuscitators Manual self-inflating resuscitators designed for single patient use. These resuscitators are inexpensive when compared with permanent ones and eliminate the need for cleaning and processing following use.

Double Circuit A classification of mechanical ventilator circuits in which the gas that drives the ventilator is separate from the gas that is delivered to the patient. The Bennett MA-2+2 and Monaghan 225/SIMV ventilators are examples of double circuit ventilators.

Downs' Valve   A type of PEEP/CPAP valve that operates using a spring and a diaphragm to generate an expiratory resistance.

Drive Mechanism   The system utilized by the ventilator to transmit or convert the input power to useful ventilatory work.

Dry Rolling Seal Spirometer   A type of spirometer that employs a piston in the measurement of lung volumes. The *rolling seal* term is derived from the fine plastic seals that seal the piston against the cylinder wall.

Ducted Ejector   A device using a nozzle and viscous shearing and vorticity to increase total flow. The nozzle exit is directed into a duct to control gas flow and increase the total flow from the device.

Dysfunctional Hemoglobin   Hemoglobin, which is not capable of reversibly binding with oxygen. These hemoglobin variants include carboxyhemoglobin and methemoglobin.

Endotracheal Tube   An endotracheal tube is an artificial airway that is passed through the mouth or nose and advanced into the trachea. Endotracheal tubes may be cuffed or uncuffed, depending upon their size.

Endtidal CO_2 Monitor   An infrared monitor that analyzes an exhaled gas sample and displays the partial pressure of carbon dioxide.

Evaporation   The process of liquid water changing to a vapor as a result of molecular kinetic activity. Some molecules in a liquid have sufficient energy to escape the cohesive forces of the liquid and change state to a vapor.

Exhalation Valve   The exhalation valve is a mushroom or diaphragm type valve, located on the patient circuit. During inspiration the valve is pressurized, closing it so that pressure can build in the patient circuit. Many acute care ventilators incorporate the exhalation valve inside the ventilator to more accurately control flows PEEP pressures.

Fenestrated Tracheostomy Tube   A fenestrated tracheostomy tube is a specialized tracheostomy tube with a fenestration (hole) located at the curve of the tube above the cuff, which, when placed correctly, is in the trachea. By removing the inner cannula a patient can be allowed to breathe spontaneously through the natural airway, providing a means of weaning from the tracheostomy tube.

Fiber-Optic Laryngoscope   A type of laryngoscope that uses fiber-optic bundles to conduct light and images to the handheld eyepiece. Like a bronchoscope, the tip of a fiber-optic laryngoscope can be manipulated up or down.

Fick's Law   The rate of diffusion of a gas into another gas is proportional to its concentration. The greater the concentration, the faster the rate of diffusion.

Fixed Orifice Flowmeter   A type of flowmeter that utilizes an orifice of a fixed size to regulate gas flow. Due to choked flow, gas velocity cannot increase beyond what the size of the orifice will pass at a given pressure (typically 50 psi).

Fleisch Pneumotachometer   A pneumotachometer that uses a heated capillary tube network to measure flow. The heated capillary tubes cause a resistance to gas flowing through the pneumotachometer. The resistance grid is heated to prevent moisture from condensing on the grid, altering the resistance to gas flow.

Flip-Flop   A fluidic element that is a bi-stable element; often utilized to control ventilator phasing (inspiration or expiration).

Flow-By   A mode of continuous flow ventilation that functions in CPAP and SIMV modes (Puritan-Bennett 7200a only). If flow decreases from the baseline value to the sensitivity level set by the respiratory care practitioner, the microprocessor interprets the change as a patient effort. Flow-by is a flow-activated mode.

Flow Cycling   If inspiration is terminated when a specified flow is reached, the ventilator is said to be flow cycled. An example of a flow-cycled ventilator is the Bennett PR-2.

Flow-Inflating Manual Resuscitator   A flow-inflating manual resuscitator is a type of manual resuscitator that depends upon gas flow to inflate it. It is commonly used in the anesthesia and critical care settings.

Fluidics   Fluidics is the application of specialized pneumatic logic devices to control and regulate a ventilator's operation. All fluidic elements utilize the coanda effect and beam deflection in their operation.

Flutter Valve   A positive expiratory pressure device that operates using a weighted ball resting against a conical valve seat. Expiratory flow causes the ball to open and close the conical valve seat causing an oscillating pressure waveform during exhalation.

Flutter Valve Therapy   A form of hyperinflation therapy that utilizes a threshold resister consisting of a weighted ball resting on a conical seat. As the patient's expiratory flow passes through the valve, the weighted ball rises and falls, creating pressure pulses in the airway. The patient is encouraged to exhale actively to FRC using the device.

Fraction of Inspired Oxygen (F_IO_2)   The fraction of inspired oxygen (F_IO_2) is the oxygen concentration delivered to the patient expressed as a decimal.

Fractional SaO_2   The percentage of oxygen saturation when compared to the total of all hemoglobin variants (functional and dysfunctional).

Frequency   The frequency refers to the number of times a periodic function (waveform) repeats in a unit of time. For ultrasonic nebulizers, frequency is expressed in hertz (Hz) or "cycles per second."

Functional Hemoglobin   The combination of oxyhemoglobin and deoxyhemoglobin in the blood. This constitutes the portion of hemoglobin capable of reversibly binding with oxygen.

Functional SaO_2   The percentage of oxygen saturation when compared to the functional hemoglobin.

Galvanic Oxygen Analyzer   An oxygen analyzer that is dependent upon an electrochemical reaction forming free electrons. Electrical current is proportional to oxygen concentration.

Gay-Lussac's Law   Gay-Lussac's law relates the pressure and the temperature of a gas when the volume remains constant. The law states that when temperature increases, the pressure will also increase ($P_1/T_1 = P_2/T_2$).

Graham's Law   The rate of gas diffusion through a liquid is proportional to the solubility of the gas and is inversely proportional to the square root of its gram molecular weight.

Head Box   A type of enclosure used for infants that encloses the head and neck. This facilitates the delivery of oxygen while allowing body access for patient care.

Head Tilt Maneuver   The head tilt maneuver is performed by tilting the head backward, hyperextending the neck slightly to open the airway. This maneuver should not be performed if a cervical spine injury is suspected.

Heat and Moisture Exchanger   A tubular-shaped device that contains a hygroscopic element, which is placed in-line with the patient's airway. Humidity condenses during exhalation on the hygroscopic element and then evaporates during inspiration, humidifying the inspired gas.

Heated Wire Grid   A method used to measure flow. A wire grid placed in a stream of flowing gas is heated to a constant temperature. As gas flow cools the wire grid, more current must be added to maintain a constant temperature. Therefore, gas flow becomes proportional to current.

Hemoglobin   A protein-iron compound contained in the red blood cell. Hemoglobin is responsible for the majority of oxygen transport in the blood.

Henry's Law   The rate of diffusion of a gas into or out of a liquid is proportional to the partial pressure of that gas at a given temperature. The greater the partial pressure, the faster the rate of diffusion.

Hertz   A unit of measure for frequency or rate in cycles per second. Units of frequency were named after German physicist Heinrich Rudolf Hertz (1857–1894).

High Air Flow with Oxygen Entrainment (HAFOE)   Devices that employ viscous shearing and vorticity to entrain room air into a stream of high velocity oxygen. These devices precisely mix the air and oxygen to deliver consistent concentrations of oxygen.

High-Flow Oxygen Delivery System   An oxygen delivery device that meets all of the patient's inspiratory needs. Using this device, the patient does not entrain any room air.

High Frequency Chest Wall Oscillation Therapy (HFCWO)   HFCWO is the application of pressure pulses to the thoracic cage via a pneumatic inflatable vest. It is a form of therapy that the patient may self administer following adequate instruction and demonstration.

High-Frequency Flow Interrupter (HFFI)   A type of ventilator that delivers small bursts of gas by interrupting a high-pressure or high-flow gas source. This is most commonly performed by using a rotating ball device that has a single gas port or pathway. These ventilators do not employ an injector cannula or catheter.

High-Frequency Jet Ventilator (HFJV)   A high-frequency jet ventilator employs short, high-pressure puffs or bursts of gas at high frequencies to accomplish gas exchange. These high-frequency bursts of gas are introduced into the airway through a small catheter at the endotracheal tube port through a special adapter or through a specialized endotracheal tube (High-Lo Jet Tracheal Tube).

High-Frequency Oscillatory Ventilators (HFOV) High-frequency oscillatory ventilators (HFOV) are active during both inspiration and exhalation. Most HFOV ventilators employ a diaphragm, piston, or modified acoustic speaker to oscillate the gas into and out of the airway.

High-Frequency Positive-Pressure Ventilator (HPPV) A type of mechanical ventilator with a modified circuit having a low compliance and compressible volume allowing tidal volume delivery at high frequencies.

Holding Chamber A specially designed valved chamber that is engineered to decrease the velocity of medication expelled from a metered dose inhaler (MDI) and act as a reservoir enhancing medication delivery to the lung.

Home Sleep Monitors Home sleep monitors are portable monitors comprised typically of four monitored channels consisting of ECG, snoring microphone, oximeter, and an airflow thermister.

Humidifier A device capable of adding water to a gas as water vapor.

Humidity Water contained in a gas as vapor. Humidity is sometimes referred to as gaseous water.

Humidity Deficit The humidity deficit is the difference between body humidity and the absolute humidity of the inspired gas expressed in mg/L.

Hygroscopic A substance that has the ability to absorb water and water vapor. Silica gel is a common compound used in medical equipment to absorb water and is sometimes termed a desiccant.

Hyperbaric Oxygen Therapy The application of oxygen at pressures greater than atmospheric pressure to treat very specific disease entities. Hyperbaric therapy may employ a multiplace (more than one patient) or monoplace (single patient) chamber.

Hypertonic A solution having a greater concentration of a solute when compared to another solution. Hypertonic solutions are capable of exerting more osmotic pressure as a result of the higher concentration of solute.

Hypotonic A solution having a lower concentration of solute when compared to another solution. Hypotonic solutions exert a lower osmotic pressure than solutions that are hypertonic.

Hypoxemia A deficiency of oxygen in the arterial blood or partial pressure of oxygen measured in mmHg.

Impedance Plethysmography The measurement or detection of ventilation by using changes in electrical impedance between two electrodes placed on the chest. As the chest expands and contracts, the electrical impedance changes between the electrodes and can be measured.

Inspiratory-to-Expiratory (I:E) Ratio The I:E ratio is the ratio of inspiratory time to expiratory time. A normal physiological I:E ratio is 1:2. When ventilating a patient, an I:E ratio of 1:2 or greater allows adequate time for the great vessels to fill during expiration, reducing the cardiovascular compromise associated with positive pressure ventilation.

Incentive Spirometry Incentive spirometry is the application of biofeedback devices (incentive spirometers) to coach and encourage patients to take deeper breaths.

Incubator A type of enclosure used with infants that encloses the entire infant's body. More commonly used for thermal and photo regulation rather than for controlling the oxygen environment.

Indirect Acting Cylinder Valve A type of cylinder valve that employs a diaphragm to open and close the valve seat. Turning the valve stem causes the diaphragm to be displaced through a spring, indirectly opening the valve seat.

Indirect Calorimetry Indirect calorimetery measure inhaled and exhaled oxygen and carbon dioxide, minute volume, and tidal volume. This data is then used to calculate the respiratory quotient (VCO_2/VO_2) and the resting energy expenditure (REE), using the Weir equation.

Inductive Plethysmography Inductive plethysmography operates using elastic bands that are positioned around the abdomen and around the chest. As the chest expands and contracts, coiled wires within the bands expand and contract. As the cross-sectional area of the bands changes with abdominal or thoracic motion, the frequency of the oscillations changes due to a change in inductance.

Inertial Impaction   The process of removing larger aerosol particles from a carrier gas due to their greater inertia (mass × velocity = inertia). The larger particles (greater mass) travel in a straight path and impact against objects placed in the path (baffles).

Input Power   The power source utilized by a ventilator to provide the energy required to support the patient's ventilation. Input power can include pneumatic, electric, or combined pneumatic and electric power.

Inspiratory Plateau   Inspiratory plateau, or inspiratory pause, is a brief pause (.5 to 2 seconds) at end inspiration. The purpose of the pause is to improve gas distribution throughout the lungs.

Inspiratory Time   Inspiratory time is the duration of inspiration during mechanical ventilation expressed in seconds. As inspiratory time increases, mean airway pressure increases, and the I:E ratio becomes lower.

Intermittent Positive Pressure Breathing (IPPB)   The application of positive pressure for short time intervals (10 to 20 minutes) to hyperinflate the lungs of a spontaneously breathing patient. Positive pressure ventilators (IPPB machines) are employed to deliver the positive pressure.

Intrapulmonary Percussive Ventilation (IPV®)   High-frequency, manually triggered, pressure-limited, time-cycled ventilation combined with aerosol administration. Designed to facilitate the mobilization and removal of pulmonary secretions.

Intubation   Intubation is the placement of an endotracheal tube into the trachea to secure an airway for positive pressure ventilation. Intubation may be performed nasally or orally.

Isotonic   A solution having the same concentration of solutes as another solution. Two solutions that are isotonic exert the same osmotic pressures.

Jackson Tracheostomy Tube   The Jackson tracheostomy tube is a cuffless sterling silver tracheostomy tube. It is intended for long-term application (months or years) and is very durable.

Kinetic Theory   The kinetic theory describes the behavior of an ideal gas. The theory states that (1) molecules are in random motion, (2) any molecular collisions are completely elastic in nature (energy is not lost, only transferred), (3) as temperature increases, kinetic activity also increases, and (4) there is no physical attraction between gas molecules.

Kistner Button   The Kistner button is similar to the trach button, only it is made from a more pliable plastic. This device does not have any provisions for mechanical ventilation or a removable plug. The Kistner button maintains the stoma as does the trach button.

Kymograph   A revolving drum that records a volume tracing providing an X-Y plot. The Y-axis represents volume while the X-axis represents time. This recorder allows the measurement of expiratory flows.

Laminar Gas Flow   Smooth uniform gas flow in one direction. Laminar flow occurs at velocities such that the Reynold's number is less than 2,000.

Lanz Tube   The Lanz tube incorporates a regulating valve and a control balloon made of latex within the large pilot balloon. The regulation valve and balloon limit cuff pressures to between 16 and 18 mmHg.

Laryngeal Mask Airway   The laryngeal mask airway is a small, triangular-shaped, inflatable mask secured to a tube. The laryngeal mask is designed to be positioned such that, when the mask is inflated, it seals the esophagus. Ventilation through the airway inflates the lungs.

Laryngoscope   An endoscopic instrument that is designed to visualize and expose the larynx.

Levey-Jennings Chart   The Levey-Jennings chart is a means of plotting quality control data graphically in relation to the mean and standard deviation. This chart facilitates the identification of out-of-control results, shifts, and trends.

Limit Variable   A variable (pressure, volume, flow, or time) that is allowed to reach a maximum value and is held at that value. Inspiration is not terminated once this value has been met.

Low-Flow Oxygen Delivery Devices   Oxygen delivery devices that only meet part of the patient's inspiratory needs. The remainder of the patient's needs are met by the inspiration of room air. Accurate oxygen concentration delivery is not possible with this type of device due to the air entrainment variation.

Lukens Trap   The Lukens trap is a specimen trap that can be placed in the vacuum circuit, when suctioning a patient, to obtain a sample for culture and analysis.

Macintosh Laryngoscope Blade   A curved laryngoscope blade that is designed to be inserted into the vallecula, and when lifted moves the epiglottis superiorly exposing the vocal cords.

Magill Forceps   Magill forceps are long curved forceps that facilitate endostracheal tube placement by allowing the practitioner who is intubating to grasp the endotracheal tube to better guide its advancement into the airway.

Magnetic Valve   A PEEP/CPAP generation device that utilizes magnetic attraction to a metal diaphragm to generate PEEP/CPAP pressures.

Mainstream Nebulizer   A small-volume nebulizer in which the aerosol is generated in the path of the carrier gas.

Mandatory Minute Ventilation (MMV)   A mode of ventilation in which the respiratory care practitioner sets a minimum minute volume, tidal volume, respiratory, peak flow, assist sensitivity, and oxygen percentage. If the patient's spontaneous ventilation falls below the minimum minute volume, the ventilator delivers mandatory breaths until that volume is reached.

Maximum Absolute Humidity   The capacity of a gas for humidity at any given temperature. In other words, the maximum water vapor content expressed in mg/L at which 100% saturation is achieved.

Mechanical Manometer   A mechanical manometer is similar in construction to an aneroid barometer. A diaphragm or evacuated container is exposed to the area where pressure measurement is desired. Gas pressure against the diaphragm or chamber causes a needle to move through a gear set, much like a mechanical watch that records the pressure.

Mechanical Percussor   A mechanical device (electrically or pneumatically powered) that is used for mechanical chest percussion. Use of mechanical percussors is less physically fatiguing and ensures uniformity in administration of chest physiotherapy.

Membrane Enricher   A membrane enricher is a type of home oxygen therapy device that utilizes a semipermeable membrane to separate the nitrogen from the oxygen in room air.

Mercury Barometer   A device used to measure air pressure that employs a column of mercury inverted into a mercury reservoir. Gas pressure against the surface of the reservoir causes the mercury column to rise or fall.

Metered Dose Inhaler (MDI)   A small, compact, pressurized cartridge containing medication for self-administration. Each time the MDI is squeezed, a metered amount of medication is aerosolized, which the patient then inhales.

Miller Laryngoscope Blade   A straight laryngoscope blade that is designed to lift the epiglottis directly, exposing the larynx and vocal cords.

Minimal Leak Technique   A technique of inflating an artificial airway cuff to the point where a small leak can be auscultated at the trachea.

Minimal Occlusion Volume (MOV)   A technique of inflating an artifical airway cuff to the point where no leak can be auscultated at the trachea.

Mist Tents   A type of enclosure typically used for pediatric patients that encloses the entire body. The patient may have cool aerosol and oxygen introduced into the tent to control both humidity and oxygen concentration.

Molecular Diffusion   The theory stating that the increased frequencies associated with high-frequency ventilation will enhance the kinetic activity of gas molecules in the alveoli, increasing their diffusion across the alveolar capillary membrane.

Molecular Sieve Concentrator   A molecular sieve oxygen concentrator is a home oxygen therapy device that separates nitrogen from room air and passes oxygen. It works by means of adsorption using a sieve bed composed of Zeolite.

Mouth-to-Mask Ventilation Device   A mask and one-way valve or filter assembly used for cardiopulmonary resuscitiation as a barrier device to protect the caregiver.

Murphy Eye   The Murphy eye is a small-diameter hole that provides an alternate pathway for gas to flow in the event the proximal tip becomes obstructed. If the tip becomes obstructed, air will continue to flow, but resistance will increase due to the decreased airway diameter.

Nasal Cannula   A type of oxygen delivery device that delivers oxygen to prongs that rest in the nares of the nose. This is a low-flow oxygen delivery device that is readily tolerated by most patients.

Nasal Catheter   A type of low-flow oxygen delivery device that consists of a small catheter that is passed through one nare and advanced to the posterior pharynx at the level of the uvula.

Nasopharyngeal Airway   The nasopharyngeal airway is an airway that is designed to be inserted through the nose into the posterior pharynx to relieve upper airway obstruction. The airway separates the tongue from the posterior pharynx.

Nebulizer   A device that produces an aerosol. Pneumatic nebulizers contain baffles to help stabilize and reduce particle sizes.

Needle Valve   A needle valve is one means of controlling gas flow and pressure. As the valve is opened more, more flow and pressure are allowed past the valve seat. A common application of a needle valve in plumbing is the faucet on a sink.

Negative Pressure Ventilators   A classification of ventilators that cause lung expansion by applying a negative pressure outside of the chest. An iron lung is an example of this type of ventilator.

Non-Constant Flow Generator   An inspiratory phase classification for a ventilator that produces a sine-wave-shaped flow pattern during inspiration. These ventilators typically use a rotary-driven piston to produce this flow pattern.

Non-invasive Positive-Pressure Ventilation (NPPV)   Non-invasive Positive-Pressure Ventilation (NPPV) is the application of positive pressure to the airway without the use of an endotracheal tube, or tracheostomy tube (artificial airway). Rather, positive pressure is applied to the airway via a full face or nasal mask.

Non-Rebreathing Mask   A type of low-flow delivery device that attempts to limit room air entrainment by the placement of one-way valves along the side of the mask and at the opening to the reservoir bag. Most are disposable devices and rarely meet the requirements of no air entrainment.

Olympic Trach-Talk™   The Olympic Trach-Talk™ is a specialized aerosol T with a spring-loaded, one-way valve. It is placed onto a

tracheostomy tube (with the cuff deflated). A humidifier or aerosol generator provides oxygen and humidification to the airway.

Open Loop Control Circuit   An open loop control circuit is one where the desired output is selected and the ventilator achieves the desired output without any further input from the clinician or the ventilator itself.

Operator Activation   Operator activation occurs when the respiratory care practitioner delivers a manual mandatory (ventilator) breath to the patient by activating the appropriate control.

Or/Nor Gate   A monostable, fluidic element with two control ports.

Oral and Nasal RAE® Endotracheal Tubes   These specialized endotracheal tubes have a preformed bend in their design. This bend is designed to remove the anesthesia/ventilator circuit from the patient's head. The preformed bend allows this positioning of the circuit without the risk of kinks or disconnects.

Oropharyngeal Airway   The oropharyngeal airway is an airway designed to be inserted into the mouth, separating the tongue from the posterior pharynx. It is designed specifically to relieve upper airway obstruction.

Oxygen Concentrator   A device that separates oxygen from room air for delivery of oxygen-rich gas to the patient. Most concentrators operate using molecular sieves, which adsorb the nitrogen from the air and pass the oxygen.

Oxygen Conserving Device (OCD)   A oxygen conserving device (OCD) is a type of regulator that senses inspiration, only delivering oxygen during the inspiratory phase. The device may be electronic or pneumatic in its operation. Use of an OCD can easily double the duration of a compressed gas cylinder.

Oxyhood   A type of enclosure used for infants that encloses the head and neck. This facilitates the delivery of oxygen while allowing body access for patient care. This device is synonymous with a head box.

Oxygen Proportioner   A device designed to mix oxygen and air in precise concentrations, using proportioning valves. These devices are sometimes referred to as blenders. An oxygen proportioner provides precise concentrations of gas at 50 psi to operate other equipment.

Paramagnetic Principle The physical principle that some gases are attracted to the strongest portion of a magnetic field (oxygen is a paramagnetic gas). This principle is employed in the operation of a physical oxygen analyzer.

Partial Rebreathing Mask A type of disposable low-flow oxygen mask that incorporates a reservoir bag into its design, increasing oxygen delivery when compared with a simple mask. The patient rebreathes about ⅓ of the reservoir's volume with each breath, hence the term partial rebreathing.

Pascal's Law A fluid confined within a container will transmit pressure uniformly in all directions, with the net forces acting perpendicular to the container surface.

Passy-Muir Tracheostomy Valve A tracheostomy valve designed to facilitate the use of the upper airway when the tracheostomy tube cuff is deflated. It is a one-way valve that forces air on exhalation through the upper airway.

Patient Activation Patient activation occurs when the ventilator sensitivity system detects a patient's spontaneous effort and delivers a mandatory (ventilator) breath.

Peak Flowmeter A device that is used to measure a patient's peak expiratory flow rate. This is commonly done to assess the effectiveness of bronchodilator therapy.

Pendelluft A world of German origin which means "air swinging freely." Due to differing time constants, not all areas of the lung fill and empty at the same rates. Therefore, the unequal filling and emptying results in air moving from one lung region to another, making gas distribution more uniform.

Pendant Cannula A type of oxygen conserving device which incorporates a small reservoir between the delivery tubing and the cannula. The reservoir enhances oxygen delivery, conserving the amount of oxygen used.

Percussionator® A pneumatically-powered pressure controller that is time cycled. The percussionator cycles at a rate of 100 to 250 cycles per minute. It is employed by the Percussionaire Corporation's IPV devices.

Percussors Percussors are mechanical devices (electric or pneumatic) that produce vibrations when applied to the chest wall. Percussors help to improve the effectiveness of chest physiotherapy by relieving the muscle fatigue experienced by respiratory care practitioners when performing manual percussion.

pH Glass A special type of glass that is permeable to hydrogen ions. This glass is used to develop a potential (voltage) between two solutions of differing pH.

Phase Variable A variable (pressure, volume, flow, or time) that is measured and used to initiate a phase of the ventilatory cycle. For example, a variable used to initiate the change from expiration to inspiration, inspiration, the change from inspiration to expiration, or the expiratory phase.

Phasitron® The phasitron is the mechanical and pneumatic interface between the patient and the percussionator. It is a sliding venturi, which is spring loaded in the closed position. Gas flow during inspiration from the percussionator opens the Phasitron®, delivering a pulsed gas flow to the patient.

Piezoelectric Crystal A crystal that is capable of converting electrical energy (RF energy) to mechanical energy (vibrations). The crystal resonates at the same frequency as the electrical energy driving it.

Pilot Balloon The pilot balloon is an inflatable chamber near the distal end of the pilot tube, which supplies gas pressure and volume to inflate the cuff of an artificial airway. Inflation of the balloon indicates that the cuff contains air. Cuff pressures should be monitored to help prevent pressure necrosis rather than solely relying on the "feel" of the pilot balloon.

Pilot Tube The pilot tube is the line that supplies pressure to the cuff of an artificial airway. It is a small-diameter line connected to the artificial airway, and it terminates inside the cuff.

Pin Index Safety System (PISS) PISS is a safety system designed by the Compressed Gas Association for small cylinders using yoke-type valve connections. Two pins are positioned in two of six positions to prevent the mismatching of regulators or cylinder yokes with the incorrect gas cylinder.

Piston Drive Mechanism A ventilator that uses a piston as the drive mechanism to convert its input power to ventilatory work. The piston may be rotary or linearly driven, which determines its waveform characteristics.

Pitot Tube Flow Sensor Pitot tube flow sensors measure flow based upon a differential pressure. One set of ports is directly exposed to the on-coming gas, while the other set measures static pressure. The pressure difference between the two sets of ports is proportional to flow.

Pitt Speaking Tube/Communi-Trach The Pitt speaking tube/Communi-Trach is a specialized tracheostomy tube that facilitates speech when the cuff is inflated. A separate tube supplies a flow of oxygen above the cuff, permitting gas flow through the vocal cords.

Pneumatic Splinting Maintenance of a patient airway using positive pressure (CPAP or Bi-Level Positive Airway Pressure) to separate the tongue from the soft palate.

Pneumotachometers Devices that are used to measure flow rates. Pneumotachometers typically operate by measuring a pressure difference across a resistance or by creating a pressure difference using a Venturi tube.

Poiseuille's Law Poiseuille's law describes the relationship between volumetric flow, viscosity, pressure, length, and velocity of a gas flowing through a tube. Poiseuille's law only applies for laminar flow. One important relationship of Poiseuille's law is that as the radius of a tube is decreased by ½, the resistance to gas flow increases by 16 times.

Polarographic Oxygen Analyzer An oxygen analyzer that uses a Clark electrode to measure oxygen. Oxygen reacts electrochemically to form free electrons, resulting in current flow being proportional to oxygen concentration. This analyzer differs from a galvanic type by the addition of a battery.

Positive End Expiratory Pressure (PEEP) The application of positive pressure during the expiratory phase of positive pressure ventilation.

Positive-Expiratory-Pressure (PEP) Therapy A form of hyperinflation therapy in which the patient exhales actively against a fixed resistance to FRC, which maintains positive pressure in the airways during exhalation. This therapy mechanically splints the airways open during exhalation through the application of pressure.

The application of positive pressure ($10-15$ cmH$_2$O) during active exhalation to increase the functional residual capacity (FRC) following a larger than normal tidal breath. PEP therapy sessions (10 breaths) are followed by coughing to promote secretion clearance.

Positive Pressure Ventilator A positive pressure ventilator applies pressure inside the chest to expand it. This type of ventilator requires the use of a tight-fitting mask, or more commonly, an artificial airway.

Potentiometer A wire-wound variable resister that operates by changing its effective length, altering its total resistance.

Pressure Pressure is a measure of force divided by surface area.

Pressure Controlled Ventilation A form of continuous mandatory ventilation in which all breaths are pressure limited and time cycled. This form of ventilation may also be combined with inverse I:E ratios (4:1 to 1.1:1), which are then termed pressure-controlled inverse ratio ventilation (PCIRV).

Pressure Cycling A means of terminating inspiration when a preset pressure is achieved. The Bird Mark 7 is an example of a pressure cycled ventilator.

Pressure Limited A pressure-limited breath occurs when a volume, flow, or time cycled inspiration is terminated when an operator-set pressure is reached (pressure limit). A type of breath delivery where pressure rises to a preset value and is maintained at that value until the breath ends.

Pressure Support A spontaneous mode of ventilation in which a constant pressure is applied during the inspiratory phase. Inspiration is terminated when a specific flow rate is reached.

Pressure Transducer An electrical component that converts a pressure change into an electrical signal. Two common types of pressure transducers are strain gauge and variable reluctance transducers.

Proportional Scissor Valve A proportionally controlled valve that use moveable arms, which function like a scissors compressing or opening a rubber tube, thereby opening and closing the valve.

Proportional Solenoid Valve A type of solenoid valve that is able to open or close in discrete steps or positions. Proportional solenoid valves are typically microprocessor controlled.

Proportioning Valve A device that mixes oxygen and air in precise concentrations. These devices operate using a proportioning valve. Sometimes proportioning valves are referred to as blenders.

Pulsation Dampener   A small, rigid reservoir (less than 1 liter) used by ventilator manufacturers to reduce pressure changes due to changes in flow.

Pulse Oximeter   A monitoring device that measures oxygen saturation noninvasively using red and infrared light.

Quality Control   The use of statistical analysis in conjunction with known standards to assess an instrument's accuracy, reliability, and reproducibility. Quality control programs also identify technical and random errors that may occur in the operation of the instrument.

Reducing Valve   A specialized valve that is designed to reduce gas pressure. Reducing valves may reduce pressure in one step (single-stage) or many steps (multistage). All reducing valves operate by balancing spring tension and gas pressure across a diaphragm.

Reducing Valve Drive Mechanism   A ventilator which employs a reducing valve to convert its input power to ventilatory work. The Bennett PR-2 is an example of a ventilator using a reducing valve drive mechanism.

Regulator   A regulator is a combination of a reducing valve and a flowmeter into one device. Regulators may employ Bourdon flowmeters or Thorpe tube flowmeters, depending upon their design.

Relative Humidity   Relative humidity is the result of the absolute humidity divided by the capacity multiplied by 100 (absolute ÷ capacity × 100 = relative humidity). This percentage relates the humidity of a gas to the capacity of that gas at a given temperature.

Reservoir Cannula   A type of oxygen-conserving cannula that incorporates a small reservoir that rests on the patient's lip. The reservoir reduces the flow needed to achieve a desired oxygen concentration.

Respironics PressureEasy   The Pressure-Easy consists of a diaphragm spring assembly with a line that connects to the endotracheal tube via a T-piece assembly. The purpose of the PressureEasy is to maintain a low pressure in the endotracheal tube cuff during positive pressure ventilation.

Reynold's Number   The Reynold's number equation is used to predict whether gas flow will be laminar or turbulent. The calculation accounts for the gas' velocity, viscosity, density, and the diameter of the tube. If the number is less than 2,000, flow will be laminar.

Robertshaw Tube   The Robertshaw tube is made for selective entry into either the right (Robertshaw right) or left (Robertshaw left) bronchus. Like the Carlens tube, it is a double-cuffed endotracheal tube.

Schmidt Trigger   A fluidic element consisting of three proportional amplifiers and two flip-flop elements. This device is often used to detect small pressure changes.

Self-Inflating Manual Resuscitator   A self-inflating manual resuscitator is one that does not depend upon gas flow for inflation. The elasticity of the bag causes it to inflate once it is released after applying a breath.

Sensitivity   Sensitivity refers to the ventilator's ability to sense a patient's spontaneous breathing effort. Most sensitivity systems employ a pressure sensing device, while others use a flow sensing device. If a ventilator's sensitivity system is adjusted properly, very little patient effort is required to initiate ventilation.

Servo Controlled   The application of a closed-loop feedback control system to adjust the output of a heater or valve to regulate temperature, flow, pressure, or volume.

Servo Feedback Control   A form of ventilator control that uses sensors that monitor pressure, flow, and sometimes F_1O_2 inside the ventilator, in the patient circuit, or in both. Signals from these sensors are compared to reference values set by the operator who adjusts the controls.

Severinghaus Electrode   The PCO_2 electrode in a blood gas system or transcutaneous electrode.

Shift   A change in quality control values such that all values change from one side of the mean to the other.

Sidestream Nebulizer   A small-volume nebulizer in which aerosol is generated adjacent to the flow of carrier gas.

Sigh Mode   The periodic delivery of a larger than normal tidal volume to mimic a spontaneous sigh breath.

Silver Jackson (or Hollinger) Tracheostomy Tube   The silver Jackson (or Hollinger) tracheostomy tube is a nondisposable, reusable tracheostomy tube with a removable inner cannula. Made of sterling silver, it is more durable than a PVC tracheostomy tube and is also cuffless.

Simple Oxygen Mask   A type of low-flow oxygen delivery device that incorporates a mask covering the patient's mouth and nose. The mask increases the reservoir volume over the anatomic reservoir, thereby increasing oxygen delivery.

Single Circuit   A classification of ventilator circuits in which the gas that drives the ventilator is the same gas that is delivered to the patient. The Puritan-Bennett 7200a is one example of a single-circuit ventilator.

Small Particle Aerosol Generator (SPAG) A pneumatically-powered nebulizer designed specifically for the administration of Ribaviran for the treatment of respiratory syncytial virus (RSV). The SPAG nebulizer utilizes a secondary gas flow and a drying chamber to further reduce particle size.

Soft Tissue Obstruction   Soft tissue obstruction is upper airway obstruction caused by the tongue and the soft tissues of the posterior pahrnyx. Soft tissue obstruction is the most common type of airway obstruction.

Solenoid Valve   A type of electromechanical valve that operates using an electromagnet to open the valve. Spring tension usually returns the valve to the closed position.

Spacer   A small hollow chamber designed for use with metered dose inhalers (MDI). The spacer enhances medication delivery and helps to alleviate coordination problems for patients using MDIs.

Stead-Wells Water-Seal Spirometer   A Stead-Wells water seal spirometer is a type of water seal spirometer that incorporates a lightweight plastic bell into its design. The lightweight plastic bell helps to overcome the inertial effects on other water seal spirometers having metal bells incorporated into their designs. This allows more accurate measurement of subtle flow rates and a better frequency response.

Stepper Motor   A type of electric motor that moves in discrete positions or steps in response to an input voltage. The voltage applied to the motor determines how far it will move.

Strain Gauge   An electrical device consisting of a thin coil of wire bonded to a paper or plastic substrate. As the gauge is stretched (strained), electrical resistance increases due to the greater length of the wires.

Strain Gauge Pressure Transducer   A form of pressure transducer that uses a strain gauge

imbedded on a flexible diaphragm. As pressure changes the position of the diaphragm, electrical resistance changes due to changes in the length of the strain gauge.

Stylet   The stylet is a semi-rigid protected wire guide that is used to assist in the placement of an endotracheal tube during intubation.

Suction Catheter   A suction catheter is a small-diameter tube that is used to aspirate the airway while removing secretions or foreign material. It may be used with artificial airways as well as with the natural airway.

Suction Regulator   A suction regulator is a device that adjusts the vacuum level applied to another piece of equipment. Suction regulators are employed when performing artificial airway aspiration, using chest tubes and other applications.

Synchronized Intermittent Mandatory Ventilation   A mode of ventilation in which the patient is allowed to breathe spontaneously between mandatory (machine) breaths.

Taylor Dispersion   A model of gas exchange describing that the addition of convective flow to a diffusive process enhances gas distribution. Fredburg expanded upon Taylor's theories and hypothesized that flow and turbulence may be augmented by increasing the ventilatory frequency.

Thermal Anemometer   A type of flow measuring device, which operates by gas flow cooling a thermistor bead, wire grid, or other electrically heated element. Gas flow is proportional to changes in temperature (electrical current).

Thorpe Tube Flowmeter   A Thorpe tube flowmeter is a type of flowmeter that incorporates a tapered tube and a float to measure gas flow. This type of flowmeter may be uncompensated or compensated for back pressure. Compensation is determined by the placement of the needle valve in relationship to the Thorpe tube.

Tidal Volume   Tidal volume is the amount of gas inhaled or exhaled during a normal spontaneous breath. When mechanically ventilating a patient, tidal volume refers to the volume of gas delivered during the inspiratory phase.

Time Activation   Time activation occurs when inspiration begins following the passage of a specified time.

Time Cycling   Time cycling occurs when inspiration ends following the passage of a specified time.

Tonicity   Tonicity reflects the degree of osmotic pressure between two solutions. A solution may have greater tonicity (hypertonic), less tonicity (hypotonic), or no tonicity (isotonic).

Tonometry   The equilibration of whole blood with known gas samples for the purpose of quality control. An instrument known as a tonometer is used to mix the whole blood with the known gas samples.

Torr   Torr is a unit of pressure named for Evangelista Torricelli, the inventor of the barometer. The units in the SI system are mmHg.

Trach Button   The trach button is a specialized tracheostomy weaning device that is designed to temporarily occlude the tracheostomy stoma. Once it is in place and plugged, the patient must use his or her normal airway to breathe.

Tracheostomy Tube   The tracheostomy tube is an airway that is designed to be surgically placed below the larynx at the second tracheal ring. It will relieve upper airway obstruction and may be cuffed or cuffless.

Transcutaneous Electrode   An electrode that samples PO_2 or PCO_2 transcutaneously or across the skin.

Transducer   A device that converts one form of energy to another. Transducers commonly convert a pressure, flow, or temperature to an electrical signal that can be measured.

Transtracheal Catheter   A low-flow delivery device that is invasive and consists of a cannula that is surgically placed at the second cartilaginous ring. By introducing oxygen directly into the trachea, oxygen flow may be reduced to achieve a desired oxygen concentration.

Trend   A group of six or more quality control results that display an increasing or decreasing pattern from the normal random distribution.

Trigger Variable   A variable (pressure, volume, flow, or time) that is measured and used to initiate inspiration.

Tubing Compliance   A measure of the distensibility of a ventilator circuit expressed in mL/cmH_2O.

Turbulent Gas Flow   Turbulent gas flow is erratic and irregular, having multiple vectors of direction. This type of flow requires more energy to sustain.

Ventilator   A mechanical device that moves gas into the lungs by applying positive pressure within the lungs or negative pressure outside the chest.

Venturi Masks   A type of air entrainment mask that has been misnamed. This mask works using the principles of viscous shearing and vorticity and is also referred to as a High Air Flow with Oxygen Enrichment (HAFOE) device.

Venturi Pneumotachometer   A venturi pneumotachometer measures flow by measuring a pressure differential before the throat of a venturi and the pressure at the venturi throat. The flow through the venturi is proportional to the pressure difference.

Venturi's Principle   A principle that relates a pressure reduction within a diverging duct to the velocity of the gas flowing through it. As velocity increases, the pressure at the tube's restriction decreases. Venturi's principle applies when the gas flow is noncompressible and is laminar.

Viscous Shearing and Vorticity   A phenomenon by which gas or a liquid may be entrained into a high-velocity gas stream by shear forces and vortices or eddies.

Volume Assisted Pressure Support (VAPS)   A form of pressure support that ensures that the patient will receive a specific minimum tidal volume with each pressure-supported breath.

Volume-Controlled Ventilation   A form of continuous mandatory ventilation in which all breaths are volume controlled (the ventilator may be a flow controller).

Volume Cycling   The termination of inspiration after a preset volume has been delivered.

Vortex Sensor   A flow measuring device which relies on the vortex shedding principle to detect flow. Struts placed in the gas flow pathway cause turbulence, which is detected by ultrasonic energy transmission.

Water Column   A type of PEEP/CPAP device that uses a container of water, which generates the expiratory resistance to provide positive pressure. In a water column system, the expiratory limb is simply immersed into a container of water.

Water Seal Spirometer   A type of spirometer that employs a bell that is immersed in a water bath to measure lung volumes. As the patient's inhaled and exhaled gases move into and out of the bell, the bell rises or falls, allowing accurate volume determination.

Water-Weighted Diaphragm   A type of PEEP/CPAP device that utilizes a water column pressing on a diaphragm to generate PEEP/CPAP pressures.

Wheatstone Bridge   A sensitive electrical circuit composed of four resisters in series that allows the measurement of small changes in voltage or current. These are used in conjunction with transducers to measure pressure or flow changes.

Wire-Wrapped Reinforced Endotracheal Tube   This specialized endotracheal tube facilitates intubation of a tortuous airway or in a case when intubation is only possible with a smaller-diameter endotracheal tube. Kinking of the tube can become problematic. Endotracheal tubes can be reinforced with a heilical reinforcing wire imbedded into the PVC material such that the wire wrap helps to prevent kinking.

Wright Respirometer   A portable, vane-type respirometer that measures volumes. The spirometer has a narrow accuracy range of gas flow (10 to 20 L/min) and is easily damaged by excessive flow (greater than 300 L/min).

Yankauer Suction   A Yankauer suction (tonsil tip) catheter is a rigid large-diameter plastic or metal catheter designed to quickly remove large amounts of liquid material from the airway.

Zone Valve   A safety valve that is placed in an oxygen piping system such that gas flow may be shut off in the event of a fire or other emergency.

INDEX

Page numbers followed by "f" denote figures; page numbers followed by "t" denote tables.